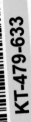
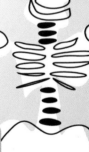
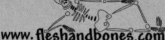

*Saunders' Pocket Essentials of*

# Clinical
# MEDICINE

*Saunders' Pocket Essentials*

*Series Editors*

# Parveen Kumar and Michael Clark

Barts and the London, Queen Mary's School of
Medicine and Dentistry, University of London, UK

*Commissioning Editor:* Ellen Green
*Project Development Manager:* Hannah Kenner
*Project Manager:* Nancy Arnott
*Designer:* Sarah Russell
*Illustrator:* Hardlines and Richard Morris

*Saunders' Pocket Essentials of*

# Clinical THIRD EDITION
# MEDICINE

## Anne Ballinger MD FRCP

Senior Lecturer,
Digestive Diseases Research Centre,
Barts and the London,
Queen Mary's School of Medicine and Dentistry,
University of London,
UK

## Stephen Patchett MD FRCPI

Consultant Physician/Gastroenterologist,
Beaumont Hospital,
Dublin,
Ireland

*Series Editors*
**Parveen Kumar** and **Michael Clark**

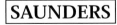

An Imprint of Elsevier

EDINBURGH LONDON NEW YORK PHILADELPHIA ST LOUIS
SYDNEY TORONTO 2003

SAUNDERS
An imprint of Elsevier Limited

First edition 1995
Second edition 2000
Third edition 2003

Standard Edition ISBN: 0 7020 2645 X
  Reprinted 2003, 2004, 2005
International Edition ISBN: 0 7020 2701 4
  Reprinted 2003, 2005

Book + CD of PDA version (pack) ISBN: 0 7020 2728 6
CD of PDA version ISBN: 0 7020 2727 8
Web download of PDA version ISBN: 0 7020 2731 6

**British Library Cataloguing in Publication Data**
A catalogue record for this book is available from the British Library

**Library of Congress Cataloging in Publication Data**
A catalog record for this book is available from the Library of Congress

**Note**
Medical knowledge is constantly changing. As new information becomes available, changes in treatment, procedures, equipment and the use of drugs become necessary. The editors and the publishers have taken care to ensure that the information given in this text is accurate and up to date. However, readers are strongly advised to confirm that the information, especially with regard to drug usage, complies with the latest legislation and standards of practice.

 your source for books, journals and multimedia in the health sciences

**www.elsevierhealth.com**

Printed in China

The publisher's policy is to use paper manufactured from sustainable forests

# Series preface

Medical students and doctors in training are expected to travel to different hospitals and community health centres as part of their education. Many books are too large to carry around, but the information they contain is often vital for the basic understanding of disease processes.

The *Saunders' Pocket Essentials* series is designed to provide portable, pocket-sized companions to larger texts such as our own *Clinical Medicine*. They are most useful for clinical practice, whether in hospital or the community, and for exam revision.

All the books in the series have the same helpful features:

- Succinct text
- Simple line drawings
- Emergency and other boxes
- Tables that summarize causes and clinical features of disease
- Exam questions and explanatory answers
- Dictionary of terms

They contain core material for quick revision, easy reference and practical management. The modern format makes them easy to read, providing an indispensable 'pocket essential.'

**Parveen Kumar** and **Michael Clark**
*Series Editors*

# Preface

This new third edition of *Pocket Essentials of Clinical Medicine*, based on Kumar and Clark's *Clinical Medicine*, has been thoroughly revised and updated, in line with changes in medicine and in the parent text.

We've improved and expanded the popular features associated with the *Pocket Essentials* series, such as emergency boxes, tables, exam questions and answers, while maintaining the core attribute of a succinct and highly portable text. We've also added some new features for this edition. There is now a list of useful websites, a new chapter on ethics and communication, and an enlarged dictionary of terms that gives brief descriptions of some rare conditions and explanations of some key medical terms. The index has also been greatly expanded, in response to requests from readers for a fully searchable book.

The appearance of the text has also been greatly improved for this third edition, with the use of full colour throughout. The colour has been used in two ways: to make the text more attractive and therefore easier to read and navigate, and to relate it to the parent text, *Clinical Medicine 5e*, by using the same 'colour coding' scheme for specific chapters. Readers will also find more cross references to *Clinical Medicine 5e*, identified by the use of *K&C* with the page number, thus making it easier to look up information in the larger book.

Finally, we are delighted that the book is now available in two forms: as a pocket textbook and as an electronic product for use on hand-held computers or 'palm-tops'/PDAs. We hope students and qualified doctors will welcome this choice in formats.

We would again like to thank Mike Clark and Parveen Kumar for their support and assistance in the preparation of this third edition of *Pocket Essentials*, and to express our indebtedness to the contributors of the parent text, *Clinical Medicine*. Finally without the continued help, support and hard work of Hannah Kenner, Project Development Manager at Elsevier, this book would not have been completed in its present form.

**Anne Ballinger** and **Stephen Patchett**

# Contents

Medical emergencies   *Inside front cover*

Series preface   vii

Preface   ix

Abbreviations   xiii

Significant websites   xvii

1   **Ethics and communication**   1
2   **Infectious diseases and tropical medicine**   7
3   **Gastroenterology and nutrition**   53
4   **Liver, biliary tract and pancreatic disease**   113
5   **Diseases of the blood and haematological malignancies**   165
6   **Rheumatology**   235
7   **Water and electrolytes**   283
8   **Renal disease**   309
9   **Cardiovascular disease**   365
10   **Respiratory disease**   443
11   **Intensive care medicine**   505
12   **Poisoning, drug and alcohol abuse**   523
13   **Endocrinology**   541
14   **Diabetes mellitus and other disorders of metabolism**   599
15   **Neurology**   635
16   **Dermatology**   723
17   **Practical procedures**   733
    **Examination questions**   757
    **Dictionary of terms**   799

Index   815

Normal values   *Inside back cover*

# Abbreviations

ACE      angiotensin-converting enzyme
ACTH     adrenocorticotrophic hormone
ADH      antidiuretic hormone
AF       atrial fibrillation
AIDS     acquired immunodeficiency syndrome
ANA      antinuclear antibodies
ANCA     antineutrophil cytoplasmic antibodies
ANF      antinuclear factor
ARDS     adult respiratory distress syndrome
AST      aspartate aminotransferase
AV       atrioventricular
AXR      abdominal X-ray

BCG      bacille Calmette–Guérin
BMI      body mass index
BNF      *British National Formulary*
BP       blood pressure

CAL      chronic airflow limitation
CAPD     continuous ambulatory peritoneal dialysis
CCF      congestive cardiac failure
CCU      coronary care unit
CLL      chronic lymphatic leukaemia
CML      chronic myeloid leukaemia
CNS      central nervous system
CRP      C-reactive protein
CSF      cerebrospinal fluid
CT       computerized tomography
CVP      central venous pressure
CXR      chest X-ray

DIC      disseminated intravascular coagulation
DNA      deoxyribonucleic acid
DVT      deep venous thrombosis

ECG      electrocardiogram
EEG      electroencephalogram
ELISA    enzyme-linked immunosorbent assay

| ERCP | endoscopic retrograde cholangiopancreatography |
|---|---|
| ESR | erythrocyte sedimentation rate |
| FBC | full blood count |
| GABA | γ-aminobutyric acid |
| γ-GT | γ-glutamyltranspeptidase |
| GFR | glomerular filtration rate |
| GORD | gastro-oesophageal reflux disease |
| Hb | haemoglobin |
| 5-HIAA | 5-hydroxyindoleacetic acid |
| HIV | human immunodeficiency virus |
| HLA | human leucocyte antigen |
| Ig | immunoglobulin (e.g. IgM = immunoglobulin the M class) |
| i.m. | intramuscular |
| INR | international normalized ratio |
| iu/IU | international unit |
| i.v. | intravenous |
| IVP | intravenous pyelogram |
| JVP | jugular venous pressure |
| K&C | Kumar & Clark: *Clinical Medicine 5e* (Saunders 2002) |
| LP | lumbar puncture |
| LVF | left ventricular failure |
| MCV | mean corpuscular volume |
| ME | myalgic encephalomyelitis |
| MRI | magnetic resonance imaging |
| MRSA | methicillin-resistant *Staphylococcus aureus* |
| MSU | mid-stream urine |
| ND | Notifiable disease |
| NSAIDs | non-steroidal anti-inflammatory drugs |
| $Pa_{CO_2}$ | partial pressure of carbon dioxide in arterial blood |
| $Pa_{O_2}$ | partial pressure of oxygen in arterial blood |
| PCR | polymerase chain reaction |
| PCV | packed cell volume |
| PPI | proton pump inhibitor |

| | |
|---|---|
| PR | per rectum (rectal instillation) |
| PT | prothrombin time |
| PTC | percutaneous transhepatic cholangiography |
| PTCA | percutaneous transluminal coronary angioplast |
| PTTK | partial thromboplastin time with kaolin |
| RCC | red cell count |
| RhF | rheumatoid factor |
| RIA | radioimmunoassay |
| RNA | ribonucleic acid |
| s.c. | subcutaneous |
| SLE | systemic lupus erythematosus |
| STI | sexually transmitted infection |
| SVC | superior vena cava |
| SVT | supraventricular tachycardia |
| TIA | transient ischaemic attack |
| TNM | tumour, node, metastasis classification |
| TPN | total parenteral nutrition |
| TRH | thyrotrophin-releasing hormone |
| TSH | thyroid-stimulating hormone |
| VDRL | Venereal Disease Research Laboratory (test for syphilis) |
| VF | ventricular fibrillation |
| VIP | vasoactive intestinal polypeptide |
| VT | ventricular tachycardia |
| WBC | white blood (cell) count |
| WCC | white cell count |
| WE | Wernicke's encephalopathy |

# Significant websites

## General websites

http://www.ncbi.nlm.nih.gov/PubMed
PubMed: Medline on the Web

http://www.nih.gov/health
US National Institutes of Health website (biomedical research, free)

http://www.nice.org.uk
UK National Institute for Clinical Excellence

http://www.chi.nhs.uk/
Commission for Health Improvement

http://www.nelh.nhs.uk/guidelinesfinder/
Details of UK national guidelines with links to Internet versions

http://gungadin.cs.brandeis.edu/~weiluo/main3.htm
Lists biomedical acronyms and their meanings

## Healthcare journal and magazines

http://www.jr2.ox.ac.uk/bandolier/
Bandolier (free abstracts and good links)

http://www.bmj.com/index.shtml
British Medical Journal

http://www.doh.gov.uk/cmo/publications.htm
Chief Medical Officer's publications

## Medical societies and organizations

http://www.gmc-uk.org/
UK General Medical Council

### 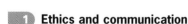 Ethics and communication

http://www.nih.gov/sigs/bioethics/
US National Institutes of Health website: bioethics pages

### 2 Infectious diseases and tropical medicine

http://www.idlinks.com
General starting point for infectious disease links

http://www.phls.co.uk/
UK Public Health Laboratory Service: UK regional information on infections

http://www.hivatis.org/
Centers for Disease Control and Prevention: HIV/AIDS treatment/information service

http://www.doh.gov.uk/eaga/
Department of Health Expert Advisory Group on AIDS: information about post-exposure prophylaxis, guidelines for pre-test discussion on HIV testing and risks of transmission

http://www.nfid.org/factsheets/
National Foundation for Infectious Diseases, USA: fact sheets on infectious diseases

## 3 Gastroenterology and nutrition

http://www.who.int/nutgrowthdb/
World Health Organization site, provides information on world-wide nutritional issues, resources and research

http://www.digestivedisorders.org.uk/leaflets/ibs.html
Irritable bowel syndrome

http://www.coeliac.co.uk
Coeliac disease

## 4 Liver, biliary tract and pancreatic disease

http://www-micro.msb.le.ac.uk/335/Hepatitis.html
Viral hepatitis

## 5 Diseases of the blood and haematological malignancies

http://www.hemophilia.org
US National Hemophilia Foundation

## 6 Rheumatology

http://www.arc.org.uk
UK Arthritis Research Campaign

http://www.rheumatology.org.uk/
British Society of Rheumatology: useful, patient-oriented information

**7** **Water and electrolytes &**
**8** **Renal disease**

http://www.nephronline.org
For healthcare professionals involved in the management of
patients with kidney disease

http://www.kidney.org.uk/
UK charity run by and for patients

**9** **Cardiovascular disease**

http://www.resus.org.uk
UK Resuscitation Council

**10** **Respiratory disease**

http://www.quitsmokinguk.com
Good site for those wanting to quit or to help patients to quit

http://www.brit-thoracic.org.uk
British Thoracic Society: guidelines for the management of many
respiratory diseases including asthma. UK National Asthma
Campaign

http://www.goldcopd.com
WHO global initiative for COPD: diagnosis, treatment and prevention
of COPD

**11** **Intensive care medicine**

http://www.ics.ac.uk
UK Intensive Care Society

**12** **Poisoning, drug and alcohol abuse**

http://www.doh.gov.uk/cmo/cmo0202.htm
Department of Health: detailed information on CO poisoning

http://www.drinksafely.info
Patient-based website: useful information about harmful effects of
alcohol and guidelines for safe drinking

**13** **Endocrinology**

http://www.niddk.nih.gov/health/endo/endo.htm
US National Institutes of Health, National Institute of Diabetes
& Digestive & Kidney Diseases

http://www.endocrineweb.com
Endocrine web resource

http://www.pituitary.org.uk
The Pituitary Foundation (UK charity)

## 14 Diabetes mellitus and other disorders of metabolism

http://www.sign.ac.uk/guidelines/index.html
Scottish Intercollegiate Guidelines Network: guidelines on a range of subjects including diabetes

http://www.diabetes.org.uk
Diabetes UK charity (formerly the British Diabetic Association): information for patients, researchers and health professionals

http://www.jdf.org.uk
Juvenile Diabetes Foundation (UK)

## 15 Neurology

http://www.stroke.org.uk
UK Stroke Association

http://www.parkinsons.org.uk
Parkinson's Disease Society

http://www.epilepsy.org.uk
The British Epilepsy Association

http://www.mssociety.org.uk
The Multiple Sclerosis Society

http://www.gbs.org.uk
Guillain–Barré Syndrome Support Group: past patients offer visiting and counselling services

## 16 Dermatology

http://www.bad.org.uk
British Association of Dermatologists

http://tray.dermatology.uiowa.edu/Dermlmag.htm
Dermatologic image database (adult)

http://www.eczema.org
UK National Eczema Society (atopic eczema)

# Ethics and communication

Ethical and moral issues are an important part of medical care, particularly with respect to controversial topics such as euthanasia, organ donation and genetic technology. A doctor with clinical responsibility for a patient has three corresponding duties of care:

- *Protect life and health.* Clinicians should practise medicine to a high standard and not cause unnecessary suffering or harm. Treatment should only be given when it is thought to be beneficial to that patient. Competent patients have the right to refuse treatment, but decisions not to provide life-sustaining treatment should only be taken with their informed consent on the basis of a clear explanation about the consequences of their refusal.

- *Respect autonomy.* Clinicians must respect the need to maintain the autonomy and self-determination of patients and thus recognize that the patient has the ability to reason, plan and make choices about the future. Wherever possible patients should remain responsible for themselves. Informed consent and confidentiality are fundamental parts of good medical practice and respect for human dignity. Medical information belongs to the patient and should not be disclosed to any other parties, including relatives, without the informed consent of the patient. However, the right to privacy does not entail the right to harm others in exercising it, and in certain circumstances clinicians must breach confidentiality, e.g. infectious patients who pose a threat to specific individuals through undisclosed risks. Breach of confidentiality in these circumstances is usually only done after informing the patient of the intent to do so.

- *Protect life and health and respect autonomy with fairness and justice.* All patients have the right to be treated

equally regardless of race, fitness, social worth, class
or any other arbitrary prejudice or favouritism.

Various regulatory bodies, common law and the Human
Rights Act 1998 regulate medical practice and ensure that
doctors take their duties of care seriously. The standards
expected of healthcare professionals by their regulatory
bodies (including the General Medical Council (GMC), the
Royal College of Physicians and British Medical
Association) may at times be higher than the minimum
required by law.

# Legally valid consent

It is a general legal and ethical principle that valid consent
must be obtained before starting treatment or physical
investigation, or providing personal care, for a patient. This
principle reflects the right of patients to determine what
happens to their own bodies. For instance common law has
established that touching a patient without valid consent
may constitute the civil or criminal offence of battery.
Furthermore, failure to obtain adequate consent may be a
factor in a claim of negligence against the health profes-
sional involved, particularly if the patient suffers harm as a
result of treatment.

## Obtaining consent

For consent to be valid it must be given voluntarily after providing the patient with a reasonable amount of information
about the risks of the proposed treatment or investigation. In
addition, the patient must have the capacity to consent to the
treatment in question, i.e. the patient must be able to com-
prehend and retain information about the treatment and use
this information in the decision-making process. In the case
of adults who cannot give informed consent because of brain
damage the doctor must decide if the proposed treatment is
in the best interests of the patient. The treatment should be
discussed with the relatives but they should not be asked to
provide consent. Treatment can only be given legally to adult

patients without consent if they are temporarily or permanently incompetent to provide it and the treatment is necessary to save their life, or to prevent them from incurring serious and permanent injury. In the UK, the legal age of presumed competence to consent to treatment is 16 years. Below this age, those with parental responsibility are the legal proxies of their children and usually consent to treatment on their behalf. The clinician providing the treatment or investigation is responsible for ensuring that the patient has given valid consent before treatment begins.

# Communication

Communication is the way in which clinicians integrate clinical science with patient-centred, evidence-based shared healthcare. It is the process of exchanging information and ideas and also making a trusting relationship upon which the collaborative partnership between patients and their families and healthcare workers depends. Good communication improves health outcomes, including symptom resolution, reduction in adverse psychological outcomes, improved pain control and reduced patient anxiety. Failure of communication leads to poor delivery of information, lack of patient understanding and ultimately the patient feeling deserted and devalued. The majority of complaints against doctors are not based on failures of biomedical practice but on poor communication. Patients have identified qualities used by the doctor in the interview which lead to good relationships. Doctors who were considered to have communicated well:

- orientated patients to the process of the visit, e.g. introductory comments: 'We are going to do this first and then go on to that'
- used facilitative comments
- asked patients their opinion
- used active listening
- used humour and laughter
- conducted slightly longer visits (18 versus 15 minutes).

# The medical interview

Clinicians must use their time to the greatest benefit of their patients. It is essential to find out not only the medical facts in detail but also what patients have experienced and what impact this experience has had upon them. There are three phases to an interview:

***Opening*** The start of the interview will be helped by well-organized arrangements for appointments, reception and punctuality. The physician should come out of the room to greet the patient, establish eye contact and shake hands if appropriate. Clinicians should introduce themselves by telling patients their name, status and responsibility to the patient; a name badge will reinforce this information. The patient should sit beside the clinician and not on the far side of a desk.

***Exploring and focusing*** In addition to obtaining a complete history the clinician should also determine the impact of the problem on the patient's life, the patient's ideas and fears and the patient's attitude to similar problems in others. The clinician will obtain more information by starting with open questions and then guiding the history by using closed questions for further detail. An open question such as 'What has brought you to see me today?' allows the patient to speak freely and the clinician will obtain more information. A closed question such as 'What date exactly did the headache start?' will not allow patients to address all their concerns and they will not speak freely. During the interview a smile and eye contact from the physician will let the patient know that the doctor is listening attentively. Demonstrating empathy is a key skill in building the patient–clinician relationship and involves the patient's experiences being seen, heard and accepted with some feedback to demonstrate this. For instance, 'The last point made you look worried. Is there something more serious about that point you would like to tell me?' demonstrates that the patient's experiences have been seen. Patients are more likely to adhere to clinical advice if they get comprehensible information, if it makes sense of their problems, and if they can get easy access to more information if they need it. Patients must always be given information in a logical sequence, using simple language and avoiding medical terms, and if possible with the aid of simple diagrams and key words. It is useful to check that the patient understands before moving on to another point. Further aids for information such as medical support groups and reference web sites are always useful.

***Closing*** Closing the interview may start with a brief summary of the patient's agenda and then of that of the clinician. The patient should be told the arrangements for further interview and the commitment to informing other healthcare professionals involved with the patient. It is useful to make a written record in the patient's notes as to what the patient has been told and what has been understood. In some situations it is useful if the patient knows how to contact an appropriate team member as a safety net before the next interview. The interview is closed with an appropriate farewell and some words of encouragement.

## Breaking bad news

Breaking bad news can be difficult and the way that it is broken has a major psychological and physical effect upon patients. In these situations patients usually know more than anyone has guessed, welcome clear information and do not want to be drawn into a charade of deception which does not allow them to discuss their illness and the future. The clinician should begin the interview by finding out how much the patient knows and if anything new has developed since the last encounter. The clinician should give the patient a warning that the news is bad or more serious than initially thought and then pause to allow the patient to think this over and only continue when the patient gives some lead to follow. The clinician should then give small chunks of information and ensure that the patient understands before moving on. Frequent pauses allow the patient to think. The interview should be stopped and resumed at a later date if necessary. The patient should be provided with some positive information and hope tempered with realism. The patient may ask for a time frame of events but it is often impossible to give an accurate time frame for a terminal disease. The importance of maintaining a good quality of life during this time must be stressed. The patient must be given the opportunity for other family members to meet with the clinician. The interview should close with a further interview date – preferably soon, a contact name as a safety net before the next interview and details regarding further sources of information.

# 2

# Infectious diseases and tropical medicine

Infectious diseases are the most common diseases of humans and a major source of morbidity and mortality in both developed and developing countries. Upper respiratory tract infections and gastroenteritis are commonly seen in the community and do not often need admission to hospital. With increasing travel abroad more tropical diseases are now seen in the UK and, with the emergence of AIDS, opportunistic infections are seen more commonly. In the UK some infectious diseases must be notified to the local Medical Officer for Environmental Health; these are indicated by the abbreviation ND where appropriate.

## Pyrexia of unknown origin (K&C p. 2)

Pyrexia (or fever) of unknown origin (PUO) is defined as a documented fever (> 38°C) lasting more than 2 weeks in which a clinical history, repeated thorough physical examination and routine investigations have failed to reveal a cause. Occult infection remains the most common cause in adults. Collagen vascular disease, drug hypersensitivity and malignancy are other causes (Table 2.1).

### Investigations

First-line investigations should be repeated as the results may have changed since the tests were first performed:

- Full blood count, including a differential white cell count (WCC) and blood film
- Erythrocyte sedimentation rate (ESR)
- Serum urea and electrolytes, liver biochemistry and blood glucose
- Blood cultures – several sets from different sites at different times
- Microscopy and culture of urine, sputum and faeces
- Baseline serum for virology
- Chest X-ray
- Serum rheumatoid factor and antinuclear antibody.

**Table 2.1**
Some causes of pyrexia of unknown origin

**Infection (20–40%)**
Pyogenic abscess: e.g. liver, pelvic, subphrenic
Tuberculosis
Infective endocarditis
Viruses: Epstein–Barr, cytomegalovirus
Primary HIV infection
Brucellosis
Lyme disease
Malaria

**Malignant disease (10–30%)**
Lymphoma
Leukaemia
Renal cell carcinoma
Hepatocellular carcinoma

**Collagen vascular disease (15–20%)**
Adult Still's disease
Rheumatoid arthritis
Systemic lupus erythematosus
Wegener's granulomatosis
Giant cell arteritis

**Miscellaneous (10–25%)**
Drug fever
Thyrotoxicosis
Inflammatory bowel disease
Sarcoidosis
Granulomatous hepatitis: e.g. tuberculosis, sarcoidosis
Factitious fever (switching thermometers, injection of pyogenic material)
Familial Mediterranean fever

Second-line investigations are performed in patients who remain undiagnosed and when repeat physical examination is unhelpful.

- Abdominal imaging with ultrasound, CT or MRI to detect occult abscesses and malignancy
- Echocardiography for infective endocarditis
- Biopsy of liver and bone marrow; temporal artery biopsy (p. 702) should be considered in the elderly
- Determination of HIV status
- Radionuclide scanning after injection of indium- or technetium-labelled white cells (previously harvested from the patient) can localize an abscess and may be useful when other imaging is unhelpful.

## Management

The treatment is of the underlying cause. In a few patients no diagnosis is reached after thorough investigation and in most of these the fever will resolve on follow-up.

## Septicaemia (K&C p. 77)

The term bacteraemia refers to the transient presence of organisms in the blood (generally without causing symptoms) as a result of local infection or penetrating injury. The term septicaemia, on the other hand, is usually reserved for the clinical picture that results from the systemic inflammatory response to infection. Inflammation is normally intended to be a local and contained response to infection. Activated polymorphonuclear leucocytes, macrophages and lymphocytes release inflammatory mediators including tumour necrosis factor, interleukin-1 (IL-1), platelet activating factor, IL-6, IL-8, interferon and eicosanoids. In some cases, mediator release exceeds the boundaries of the local environment leading to a generalized response that affects normal tissues. This process is referred to as sepsis and the clinical features include fever, tachycardia, an increase in respiratory rate and hypotension. Septicaemia has a high mortality without treatment, and demands immediate attention. The pathogenesis and management of septic shock is discussed on pages 505 and 508.

## Aetiology

Overall, about 40% of cases are the result of Gram-positive organisms and 60% of Gram-negative ones. Fungi are much less common but should be considered, particularly in the immunocompromised. In the previously healthy adult, septicaemia may occur from a source of infection in the chest (e.g. with pneumonia), urinary tract (often Gram-negative rods) or biliary tree (commonly *Enterococcus faecalis*, *Escherichia coli*). Intravenous drug abusers frequently get septicaemia caused by *Staphylococcus aureus* and *Pseudomonas* sp. Hospitalized patients are susceptible to infection from wounds, indwelling urinary catheters and intravenous cannulae.

## Clinical features

Fever, rigors and hypotension are the cardinal features of severe septicaemia. Lethargy, headache and a minor change in conscious level may be preceding features. In elderly and immunocompromised patients the clinical features may be quite subtle and a high index of suspicion is needed.

Certain bacteria are associated with a particularly fulminating course:

- Staphylococci that produce an exotoxin called toxic shock syndrome toxin-1. The toxic shock syndrome is characterized by an abrupt onset of fever, rash, diarrhoea and shock. It is associated with the use of infected tampons in women but may occur in anyone, including children.
- Meningococci that produce the Waterhouse–Friderichsen syndrome. This is a rapidly fatal illness (without treatment), with a purpuric skin rash and shock. Adrenal haemorrhage (and hypoadrenalism) may or may not be present.

## Investigations

In addition to blood count, serum electrolytes and liver biochemistry:

- Blood cultures
- Cultures from possible source: urine, abscess aspirate, sputum
- In some cases: chest radiography, abdominal ultrasonography and CT scan.

## Management

Antibiotic therapy should be started immediately the diagnosis is suspected and after appropriate culture samples have been sent to the laboratory. The probable site of origin of sepsis will often be apparent, and knowledge of the likely microbial flora can be used to choose appropriate treatment. In cases where 'blind' antibiotic treatment is necessary, a reasonable combination would be intravenous gentamicin and piperacillin, or cefotaxime, with or without metronidazole. Therapy may subsequently be altered on the basis of culture and sensitivity results.

# Common viral infections

## Measles ND (*K&C p. 58*)

Measles is caused by infection with an RNA paramyxovirus which is spread by droplets. With the introduction of immunization policies using a live attenuated vaccine in the West the incidence has fallen, but it remains common in developing countries, where it is associated with a high morbidity and mortality. One attack confers lifelong immunity.

### Clinical features

The incubation period is 8–14 days. Two distinct phases of the disease can be recognized.

***The infectious pre-eruptive and catarrhal stage*** There is fever, cough, rhinorrhoea, conjunctivitis and Koplik's spots in the mouth (small grey irregular lesions on an erythematous base, commonly on the inside of the cheek).

***The non-infectious eruptive or exanthematous stage*** Characterized by the presence of a maculopapular rash which starts on the face and spreads to involve the whole body. The rash becomes confluent and blotchy.

### Complications (*uncommon in the healthy child*)

Gastroenteritis, pneumonia, otitis media, encephalitis, myocarditis, subacute sclerosing panencephalitis (rare).

### Management

The diagnosis is usually clinical and treatment is symptomatic. Measles vaccine is given to children between 12 and 18 months of age, in combination with mumps and rubella vaccine (MMR) to prevent infection.

## Mumps ND (*K&C p. 59*)

Mumps is also caused by infection with a paramyxovirus, spread by droplets. The incubation period averages 18 days.

### Clinical features
Mumps is predominantly an infection of school-aged children and young adults. There is fever, headache and malaise, followed by the development of parotid gland swelling. Less common features are orchitis, meningitis, pancreatitis, oophoritis, myocarditis and hepatitis.

### Management
Diagnosis is usually clinical. In doubtful cases demonstration of a rise in serum antibody titres is necessary for diagnosis. Treatment is symptomatic. The disease is prevented by administration of a live attenuated mumps virus vaccine.

## Rubella ND *(K&C p. 54)*
Rubella ('German measles') is caused by an RNA virus and has a peak age of incidence of 15 years. The incubation period is 14–21 days. During the prodrome the patient complains of malaise, fever and lymphadenopathy (suboccipital, postauricular, posterior cervical nodes). A pinkish macular rash appears on the face and trunk after about 7 days and lasts for up to 3 days.

### Diagnosis
The diagnosis may be suspected clinically and a definitive diagnosis is made by demonstrating a rising serum antibody titre in paired samples taken 2 weeks apart, or by the detection of rubella-specific IgM.

### Management
Treatment is symptomatic. Complications are uncommon but include arthralgia, encephalitis and thrombocytopenia.

### Congenital rubella syndrome
Maternal infection during pregnancy may affect the fetus, particularly if infection is acquired in the first trimester. Congenital rubella syndrome is characterized by the presence of congenital cardiac defects, eye lesions (particularly cataracts), microcephaly, mental handicap and deafness. There may also be persistent viral infection of the liver, lungs and heart, with hepatomegaly, pneumonitis and myocarditis. The teratogenic effects of rubella underlie the importance of preventing maternal infection with immunization.

# Herpes viruses

## Herpes simplex virus (HSV) infection (*K&C* p. 46 & p. 1276)

HSV-1 causes:

- Herpetic stomatitis with buccal ulceration, fever and local lymphadenopathy
- Herpetic whitlow: damage to the skin over a finger allows access of the virus, with the development of irritating vesicles
- Keratoconjunctivitis
- Encephalitis
- Systemic infection in immunocompromised patients.

HSV-2 is transmitted sexually and causes genital herpes, with painful genital ulceration, fever and lymphadenopathy. There may be systemic infection in the immunocompromised host and in severe cases death may result from hepatitis and encephalitis. These divisions are not rigid, because HSV-1 can also give rise to genital herpes.

Recurrent HSV infection occurs when the virus lies dormant in ganglion cells and is reactivated by trauma, febrile illnesses and ultraviolet irradiation. This leads to recurrent labialis ('cold sores') or recurrent genital herpes.

### Investigations

The diagnosis is often clinical but the virus may be cultured from lesions. Herpes simplex encephalitis is discussed on page 691.

### Management

Aciclovir is used topically and systemically for both primary and recurrent infection of the skin and mucous membranes. Penciclovir is used topically as a cream for herpes labialis.

## Herpes zoster (*K&C* p. 48 & p. 1277)

**Varicella (chickenpox)** Primary infection with this virus causes chickenpox, which may produce a mild childhood illness, although this can be severe in adults and immunocompromised patients.

## Clinical features

After an incubation period of 14–21 days there is a brief pro-dromal period of fever, headache and malaise. The rash, predominantly on the face, scalp and trunk, begins as macules and develops into papules and vesicles, which heal with crusting. Complications include pneumonia and central nervous system involvement.

## Investigations

The diagnosis is usually clinical. Electron microscopy of vesicle fluid may reveal the virus.

## Management

Healthy children require no treatment. Immunocompromised patients are treated with intravenous aciclovir and zoster-immune immunoglobulin (ZIG). Anyone over the age of 16 is given antiviral therapy with aciclovir because they are more at risk of severe disease. Because of the risk to both mother and fetus during pregnancy, pregnant women exposed to varicella zoster virus should receive prophylaxis with ZIG and treatment with aciclovir if they develop chickenpox.

**Herpes zoster (shingles)** After the primary infection herpes zoster remains dormant in dorsal root ganglia and reactivation causes shingles.

## Clinical features

Pain and tingling in a dermatomal distribution precede the rash by a few days. The rash consists of papules and vesicles in the same dermatome. The most common sites are the lower thoracic dermatomes and the ophthalmic division of the trigeminal nerve (pages 654 and 655).

## Management

Treatment is with oral famciclovir given as early as possible. The main complication is postherpetic neuralgia, which can be severe and last for years. Treatment is with carbamazepine or phenytoin.

# Infectious mononucleosis (K&C p. 49)

Infectious mononucleosis is caused by the Epstein–Barr virus (EBV) and predominantly affects young adults. EBV is transmitted in saliva and by aerosol.

## Clinical features

Many infections are asymptomatic. In symptomatic patients the main features are fever, headache, sore throat and a transient macular rash. There may be palatal petechiae, cervical lymphadenopathy, splenomegaly and mild hepatitis. Rare complications include splenic rupture, myocarditis and meningitis.

## Investigations

Atypical lymphocytes on a peripheral blood film strongly suggest infection. The diagnosis is confirmed by a positive Paul–Bunnell reaction (agglutination of sheep red cells by heterophile antibodies) and serum IgM antibodies to EBV.

## Management

Most cases require no treatment. Corticosteroids are given if there are systemic complications. Infection with *Toxoplasma gondii* or cytomegalovirus may produce a similar clinical picture in immunocompetent adults.

# Other infections

## Lyme borreliosis (Lyme disease) (K&C p. 81)

Lyme disease is a multisystem inflammatory disease caused by the spirochaete *Borrelia burgdorferi*. Infection is spread from deer and other wild mammals by *Ixodes* ticks.

### Clinical features

The clinical manifestations of Lyme disease are divided into three phases. Not all stages need appear and, conversely, clinical stages may overlap.

- Early localized disease includes erythema migrans (EM) and associated non-specific complaints of fever, malaise, headache or myalgia. EM usually occurs within 1 month of the tick bite, is usually asymptomatic and expands over the course of several days with central clearing.

- Early disseminated disease occurs days to months after the tick bite and consists of neurological (meningoencephalitis or polyneuropathy) or cardiac (myocarditis or conduction defects) problems.
- Late disease occurs months to years after the onset and consists of chronic and persistent neurological disease and/or arthritis.

### Investigations

The diagnosis can be made on the basis of typical clinical features in a patient living or visiting an endemic area.

*Serology* will show IgM antibodies in the first month and IgG antibodies late in the disease.

### Management

Amoxicillin, doxycycline or cephalosporins are the treatments of choice in the early stages of disease. Intravenous benzylpenicillin should be given for later stages of disease. To prevent infection in tick-infested areas, repellants and protective clothing should be worn and ticks removed promptly from the site of a bite. A vaccine is available and should be offered to those at high risk of infection.

## Leptospirosis (K&C p. 80)

This zoonosis is caused by a Gram-negative organism, *Leptospira interrogans*, which is excreted in animal urine and enters the host through a skin abrasion or intact mucous membranes. Individuals who work with animals or take part in water sports which bring them into close contact with rodents (e.g. boating lakes, diving) are most at risk.

### Clinical features

Following an incubation period of about 10 days, the initial leptospiraemic phase is characterized by fevers, headache, malaise and myalgia, followed by an immune phase, which is most commonly manifest by meningism. Most recover uneventfully at this stage. A small proportion go on to develop tender hepatosplenomegaly, jaundice, haemolytic anaemia, myocardial involvement and oliguric renal failure with microscopic haematuria (Weil's disease).

### Investigations
*Blood or CSF culture* can identify the organisms in the first week of the disease. The organism may be detected in the urine during the second week.

*Serology* will show specific IgM antibodies by the end of the first week.

### Management
Penicillin or erythromycin is most commonly used. The complications of the disease are treated appropriately.

## Tropical medicine

### Fever in the returned traveller
Fever is a common problem in travellers returning from tropical countries. Malaria is the single most common cause of fever in recent travellers from the tropics. Falciparum malaria has the potential to be rapidly fatal, and so evaluation of fever in this group of patients is often regarded as a medical emergency. Table 2.2 lists the causes of fever in travellers from the tropics; in about 25% of cases no specific cause is found. The most common causes are discussed in greater detail below.

### Approach to diagnosis
An accurate history and physical examination will help formulate an appropriate differential diagnosis and guide initial investigations. In addition to a full medical history an accurate travel history must be obtained:

- Countries visited, arrival and departure dates (for assessment of incubation period; Table 2.3)
- Travel in rural (where infection may be more common) or urban areas
- Exposure to vectors: mosquitoes, ticks, flies and fresh water infested with snails containing schistosomes

- Needle and blood exposure, e.g. blood transfusion or surgery, shared needles, acupuncture
- Vaccination and prophylaxis: recent vaccination against yellow fever and hepatitis A and B is extremely effective; subsequent infection with these agents is very unlikely. Vaccination against typhoid is only partially effective, therefore infection is still a possibility. Malaria is always a possibility, even in those who have taken chemoprophylaxis

**Table 2.2**
Causes of fever after travel to the tropics

| | |
|---|---|
| Malaria | |
| Viral hepatitis | |
| Febrile illness unrelated to foreign travel* | 80% of specific infections |
| Dengue fever | |
| Enteric fever (typhoid and paratyphoid fevers) | |
| Gastroenteritis | |
| Rickettsia | |
| Amoebic liver abscess | |
| Tuberculosis | |
| Acute HIV infection | |
| Others | |

* Includes respiratory and urinary tract infection

**Table 2.3**
Typical incubation periods for tropical infections

| Incubation period | Infection |
|---|---|
| Short (< 10 days) | Arboviral infections (including dengue fever), enteric bacterial infections, paratyphoid, plague, typhus, haemorrhagic fevers |
| Medium (10–21 days) | Malaria (but may be much longer), typhoid fever (rarely 3–60 days) scrub typhus, African trypanosomiasis, brucellosis, leptospirosis |
| Long (> 21 days) | Viral hepatitis, tuberculosis, HIV, schistosomiasis, amoebic liver abscess, visceral leishmaniasis, filariasis |

- History of unprotected sexual intercourse may suggest an acute HIV or hepatitis B seroconversion illness (p. 125).

## Investigations

The initial work-up of a febrile patient who has travelled to the tropics is listed below. Additional studies depend upon exposure and other factors.

- Full blood count with differential white cell count, and thick and thin blood malaria films; repeat after 12–24 hours if initial films negative and malaria suspected
- Liver biochemistry – abnormal results found in many tropical infections
- Cultures of blood and stool
- Microscopy and culture of urine
- Chest X-ray
- 'Acute' serum for storage and subsequent antibody detection with paired convalescent serum at a later date.

## Malaria ND (K&C p. 98)

Malaria is a protozoan parasite widespread in the tropics and subtropics (Fig. 2.1). Each year 300 million people are affected, with a mortality rate of 1%.

### Aetiology

Travellers abroad are infected following the bite of an infected female mosquito of the genus *Anopheles*. Rarely the parasite is transmitted by importation of infected mosquitoes by air (airport malaria).

Four malaria parasites may infect humans; by far the most hazardous is *Plasmodium falciparum*, the symptoms of which can rapidly progress from an acute fever with rigors to severe multiorgan failure, coma and death. Once successfully treated this form does not relapse. The other malaria parasites, *P. vivax*, *P. ovale* and *P. malariae*, cause a more benign illness. However, *P. ovale* and *P. vivax* may relapse and *P. malariae* may run a chronic course over months or years.

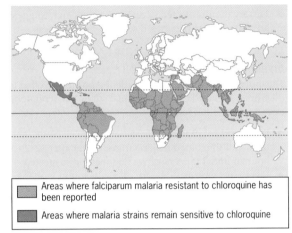

Areas where falciparum malaria resistant to chloroquine has been reported

Areas where malaria strains remain sensitive to chloroquine

**Fig. 2.1 Malaria – geographical distribution.**

20

## Pathogenesis

The infective form of the parasite (sporozoites) passes through the skin and via the bloodstream to the liver. After a variable number of days they invade red blood cells and pass through further stages of development, which terminate with the rupture of the red cell. Rupture of red blood cells contributes to anaemia and releases pyrogens, causing fever. Red blood cells infected with *P. falciparum* adhere to the endothelium of small vessels and the consequent vascular occlusion causes severe organ damage, chiefly in the kidney, liver and brain. *P. ovale and P. vivax* may remain latent in the liver, and this is believed to be responsible for the relapses that may occur.

## Clinical features

The incubation period varies:

- 10–14 days in *P. vivax, P. ovale* and *P. falciparum* infection
- 18 days to 6 weeks in *P. malariae* infection.

The onset of symptoms may be delayed in the partially immune or after prophylaxis. There is an abrupt onset of fever (> 40°C), tachycardia and rigors, followed by profuse sweating some hours later. This may be accompanied by anaemia and hepatosplenomegaly.

*P. falciparum* (Table 2.4) should be considered a medical emergency because patients may deteriorate rapidly. The following clinical forms are recognized and are more likely to occur when more than 1% of the red blood cells (RBC) are parasitized:

- *Cerebral malaria* is characterized by a high fever, convulsions, coma and eventually death. Hypoglycaemia, a complication of severe malaria, may present in a similar way and must be excluded.
- *Blackwater fever*, so called because of the production of dark brown-black urine (haemoglobinuria) resulting from severe intravascular haemolysis.

## Investigations

The conventional method for diagnosing malaria is light microscopy of a Giemsa-stained thick and/or thin blood smear. The smears also allow quantification of the percentage of parasitized red cells and may be helpful for species identification. Antigen-capture test kits use a rapid simple dipstick test from a finger-prick blood sample to give a result in 10–15 minutes and are used in the field in

**Table 2.4**
Possible features of falciparum malaria

| | |
|---|---|
| Central nervous system | Impaired consciousness and fits |
| Renal | Haemoglobinuria (Blackwater fever) Oliguria Uraemia (acute tubular necrosis) |
| Blood | Severe anaemia Disseminated intravascular coagulation |
| Respiratory | Acute respiratory distress syndrome/acute lung injury |
| Metabolic | Hypoglycaemia Metabolic acidosis |
| Gastrointestinal | Diarrhoea Jaundice Splenic rupture |
| Other | Hyperpyrexia Shock |

developing countries. Other investigations include full blood count, serum urea and electrolytes, liver biochemistry and blood glucose.

## Management

The acute treatment and eradication therapy of uncomplicated malaria is summarized in Table 2.5. Antipyretics such as aspirin and paracetamol are given as necessary, and intravenous fluids may be required to combat dehydration and shock.

*Severe malaria*, indicated by the presence of any of the complications listed in Table 2.4 or if more than 1% of the RBCs are infected, constitutes a medical emergency and optimal management may require admission to the ITU. Expert advice should be sought from a malaria reference centre.

**Table 2.5**
Treatment of an acute uncomplicated attack of malaria

| Type of malaria | Drug treatment |
| --- | --- |
| *Plasmodium vivax,* P. ovale, P. malariae | Chloroquine: 600 mg<br>300 mg 6 hours later |
| Chloroquine-sensitive P. falciparum | 300 mg 24 hours later<br>300 mg 24 hours later |
| Chloroquine-resistant, Fansidar-sensitive P. falciparum | Fansidar: 3 tablets as a single dose |
| Chloroquine and Fansidar-resistant P. falciparum | Quinine: 600 mg 3 times daily for 7 days *plus*<br>Tetracycline: 500 mg 4 times daily for 7 days or Fansidar: 3 tablets as a single dose at the end of 7 days |
|  | Alternative therapy<br>Mefloquine: 20 mg/kg in 2 doses 8 hours apart |
|  | Alternative therapy<br>Malarone: 4 tablets daily for 3 days |
| **Eradication**<br>For P. vivax, P. ovale | Oral primaquine* 15 mg daily for 14 days |

Chloroquine doses quoted are for the base drug; Fansidar = pyramethamine/sulfadoxine

* Check for glucose-6-phosphate dehydrogenase deficiency first (p. 189)

Intravenous chloroquine is given for patients from chloroquine-sensitive areas and quinine or artesunate for patients
from chloroquine-resistant areas. In developing countries
where facilities are not available for intravenous infusion,
alternative routes are by intramuscular injection (chloroqui-
nine and quinine), nasogastric tube (chloroquine) or rectally
(artemisinin). Intravenous glucose is given for hypoglycaemia and benzodiazepines for seizures. Early dialysis
for acute renal failure should be commenced and positive-
pressure ventilation for non-cardiogenic pulmonary oedema.

## Prevention and control

Effective prevention of malaria includes the following
elements:

- Awareness of risk
- Use of mechanical barriers such as insecticide-
  impregnated nets and mosquito repellents
- Chemoprophylaxis.

As a result of changing patterns of resistance, advice about
chemoprophylaxis should be sought before leaving for a
malaria-endemic area. Further details can be found in the
*British National Formulary* or from travel advice centres.
Prophylaxis does not afford full protection. Drug regimens
should be started at least 1 week before departure and continued without interruption for 4 weeks after return. The
rationale for this advice is to ensure therapeutic drug levels
before travelling and to enable unwanted effects to be dealt
with before departure. The continued use of drugs after
returning home will deal with infection contracted on the
last day of exposure.

*Chloroquine* 300 mg weekly is recommended in travellers
to chloroquine-sensitive areas. In areas of limited chloroquine resistance this is combined with proguanil 200 mg
daily. This regimen has few side-effects and is safe in
pregnancy.

*Mefloquine* 250 mg weekly is used in areas where falciparum malaria is highly resistant to chloroquine. With the
now widespread geographic prevalence of chloroquine-
resistant *P. falciparum*, mefloquine is for many travellers the

mainstay of malarial chemoprophylaxis. An alternative is malarone (proguanil/atovaquone) or doxycycline.

## Dengue fever (K&C p. 56)

Dengue fever is caused by a flavivirus. It is found mainly in Asia, Africa, Central and South America where it is a common cause of fever and may be fatal. The virus is transmitted by the mosquito *Aedes aegypti*. After an incubation period of 5–6 days there is an abrupt onset of fever, headache, retro-orbital pain and severe myalgia, often with a skin rash. Rare complications include shock and haemorrhagic manifestations, including purpura, epistaxis and melaena. Diagnosis is clinical and confirmed by acute and convalescent serum samples. Treatment is supportive.

## Enteric fever (K&C p. 71 & p. 88)

Typhoid fever and paratyphoid fever are caused by *Salmonella typhi* and *Salmonella paratyphi* (types A, B and C), respectively.

## Typhoid fever ND (K&C p. 71 & p. 88)

Humans are the only known reservoir of infection, and the spread is faecal–oral.

### Clinical features

After an incubation period of 10–14 days there is an insidious onset of headache, dry cough and constipation, and a rising fever with relative bradycardia. In the second week of the illness an erythematous maculopapular rash that blanches on pressure and is referred to as 'rose spots' appears, chiefly on the upper abdomen and thorax, lasting for only 2–3 days. There is splenomegaly (75%), cervical lymphadenopathy and hepatomegaly (30%). Diarrhoea may develop. Complications, usually occurring in the third week, are pneumonia, meningitis, acute cholecystitis, osteomyelitis, intestinal perforation and haemorrhage. Recovery occurs in the fourth week.

### Investigations

The diagnosis of enteric fever requires the culture of the causative microorganism from the patient. Organisms can be cultured from the blood, faeces, and urine depending on the stage in the illness that individuals present for medical attention. In complicated cases or where the diagnosis remains in doubt bone marrow cultures may be positive even after starting antibiotics.

*Blood count* shows leucopenia.

*Serologic tests* (Widal test) are of limited clinical utility.

### Management
Quinolone antibiotics, e.g. ciprofloxacin, are the treatment of choice. Infection is cleared when consecutive cultures of urine and faeces are negative. Some patients become chronic carriers, with the focus of infection in the gall bladder. Treatment is with amoxicillin and probenecid for 6 weeks. The most common method of prophylaxis for travellers is by intramuscular administration of a capsular polysaccharide vaccine.

## Paratyphoid ND (*K&C* p. 71 & p. 88)
Paratyphoid results in a milder illness that is otherwise clinically indistinguishable from typhoid fever. Treatment is with co-trimoxazole for 2 weeks.

## Entercolitis ND
Other *Salmonella* species (*S. choleraesuis* and *S. enteritidis*) cause a self-limiting infection presenting with diarrhoea and vomiting (Table 2.6).

## Amoebiasis ND (*K&C* p. 106)
Amoebiasis is caused by infection of the human gastrointestinal tract with the protozoal organism *Entamoeba histolytica*. Infection occurs world-wide, although much higher incidence rates are found in the tropics and subtropics. The modes of transmission are:

- Ingestion of cysts in contaminated food and water
- Person-to-person contact
- Sexual transmission among homosexual men.

**Table 2.6**
Pathogenic mechanisms of bacterial gastroenteritis

| Pathogenesis | Mode of action | Clinical presentation | Examples |
|---|---|---|---|
| **Mucosal adherence** | Effacement of intestinal mucosa | Moderate watery diarrhoea | Enteropathogenic *E. coli* (EPEC) |
| **Mucosal invasion** | Penetration and destruction of mucosa | Bloody diarrhoea | *Shigella* spp.<br>*Campylobacter* spp.<br>Enteroinvasive *E. coli* (EIEC) |
| **Toxin production**<br>Enterotoxin | Fluid secretion without mucosal damage | Profuse watery diarrhoea | *Vibrio cholerae*<br>*Salmonella* spp.<br>*Campylobacter* spp.<br>Enterotoxigenic *E. coli* (ETEC) |
| Neurotoxin | Paralysis of autonomic nervous system | Variable diarrhoea and vomiting | *Bacillus cereus*<br>*Staphylococcus aureus* producing enterotoxin B |
| Cytotoxin | Damage to the mucosa | Bloody diarrhoea | *Salmonella* spp.<br>*Campylobacter* spp.<br>Enterohaemorrhagic *E. coli* (EHEC) |

## Clinical features

**Intestinal amoebiasis (amoebic dysentery)** Invasion of the colonic epithelium by *E. histolytica* leads to tissue necrosis and ulceration. Ulceration may deepen and progress under the mucosa to form typical flask-like ulcers. The presentation varies from mild bloody diarrhoea to fulminating colitis, with the risk of toxic dilatation, perforation and peritonitis. In 10% of cases an amoeboma (inflammatory fibrotic mass) develops, commonly in the caecum or rectosigmoid region, which may bleed, cause obstruction or intussusception, or be mistaken for a carcinoma.

**Amoebic liver abscess** An amoebic liver abscess develops when organisms invade through the bowel serosa, enter the portal vein and pass into the liver. The abscess is usually single and in the right lobe of the liver. There is tender hepatomegaly, a high swinging fever and profound malaise. There may not be a history of colitis.

## Investigations

**Serology** Amoebic fluorescent antibody test (FAT) is positive in 90% of patients with liver abscess and in 60–70% of patients with active colitis.

**Colonic disease** Microscopic examination of fresh stool or colonic exudate obtained at sigmoidoscopy shows the motile trophozoites which contain red blood cells.

**Liver disease** Liver abscesses should be considered when the serum alkaline phosphatase is elevated. Liver ultrasonography or CT scan will confirm the presence of an abscess.

## Differential diagnosis

Amoebic colitis must be differentiated from the other causes of bloody diarrhoea: inflammatory bowel disease, bacillary dysentery, *E. coli*, *Campylobacter* sp., salmonellae and, rarely, pseudomembranous colitis. Amoebic liver abscess must be differentiated from a pyogenic abscess and/or a hydatid cyst.

## Management

Metronidazole is given for 5 days in amoebic colitis and a more prolonged course (10–14 days) in liver abscess. A large tense abscess may require percutaneous drainage under ultrasound guidance. After treatment of the invasive disease, the bowel should be cleared of parasites with a luminal amoebicide such as diloxanide furoate.

## Control and prevention

Improved standards of personal hygiene and water supply are required. Travellers are advised to drink bottled water. Individual chemoprophylaxis is not advised because the risk of acquiring infection is low. There is no effective vaccine.

# Shigellosis (bacillary dysentery) ND

(K&C p. 71)

Shigellosis is an acute self-limiting intestinal infection which occurs world-wide but is more common in tropical countries and in areas of poor hygiene. Transmission is by the faecal–oral route. The four *Shigella* species (*S. dysenteriae*, *S. flexneri*, *S. boydii* and *S. sonnei*) invade and damage the intestinal mucosa. Some strains of *S. dysenteriae* secrete a cytotoxin which results in diarrhoea.

## Clinical features

After an incubation period of about 2 days there is an abrupt onset of fever, malaise, abdominal pain and watery diarrhoea, which may progress to bloody diarrhoea with mucus and tenesmus.

## Investigations

The diagnosis is made on the basis of the stool culture.

## Differential diagnosis

This is from other causes of bloody diarrhoea (see above). Sigmoidoscopic appearances may be the same as those in inflammatory bowel disease.

## Management

The treatment of choice is ciprofloxacin 500 mg twice daily.

# Cholera ND (*K&C* p. 70 & p. 87)

Cholera is caused by the Gram-negative bacillus, *Vibrio cholerae*. Infection is common in tropical and subtropical countries in areas of poor hygiene. Infection is by the faecal–oral route, and spread is predominantly by ingestion of water contaminated with the faeces of infected humans. There is no identified animal reservoir.

Following attachment and colonization of the small intestinal epithelium *V. cholerae* produces its major virulence factor, cholera toxin. The B subunit of the toxin attaches to the enterocyte surface receptor, the ganglioside GM1; this allows migration of the A subunit into the cell to stimulate adenylate cyclase activity and increase cAMP levels. This produces massive secretion of isotonic fluid into the intestinal lumen. Cholera toxin also increases serotonin release from enterochromaffin cells in the gut, which contributes to the secretory activity and diarrhoea. Additional enterotoxins have been described in *V. cholerae* which may contribute to its pathogenic effect.

29

## Clinical features

The incubation period varies from a few hours to 6 days. The illness varies from mild diarrhoea to profuse watery diarrhoea ('rice-water stools') resulting in dehydration, hypotension and death.

## Investigations

The diagnosis is largely clinical. Fresh stool microscopy may show the motile vibrios.

## Management

Management is aimed at effective rehydration, which is mainly oral but in severe cases intravenous fluids are given. Oral rehydration solutions (ORS) depend on the fact that there is a glucose-dependent sodium absorption mechanism not related to cAMP and thus unaffected by cholera toxin. The traditional World Health Organization ORS contains sodium (90 mmol/L) and glucose (111 mmol/L), along with potassium, chloride and citrate. New ORS solutions based on rice water may be more effective and are being evaluated.

Tetracycline for 3 days helps to eradicate the infection, decrease stool output and shorten the duration of the illness.

### Prevention and control
Good hygiene and sanitation are the most effective measures for the reduction of infection. Oral cholera vaccines are under development.

## Giardiasis (*K&C* p. 107)
*Giardia intestinalis* is a flagellated protozoan that is found world-wide but is more common in tropical areas. It is a cause of traveller's diarrhoea (see later).

### Clinical features
The clinical features are the result of damage to the small intestine, with subtotal villous atrophy in severe cases. There is diarrhoea, nausea, abdominal pain and distension, with malabsorption and steatorrhoea in some cases. Repeated infections can result in growth retardation in children.

### Investigations
Treatment is often given based on clinical suspicion. If necessary, the diagnosis is made by finding cysts on stool examination or parasites in duodenal aspirates or biopsies.

### Management
Metronidazole 2 g as a single dose daily for 3 days will cure most infections; some patients need two or three courses.

## Gastroenteritis and food poisoning ND

The most common form of acute gastrointestinal infection is gastroenteritis, causing diarrhoea with or without vomiting. Not all cases of gastroenteritis (*K&C* p. 70) are food poisoning (*K&C* p. 75), as the pathogens are not always food- or water-borne. Individuals at increased risk of infection include infants and young children, the elderly,

travellers (principally to developing countries), the immunocompromised and those with reduced gastric acid secretion. Viral gastroenteritis is a common cause of diarrhoea
and vomiting in young children but is rarely seen in adults.
Protozoal and helminthic gut infections are rare in the West
but relatively common in developing countries.

Bacteria can cause diarrhoea in three different ways
resulting in two broad clinical syndromes: watery diarrhoea and bloody diarrhoea i.e. dysentery (Table 2.6).

The clinical features associated with the causative organisms of food poisoning are summarized in Table 2.7.
Listeriosis (infection with *Listeria monocytogenes*) is associated with contaminated coleslaw, non-pasteurized soft
cheeses and other packaged chilled foods. The main feature
of listeria infection is meningitis, occurring perinatally and
in immunocompromised adults (see p. 688).

## Traveller's diarrhoea

Acute gastrointestinal infection affects 30–50% of travellers
from western countries to the developing world. Typically
abdominal cramps and diarrhoea begin 4–6 days after
arrival and last 1–3 days. Less commonly diarrhoea persists
and may last for weeks. Infection is most commonly due to
enterotoxigenic *E. coli* (ETEC, Table 2.8). To reduce the risk
of infection, travellers are advised to drink bottled water,
peel fruit before eating it and avoid salads because the
ingredients may have been washed in contaminated water.
Antibiotic prophylaxis, e.g. with ciprofloxacin, is not routinely recommended but is considered for patients with
inflammatory bowel disease, immunosuppression and
coexistent medical disease which would be compromised
by dehydration, e.g. renal failure. Treatment of traveller's
diarrhoea is with rehydration, antibiotics, e.g. ciprofloxacin,
for moderate to severe symptoms, and antidiarrhoeal
agents, e.g. loperamide, for watery diarrhoea. Investigation,
with microscopy and culture of three serial stool specimens,
is usually only necessary for individuals with dysentery
when invasive organisms are involved, or when diarrhoea
persists in the returning traveller. Colonoscopy and biopsy
are occasionally necessary in this latter group, particularly
if an alternative diagnosis is considered, such as inflammatory bowel disease.

**Table 2.7**
Bacterial causes of food poisoning ND

| Organism | Source/vehicles | Incubation period | Symptoms | Diagnosis | Recovery |
|---|---|---|---|---|---|
| Staphylococcus aureus | Man – contaminated food and water | 2–4 h | Diarrhoea, vomiting and dehydration | Culture organism in vomitus or remaining food | < 24 h |
| E. coli O157:H7 | Cattle – meat, milk | 12–48 h | Watery diarrhoea ± haemorrhagic colitis, HUS | Stool culture | 10–12 days |
| Bacillus cereus | Environment – contaminated food | 1–6 h | Diarrhoea, vomiting and dehydration | Culture organism in faeces and food | 2–3 days |
| Clostridium perfringens | Environment – contaminated food | 8–22 h | Watery diarrhoea and cramping pain | Culture organism in faeces and food | 2–3 days |
| Clostridium botulinum | Environment – bottled or canned food | 18–24 h | Brief diarrhoea and paralysis due to neuromuscular blockade | Demonstrate toxin in food or faeces | 10–14 days |
| Salmonella spp. | Cattle and poultry – eggs, meat | 12–48 h | Abrupt diarrhoea, fever and vomiting | Stool culture | Usually 3–6 days, but may be up to 2 weeks |

**Table 2.7**
(continued)

| Organism | Source/vehicles | Incubation period | Symptoms | Diagnosis | Recovery |
|----------|-----------------|-------------------|----------|-----------|----------|
| *Campylobacter jejuni* | Cattle and poultry – meat, milk | 48–96 h | Diarrhoea + blood, fever, malaise and abdominal pain | Stool culture | 3–5 days |
| *Shigella* spp. | Man – contaminated food and water | 24–48 h | Acute watery, bloody diarrhoea | Stool culture | 7–10 days |

HUS, haemolytic uraemic syndrome characterized by the triad of acute renal failure, haemolytic anaemia and thrombocytopenia. Patients who also have neurological symptoms are considered to have the related disorder thrombotic thrombocytopenic purpura (TTP)

**Table 2.8**
Causes of traveller's diarrhoea

**Bacteria – 70–90% of cases**
Enterotoxigenic *Escherichia coli*
*Shigella* sp.
*Salmonella* sp.
*Campylobacter jejuni*
*Aeromonas* and *Plesimonas* spp.

**Viruses – 10%**
Rotavirus
Norwalk virus family

**Protozoa – < 5%**
*Giardia intestinalis*
*Entamoeba histolytica*
*Cryptosporidium parvum*
*Cyclospora cayetanensis*

# Helminths (*K&C* p. 109)

The helminths or worms that may infect man are of three classes (Table 2.9). In the UK only three species are commonly encountered: *Enterobius vermicularis*, *Ascaris lumbricoides* and *Taenia saginata*. Occasionally other species are imported from abroad, where they occur mainly in tropical and subtropical countries. A raised blood eosinophil count (eosinophilia) occurs at some stage in nearly all helminth infections.

# Sexually transmitted infections
(*K&C* p. 120)

Sexually transmitted infections (STIs) remain endemic in all societies, and the range of diseases spread by sexual activity continues to increase. The three common presenting symptoms are:

- Urethral discharge (see below)
- Genital ulcers (see below)
- Vaginal discharge caused by *Candida albicans*,
  *Trichomonas vaginalis*, *Neisseria gonorrhoeae*, *Chlamydia*

Table 2.9
Summary of intestinal diseases caused by helminths (parasitic worms)

| | Helminth | Clinical manifestations | Diagnosis | Treatment of choice |
|---|---|---|---|---|
| **Nematodes (roundworms)** | | | | |
| Small intestine | *Strongyloides stercoralis* | Local dermatitis at site of skin penetration, diarrhoea, malabsorption, disseminated disease. Symptoms may continue for years as a result of autoinfection | Larvae in fresh stool. Detection of specific serum antibodies (serology) | Tiabendazole |
| | Hookworm: *Ancylostoma duodenale*, *Necator americanus* | Local dermatitis at the site of skin penetration, nausea, epigastric pain, iron deficiency anaemia | Detection of eggs in faeces | Mebendazole |
| | Roundworm: *Ascaris lumbricoides* | Often asymptomatic. Vomiting, abdominal discomfort, anorexia, intestinal obstruction. Pulmonary eosinophilia after migration to the lungs | Detection of eggs in faeces | Levamisole |

(continued)

Table 2.9
(continued)

|  | Helminth | Clinical manifestations | Diagnosis | Treatment of choice |
|---|---|---|---|---|
|  | *Trichinella spiralis* | Abdominal pain and diarrhoea. Larvae penetrate the bowel wall and invade striated muscle causing pain | Serology, muscle biopsy | Albendazole |
|  | *Toxocara canis* | Penetration of small intestine to lungs (bronchospasm), liver (hepatomegaly), heart, brain and eye | Serology | Albendazole |
| Large intestine | Whipworm: *Trichuris trichiura* | Often asymptomatic. Mucosal damage may result in bloody diarrhoea | Detection of eggs in faeces | Pyrantel pamoate |
|  | Threadworm: *Enterobius vermicularis* | Pruritus ani | Apply adhesive tape to perineum and identify eggs microscopically | Mebendazole |

**Table 2.9**
(continued)

| | | | |
|---|---|---|---|
| **Trematodes (flukes)** | | | |
| Blood flukes | Schistosoma species | Snail vectors release cercariae which penetrate human skin (causing swimmer's itch) during swimming and paddling. Worms migrate to pelvic veins and bladder (S. haematobium) causing haematuria, hydronephrosis and renal failure. S. mansoni and S. japonicum migrate to the mesenteric veins and bowel causing bloody diarrhoea, intestinal strictures, hepatic fibrosis and portal hypertension | Detection of eggs in urine, stool or rectal biopsy. Serology. | Praziquantel |
| Liver flukes | Clonorchis sinensis Opisthorchis felineus and O. viverrini Fasciola hepatica | Cholangitis, biliary carcinoma | Detection of eggs on stool microscopy | Praziquantel Tiabendazole |

(continued)

Table 2.9
(continued)

| Helminth | Clinical manifestations | Diagnosis | Treatment of choice |
|---|---|---|---|
| **Cestodes (tapeworms)** | | | |
| *Taenia saginata* | Beef tapeworm acquired by eating insufficiently cooked beef. Causes abdominal pain and malabsorption | Detection of eggs on stool microscopy | Praziquantel |
| *Taenia solium* | Pork tapeworm from undercooked pork. Larvae penetrate the intestinal wall and cause disseminated disease involving skin, skeletal muscle and brain (fits, focal signs) | Serology, imaging of cysts in muscle and brain by X-ray, CT or MRI | Albendazole |
| *Echinococcus granulosus* | Hydatid disease acquired by eating meat (from sheep, cattle) contaminated with ova excreted by dogs. Large cysts develop in liver, lung and brain. Anaphylactic reactions if cyst contents escape | Ultrasound, CT and MRI show the cysts and daughter cysts. Diagnosis by serology | Surgical excision and albendazole |

*trachomatis*, herpes simplex, cervical polyps, neoplasia, retained tampon, chemical irritants. Bacterial vaginosis is also characterized by a vaginal discharge but it is not clear to what extent this is a sexually transmitted infection. It occurs when the normal lactobacilli of the vagina are replaced by a mixed flora of *Gardnerella vaginalis* and anaerobes, resulting in an offensive discharge.

STIs predominantly seen in the tropics are chancroid, granuloma inguinale and lymphogranuloma venereum. They may present with genital ulceration and inguinal lymphadenopathy.

The aspects of management of all the STIs are:

- Accurate diagnosis and effective treatment
- Screening for other STIs (multiple STIs may coexist)
- Patient education
- Contact tracing: the patient's sexual partners must be traced so that they can be treated, thereby preventing the disease from spreading further
- Follow-up to ensure that infection is adequately treated.

## Urethritis (K&C p. 124)

Urethritis in men presents with urethral discharge and dysuria. It is often asymptomatic in women.

## Gonorrhoea (K&C p. 122)

The causative organism, *Neisseria gonorrhoeae* (gonococcus), is a Gram-negative intracellular diplococcus which infects epithelium, particularly of the urogenital tract, rectum, pharynx and conjunctivae.

### Clinical features

The incubation period ranges from 2–14 days. In men the symptoms are purulent urethral discharge and dysuria. In homosexual men proctitis may produce anal pain, discharge and itch. Women may be asymptomatic or complain of vaginal discharge, dysuria and intermenstrual bleeding. Complications include salpingitis and Bartholin's abscess in women, epididymitis and prostatitis in men, and systemic spread with a rash and arthritis (p. 252). Infants born to infected mothers may develop ocular infections (ophthalmia neonatorum).

## Diagnosis
Gram stain and culture of a swab taken from the urethra in men and the endocervix in women. Blood culture and microscopy of synovial fluid should be performed in cases of disseminated gonorrhoea.

## Management
Single-dose ciprofloxacin (500 mg by mouth) is the treatment of choice for uncomplicated anogenital infection. Longer courses are required for complicated infections. Culture tests should be repeated at least 72 hours after treatment is complete.

## Non-gonococcal urethritis (NGU)
The most common cause is infection with *Chlamydia trachomatis*, which in men presents with urethral discharge and dysuria. In women infection may be asymptomatic and only found during investigations for infertility (secondary to salpingitis and fallopian tube blockage). The diagnosis of chlamydial urethritis is best made by nucleic acid amplification tests such as the polymerase chain reaction. The new urine-based diagnostic tests avoid the patient discomfort associated with urethral sampling. Treatment is with oxytetracycline or erythromycin (in pregnancy). Other causes of NGU are *Ureaplasma urealyticum*, *Bacteroides* sp. and *Mycoplasma* sp.

## Genital ulcers
The infective causes of genital ulceration in the UK include syphilis, herpes simplex and herpes zoster. Non-infective causes are Behçet's disease, toxic epidermal necrosis (p. 729), carcinoma and trauma.

## Syphilis (K&C p. 125)
The causative organism, *Treponema pallidum*, is a motile spirochaete which enters via a skin abrasion during close

sexual contact. The organism may also pass transplacentally from mother to fetus.

## Primary infection

After an incubation period of 10–90 days a papule develops at the site of infection. This ulcerates to become a painless, firm chancre which heals spontaneously within 2–3 weeks.

## Secondary infection

This occurs 4–10 weeks after the appearance of the primary lesion. There may be one or more of the following features: fever, sore throat, arthralgia, generalized lymphadenopathy, widespread skin rash (except the face), superficial ulcers in the mouth (snail-track ulcers) and condylomata lata (warty perianal lesions). In most patients symptoms subside within 1 year.

## Tertiary syphilis

Occurs after a latent period of 2 years or more. The characteristic lesion is a gumma (granulomatous lesion) occurring in the skin, bones, liver and testes. Cardiovascular syphilis is mentioned on pages 420 and 440 and neurosyphilis is described on page 694.

Cardiovascular syphilis is mentioned on pages 420 and 440 and neurosyphilis is described on page 694.

## Congenital syphilis

This usually becomes apparent between the second and sixth weeks after birth, early signs being nasal discharge, skin and mucous membrane lesions, and failure to thrive. Signs of late syphilis appear after 2 years of age, when there are also characteristic bone and teeth abnormalities as a result of earlier damage.

## Diagnosis

- *Dark ground microscopy of fluid* taken from lesions shows organisms in primary and secondary disease. Serological tests may be negative in primary disease.
- *Serology.* The *T. pallidum* enzyme immunoassay (EIA) is the screening test of choice. A positive test is then confirmed with the *T. pallidum* haemagglutination assay (TPHA) and Venereal Disease Research Laboratory (VDRL) test. The VDRL test is detectable

within 3–4 weeks of infection; it becomes negative in treated patients and in some untreated patients with late tertiary syphilis. Other diseases, e.g. autoimmune disease and malignancy, may give false positive results. The *T. pallidum* EIA, TPHA and the fluorescent treponemal antibody test are positive in most patients with primary disease, and remain positive in spite of treatment. They do not distinguish between syphilis and other treponemes, e.g. yaws.

### Management

Intramuscular procaine benzylpenicillin (procaine penicillin) for 10 days is given for primary and secondary syphilis. For tertiary syphilis treatment is continued for 4 weeks. The Jarisch–Herxheimer reaction, characterized by malaise, fever and headache, occurs most commonly in secondary syphilis and is the result of release of TNF-$\alpha$, IL-6 and IL-8 when organisms are killed by antibiotics.

## HIV and AIDS

Human immunodeficiency virus (HIV) infection is the cause of the acquired immune deficiency syndrome (AIDS). About 34 million people are infected with HIV world-wide. Africa suffers most of the disease burden.

### Epidemiology (K&C p. 131)

Transmission is by:

- *Sexual intercourse.* World-wide, heterosexual intercourse accounts for the vast majority of infections. Homosexual transmission accounts for about two-thirds of infections in Europe, the USA and Australia.
- *Mother to child.* Transmission can occur in utero, during childbirth and via breast milk.
- *Contaminated blood, blood products and organ donations.* The risk is now minimal in developed countries since the introduction of screening blood products in 1985.
- *Contaminated needles.* Intravenous drug addicts, needle-stick injuries in healthcare workers.

HIV infection is not spread by ordinary social or household contact.

## Pathogenesis of HIV infection (K&C p. 133)

The virus consists of an outer envelope and an inner core. The core contains RNA and the enzyme reverse transcriptase, which allows viral RNA to be transcribed into DNA and then incorporated into the host cell genome (i.e. a retrovirus). The rapid emergence of viral quasispecies (closely related but genetically distinct variants) is due to the high mutation rate of reverse transcriptase and the high rate of viral turnover. This genetic diversification has implications for the evolution of viral variants with resistance to antiviral drugs.

HIV surface glycoprotein gp120 binds to the CD4 molecule on host lymphocytes. Other cells of the immune system bearing the CD4 receptor are also affected. The interaction between CD4 and HIV surface glycoprotein together with host chemokine co-receptors CCR5 and CXCR4 is responsible for HIV entry into cells and release of viral RNA. There is a progressive and severe depletion of infected CD4 helper lymphocytes which results in host susceptibility to infections with intracellular bacteria and mycobacteria. The coexisting antibody abnormalities predispose to infections with capsulated bacteria, e.g. *Strep. pneumoniae* and *H. influenzae*. The clinical illness associated with HIV infection is due to this immune dysfunction, and also to a direct effect of HIV on certain tissues.

## Natural history of HIV infection (K&C p. 134)

The typical pattern of HIV infection is shown in Figure 2.2. Throughout the course of HIV infection viral load and immunodeficiency progress steadily, despite the absence of observed disease during the latency period.

HIV infection is divided into the following stages:

- *Category A* includes:
  - Primary HIV infection (also called acute HIV infection or acute seroconversion syndrome). Symptoms range from a mild glandular fever-like illness to an aseptic meningitis; severe symptoms are rare.

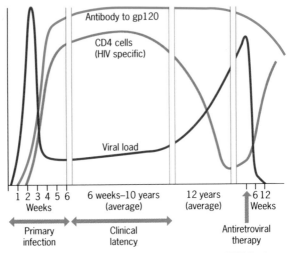

**Fig. 2.2 Schematic representation of the course of HIV infection in vivo. The effect of antiretroviral therapy is also shown.**

- Clinical latent period with or without persistent generalized lymphadenopathy defined as nodes > 1 cm in diameter at two or more extrainguinal sites for more than 3 months in the absence of causes other than HIV infection.
- *Category B.* Early symptomatic HIV infection, which includes patients who do not have conditions specific to category A or C, e.g. persistent vaginal candidiasis, oral hairy leucoplakia, herpes zoster involving more than one dermatome, idiopathic thrombocytopenic purpura and pelvic inflammatory disease.
- *Category C* includes patients with clinical conditions indicating that they have severe immunosuppression (AIDS; Table 2.10).

### Effects of HIV infection
The clinical findings resulting from direct HIV infection are summarized in Table 2.11.

**Table 2.10**
AIDS-defining conditions*

Candidiasis of bronchi, trachea or lungs
Candidiasis, oesophageal
Cervical carcinoma, invasive
Coccidioidomycosis, disseminated or extrapulmonary
Cryptococcosis, extrapulmonary
Cryptosporidiosis, chronic intestinal (1-month duration)
Cytomegalovirus (CMV) disease (other than liver, spleen or nodes)
CMV retinitis (with loss of vision)
Encephalopathy (HIV-related)
Herpes simplex, chronic ulcers (1-month duration); or bronchitis,
    pneumonitis or oesophagitis
Histoplasmosis, disseminated or extrapulmonary
Isosporiasis; chronic intestinal (1-month duration)
Kaposi's sarcoma
Lymphoma, Burkitt's
Lymphoma, immunoblastic (or equivalent term)
Lymphoma (primary) of brain
*Mycobacterium avium* complex or *M. kansasii*, disseminated or
    extrapulmonary
*Mycobacterium tuberculosis*, any site
*Mycobacterium*, other species or unidentified species,
    disseminated or extrapulmonary
*Pneumocystis carinii* pneumonia
Pneumonia, recurrent
Progressive multifocal leucoencephalopathy
*Salmonella* septicaemia, recurrent
Toxoplasmosis of brain
Wasting syndrome, due to HIV

* USA definition also includes those with a CD4 count < 200 cells/μL

## Conditions due to immunodeficiency (K&C p. 137)

Immunodeficiency allows the development of opportunistic infections. These are diseases caused by organisms that are not usually considered pathogenic, unusual presentations of known pathogens, and the occurrence of tumours that have an oncogenic viral aetiology. Susceptibility increases as the patient becomes more immunosuppressed. When patients are severely immunocompromised (CD4 count < 100 cells/μL) disseminated infections with organisms of very low virulence such as *M. avium-intracellulare* and *Cryptosporidium* are able to establish themselves. The mortality and morbidity associated with HIV infection have declined dramatically since the introduction of highly active antiviral treatment (HAART). Similarly, long-term

**Table 2.11**
**Direct HIV effects**

| | |
|---|---|
| Neurological disease | AIDS dementia complex |
| | Distal sensory peripheral neuropathy |
| | Autonomic neuropathy causing diarrhoea and postural hypotension |
| Eye | Retinal cotton wool spots – rarely troublesome |
| Mucocutaneous | Dry, itchy flaky skin |
| | Pruritic papular eruption |
| | Aphthous ulceration in the mouth |
| Haematological | Anaemia of chronic disease |
| | Neutropenia |
| | Autoimmune thrombocytopenia |
| Gastrointestinal | Anorexia leading to weight loss in advanced disease |
| | HIV enteropathy leading to diarrhoea and malabsorption |
| Renal | Renal impairment |
| | Nephrotic syndrome |
| Respiratory | Chronic sinusitis and otitis media |
| | Lymphoid interstitial pneumonitis – lymphocytic infiltration of the lung, causing dyspnoea and a dry cough |
| Endocrine | Reduced adrenal function – infection may precipitate clear adrenal insufficiency |
| Cardiac | Myocarditis and cardiomyopathy |

secondary chemoprophylaxis for previously life-threatening infections may not be necessary when HAART maintains the CD4 count above 200 cells/$\mu$L and the viral load is low.

## Protozoal infections

*Toxoplasma gondii* most commonly causes encephalitis and cerebral abscess in AIDS patients. Clinical features include focal neurological signs, fits, fever, headache and possible confusion. Eye involvement with chorioretinitis may also be present. Diagnosis is made on the basis of positive toxoplasmosis serology and multiple ring-enhancing lesions on contrast-enhanced CT or MRI brain scan. Treatment is with pyrimethamine, sulfadiazine and folinic acid (leucovorin); lifelong maintenance may be required to prevent relapse.

*Cryptosporidium parvum* causes severe chronic watery diarrhoea and sclerosing cholangitis. Diagnosis is made by demonstrating cysts on stool microscopy or on small bowel biopsy specimens obtained at endoscopy. Treatment is symptomatic with antidiarrhoeal agents together with fluid, electrolyte and nutritional support.

Microsporidia infection (usually *Enterocytozoon bieneusi*) causes a diarrhoeal illness. Diagnosis is made by demonstrating spores in the stools. Treatment is with albendazole.

## Viruses

Cytomegalovirus (CMV) causes:

- Retinitis with floaters, loss of visual acuity and orbital pain. The diagnosis is made on fundoscopy which shows a characteristic appearance of the retina with haemorrhages and exudate. Treatment is with intravenous ganciclovir or foscarnet, continued long-term to prevent reactivation. Oral and topical forms of ganciclovir are available for maintenance treatment.
- Colitis, which presents with bloody diarrhoea and abdominal pain. Diagnosis is made by demonstrating characteristic 'cytomegalic cells' (large cells containing an intranuclear inclusion and sometimes intracytoplasmic inclusions) on light-microscopic examination of mucosal biopsy specimens. Treatment is with intravenous ganciclovir or foscarnet.
- Oesophageal ulceration, causing painful dysphagia.
- Less commonly, polyradiculopathy, encephalitis and pneumonitis.

Herpes simplex virus infection causes genital and oral ulceration, and systemic infection. Varicella zoster occurs at any stage of HIV infection, but may be more aggressive and longer lasting than in immunocompetent patients. Herpesvirus 8 is associated with Kaposi's sarcoma. Infection usually responds to aciclovir. Epstein–Barr virus (EBV) causes oral hairy leucoplakia, presenting as a pale ridged lesion on the side of the tongue. Treatment is with aciclovir. Human papilloma virus (HPV) produces genital and plantar warts. HPV infection is associated with the more rapid development of squamous cell cancer of the cervix and anal cancer. Papovavirus causes progressive multifocal leucoencephalopathy, which presents with intellectual impairment and often hemiparesis and aphasia.

## Fungi

*Pneumocystis carinii* causes pneumonia in severely immuno-compromised patients (CD4 count < 200 cells/μL). There is an insidious onset of breathlessness, a non-productive cough, fever and malaise. The chest X-ray may be normal or show bilateral perihilar interstitial infiltrates, which can progress to more diffuse shadowing. Definitive diagnosis is made by demonstrating the organisms in specimens obtained at bronchoalveolar lavage. Treatment is with intravenous co-trimoxazole, intravenous pentamidine or dapsone and trimethoprim. Systemic corticosteroids reduce mortality in severe cases ($P_aO_2$ < 9.5 kPa). Long-term pro-phylaxis is required in patients whose CD4 count is below 200 cells/μL.

Cryptococcus most commonly causes meningitis in AIDS patients. There is an insidious onset of fever, nausea and headache, eventually with impaired consciousness and change in affect. Diagnosis is made by CSF microscopy (Indian ink staining shows the organisms directly) and culture. Treatment is with intravenous amphotericin B or fluconazole, and oral fluconazole and continued long-term in the absence of HAART.

Mucosal infection with candida (usually *Candida albicans*) presents as creamy plaques in the mouth, vulvovaginal region and oesophagus (producing dysphagia and retro-sternal pain). Infection usually responds to treatment with fluconazole or itraconazole. Disseminated infection with *Aspergillus fumigatus* occurs in advanced HIV infection. The prognosis is poor, with amphotericin B being the mainstay of therapy.

## Bacterial infection

This may present early in HIV infection, is often dissemi-nated and frequently recurs. *Mycobacterium tuberculosis* (TB) can cause disease at all stages of HIV infection, but extrapulmonary TB is more common with advanced disease. *Mycobacterium avium-intracellulare* (MAI) occurs in patients with advanced AIDS (CD4 count < 50 cells/μL). Clinical features include fever, anorexia, weight loss, diarrhoea and anaemia with bone marrow involvement. MAI is typically resistant to standard antituberculous therapies. A combination of ethambutol, rifabutin and clarithromycin reduces the burden of organisms and provides symptomatic benefit. Other infections include *Strep. pneumoniae, H. influenzae*, staphylococcal skin infection and salmonella.

## Neoplasia

The commonest tumours are Kaposi's sarcoma and non-Hodgkin's lymphoma.

- Kaposi's sarcoma is a vascular tumour which appears as red-purple, raised, well-circumscribed lesions on the skin, hard palate and conjunctivae, and in the gastrointestinal tract. The lungs and lymph nodes may also be involved. Human herpesvirus 8 is implicated in the pathogenesis. Localized disease is treated with radiotherapy; systemic disease is treated with chemotherapy.
- Non-Hodgkin's lymphoma occurs in the brain, gut and lung. It is an aggressive tumour with a poor prognosis.
- Squamous cell carcinoma of the cervix and anus is associated with HIV. Human papillomavirus may play a part in the pathogenesis.

### Diagnosis and monitoring (K&C p. 144)

Testing for HIV infection must only be undertaken with informed consent, and the patient should receive advice from a trained counsellor about the implications of a positive test (e.g. difficulties in obtaining life insurance, mortgages).

HIV infection is diagnosed by the following tests:

- IgG antibodies in the serum may not appear for up to 3 months after infection. They are the most commonly used marker of HIV infection
- Measurement of HIV RNA (viral load) in plasma

- Measurement of viral p24 antigen (p24ag) in plasma if RNA assay is unavailable. Antigen disappears 8–10 weeks after exposure.

Following a diagnosis of HIV infection the numbers of circulating CD4 lymphocytes are measured 3-monthly; patients with counts below 200 cells/μL are at greatest risk of HIV-related pathology. Plasma levels of HIV RNA ('viral load', measured in copies of RNA per mL) is a measure of viral replication. The viral load is the best indicator of long-term prognosis, and levels fall with effective antiretroviral medication.

The diagnosis of AIDS is made when an HIV-positive patient develops one or more of a defined list of opportunistic infections, malignancies or HIV-associated illnesses (Table 2.10) in the absence of other causes of immunosuppression, e.g. leukaemia, immunosuppressive drugs.

## *Management* (K&C p. 146)

Management involves treatment with antiretroviral drugs, social and psychological care, prevention of opportunistic infections and prevention of transmission of HIV. HIV infection cannot be cured and the aim of treatment is to suppress viral replication to as low a level as possible for as long as possible. Table 2.12 lists the antiretroviral drugs.

In the UK indications to consider the initiation of antiretroviral therapy include:

- Symptomatic HIV disease
- CD4 count < 200 cells/μL
- Patients with a CD4 count between 200 and 350 cells/μL who have a very high viral load (> 10 000 copies/mL of plasma) or rapidly falling CD4.

Treatment is initiated with a combination of drugs started simultaneously. The preferred regimen is two nucleoside reverse transcriptase inhibitors in combination with either a non-nucleoside reverse transcriptase inhibitor, a protease inhibitor, or with abacavir as a third drug. The goal is to achieve a viral load below the limits of detection within 6–9 months of starting treatment. Patients may need to change therapy because of virologic failure or side-effects.

50

Table 2.12
Antiretroviral drugs

| Class of drug | Mechanism of action | Drug | Side-effects |
|---|---|---|---|
| **Reverse transcriptase inhibitors** | | | |
| Nucleoside analogues | Bind to viral DNA and inhibit reverse transcriptase, also act as DNA chain terminators | Abacavir Didanosine Lamivudine Stavudine Zalcitabine Zidovudine | Nausea, mitochondrial dysfunction, lactic acidosis and polyneuropathy may occur with any of these drugs. In addition pancreatitis with didanosine, myelosuppression with lamivudine and zidovudine, myelopathy with zidovudine |
| Non-nucleoside reverse transcriptase inhibitors | Bind directly to, and inhibit reverse transcriptase | Efavirenz Nevirapine | Rash and Stevens–Johnson syndrome. Hepatic toxicity with nevirapine, CNS effects with efavirenz |
| Nucleotide analogues | Competitive reverse transcriptase inhibitors | Tenofovir (available in Europe on named-patient basis only) | |
| **Protease inhibitors** | Act competitively on HIV aspartyl protease enzyme which is involved in production of functional viral proteins and enzymes | Amprenavir Indinavir Nelfinavir Ritonavir Saquinavir | Nausea, diarrhoea, abnormalities of fat distribution, raised plasma lipids, hyperglycaemia, abnormal liver biochemistry/hepatotoxicity. Perioral paraesthesia with amprenavir and ritonavir |

## Prevention and control

- The average risk of HIV transmission following a needle-stick injury involving contaminated blood is about 0.3%; post-exposure prophylaxis with zidovudine, lamivudine and indinavir for 4 weeks reduces the risk by about 80%. Prophylaxis should be started as soon as possible after exposure.
- Pregnant HIV-positive women should receive antiviral therapy to reduce the risk of vertical transmission. They should be advised against breast-feeding.
- The use of condoms reduces sexual transmission of HIV.
- Advise drug addicts not to share needles; some areas provide free sterile needles.

## Prognosis

The rate of progression among patients infected with HIV varies greatly. The average life expectancy for an HIV-infected patient in the absence of treatment is approximately 10 years. The mean survival following a CD4 count of 200 cells/$\mu$L is about 3 years. The introduction of HAART has resulted in a dramatic decrease in mortality and opportunistic infections in patients with HIV.

**USEFUL WEBSITES**

http://www.hivatis.org/
Centers for Disease Control and Prevention: HIV/AIDS treatment/information service

http://www.doh.gov.uk/eaga/
Department of Health Expert Advisory Group on AIDS: information about post-exposure prophylaxis, guidelines for pre-test discussion on HIV testing and risks of transmission

http://www.nfid.org/factsheets/
National Foundation for Infectious Diseases, USA: fact sheets on infectious diseases

http://www.phls.co.uk/advice/index.htm
Public Health Laboratory Service, UK: advice and guidelines for infectious diseases

# 3

# Gastroenterology and nutrition

## Symptoms of gastrointestinal disease

### Abdominal pain

Acute abdominal pain is discussed on page 102.

### Dysphagia

Dysphagia is difficulty in swallowing. The causes are listed on page 57.

### Heartburn

Heartburn is a retrosternal burning discomfort which spreads up towards the throat and is a common symptom of acid reflux (p. 58). The pain can sometimes be difficult to distinguish from the pain of ischaemic heart disease, although a careful history will usually differentiate between the two (pp. 58 and 366).

### Dyspepsia

Dyspepsia describes a range of symptoms referable to the upper gastrointestinal tract, e.g. nausea, heartburn, acidity, pain or distension. Patients are more likely to use the term 'indigestion' for these symptoms.

### Flatulence

Flatulence describes excessive wind, presenting as belching, abdominal distension and the passage of flatus per rectum. It is rarely indicative of serious underlying disease.

### Vomiting

Vomiting occurs as a result of stimulation of the vomiting centres in the lateral reticular formation of the medulla. This may result from stimulation of the chemoreceptor trigger zones in the floor of the fourth ventricle or from vagal afferents from the gut. It is associated with many gastrointestinal conditions, but nausea and vomiting without pain are frequently non-gastrointestinal in origin. Non-gastrointestinal causes of vomiting include CNS disease (e.g. raised intracranial pressure, migraine), drugs especially chemotherapeutic agents, metabolic conditions (e.g. uraemia, diabetic ketoacidosis) and pregnancy. Persistent nausea and vomiting is often functional in origin (p. 100).

## Constipation

Constipation is difficult to define because there is considerable individual variation, but it is usually taken to mean infrequent passage of stool (< twice weekly) or the difficult passage of hard stools.

## Diarrhoea

Diarrhoea implies the passage of increased amounts of loose stool (stool weight > 250 g/24 h) (p. 97). This must be differentiated from the frequent passage of small amounts of stool (which patients often refer to as diarrhoea), which is commonly seen in functional bowel disorders.

## Steatorrhoea

Steatorrhoea is the passage of pale bulky stools that contain fat (> 18 mmol/24 h) and indicates fat malabsorption as a result of small bowel, pancreatic or biliary disease. The stools often float because of increased air content and are difficult to flush away.

# The mouth

Problems in the mouth are common and often trivial, although they can cause severe symptoms.

## Mouth ulcers (K&C p. 259)

### Non-infective

- Recurrent aphthous ulceration is the most common cause of mouth ulcers and affects at least 20% of the population; in most cases the aetiology is unknown.

The history is of recurrent self-limiting episodes of painful oral ulcers (rarely on the palate). Topical corticosteroids are used for symptomatic relief but they have no effect on the natural history. In a few cases ulcers are associated with trauma or gastrointestinal and systemic diseases, e.g. anaemia, inflammatory bowel disease, coeliac disease, Behçet's disease, Reiter's disease, systemic lupus erythematosus, pemphigus, pemphigoid, and fixed drug reactions.

- Squamous cell carcinoma presents as an indolent ulcer, usually on the lateral borders of the tongue or floor of the mouth. Aetiological factors include tobacco (smoking and chewing) and alcohol. Treatment is with surgery, radiotherapy or a combination of both.

### Infective
Many infections can affect the mouth, though the most common are viral and include:

- Herpes simplex virus type 1
- Coxsackie A virus
- Herpes zoster virus.

## Oral white patches
Oral white patches are associated with smoking, *Candida* infection, lichen planus, trauma and syphilis. Leucoplakia is the term used to describe oral white patches or plaques for which no local cause can be found (i.e. a diagnosis of exclusion). Leucoplakia is occasionally a premalignant lesion and thus oral white patches must be biopsied to exclude malignancy. Hairy leucoplakia is an Epstein–Barr-related white patch on the side of the tongue, which is almost pathognomonic of HIV infection; it is not premalignant.

## Atrophic glossitis
A smooth sore tongue with loss of filiform papillae may occur in patients with iron, vitamin $B_{12}$ or folate deficiency.

## Geographical tongue
This affects 1–2% of the population and describes discrete areas of depapillation on the dorsum of the tongue. This

may be asymptomatic or produce a sore tongue. The aetiology is unknown and there is no specific treatment.

## Periodontal disorders

Gum bleeding is most commonly caused by gingivitis, an inflammatory condition of the gums associated with dental plaque. Bleeding may also be associated with generalized conditions such as bleeding disorders and leukaemia. Acute ulcerative gingivitis (Vincent's infection) is characterized by the development of crater-like ulcers, with bleeding, involving the interdental papillae, followed by lateral spread along the gingival margins. It is thought to be the result of spirochaetal infection occurring in the malnourished and immunocompromised. Treatment is with oral metronidazole and good oral hygiene.

## Salivary gland disorders (*K&C* p. 261)

Xerostomia (mouth dryness) may be caused by anxiety, drugs such as tricyclic antidepressants, Sjögren's syndrome and dehydration.

Infection (parotitis) may be viral, i.e. mumps virus, or bacterial (staphylococci or streptococci).

Sarcoidosis produces enlargement of the parotid glands and, if combined with lacrimal gland enlargement, is known as the Mikulicz syndrome.

Calculus formation usually occurs in the duct of the submandibular gland, and causes painful swelling of the gland before or during mastication.

Tumours most commonly affect the parotid gland and are usually benign, e.g. pleomorphic adenoma. Treatment is with surgical resection. Involvement of the VIIth cranial nerve raises the suspicion of malignancy.

## The oesophagus

The main oesophageal symptoms are dysphagia, heartburn and painful swallowing (odynophagia).

- Dysphagia is usually investigated with a barium swallow, followed by upper gastrointestinal endoscopy where appropriate. The causes are listed in Table 3.1. The commonest causes are peptic or malignant strictures and bulbar palsies. Typically, mechanical narrowing of the oesophagus, particularly in oesophageal malignancy, produces progressive dysphagia, initially for solids and eventually for liquids. Motor disorders, e.g. achalasia and scleroderma, produce dysphagia for both solids and liquids together.

- Heartburn is a retrosternal or epigastric burning sensation produced by the reflux of gastric acid into the oesophagus. The pain may radiate up to the throat and be confused with chest pain of cardiac origin. It is often aggravated by bending or lying down.

- Painful swallowing occurs with infections of the oesophagus (herpes simplex virus, *Candida*) or in gastro-oesophageal reflux disease, particularly with alcohol and hot liquids.

57

**Table 3.1**
Causes of dysphagia

**Intrinsic lesion**
Foreign body
Benign (peptic) stricture
Malignant stricture
Oesophageal ring or web
Pharyngeal pouch

**Neuromuscular disorders**
Bulbar palsy
Pharyngeal disorders
Myasthenia gravis

**Motility disorders**
Achalasia
Scleroderma
Diffuse oesophageal spasm
Presbyoesophagus (oesophagus of old age)
Diabetes mellitus
Chagas' disease

**Extrinsic pressure**
Goitre
Mediastinal glands
Enlarged left atrium in mitral valve disease

The oesophagus

# Gastro-oesophageal reflux disease (GORD) (K&C p. 263)

Reflux of gastric contents into the oesophagus is a normal event and clinical symptoms occur only when there is prolonged contact of gastric contents with the oesophageal mucosa.

## Pathophysiology

The lower oesophageal sphincter (LOS) tone is reduced, and there are frequent transient LOS relaxations. There is increased mucosal sensitivity to gastric acid and reduced oesophageal clearance of acid. Delayed gastric emptying and prolonged postprandial and nocturnal reflux also contribute. Mechanical or functional aberrations associated with a hiatus hernia may contribute to GORD in some patients, but patients may also have reflux in the absence of a hiatus hernia.

## Clinical features

Heartburn (p. 53) is the major symptom of GORD. The burning is aggravated by bending, stooping and lying down, and may be relieved by antacids. There may be pain on drinking hot drinks. Cough and nocturnal asthma can occur from aspiration of gastric contents into the lungs. Symptoms do not correlate well with the severity of oesophagitis.

## Investigations

The diagnosis is clinical and investigation is not usually required in patients less than 45 years without 'alarm' symptoms (weight loss, dysphagia, anaemia).

**Oesophagoscopy** shows the presence of oesophagitis. The mucosa can, however, be normal in patients with symptoms of reflux.

**Barium swallow** This may show an ulcerated lower oesophagus and demonstrate a hiatus hernia if present.

**24-hour intraluminal pH monitoring** Insertion of a pH probe into the lower oesophagus via the nose allows continual monitoring of acid reflux over 24 hours. This is performed to confirm GORD prior to surgery or in difficult diagnostic cases.

## Management

Conservative measures with weight loss, a reduction in alcohol intake, cessation of smoking and simple antacids are often sufficient for mild symptoms.

- *Alginate-containing antacids* are usually first-line treatments; they prevent reflux by forming a 'foam raft' on gastric contents.
- *$H_2$-receptor antagonists* (e.g. ranitidine) improve the symptoms of heartburn.
- *Prokinetic agents,* such as metoclopramide and domperidone, are occasionally helpful.
- *Proton pump inhibitors* (PPIs) (e.g. omeprazole, esomeprazole, lansoprazole, pantoprazole) inhibit gastric hydrogen–potassium-ATPase and block the luminal secretion of gastric acid. They are potent acid blockers and the drugs of choice for all but mild cases.
- *Endoscopic therapy.* Endoscopic gastroplasty (sutures are placed endoscopically in the lower oesophagus), the Stretta procedure (radiofrequency energy is delivered to the LOS to induce fibrosis), and endoscopic injection of submucosal polymers to bolster the LOS are being increasingly employed in patients dependent on PPIs.
- *Surgery* may be necessary for the few patients who continue to have symptoms in spite of full medical therapy, or in young people whose symptoms return rapidly on stopping treatment. The fundus of the stomach is sutured around the lower oesophagus to produce an antireflux valve (Nissen fundoplication). This procedure is performed laparoscopically which reduces length of hospital stay and the time taken to return to work, compared to open operation.

## Complications

Oesophageal stricture formation is the major complication of reflux and presents with intermittent dysphagia. It is treated with endoscopic dilatation. Long-standing acid reflux may cause metaplasia from squamous to columnar epithelium in the lower oesophagus, a change known as Barrett's oesophagus. The diagnosis is made at endoscopy when the pale glossy squamous epithelium is replaced by red-coloured columnar epithelium. Barrett's oseophagus is premalignant for adenocarcinoma of the oesophagus and patients with this condition should undergo regular endoscopic surveillance with multiple biopsies to look for dysplasia or carcinoma.

## Achalasia (*K&C* p. 266)

Achalasia is a disease of unknown aetiology, characterized by aperistalsis and non-propulsive tertiary contractions in the body of the oesophagus, and the failure of relaxation of the LOS on initiation of swallowing.

### Pathology

There is a decrease in ganglionic cells in the nerve plexus of the oesophageal wall and degeneration in the vagus nerve.

### Clinical features

The disease can present at any age but is rare in childhood. There is usually a long history of dysphagia for both liquids and solids, which may be associated with regurgitation. Severe retrosternal chest pain may occur, particularly in younger patients.

### Investigations

- Barium swallow will show dilatation of the oesophagus, lack of peristalsis, a gradually tapering lower end (beak deformity) and asynchronous contractions of the oesophagus.
- Oesophagoscopy may be necessary to exclude a carcinoma which can produce similar symptoms and X-ray appearance.
- Oesophageal manometry (measurement of intra-oesophageal pressure during swallowing) demonstrates aperistalsis and failure of LOS relaxation.
- Chest X-ray may show a dilated oesophagus with a fluid level behind the heart. The fundal gas shadow is not present.

## *Management*

Endoscopic pneumatic dilatation of the LOS, under X-ray screening, is the procedure of choice and is successful in 80% of cases. Endoscopic injection of botulinum toxin into the LOS has been advocated, with variable success rates. Surgical division of the sphincter (Heller's cardiomyotomy) is used in resistant cases and is performed laparoscopically. GORD is a complication of all treatments, particularly surgery.

## *Complications*

There is a slight increase in the incidence of carcinoma of the oesophagus, which is typically squamous in type. This increase is regardless of the treatment undertaken.

## Systemic sclerosis (*K&C* p. 267)

There is oesophageal involvement in over 90% of patients with systemic sclerosis. The smooth muscle layer is replaced by fibrous tissue. The LOS pressure is reduced, thereby permitting reflux. Patients may be asymptomatic or complain of reflux and dysphagia. Dysphagia is caused by stricture formation complicating reflux. Treatment is as for reflux and stricture formation.

## Diffuse oesophageal spasm (*K&C* p. 267)

This is a severe form of abnormal oesophageal motility which most commonly presents in middle age, and can produce chest pain and dysphagia. A 'corkscrew' appearance may be seen on barium swallow. 'Nutcracker oesophagus' is a variant characterized by high-amplitude peristaltic waves in the oesophagus. Treatment of these disorders is difficult, but calcium-channel blockers, e.g. oral nifedipine, may be helpful. Treatment of GORD may help.

## Hiatus hernia

On its own a hiatus hernia is not responsible for symptoms unless there is associated reflux. There are two main forms:

- *Sliding*. The gastro-oesophageal junction slides through the hiatus and lies above the diaphragm.

- *Para-oesophageal.* A part of the stomach rolls up through the hiatus alongside the oesophagus, the sphincter remaining below the diaphragm.

## Malignant oesophageal tumours (*K&C* p. 268)

### Pathology
- Squamous cell, usually of the middle third of the oesophagus
- Adenocarcinoma of the lower third of the oesophagus.

### Epidemiology

**Squamous carcinoma** The incidence is 5–10 per 100 000 in the UK, although it varies greatly throughout the world, being particularly high in China and parts of Africa and Iran. It is most common in the 60–70-year age group. It is associated with heavy alcohol intake, heavy smoking and a high intake of salted fish and pickled vegetables. Other predisposing factors include achalasia and coeliac disease.

**Adenocarcinoma** This arises from the columnar-lined epithelium of the lower oesophagus (Barrett's oesophagus) which results from long-standing reflux.

### Clinical features
Symptoms include progressive dysphagia (initially for solids and later for liquids), weight loss, and chest pain, which may be due to bolus food impaction or local infiltration. Physical signs are usually absent.

### Investigations
- Barium swallow or oesophagoscopy are the initial investigations.
- CT, MRI and endoscopic ultrasonography may be helpful in staging the lesion for surgery.

### Management
In many patients only symptomatic treatment to relieve the dysphagia is possible. This is usually done endoscopically:

- Dilatation of the stricture and insertion of an expanding metal stent to keep the oesophagus open

- Laser to photocoagulate the tumour
- Alcohol injections into the tumour to cause local necrosis.

Surgical resection may be carried out in the few patients when staging has shown that the tumour has not infiltrated outside of the oesophageal wall. The combination of chemotherapy and radiotherapy prior to surgery (neoadjuvant chemotherapy) may increase survival. Radiation alone is sometimes employed with limited success in both squamous cell carcinoma and adenocarcinoma.

### Prognosis
The prognosis overall is poor (9% 5-year survival) as most patients can only be treated palliatively.

## Benign oesophageal tumours
Leiomyomas are the most common benign tumours. They are usually discovered incidentally and do not often produce symptoms.

## Oesophageal perforation
The commonest cause of oesophageal perforation is iatrogenic and occurs after endoscopic dilatation of oesophageal strictures (usually malignant) or achalasia. It may also occur after forceful vomiting (Boerhaave's syndrome), when there is also usually severe chest pain and collapse. On examination there may be fever, hypotension and surgical emphysema. Diagnosis is by chest X-ray, which may be normal or show air in the mediastinum and neck, and a pleural effusion. A gastrografin swallow (not barium) will confirm the diagnosis. Treatment is with intravenous antibiotics, nil by mouth and intravenous fluids. Surgical repair is needed for patients with large tears or who fail to settle with conservative management.

## The stomach and duodenum
## Gastropathy and gastritis (K&C p. 276)
*Gastropathy* is the term used when there is injury to the gastric mucosa associated with epithelial cell damage and

regeneration. There is little or no accompanying inflammation. *Gastritis* is inflammation of the gastric mucosa. This distinction has caused considerable confusion, since gastritis is often used to describe endoscopic or radiological characteristics of the gastric mucosa rather than specific histological findings.

## Gastropathy

The commonest cause of gastropathy is mucosal damage associated with the use of aspirin or other non-steroidal anti-inflammatory drugs (NSAIDs). These drugs deplete mucosal prostaglandins, by inhibiting the cyclo-oxygenase pathway, which leads to mucosal damage (p. 239). Other causes include infections, e.g. cytomegalovirus and herpes simplex virus, and alcohol in high concentrations. Gastric erosions can also be seen after severe stress (stress ulcer), burns (Curling's ulcer), and in renal and liver disease. Common symptoms include indigestion, vomiting and haemorrhage, although these correlate poorly with endoscopic and pathological findings. Erosions (superficial breaks in the mucosa < 3 mm) and subepithelial haemorrhage are most commonly seen at endoscopy. Treatment is with a proton pump inhibitor with removal of the offending cause if possible. Prophylaxis is also given to prevent future damage in patients who continue to take aspirin or NSAIDs.

## Gastritis

The commonest cause of gastritis is *Helicobacter pylori* infection (p. 65). Other causes are autoimmune gastritis (the cause of pernicious anaemia associated with antibodies to gastric parietal cells and intrinsic factor), viruses and duodenogastric reflux. Gastritis is a histological diagnosis and is usually discovered incidentally when a gastric mucosal biopsy is taken for histology at endoscopy. It is classified as acute or chronic. Acute inflammation is associated with neutrophilic infiltration, while chronic inflammation is characterized by mononuclear cells, chiefly lymphocytes, plasma cells, and macrophages. Gastritis is usually asymptomatic; whether *H. pylori* gastritis itself produces functional dyspepsia is controversial (p. 101). At endoscopy the mucosa may appear reddened or normal. No specific

treatment is required although eradication treatment for
*H. pylori* is often given.

## *Helicobacter pylori* and the upper gastrointestinal tract (*K&C* p. 271)

*Helicobacter pylori* is a Gram-negative urease-producing
spiral-shaped bacterium found predominantly in the
gastric antrum and in areas of gastric metaplasia in the duodenum. It is closely associated with chronic active gastritis,
peptic ulcer disease, and gastric cancer and gastric B cell
lymphoma. However, most patients with the infection are
asymptomatic. Some strains of *H. pylori* (CagA-positive
strains) are particularly associated with gastroduodenal
disease.

### Epidemiology

The incidence of *H. pylori* infection is higher in the older
age groups and associated with lower socio-economic
status. Most cases of infection probably occur in childhood,
and transmission is most likely via the oral–oral or
faecal–oral routes.

### Clinicopathological features

*H. pylori* infection produces a gastritis mainly in the antrum
of the stomach. In some individuals gastritis can involve
the body of the stomach leading to atrophic gastritis and in
some cases intestinal metaplasia which is a premalignant
condition.

### Investigations

#### Invasive tests (endoscopy)

- Rapid urease test (an antral biopsy which contains
  *H. pylori* when added to a urea-containing solution
  breaks down urea to release ammonia and produces a
  pH-dependent colour change in the indicator present).
- Histology with direct visualization of the organism.
- Gram stain and culture.

#### Non-invasive tests

- Urea breath test. $^{13}C$ (or $^{14}C$) labelled urea is given by
  mouth; the detection of $^{13}C$ in expired air indicates

infection with urease-producing *H. pylori*. The breath test is particularly useful to confirm eradication of the organism after appropriate treatment.

- Serological tests detect IgG antibodies to *H. pylori*. They are used to diagnose infection but are not useful for confirming eradication because patients may have antibodies for years after eradication of the organism.
- Stool tests. A specific immunoassay for qualitative detection of *H. pylori* is available with a sensitivity and specificity of greater than 90%.

## Management

Eradication of *H. pylori* is indicated for all patients with proven peptic disease. Recurrence is very uncommon in those in whom the infection is successfully eradicated. Several treatment regimens are available, although proton-pump inhibitor (PPI)-based triple therapy regimens are favoured, e.g.

- PPI (e.g. omeprazole 20 mg) plus metronidazole 400 mg and clarithromycin 500 mg all twice daily for 1 week
- PPI (e.g. omeprazole 20 mg) plus amoxicillin 1 g and clarithromycin 500 mg all twice daily for 1 week.

## Peptic ulcer disease (K&C p. 272)

A peptic ulcer is an ulcer of the mucosa in or adjacent to an acid-bearing area. Most occur in the stomach or proximal duodenum.

### Epidemiology

Duodenal ulcers are three to four times more common than gastric ulcers and occur in 15% of the population at some time. They are more common in men than in women (4:1) and both are more common in elderly people. There is a significant geographical variation.

### Aetiology

The precise mechanism of how peptic ulceration occurs is unclear though infection with *H. pylori* plays a central role. Potential pathogenic mechanisms are listed in Table 3.2.

**Table 3.2**
Proposed pathogenic mechanisms of *H. pylori*

Increased gastric acid secretion due to:
  increased fasting and meal-stimulated serum gastrin
  increased parietal cell mass
  decreased somatostatin (D) cells in the antrum

Increased pepsinogen-1

Disruption of mucous protective layer

Production of virulence factors
  Vacuolating toxin (Vac A)
  Cytotoxic associated protein (CagA)
  Urease
  Adherence factors

Genetic factors may have a role to play. Aspirin and NSAIDs
are also a cause of gastric ulceration, though less commonly
duodenal ulcers. Peptic ulceration is also seen in hyperparathyroidism and the Zollinger–Ellison syndrome (p. 164).

## Clinical features
Epigastric pain is the most common presenting symptom.
This is typically relieved by antacids but has a variable relationship to food. Duodenal ulcer pain, however, often
occurs when the subject is hungry and classically occurs at
night. Other symptoms, such as nausea, heartburn and
flatulence, may occur. Occasionally ulcers may present with
the complications of perforation or painless upper gastrointestinal haemorrhage.

## Investigations
Young patients (< 45 years) with ulcer-type symptoms
should undergo screening for *H. pylori* infection by either
serology, breath test or stool test; upper gastrointestinal
endoscopy is not usually necessary (see Management of dyspepsia, p. 69). Older patients should undergo endoscopy. In
patients found to have a gastric ulcer at endoscopy, multiple biopsies from the centre and edge of the ulcer must be
taken, because it is often impossible to distinguish by naked
eye a benign from malignant gastric ulcer. A barium meal
is useful if gastric outlet obstruction is suspected.

## Management

*Ulcers associated with H. pylori* Treatment regimens (p. 66) that successfully eradicate *H. pylori* from the gastric antrum result in healing rates of over 90% and prevent recurrence unless reinfection occurs, which is unusual. This approach to treatment is indicated in all patients with *H. pylori*-associated peptic disease.

**H. pylori-*negative peptic ulcers*** Most *H. pylori*-negative peptic ulcers are associated with aspirin and NSAID ingestion. Treatment involves the use of acid-suppressing drugs and stopping the NSAID if at all possible. PPIs (p. 59) heal most ulcers and are the drugs of choice. After ulcer healing NSAIDs can only be continued with ulcer prophylaxis (such as with a PPI or misoprostil (a prostaglandin agonist)) or therapy is switched to a selective COX-2 inhibitor (p. 239).

Follow-up endoscopy plus biopsy should be performed for all gastric ulcers to demonstrate healing and exclude malignancy (initial biopsies may be false negatives).

*Surgery* With the introduction of modern drugs, surgery is rarely performed for peptic ulceration but is reserved for the treatment of complications, namely recurrent haemorrhage, perforation and outflow obstruction.

## Complications

*Perforation* is uncommon. Duodenal ulcers perforate more commonly than gastric ulcers, usually into the peritoneal cavity. Management is initially surgical, with closure of the perforation and drainage of the abdomen. *H. pylori* should subsequently be eradicated. Conservative treatment with intravenous fluids and antibiotics may be indicated in elderly or very ill patients.

*Gastric outlet obstruction* Outflow obstruction occurs because of surrounding oedema or scarring following healing. Copious projectile vomiting is the main symptom, and a succussion splash may be detectable clinically. Metabolic alkalosis may develop as a result of loss of acid.

Management is initially with nasogastric suction and replacement of fluids and electrolytes. In some cases oedema may settle with conservative management, but treatment with surgery or balloon dilatation is often required.

**Haemorrhage** See page 71.

# Management of dyspepsia in the community

Because significant GI pathology is relatively uncommon in most young people with dyspepsia, and because of the close association of *H. pylori* with peptic disease, most would agree that investigation with endoscopy is not necessary in all patients. Older patients (> 45 years) with persistent dyspepsia should be investigated with a gastroscopy or a barium meal to rule out significant disease, as should all patients with 'alarm symptoms' such as dysphagia, weight loss or gastrointestinal bleeding. In other patients *H. pylori* status should be assessed serologically and, if positive, eradication therapy instituted. Further investigation can then be reserved for those who remain symptomatic or who are *H. pylori*-negative on initial testing.

# Malignant gastric tumours (K&C p. 277)

## Epidemiology

Gastric cancer is the sixth most common fatal cancer in the UK. The incidence increases with age and is more common in men. The frequency varies throughout the world, being more common in Japan and Chile, and relatively less common in the USA. Although the incidence overall is decreasing world-wide, proximal gastric cancers are increasing in frequency.

## Aetiology

This is unknown, *H. pylori* infection is implicated, causing chronic gastritis which in some individuals leads to atrophic gastritis and intestinal metaplasia, a premalignant pathological change. Dietary factors, such as alcohol, spiced, salted or pickled foods, and nitrate ingestion may also have a role. Smoking and achlorhydria (e.g. pernicious anaemia) are also associated with gastric cancer.

## Pathology

Tumours most commonly occur in the antrum and are almost always adenocarcinomas. They may be localized ulcerated lesions with rolled edges (intestinal type), or more diffuse with extensive submucosal spread, giving the picture of linitus plastica (diffuse type).

## Clinical features

Pain similar to peptic ulcer pain is the most common symptom. With more advanced disease, nausea, anorexia and weight loss are common. Vomiting with outflow obstruction occurs if the tumour is near the pylorus, or dysphagia can occur with lesions in the cardia. Almost 50% have a palpable epigastric mass, and a lymph node is sometimes felt in the supraclavicular fossa (Virchow's node). In patients with advanced disease there may be evidence of metastatic spread to the peritoneum and liver, with ascites and hepatomegaly. Skin manifestations of malignancy, such as dermatomyositis and acanthosis nigricans, are occasionally associated.

## Investigations

Barium meal or gastroscopy and biopsy are the investigations of choice, biopsy providing histological confirmation. CT, MRI and endoscopic ultrasonography are useful in staging the tumour and guiding operability.

## Management

Surgery is the best form of treatment if the tumour is operable. Chemotherapy is sometimes used for unresectable lesions with a modest improvement in survival.

## Prognosis

The overall survival is poor (10% 5-year survival). Those patients undergoing curative operations, however, have a 5-year survival of 50%. In Japan, where the incidence of the disease is high and there is an active screening programme, earlier diagnosis and an aggressive surgical approach have resulted in a 5-year survival of 90%.

## Benign gastric tumours

The most common is a stromal tumour, which is usually asymptomatic although it can ulcerate and bleed. Gastric polyps are uncommon and usually regenerative. Adenomatous polyps can occur but are rare.

## Gastrointestinal bleeding

### Acute upper gastrointestinal bleeding
(K&C p. 280)

Haematemesis is the vomiting of blood. Melaena is the passage of black tarry stools, which is the result of altered

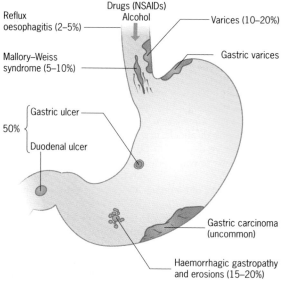

**Other uncommon causes**
Hereditary telangiectasia (Osler–Weber–Rendu syndrome)
Pseudoxanthoma elasticum
Blood dyscrasias
Dieulafoy gastric vascular abnormality
Portal gastropathy
Aortic graft surgery with fistula

**Fig. 3.1 Causes of upper gastrointestinal haemorrhage.**

blood from the upper intestine (50 mL or more is required to produce melaena).

## Aetiology

Chronic peptic ulceration is the most common cause of upper gastrointestinal bleeding (Fig. 3.1). Relative incidences vary according to patient population. Aspirin and NSAIDs may be responsible for bleeding from both duodenal and gastric ulcers, particularly in elderly people. Corticosteroids have been implicated, but in the usual therapeutic dosage they probably have no relationship to gastrointestinal bleeding.

## Management

A large-bore (16-gauge) intravenous cannula should be placed in a peripheral vein and blood taken for full blood count, liver biochemistry, urea and electrolytes, clotting screen and 'group and save'; crossmatch at least 2 units of blood if there is evidence of a large bleed (blood pressure < 100 mmHg, pulse > 100 beats per min, cool or cold extremities with slow capillary refill, Hb < 10 g/dL).

**Resuscitate** In many patients no specific treatment is required, bleeding stops spontaneously and the patient remains well compensated. In patients with large bleeds or clinical signs of shock, urgent transfusion, ideally with whole blood, is required (p. 508). Monitoring pulse rate and venous pressure will guide transfusion requirements.

**Determine site of bleeding** This may be evident from the history, e.g. bleeding from a peptic ulcer is suggested by a history of aspirin or NSAID ingestion or previous peptic ulceration. Mallory–Weiss syndrome (haematemesis from a tear in the oesophagus) is suggested by a history of vomiting preceding the haematemesis. Endoscopy should be performed as soon as possible, and preferably within 24 hours. More urgent endoscopy may be indicated if varices are strongly suspected from the history. Endoscopy can detect the site of haemorrhage in 80% or more of cases.

**Specific management** A stepwise approach to the management of upper gastrointestinal bleeding is illustrated in Emergency Box 3.1.

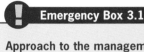

## Emergency Box 3.1

### Approach to the management of GI bleeding

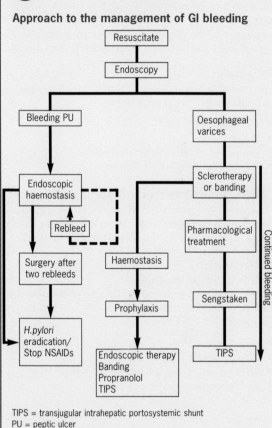

TIPS = transjugular intrahepatic portosystemic shunt
PU = peptic ulcer
Bleeding oesophageal varices is discussed on page 136.

At endoscopy varices should be treated with sclerotherapy or banding (p. 136). Ulcers that are actively bleeding or demonstrate stigmata of recent bleeding (a visible vessel or overlying clot) should be treated by injection of dilute epinephrine (adrenaline) or the vessel coagulated with the heater probe or bipole probe. In general all patients who are otherwise fit and haemodynamically stable and who at endoscopy have no stigmata of recent haemorrhage can be discharged from hospital within 24 hours. The role of intravenous uncertain proton pump inhibitors in acute peptic ulcer bleeding is, although they may reduce rebleeding rates and transfusion requirements following endoscopic therapy. Surgery may be required for persistent or recurrent bleeding from ulcers.

## Prognosis

The overall mortality rate is 5–10%. The following are associated with a poor prognosis:

- Old age (> 65 years)
- Shock
- Continued bleeding or rebleeding
- Presence of chronic liver disease.

# Lower gastrointestinal bleeding (K&C p. 283)

Massive bleeding is rare and usually the result of diverticular disease or ischaemic colitis. Minor bleeds from haemorrhoids are common. The causes are listed in Table 3.3.

## Management

With large bleeds resuscitation with intravenous fluids/whole blood may be required. The site of bleeding must then be determined using the following investigations as appropriate:

- Rectal examination, e.g. carcinoma
- Proctoscopy, e.g. haemorrhoids
- Sigmoidoscopy, e.g. inflammatory bowel disease
- Barium enema – any mucosal lesion

---

**Table 3.3**
Causes of lower GI bleeding

Haemorrhoids
Carcinoma
Colitis: ulcerative colitis, Crohn's, infective
Angiodysplasia (abnormal collections of blood vessels)
Colonic diverticula
Polyps
Meckel's diverticulum
Ischaemic colitis
Anal fissure

---

- Colonoscopy – diagnosis and removal of polyps
- Angiography – vascular abnormality, e.g. angiodysplasia.

**Specific management** Lesions should be treated as appropriate.

# Chronic gastrointestinal bleeding

Chronic gastrointestinal bleeding usually presents with iron deficiency anaemia. Blood loss producing anaemia in all men, and in women after the menopause, is always the result of bleeding from the gastrointestinal tract and requires investigation. The causes of chronic blood loss are those that cause acute bleeding (see Fig. 3.1 and Table 3.3). However, oesophageal varices, duodenal ulcers and diverticular disease very rarely bleed chronically.

## Investigations

Initial investigations are a 'top and tail', performed at the same endoscopic session, i.e. gastroscopy and colonoscopy; a distal duodenal biopsy is taken at endoscopy to look for coeliac disease as the cause of iron deficiency.

Further investigations, usually in the order listed, are reserved for difficult cases where the above tests have not identified a source of bleeding:

- Small bowel barium follow-through
- Coeliac axis and mesenteric angiography
- Technetium-labelled red cell scan
- Small bowel enteroscopy and/or wireless capsule endoscopy.

## Management

The cause of the bleeding is treated and oral iron (p. 170) is given to treat the anaemia.

## The small intestine

The small intestine has a number of functions, many of which are concerned with the digestion and absorption of nutrients. Nutrients are absorbed throughout the small intestine, with the exception of vitamin $B_{12}$ and bile salts, which have specific receptors in the terminal ileum (*K&C* p. 284).

The presenting features of small bowel disease are diarrhoea, steatorrhoea (p. 54), abdominal pain or discomfort, and weight loss, which is the result of accompanying anorexia. The two most common causes of small bowel disease in developed countries are coeliac disease and Crohn's disease. In many small bowel diseases malabsorption of specific substances occurs, but these deficiencies do not dominate the clinical picture. An example is Crohn's disease, in which malabsorption of vitamin $B_{12}$ can be demonstrated, but this is not usually a clinical problem. The major disorders of the small intestine that cause malabsorption are shown in Table 3.4.

## Coeliac disease (gluten-sensitive enteropathy) (K&C p. 291)

Coeliac disease is a condition in which there is an abnormal jejunal mucosa that improves morphologically when the patient is treated with a gluten-free diet and relapses when gluten is reintroduced. Gluten is contained in wheat, rye and barley. Pure oats are not harmful.

### Epidemiology

World-wide distribution, but it is rare in African people and more common in Ireland (incidence 1 in 100; 1 in 300 in UK).

### Aetiology

The toxic portion of gluten is the peptide α-gliadin. The exact mechanism by which gluten causes damage to the intestinal mucosa is not known. The strong association with the haplotypes HLA-A1, -B8, -DR3, -DR7 and -DQ2 suggests

---

**Table 3.4**
Disorders of the small intestine causing malabsorption

Coeliac disease
Crohn's disease
Dermatitis herpetiformis
Tropical sprue
Small bowel bacterial overgrowth
Intestinal resection
Whipple's disease
Radiation enteritis
Parasite infection, e.g. *Giardia intestinalis*

an immunological origin. It is thought that gluten-sensitive T lymphocytes recognize gluten-derived peptide epitopes when presented in association with DQ2. Upon activation these gluten-sensitive T cells develop a Th1/Th0-type inflammatory response which produces the observed mucosal damage. The enzyme tissue transglutaminase (tTG) modifies gluten, which increases its stimulating effect on gluten-sensitive T-cells.

## Pathology

There are absent or stunted small intestinal villi with elongation of crypts (subtotal villous atrophy). There is a chronic inflammatory cell infiltrate in the lamina propria, with an increase in intraepithelial cell lymphocytes.

## Clinical features

Coeliac disease can present at any age but there are two peaks in incidence: in infancy, after weaning on to gluten-containing foods, and in adults at 30–40 years. It often presents with non-specific symptoms of tiredness and malaise, or symptoms of small intestinal disease (see above).

Physical signs are usually few and non-specific, and related to anaemia and nutritional deficiency. There is an increased incidence of atopy and autoimmune disease.

## Investigations

**Jejunal mucosal biopsy** obtained via the endoscope. The mucosa shows the histological features described above. Other causes of villous atrophy (Table 3.5) are rare in adults in the Western world.

| Table 3.5 |
| --- |
| Causes of villous atrophy in adults |
| Coeliac disease |
| Dermatitis herpetiformis |
| Giardiasis |
| Malnutrition |
| Ischaemia |
| Lymphoma |
| Whipple's disease |
| Tropical sprue |

**Serum antibodies** Endomysial (EMA) and tissue trans-glutaminase (tTG) antibodies have a very high sensitivity and specificity for coeliac disease and can also be used to screen patients who have non-specific symptoms or an associated autoimmune condition such as type I diabetes mellitus. Antigliadin and antireticulin antibodies are less commonly used owing to lower sensitivity and specificity.

**Blood count** A mild anaemia is present in 50% of cases. There is almost always folate deficiency, commonly iron deficiency and, rarely, vitamin $B_{12}$ deficiency.

**Radiology** Small bowel follow-through may show a dilated bowel with thickened folds.

**Bone densitometry** (DXA scan, p. 279) should be performed in all patients because of the increased risk of osteoporosis in these patients.

## Management
Treatment is with a gluten-free diet, which should be continued lifelong. A repeat biopsy after treatment shows morphological improvement in the mucosa and confirms the diagnosis.

## Complications
There is an increased incidence of malignancy, particularly intestinal lymphoma, small bowel and oesophageal cancer. The incidence may be reduced by a gluten-free diet.

# Dermatitis herpetiformis (K&C p. 293 & 1303)
Dermatitis herpetiformis is an itchy, symmetrical eruption of vesicles and crusts over the extensor surfaces of the body. Most patients also have a gluten-sensitive enteropathy, which is usually asymptomatic. The skin condition responds to dapsone, but both the gut and the skin will improve on a gluten-free diet.

# Tropical sprue (K&C p. 293)
Tropical sprue is a progressive small intestinal disorder presenting with malabsorption which occurs in residents or

visitors to a tropical area where the disease is endemic (Asia, some Caribbean islands, Puerto Rico, parts of South America).

## Aetiology

The aetiology is unknown but the disease occurs in epidemics and improves with antibiotics, suggesting an infectious aetiology.

## Clinical features

The disease may present many years after patients have been in the tropics. There is diarrhoea, anorexia and abdominal distension. Nutritional deficiencies develop over a variable period of time.

## Investigations

Malabsorption should be demonstrated, particularly of fat and vitamin $B_{12}$. The intestinal mucosa shows partial villus atrophy affecting the whole small bowel. Infective causes of diarrhoea, particularly *Giardia intestinalis*, should be excluded.

## Management

Treatment is with a combination of folic acid and tetracycline, which may be required for up to 6 months. Nutritional deficiencies must also be corrected.

# Bacterial overgrowth (K&C p. 294)

The upper small intestine is almost sterile. Bacterial overgrowth may occur when there is stasis of intestinal contents as a result of abnormal motility, e.g. systemic sclerosis, or a structural abnormality, e.g. previous small bowel surgery or a diverticulum.

## Clinical features

There may be diarrhoea and/or steatorrhoea caused by the deconjugation of bile salts by bacteria. Vitamin $B_{12}$ deficiency, resulting from its metabolism by bacteria, can also occur.

## Diagnosis

**Breath tests** The hydrogen or $^{14}C$ breath tests are the investigations of choice. These depend on the ability of the organisms to metabolize either glucose or labelled bile salts, given by mouth, with the production of either hydrogen (from glucose) or $^{14}CO_2$ (from bile salts), which are then absorbed and can be measured in the exhaled air.

***Proximal small intestinal aspirates*** Proximal small intestinal aspirates (obtained via the endoscope) will reveal high numbers of coliforms and *Bacteroides* sp. on culture.

### Management
If possible the underlying cause should be corrected. This may not be possible and rotating courses of antibiotics are then necessary, such as tetracycline and metronidazole.

## Whipple's disease (K&C p. 295)
Whipple's disease is a rare systemic disease which almost always involves the small intestine. Common clinical features include steatorrhoea, abdominal pain, fever, lymphadenopathy, arthritis and neurological involvement. Intestinal biopsy shows periodic acid–Schiff (PAS)-positive macrophages. On electron microscopy the macrophages are seen to contain bacteria called *Tropheryma whippei*. Treatment of the disease is with co-trimoxazole for 6 months.

## Intestinal resection (K&C p. 294)
The effects of small intestinal resection depend on the extent and the area involved. Resection of the terminal ileum leads to malabsorption of:

- Vitamin $B_{12}$, leading to megaloblastic anaemia
- Bile salts, which overflow into the colon and interfere with salt and water absorption, producing diarrhoea. Bile salts in the colon also increase oxalate absorption, which may result in renal oxalate stones (p. 333).

If there is extensive resection increased hepatic bile salt synthesis cannot compensate for faecal loss and there is steatorrhoea secondary to bile salt deficiency. After massive intestinal resection there is severe loss of water and electrolytes, with malnutrition.

# Miscellaneous intestinal conditions

(*K&C p. 296*)

## Tuberculosis (TB) (*K&C p. 296 & p. 333*)

This results from reactivation of the primary disease caused by *Mycobacterium tuberculosis* (p. 478) and in the UK is most commonly seen in Asian immigrants. The ileocaecal valve is the most common site affected.

### Clinical features

There is abdominal pain, diarrhoea, anorexia, weight loss and fever. A mass may be palpable. The symptoms, signs and radiology (see below) can be similar to those of Crohn's disease, and TB must always be considered in the differential diagnosis of Asians presenting with apparent Crohn's disease.

### Diagnosis

**Radiology** The chest X-ray will show evidence of pulmonary tuberculosis in 50% of cases. The small bowel follow-through may show features similar to those of Crohn's disease (p. 87). Abdominal ultrasonography shows mesenteric thickening and lymphadenopathy.

**Endoscopy** Colonoscopy with terminal ileal biopsies is usually performed. It is not always possible to obtain bacteriological confirmation on tissue culture, and treatment is started if there is a high degree of suspicion.

**Surgery** Laparotomy is rarely needed for diagnosis.

### Management

Treatment is similar to that for pulmonary tuberculosis, i.e. isoniazid, rifampicin and pyrazinamide, although 1 year's treatment is required.

## Protein-losing enteropathy (*K&C p. 296*)

This involves increased protein loss across an abnormal intestinal mucosa. If there is inadequate hepatic synthesis of albumin to compensate for the intestinal loss, patients develop hypoalbuminaemia and oedema. Causes include Crohn's disease, Ménétrièr's disease (thickening and enlargement of gastric folds), coeliac disease and lymphatic disorders, e.g. lymphangiectasia.

## Meckel's diverticulum (K&C p. 296)

This is a congenital abnormality affecting 2–3% of the population. A diverticulum projects from the wall of the ileum approximately 60 cm from the ileocaecal valve. About half will contain gastric mucosa which secretes acid, and peptic ulceration may occur, with complications of bleeding or perforation. Diverticula may also become inflamed and present similarly to appendicitis. Treatment is surgical removal.

## Chronic intestinal ischaemia (K&C p. 297)

This is rare and results from atheromatous occlusion of mesenteric vessels in elderly people. The characteristic symptom is abdominal pain occurring after food. Diagnosis is made using angiography.

## Malignant small intestinal tumours

These are rare and present with abdominal pain, diarrhoea, anorexia and anaemia. Carcinoid tumours have additional clinical features, described below.

## Carcinoid tumours (K&C p. 299)

### Pathology

These originate from enterochromaffin cells (serotonin producing) of the intestine. The most common sites are the appendix, terminal ileum and rectum. *Carcinoid syndrome* is the term applied to the symptoms that arise as a result of products synthesized and released into the circulation by the tumour. These mediators include serotonin (5-hydroxytryptamine, or 5-HT), kinins, histamine and prostaglandins. The liver normally inactivates these mediators.

### Clinical features of the carcinoid syndrome

Patients with gastrointestinal carcinoid tumours have the carcinoid syndrome only if they have liver metastases because tumour products are able to drain directly into the hepatic vein (without being metabolized) and then into the systemic circulation, where they produce a variety of effects resulting in the carcinoid syndrome: flushing, wheezing, diarrhoea and abdominal pain, and right-sided cardiac valvular fibrosis causing stenosis and regurgitation.

## Investigations

A high level of 5-hydroxyindoleacetic acid (5-HIAA), the breakdown product of serotonin, is found in the urine in the carcinoid syndrome. Ultrasonographic examination of the liver confirms the presence of secondary deposits.

## Management

Treatment of the carcinoid syndrome is symptomatic and aimed at:

- Inhibition of tumour products with 5-HT antagonists, e.g. cyproheptadine or octreotide (a long-acting somatostatin analogue)
- Reducing tumour mass through surgical resection, hepatic artery embolization or chemotherapy.

## Adenocarcinoma (K&C p. 298)

Adenocarcinoma accounts for 50% of malignant small bowel tumours; there is an increased incidence in coeliac disease and Crohn's disease.

## Lymphoma (K&C p. 298)

Non-Hodgkin's lymphoma constitutes 15% of malignant small bowel tumours and may be B cell or T cell in origin. The latter occur with increased frequency in coeliac disease.

## Benign small bowel tumours (K&C p. 299)

- The Peutz–Jegher syndrome is an autosomal dominant condition with mucocutaneous pigmentation (circumoral, hands and feet) and hamartomatous gastrointestinal polyps. Polyps may occur anywhere in the gastrointestinal tract, but are most common in the small bowel. They may bleed or cause intussusception, and may undergo malignant change.
- Adenomas, leiomyomas and lipomas are rare. They are usually asymptomatic and discovered incidentally.
- Familial adenomatous polyposis (p. 94).

# Inflammatory bowel disease (K&C p. 300)

Two main forms are recognized: Crohn's disease, which affects any part of the gastrointestinal tract, and ulcerative colitis (UC), which affects the large bowel only.

## Epidemiology

Inflammatory bowel disease (IBD) is more common in the western world, occurring at any age but most commonly between the ages of 20 and 40 years. Both sexes are affected. In western populations the prevalence of UC is approximately 1 in 1000 and of Crohn's disease 1 in 1500 of the population.

## Aetiology

It is probable that environmental factors operate in a genetically predisposed individual. It is proposed that disruption of the intestinal epithelial integrity allows bacteria and luminal antigens to trigger an immune response. In the genetically predisposed individual, there is an exaggerated immune response. In Crohn's disease, the T cell immune response is T helper cell 1 (Th1) dominant as manifested by increased production of the pro-inflammatory cytokines, interferon-$\gamma$ and tumour necrosis factor-$\alpha$ (TNF-$\alpha$) and reduced production of the anti-inflammatory cytokines, interleukin-4 (IL-4) and IL-10. In contrast, in UC there is a Th2-dominant response with increased production of IL-5. There is also activation of other cells (neutrophils, mast cells and eosinophils) which leads to increased production of a wide variety of inflammatory mediators all of which can lead to cell damage.

### Environmental

- *Infective agents.* Measles virus and *Mycobacterium paratuberculosis* have been put forward as possible causes of Crohn's disease, but a causal relationship has not been established.
- *Smoking.* Crohn's disease is more common in smokers and UC less common. In Crohn's disease smoking doubles the risk of postoperative recurrence.

**Genetic** There is a familial tendency in both UC and Crohn's disease; twin studies suggest a stronger genetic influence in Crohn's disease than UC. Mutations within the *NOD2* gene (CARD15) present on chromosome 16 confer susceptibility to Crohn's disease but this is likely to be one of many genes that contribute to the Crohn's phenotype. The wild-type NOD2 protein regulates macrophage activation in response to bacterial lipopolysaccharides and it is not known how mutations lead to sustained activation of inflammatory pathways in Crohn's disease. There is an increased incidence of HLA-B27 in inflammatory bowel disease with ankylosing spondylitis.

## Pathology

UC and Crohn's disease have differences at both macroscopic and microscopic levels, and immunologically (Table 3.6).

## Clinical features

Crohn's disease is a progressive chronic disease with symptomatology depending on the region(s) of involved bowel; the commonest site is ileocaecal (in 40% of patients). The main feature in patients with small bowel disease is abdominal pain, usually with weight loss. Less commonly terminal ileal disease presents as an acute abdomen with right iliac fossa pain mimicking appendicitis. Colonic disease presents with diarrhoea, bleeding and pain related to defecation. In perianal disease there are anal tags, fissures, fistulae and abscess formation.

UC presents with diarrhoea, often containing blood and mucus. The clinical course may be one of persistent diarrhoea, relapses and remissions, or severe fulminating colitis (Table 3.7).

Patients with IBD may have one or more extraintestinal manifestations, and these are listed in Table 3.8.

## Investigations

The purpose of investigations is to define the nature of the disease and the extent and severity of bowel involvement.

**Blood count** Anaemia is common and is usually the normochromic, normocytic anaemia of chronic disease,

**Table 3.6**
Differences between Crohn's disease and ulcerative colitis

| | Crohn's disease | Ulcerative colitis |
|---|---|---|
| Macroscopic | Affects any part of the gut from mouth to anus | Affects only the colon |
| | Oral and perianal disease | Begins in the rectum and extends proximally in varying degrees |
| | Discontinuous involvement ('skip lesions') | Continuous involvement |
| | Deep ulcers and fissures in the mucosa: 'cobblestone appearance' | Red mucosa which bleeds easily |
| | | Ulcers and pseudopolyps (regenerating mucosa) in severe disease |
| Histology/immunology | Transmural inflammation | Mucosal inflammation |
| | Granulomata may be present | No granulomata but goblet cell depletion and crypt abscesses |
| | Th1 response | Th2 response |

**Table 3.7**
Definition of a severe attack of ulcerative colitis

| | |
|---|---|
| Bloody diarrhoea | > 6/day |
| Fever | > 37.5°C |
| Tachycardia | > 90/min |
| ESR | > 30 mm/h |
| Anaemia | Hb < 10 g/dL |
| Serum albumin | < 30 g/L |

**Table 3.8**
Non-gastrointestinal manifestations of inflammatory bowel disease

| | |
|---|---|
| Eyes | Uveitis, episcleritis, conjunctivitis |
| Joints | Small joint arthritis,* monoarticular arthritis (knees and ankles), ankylosing spondylitis,* sacroileitis |
| Skin | Erythema nodosum, pyoderma gangrenosum (necrotizing ulceration of the skin, commonly on the lower legs) |
| Liver* | Fatty change, primary sclerosing cholangitis, chronic hepatitis, cirrhosis |
| Calculi* | Increased incidence of gall bladder and renal calculi |
| Venous thrombosis | |
| Vasculitis | (Rare) |
| Amyloidosis | (Rare) |

* These manifestations are not related to disease activity
Biochemical abnormalities are common; clinically overt disease is uncommon

although iron deficiency anaemia may occur. The platelet count, ESR and C-reactive protein are often raised, and the serum albumin may be low in severe disease.

**Radiology** In Crohn's disease a small bowel follow-through shows an asymmetrical alteration in the mucosal pattern, with deep ulceration and areas of narrowing (string sign) commonly confined to the ileum. Skip lesions may be seen. Ultrasonography and CT scanning are particularly helpful in delineating abscesses, and will show thickened bowel in involved areas. MRI may be useful in perianal disease.

A plain X-ray should be performed during a severe attack of colitis to look for toxic dilatation of the colon.

**Endoscopy**  Rigid or flexible sigmoidoscopy will establish the diagnosis of UC and, less commonly, Crohn's disease. A rectal biopsy can be taken for histological examination to determine the nature of the inflammation. Colonoscopy allows the exact extent and severity of colonic and terminal ileal inflammation to be determined, and biopsies to be taken.

## Differential diagnosis

Crohn's disease must be differentiated from other causes of chronic diarrhoea, malabsorption and malnutrition. In children it is a cause of short stature. Other causes of terminal ileitis are TB and *Yersinia enterocolitica* infection (causing an acute illness). IBD affecting the colon must be differentiated from other causes of colitis: infection (p. 32), ischaemia and microscopic colitis. The latter presents with watery diarrhoea and at endoscopy the mucosa is macroscopically normal but mucosal inflammation is detected histologically.

## Management (Table 3.9)

**Medical**  Patients with Crohn's disease who smoke should be advised to stop, as this will decrease the number of relapses and reduce postoperative recurrence. The precise mechanisms responsible for the clinical efficacy of many of these treatments is not known. In general they have many anti-inflammatory and immunosuppressive properties combined with an antibacterial action in some cases (e.g. metronidazole).

**Table 3.9**
Summary of treatments used in inflammatory bowel disease

5-Aminosalicyclic acid preparations
Corticosteroids
Liquid enteral nutrition
Metronidazole
Methotrexate
Ciclosporin
Azathioprine
Anti-TNF-α (infliximab)

- 5-Aminosalicylic acid (5-ASA) tablets (mesalazine, olsalazine, balsalazide) will induce a remission in mild attacks of UC and in colonic Crohn's disease. In lower doses they are useful as a maintenance treatment to reduce the number of relapses. 5-ASA preparations can also be administered as an enema or suppository to treat proctosigmoiditis (i.e. inflammation of the rectum and sigmoid colon).

- Corticosteroids: oral steroids are used to treat acute attacks and the dose is tailed off as symptoms improve. In severe attacks intravenous steroids are necessary (Emergency Box 3.2). Proctosigmoiditis can be treated locally with steroid enemas and suppositories. Budesonide is a topically acting steroid which is poorly absorbed from the gastrointestinal tract and has fewer systemic effects than other steroids. A coated preparation allows delayed release of the drug after oral administration, and is used in the treatment of mild/moderate ileocaecal Crohn's disease.

- Azathioprine or its metabolite 6-mercaptopurine is used in patients with Crohn's disease and UC who

!  **Emergency Box 3.2**

## Management of acute severe colitis

**Admit to hospital**
Joint inpatient management between gastroenterologist and colorectal surgeon

**Investigations**
Full blood count, C-reactive protein
Serum albumin
Serum urea and electrolytes
Blood cultures (Gram-negative sepsis is common)
Plain abdominal X-ray looking for toxic dilatation (diameter, colon > 5 cm), mucosal islands, and/or perforation
Stool cultures (×3) to exclude coincidental infection

**Treatment**
Intravenous steroids: hydrocortisone 100 mg 6-hourly
Correct electrolyte and fluid imbalance
Consider i.v. ciclosporin in patients not responding to steroids
Low-molecular-weight heparin to prevent venous thrombosis

continue to have frequent relapses despite taking an adequate dose of 5-ASAs.

- Liquid enteral nutrition with an elemental (liquid preparation of amino acids, glucose and fatty acids) or polymeric diet will induce a remission in a relapse of small bowel Crohn's disease. The exact mode of action is not known. These diets are unpalatable and often have to be given via a nasogastric tube.
- Metronidazole is useful in severe perianal Crohn's disease resulting from its antibacterial action.
- Methotrexate is used in the minority of patients with active Crohn's disease which is resistant to conventional treatment with steroids. The long-term efficacy of this treatment is not known.
- Ciclosporin is occasionally used in patients with severe acute UC who fail to improve after treatment with intravenous steroids. The management of severe colitis is summarized in Emergency Box 3.2. Management should be in conjunction with the appropriate surgical team because patients not responding to medical therapy will need to undergo colectomy.
- Anti-TNF-α antibodies (infliximab) given as single infusion produces clinical improvement in 60% of patients with steroid-resistant Crohn's disease. Further infusions may be given at 8-weekly intervals to maintain remission though the optimal duration of treatment is unclear at present.

**Surgery**   Surgery is indicated for:
- Failure of medical therapy
- Complications (Table 3.10)
- Failure to grow in children.

In Crohn's disease resections are kept to a minimum as recurrence is almost inevitable in the remaining bowel. In some patients with small bowel disease, strictures can be widened (stricturoplasty) without resection.

The surgical options in UC are:

- Ileoanal anastomosis, in which the terminal ileum is used to form a reservoir (a 'pouch'), and the patient is

---

**Table 3.10**
Complications of inflammatory bowel disease

Toxic dilatation of the colon + perforation
Stricture formation*
Abscess formation (Crohn's disease)
Fistulae and fissures (Crohn's)*
Colon cancer

---

* Surgical intervention only necessary if symptomatic and not responding to medical treatment

continent with a few bowel motions per day. The pouch may become inflamed ('pouchitis'), leading to bloody diarrhoea which is treated initially with metronidazole.

- Panproctocolectomy with ileostomy (the whole colon and rectum is removed and the ileum brought out on to the abdominal wall as a stoma).
- Colectomy with an ileorectal anastomosis (diseased rectum left in situ and diarrhoea may still occur).

## Cancer in inflammatory bowel disease

Patients with extensive UC of more than 10 years' duration are at an increased risk of colorectal cancer (cumulative risk 12% after 25 years). Patients with long-standing Crohn's colitis are also at risk although less so than with UC. These patients are usually offered surveillance colonoscopy at intervals of 1–2 years. Colectomy is recommended if high-grade dysplasia is discovered.

### Prognosis

Both diseases are characterized by relapses and remissions. Almost all patients with Crohn's disease have a significant relapse over a 20-year period. The mortality rate is twice as high as that of the general population. The prognosis of UC is variable. Only 10% of patients with proctitis develop more extensive disease, but with severe fulminant disease there is a risk of colonic perforation and death.

# The colon and rectum

## Diverticular disease (*K&C* p. 312)

Pouches of mucosa extrude through the muscular wall through weakened areas near blood vessels to form diverticula. The term diverticulosis means the presence of diverticula. Diverticulitis implies inflammation, which occurs when faeces obstruct the neck of the diverticulum. Diverticula are common, affecting 50% of the population over 50 years of age.

### Aetiology

The precise cause of diverticular disease is unknown, although it appears to be related to the low-fibre diet eaten in western populations. It is thought that insufficient dietary fibre leads to increased intracolonic pressure, which causes herniation of the mucosa at sites of weakness.

### Clinical features

It is asymptomatic in 90% and usually discovered incidentally when a barium enema or colonoscopy is performed for other reasons. Symptoms are the result of bleeding or acute diverticulitis (left iliac fossa pain, fever, nausea, vomiting). Complications include abscess formation, perforation, haemorrhage, fistula formation and intestinal obstruction. Acute diverticulitis is diagnosed by CT scan or in some cases by ultrasound.

### Management

Acute attacks are treated with antibiotics (ciprofloxacin and metronidazole). Surgery is indicated rarely for complications and for frequent attacks of diverticulitis.

## Constipation (Table 3.11) (*K&C* p. 306)

This is a very common problem in the general population, and often requires no more than dietary advice and reassurance. It is particularly common in elderly people, in whom it is often associated with immobility and poor diet, and in young women in whom it may be associated with slow colonic transit or postpartum pelvic floor abnormalities. In many patients it is part of the irritable bowel syndrome (p. 101). Colorectal cancer should always be excluded in middle-aged and elderly people.

---

**Table 3.11**
Causes of constipation

Irritable bowel syndrome
Idiopathic slow transit
Pelvic floor dyssynergia
Intestinal obstruction, e.g. by colon cancer
Intestinal pseudo-obstruction
Painful anal conditions
Drugs, e.g. opiates, aluminium antacids
Hypothyroidism
Hypercalcaemia
Spinal cord lesion
Depression
Immobility
Hirschsprung's disease

---

### *Management*

A high-fibre diet and bulking agents should be the first line of treatment. Long-term laxatives (e.g. magnesium sulphate) should only be used in severe cases.

## Miscellaneous conditions

### Megacolon (*K&C* p. 311)

This term describes a number of conditions in which the colon is dilated. The most common cause is chronic constipation. Other causes are Chagas' disease and Hirschsprung's disease (congenital aganglionic segment in the rectum). Treatment is with laxatives, although Hirschsprung's disease responds to surgical resection.

### Ischaemic colitis (*K&C* p. 314)

This usually presents in the older age groups, with abdominal pain and rectal bleeding, and occasionally shock. Sigmoidoscopy is often normal apart from blood. Treatment is symptomatic, although surgery may be required for gangrene, perforation or stricture formation.

## Colon polyps and the polyposis syndromes (*K&C* p. 315)

A polyp is an elevation above the mucosal surface. They may be single or multiple, usually asymptomatic and 70–80% are adenomas. In the polyposis syndromes hundreds of polyps may be present.

**Hamartomatous polyps** Hamartomas are benign tumours composed of an overgrowth of mature cells and tissues that normally occur in the affected part, in this case the colon. They may be one of two types:

- *Juvenile polyps.* These are dominantly inherited polyps which occur in children and teenagers, and present early with diarrhoea, bleeding or intussusception.
- *Peutz–Jeghers polyps* (p. 83).

**Adenomatous polyps** are tumours of benign neoplastic epithelium. They are common, occurring in about 10% of the population. The aetiology is unknown, although genetic and environmental factors have been implicated. They rarely produce symptoms, although large polyps can bleed and cause anaemia, and villous adenomas can occasionally present with diarrhoea and hypokalaemia. Adenomatous polyps carry a malignant risk which increases with polyp size. Treatment is by endoscopic removal.

**Familial adenomatous polyposis (FAP)** is an autosomal dominantly inherited condition in which individuals usually develop hundreds of adenomatous polyps throughout the gastrointestinal tract at an early age, resulting inevitably in colon cancer unless the large bowel is removed. FAP arises from germline mutations of the *APC* gene (adenomatous polyposis coli) located on chromosome 5. Gene testing is offered to unaffected members of FAP families to establish whether or not they carry the gene. Many of these patients have congenital hypertrophy of the retinal pigment epithelium (CHRPE) and this, along with genetic analysis, facilitates screening of young patients. Carriers of the gene are counselled and offered prophylactic colectomy in young adulthood. After colectomy these patients remain at risk of small bowel cancer, particularly of the duodenum.

## Colorectal cancer (K&C p. 316)

Most colorectal cancers occur sporadically. In 5–10% of patients they occur in patients with HNPCC (see p. 97) or FAP. Colorectal cancer may also occur on a background of long-standing UC or colonic Crohn's disease.

# Sporadic colorectal cancer

## Epidemiology

This is the second most common cause of cancer death in the UK, and the incidence increases with age: most patients are over 50 years. Colon cancer is rare in Africa and Asia, largely because of environmental differences. A diet high in meat and animal fat and low in fibre is thought to be an important aetiological factor. In the west, the lifetime risk is 1 in 50, increasing to 1 in 17 in those with one affected first-degree relative.

## Inheritance

Multiple molecular genetic abnormalities are now thought to be involved in the development of sporadic colon cancer. These include the activation of tumour-promoting genes or oncogenes (K-*ras*, c-*myc*) and the inactivation of tumour suppressor genes (*MCC*, *DCC*, *p53*). The risk of a tumour developing increases with increasing number of genetic abnormalities.

95

## Pathology

It is likely that most carcinomas (other than on a background of IBD) start as a benign adenoma, the so-called 'adenoma–carcinoma' sequence. Spread is by direct invasion through the bowel wall, with later invasion of blood vessels and lymphatics and spread to the liver. The mortality of colorectal cancer is directly related to the stage at presentation, and the stage is classified according to the modified Dukes' (Table 3.12) or TNM (tumour, node, metastases) classification. Synchronous (i.e. more than one tumour) tumours are present in 2% of cases.

**Table 3.12**
Modified Dukes' grading of colon cancer

| | |
|---|---|
| Dukes' A | Tumour confined to the bowel wall |
| Dukes' B | Tumour extending through the bowel wall |
| Dukes' C | Regional lymph nodes involved |
| Dukes' D | Distant metastases |

## Clinical features

Most tumours are in the left side of the colon. They cause rectal bleeding and stenosis, with symptoms of increasing intestinal obstruction such as an alteration in bowel habit and colicky abdominal pain. Carcinoma of the caecum and ascending colon often presents with iron deficiency anaemia or a right iliac fossa mass. Clinical examination is usually unhelpful, although a mass may be palpable transabdominally or in the rectum. Hepatomegaly may be present with liver metastases.

## Investigation

Examination of the colon is performed with a double-contrast barium enema or colonoscopy. A full blood count may show anaemia, and abnormal serum liver biochemistry suggests the presence of liver secondaries. Faecal occult blood tests have been used in population screening studies but are not of value diagnostically.

## Management (K&C p. 505)

Treatment is surgical, with tumour resection and end-to-end anastomosis of bowel if possible. Adjuvant chemotherapy with 5-fluorouracil and levamisole increases survival in Dukes' grade C (TNM stage III) cases, and in some cases with Dukes' B cancer. Preoperative radiotherapy improves survival in some patients with rectal cancer, and radiotherapy can also offer effective palliation in patients with locally advanced disease. Patients with up to two or three liver metastases confined to one lobe of the liver may be offered hepatic resection. Patients who have multiple hepatic metastases which cannot be resected may benefit from chemotherapy, which increases median survival and improves quality of life.

## Prognosis

The overall 5-year survival rate is 40%, but is over 95% in tumours confined to the bowel wall (Dukes' grade A).

## Screening

High-risk individuals (i.e. patients from HNPCC families or with a first-degree relative developing colon cancer < 50 years) should be offered screening colonoscopy. Mass population screening of the over-50s with faecal occult blood tests or sigmoidoscopy has been shown to reduce the mortality from colon cancer, but this strategy has not yet been widely adopted because of the cost implications and the relatively poor uptake by healthy individuals.

## Hereditary non-polyposis colorectal cancer (HNPCC) (K&C p. 316)

HNPCC has an autosomal dominant mode of transmission with incomplete penetrance. It results from a mutation in one of six DNA mismatch repair genes which in turn lead to widespread genomic instability. Mutations in two of these, *hMLH1* and *hMSH2* account for > 95% of HNPCC families. These patients have an increased risk of developing tumours at an early age, and more often develop right-sided tumours. Many of these patients also have an increased incidence of gynaecological, urinary tract, biliary, and other malignancies. Diagnostic criteria (Amsterdam criteria) to help identify those with HNPCC, based on family history have been devised (Table 3.13). A detailed family history should always be taken in any patient presenting with cancer.

## Diarrhoea (K&C p. 320)

True diarrhoea is defined as an increase in stool weight to more than 250 g in 24 hours. This must be differentiated from the frequent passage of small amounts of stool (usually functional), and this is achieved with a 3-day stool collection for faecal weight. Acute diarrhoea is usually due

---

**Table 3.13**
Modified Amsterdam criteria for diagnosis of HNPCC

- Three or more relatives with histologically verified HNPCC-associated cancer (colorectal, endometrium, small bowel, ureter, or renal pelvis), one of whom is a first-degree relative of the other and in whom FAP has been excluded

- Families with colorectal cancer involving at least two generations

- One or more cancers were diagnosed before the age of 50

to infection or dietary indiscretion; chronic diarrhoea is defined as diarrhoea persisting for more than 14 days.

There are three main mechanisms: osmotic, secretory, abnormal motility.

## Osmotic diarrhoea

This occurs when there are large quantities of non-absorbed hypertonic substances in the bowel lumen. The diarrhoea stops when the patient stops eating or the malabsorptive substance is discontinued. The causes of osmotic diarrhoea are as follows:

- Ingestion of non-absorbable substance, e.g. a laxative such as magnesium sulphate
- Generalized malabsorption so that high concentrations of solute (e.g. glucose) remain in the lumen
- Specific malabsorptive defect, e.g. disaccharidase deficiency.

## Secretory diarrhoea

Secretory diarrhoea results from the net secretion of fluid and electrolytes into the bowel lumen, and continues when the patient fasts. The causes are:

- Inflammation, e.g. ulcerative colitis, Crohn's disease
- Infection, e.g. shigella, salmonella
- Enterotoxins, e.g. from E. coli, cholera toxin
- Hormone-secreting tumours, e.g. VIPoma (p. 164)
- Bile salts (in the colon) following ileal resection
- Fatty acids (in the colon) following ileal resection
- Some laxatives.

## Motility related

Abnormal motility often produces frequency rather than true diarrhoea. Causes are thyrotoxicosis, diabetic autonomic neuropathy and post-vagotomy.

### Investigation

Acute diarrhoea lasting a few days is the result of dietary indiscretion or an infection. Investigation is not needed and treatment is symptomatic to maintain hydration. Chronic diarrhoea always requires investigation. Figure 3.2 outlines

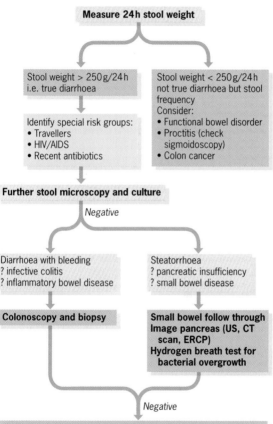

Perform outpatient sigmoidoscopy and rectal biopsy, stool cultures. If negative: Does the patient have 'true' diarrhoea?

**Measure 24h stool weight**

Stool weight > 250g/24h i.e. true diarrhoea

Identify special risk groups:
• Travellers
• HIV/AIDS
• Recent antibiotics

Stool weight < 250g/24h not true diarrhoea but stool frequency
Consider:
• Functional bowel disorder
• Proctitis (check sigmoidoscopy)
• Colon cancer

**Further stool microscopy and culture**

*Negative*

Diarrhoea with bleeding
? infective colitis
? inflammatory bowel disease

**Colonoscopy and biopsy**

Steatorrhoea
? pancreatic insufficiency
? small bowel disease

**Small bowel follow through**
**Image pancreas (US, CT scan, ERCP)**
**Hydrogen breath test for bacterial overgrowth**

*Negative*

**Neuroendocrine evaluation: Serum gastrin, VIP, calcitonin, urine 5-HIAA**
**Consider factitious diarrhoea: e.g. ingestion of laxatives**
**Determine if diarrhoea decreases with fasting (i.e. suggests osmotic diarrhoea) and i.v. fluid replacement**

VIP = vasoactive intestinal polypeptide
5-HIAA = 5-hydroxyindoleacetic acid

**Fig. 3.2 An approach to the investigation of chronic diarrhoea.**

an approach to the investigation of a patient with chronic diarrhoea. Laxative abuse, usually seen in young females, must be excluded as a cause of chronic diarrhoea. Patients taking anthraquinone purgatives, e.g. Senokot, develop pigmentation of the colonic mucosa (melanosis coli) which may be seen at sigmoidoscopy. Other laxatives may be detected in the stool or urine.

Diarrhoea is a common problem in patients with AIDS, resulting either from a specific AIDS enteropathy or from an infection (cryptosporidia, microsporidia, cytomegalovirus infection).

# Functional bowel disorders (K&C p. 324)

This is a large group of gastrointestinal disorders that are termed 'functional' because symptoms occur in the absence of any demonstrable abnormalities in the digestion and absorption of nutrients, fluid and electrolytes and no structural abnormality can be identified in the gastrointestinal tract. Functional bowel disorders are extremely common world-wide, accounting for up to 80% of patients seen in the gastroenterology clinic. Rather than a diagnosis of exclusion after normal investigations (as the definition would suggest), this is frequently a positive diagnosis made in a patient with symptoms suggestive of a functional gastrointestinal disorder (Table 3.14). It is estimated that only 25% of persons with this condition seek medical care

---

**Table 3.14**
Chronic gastrointestinal symptoms suggestive of a functional gastrointestinal disorder

Nausea alone
Vomiting alone
Belching
Chest pain unrelated to exercise
Postprandial fullness
Abdominal bloating
Abdominal discomfort/pain (right or left iliac fossa)
Passage of mucus per rectum
Frequency of bowel actions with urgency first thing in the morning

---

for it and studies suggest that those who seek care are more likely to have behavioural and psychiatric problems than those who do not seek care. Altered bowel motility, visceral hypersensitivity (they have a lower pain threshold when tested with balloon distension of the rectum), psychosocial factors, an imbalance in neurotransmitters and gastro-intestinal infection have all been proposed as playing a part in the development of functional bowel disorders. Low-dose antidepressant treatment is frequently used for these disorders if initial symptom-based treatments do not prove beneficial.

Common functional gastrointestinal disorders are:

- *Functional oesophageal disorders* occur in the absence of dysphagia, heartburn or other oesophageal disorder. They include globus (a sensation of a lump in the throat), effortless regurgitation of recently ingested food and chest pain. Sometimes these symptoms will respond to high-dose acid suppression.

- *Functional dyspepsia.* Common symptoms include indigestion, wind, nausea, early satiety and heartburn. Symptoms are sometimes very similar to peptic ulceration. Investigation is frequently unnecessary in young people (< 45 years) but endoscopy is usually required in older people or in those with alarm symptoms (see p. 69). Management is mainly by reassurance. Antacids and $H_2$-receptor antagonists are rarely of benefit. Eradication of *H. pylori* is often practised but there is little evidence that this improves symptoms. The prokinetic agents metoclopramide and domperidone are sometimes helpful, particularly in those with fullness and bloating.
- *Irritable bowel syndrome (IBS).* Crampy abdominal pain relieved by defecation or the passage of wind, altered bowel habit, a sensation of incomplete evacuation, abdominal bloating and distension are common symptoms. Symptoms are more common in women than men, and the history is usually prolonged. Characteristically the patient looks healthy. Examination is usually normal, although sigmoidoscopy and air insufflation may reproduce the pain. If frequency of defecation is a feature, a rectal

biopsy should be performed to exclude inflammatory bowel disease. Investigation depends on the individual patient. Young patients with classic symptoms do not require investigation. New symptoms in an elderly patient should prompt a search for underlying disease. Management is reassurance, with a discussion of lifestyle and diet. A high-fibre diet and antispasmodics, e.g. mebeverine, are useful in some patients. Other treatments, such as antidepressants, biofeedback and hypnotherapy, may be tried.

# The acute abdomen (K&C p. 328)

This section deals with acute abdominal conditions that cause patients to be hospitalized within a few hours of the onset of their pain. Most are admitted under the care of the surgical team, and some will need a laparotomy. Medical conditions that may present as an acute abdomen include diabetic ketoacidosis, myocardial infarction and pneumonia. The irritable bowel syndrome may also present with acute severe abdominal pain.

## History

A detailed history, which should include gynaecological symptoms, will often point to the cause of the pain.

- Acute abdominal pain may be intermittent or continuous. Intermittent (colicky) pain describes pain that occurs for a short period (usually a few minutes) and is interspersed with pain-free periods lasting a few minutes or up to half an hour. This is characteristic of mechanical obstruction of a hollow viscus, e.g. ureteric calculus or bowel obstruction (Table 3.15). Additional symptoms of bowel obstruction, which may or may not be present, are abdominal distension, vomiting and absolute constipation (i.e. failure to pass flatus or stool). Biliary pain (previously called biliary colic) resulting from obstruction of the gall bladder or bile duct is not colicky but usually a constant upper abdominal pain.

**Table 3.15**
Causes of mechanical intestinal obstruction

| | |
|---|---|
| Constriction from the outside | Bowel entrapped in a hernia<br>Adhesions<br>Volvulus, particularly of the sigmoid |
| Disease of the bowel wall | Crohn's disease<br>Carcinoma<br>Diverticular disease |
| Intraluminal obstruction | Foreign body<br>Gallstones |

Continuous pain is relentless with no periods of complete relief. It occurs in many abdominal conditions.

- The onset of pain may be sudden or gradual. Sudden onset suggests perforation of a viscus (e.g. duodenal ulcer), rupture of an organ (e.g. aortic aneurysm) or torsion (e.g. ovarian cyst). The pain of acute pancreatitis often begins suddenly.
- The site of the pain must be noted. In general, upper abdominal pain is produced by pathology of either the upper abdominal viscera – e.g. acute cholecystitis, acute pancreatitis – or the stomach and duodenum. The pain of small bowel obstruction is often in the centre of the abdomen. A common cause of acute right iliac fossa pain is acute appendicitis.
- Radiation of pain to the back suggests acute pancreatitis, rupture of an aortic aneurysm or renal tract disease.

## Examination

A general physical examination should be made and the following points noted:

- The presence of shock (pale, cool peripheries, tachycardia, hypotension) suggests rupture of an organ, e.g. aortic aneurysm, ruptured ectopic pregnancy. It may also occur in the later stages of generalized peritonitis resulting from bowel perforation (see below).
- Fever is common in acute inflammatory conditions.
- Peritonitis and bowel obstruction produce specific signs on abdominal examination.

The signs of peritonitis are tenderness, guarding and rigidity on palpation. Guarding is an involuntary contraction of the abdominal muscles when the abdomen is palpated. Peritonitis may be localized or generalized (see below). Bowel sounds are absent with generalized peritonitis.

Mechanical bowel obstruction produces distension and active 'tinkling' bowel sounds. A strangulated hernia may produce obstruction, and the hernial orifices must always be examined.

In most cases a rectal and pelvic examination should be performed.

### Investigations

- Blood tests. The white cell count may be raised in inflammatory conditions. The serum amylase may be raised in any acute abdomen, but levels greater than five times normal indicate acute pancreatitis.
- Radiology. An erect chest X-ray may show air under the diaphragm with a perforated viscus. A plain abdominal X-ray shows dilated loops of bowel and fluid levels in obstruction. Ultrasound examination is useful in the diagnosis of acute cholangitis, appendicitis and gynaecological conditions.
- Surgery. Laparoscopy or laparotomy may be required, depending on the diagnosis.

## Acute appendicitis (K&C p. 330)

Acute appendicitis occurs when the lumen of the appendix becomes obstructed by a faecolith.

### Epidemiology

It affects all age groups but is rare in the very young and very old.

### Clinical features

The typical clinical presentation is the onset of central abdominal pain which then becomes localized to the right iliac fossa (RIF), accompanied by anorexia and sometimes vomiting and diarrhoea. The patient is pyrexial, with tenderness and guarding in the RIF.

## Investigations
In many cases the diagnosis is clinical. There is a raised white cell count and ultrasonography may show an inflamed appendix. CT is also used to make the diagnosis.

## Differential diagnosis
Conditions that mimic acute appendicitis include non-specific mesenteric lymphadenitis, terminal ileitis due to Crohn's disease or *Yersinia* infection, acute salpingitis in women, inflamed Meckel's diverticulum and functional bowel diseases.

## Management
The treatment is surgical, with removal of the appendix either by open surgery or laparoscopically.

## Complications
These arise from gangrene and perforation, leading to local-ized abscess formation or generalized peritonitis.

105

# Acute peritonitis (K&C p. 330)
Localized peritonitis occurs with all acute inflammatory conditions of the gastrointestinal tract, and management depends on the underlying condition, e.g. acute appendi-citis, acute cholecystitis.

Generalized peritonitis occurs as a result of rupture of an abdominal viscus, e.g. perforated duodenal ulcer, perforated appendix. There is a sudden onset of abdominal pain which rapidly becomes generalized. The patient is shocked and lies still, as movement exacerbates the pain. A plain abdominal X-ray shows air under the diaphragm; serum amylase must be checked to exclude acute pancreatitis.

# Intestinal obstruction (K&C p. 331)
Intestinal obstruction is either mechanical or functional.

**Mechanical** (Table 3.15) The bowel above the level of the obstruction is dilated, with increased secretion of fluid into the lumen. The patient complains of colicky abdominal pain, associated with vomiting and absolute constipation.

On examination there is distension and 'tinkling' bowel sounds. Small bowel obstruction may settle with conservative management (i.e. nasogastric suction and intravenous fluids to maintain hydration). Large bowel obstruction is treated surgically.

**Functional** This occurs with a paralytic ileus, which is often seen in the postoperative stage of peritonitis or of major abdominal surgery, or in association with opiate treatment (acute colonic pseudo-obstruction, Ogilvie's syndrome). It also occurs when the nerves or muscles of the intestine are damaged, causing intestinal pseudo-obstruction. Unlike mechanical obstruction, pain is often not present and bowel sounds may be decreased. Gas is seen throughout the bowel on a plain abdominal X-ray. Management is conservative.

## The peritoneum (K&C p. 332)

The peritoneal cavity is a closed sac lined by mesothelium. It contains a little fluid to allow the abdominal contents to move freely. Conditions which affect the peritoneum are listed below.

- Infective (peritonitis)
  - secondary to gut disease, e.g. appendicitis, perforation
  - chronic peritoneal dialysis
  - spontaneous (associated with ascites)
  - tuberculous
- Neoplasia
  - secondary deposits, e.g. from ovary
  - primary mesothelioma
- Vasculitis: connective tissue disease.

## Nutrition

## Dietary requirements (K&C p. 222)

Food is necessary to provide the body with energy. The average daily requirement (Table 3.16) of a middle-aged

**Table 3.16**
Protein, energy and water requirement of normal and
hypercatabolic adults

| Metabolic state | Nutritional requirements | |
| --- | --- | --- |
| | **Normal** | **Hypercatabolic** |
| Protein (g/kg) | 1 | 2–3 |
| Nitrogen (g/kg) | 0.17 | 0.3–0.45 |
| Energy (kcal/kg) | 25–30 | 35–50 |
| Water (mL/kg) | 30–35 | 30–35 |

adult female in the UK is 8100 kJ (1940 kcal), and for a man
is 10 600 kJ (2550 kcal). This is made up of 50% carbohydrate, 35% fat and 15% protein, plus or minus 5%
alcohol. Energy requirements increase during periods of
rapid growth, such as adolescence, pregnancy and lactation, and with sepsis.

Bodyweight is maintained at a 'set point' by a precise
balance of energy intake and total energy expenditure (the
sum of the resting metabolic rate, activity energy expenditure and the thermic effect of food eaten). Weight gain is
almost always due solely to an increase in energy intake
which exceeds the total energy expenditure. Occasionally
weight gain is due to a decrease in energy expenditure, e.g.
hypothyroidism, or to fluid retention, e.g. heart failure or
ascites. On the other hand, weight loss associated with
cancer and chronic diseases is due to a reduction in energy
intake secondary to a loss of appetite (anorexia). In a few
conditions, such as sepsis and severe trauma, there is an
increase in energy requirements (hypercatabolic or hyper-
metabolic) which will result in a negative energy balance if
there is no compensatory increase in energy intake.

A balanced diet also requires sufficient amounts of minerals and vitamins. In the western world vitamin deficiency
is rare except in specific groups, e.g. alcoholics and patients
with small bowel disease, who may have multiple vitamin
deficiencies, and patients with liver and biliary tract disease
who are susceptible to deficiency of the fat-soluble vitamins
(A, D, E, K). Deficiencies of the B vitamins, riboflavin and
biotin, are rare in all patient groups and are not discussed

further. Dietary deficiency of vitamin $B_6$ (pyridoxine, pyridoxal and pyridoxamine) is also extremely rare, but drugs (e.g. isoniazid and penicillamine) that interact with pyridoxal phosphate may cause $B_6$ deficiency and a poly-neuropathy. Vitamin $B_{12}$ and folate deficiency is discussed on pages 175 and 176 and vitamin D deficiency on page 276.

There is recent evidence from epidemiological studies that β-carotene (a precursor of vitamin A) and vitamin E supplementation of western diets may protect against cancer and ischaemic heart disease by virtue of their anti-oxidant properties. However, randomized controlled trials using β-carotene supplements did not show any protective effect. There is some evidence that vitamin E may protect against the development of ischaemic heart disease, and one controlled trial has shown a reduction in the risk of non-fatal myocardial infarction when supplements were given to patients with advanced ischaemic heart disease.

## Nutritional support (K&C p. 245)

Patients should be screened for nutritional status on ad-mission to hospital and during their hospital stay. Current recommendations suggest that:

- Patients should be asked simple questions about recent weight loss, their usual weight and whether they have been eating less than usual.
- Their weight and height should be recorded and body mass index (BMI) calculated (weight [kg]/height [m]$^2$). The acceptable range of BMI is 20–25 kg/m$^2$ for men and 19–24 kg/m$^2$ for women.

Some form of nutritional supplementation is required in those patients who cannot eat, should not eat, will not eat or cannot eat enough. It is necessary to provide nutritional support for:

- All severely malnourished patients on admission to hospital. Severe malnutrition is indicated by a BMI of less than 15

- Moderately malnourished patients (BMI 15–19) who, because of their physical illness, are not expected to eat for 3–5 days
- Normally nourished patients not expected to eat for 7–10 days.

Enteral nutrition is cheaper, more physiological and has fewer complications than parenteral (intravenous) nutrition, and should be used if the gastrointestinal tract is functioning normally. With both enteral and parenteral nutrition a complete feeding regimen consisting of fat, carbohydrates, protein, vitamins, minerals and trace elements can be provided to provide the nutritional requirements of the individual (Table 3.16). Ideally a multidisciplinary nutrition support team should supervise the provision of artificial nutritional support.

## Enteral nutrition (K&C p. 246)
Foods can be given by:

- Mouth
- Fine-bore nasogastric tube for short-term enteral nutrition
- Percutaneous endoscopic gastrostomy (PEG): this is useful for patients who need feeding for longer than 2 weeks
- Percutaneous jejunostomy where a tube is inserted directly into the jejunum either endoscopically or at laparotomy.

A polymeric diet with whole protein, carbohydrate and fat is usually used; sometimes an elemental diet composed of amino acids, glucose and fatty acids is used for patients with Crohn's disease (p. 90).

## Total parenteral nutrition (TPN) (K&C p. 247)
Parenteral nutrition may be given via a feeding catheter placed in a peripheral vein or a silicone catheter placed in the subclavian vein. Central catheters must only be placed by experienced clinicians under strict aseptic conditions in a sterile environment. The risk of introducing infection is

**Table 3.17**
Complications of TPN

Catheter related: sepsis, thrombosis, embolism and pneumothorax
Metabolic, e.g. hyperglycaemia, hypercalcaemia
Electrolyte disturbances
Liver dysfunction

reduced if these catheters are only used for feeding purposes, and not the administration of drugs or blood. Peripheral feeding lines usually only last for about 5 days and are reserved for when feeding is necessary for a short period. Central lines may last for months to years. Complications of TPN are given in Table 3.17.

## Monitoring of artificial nutrition

Patients receiving nutritional support should be weighed twice weekly: they require regular clinical examination to check for evidence of fluid overload or depletion. Patients receiving nutritional support in hospital initially require daily measurements of urea and electrolytes and blood glucose. More frequent measurement of blood glucose with BM Stix is indicated in patients beginning TPN. Liver biochemistry, calcium and phosphate are measured twice weekly. Serum magnesium, zinc and nitrogen balance (see below) is measured weekly. The frequency of biochemical monitoring is adjusted according to the patient's clinical and metabolic status.

It is necessary to give 40–50 g of protein per 24 hours to maintain nitrogen balance, which represents the balance between protein breakdown and synthesis. The aim of any regimen is to achieve a positive nitrogen balance, which can usually be obtained by giving 3–5 g of nitrogen in excess of output. The amount of protein required to maintain nitrogen balance in a particular individual can be calculated from the amount of urinary nitrogen loss using the formula:

$N_2$ loss (g/24 h) = urinary urea (mmol/24 h) $\times$ 0.028 + 2

Urinary nitrogen $\times$ 6.25 = grams of protein required (most proteins contain about 16% nitrogen).

Most patients require about 12 g of nitrogen per 24 hours, but hypercatabolic patients require more, about 15 g/day.

# Disorders of bodyweight

## Obesity (*K&C* p. 241)

Obesity, defined as an excess of body fat contributing to co-morbidity is a common problem in developed countries and is becoming more common in developing countries. A BMI of 25 kg/m$^2$ or greater is a standard commonly used to define obesity. Obesity is associated with an increased prevalence of ischaemic heart disease, hypertension, diabetes mellitus, hyperlipidaemia, obstructive sleep apnoea, fatty liver and gallstones. Weight reduction can be achieved with a reduction in calorie intake and an increase in physical activity, although in practice this is difficult to achieve. Drug treatment such as orlistat, an inhibitor of pancreatic lipase and hence fat digestion, is sometimes used in the severely obese patient.

## Anorexia nervosa (*K&C* p. 1266)

Anorexia nervosa is a psychological illness, predominantly affecting young females and characterized by marked weight loss (BMI < 17.5 kg/m$^2$), intense fear of gaining weight, a distorted body image and amenorrhoea. Patients with anorexia nervosa control their body weight by a process of semi-starvation and/or self-induced vomiting (bulimia) and may develop consequences of undernutrition. Treatment is difficult and usually undertaken in a specialist eating disorders unit.

# 4

# Liver, biliary tract and pancreatic disease

The pancreas secretes the hormones insulin and glucagon (both regulate blood sugar) in addition to pancreatic enzymes involved in the digestion of fat, carbohydrate and protein in the small intestine (*K&C* p. 337). The main functions of the liver are:

- Control of synthesis and metabolism of carbohydrate, lipids, protein (including most plasma proteins and coagulation factors) and drugs. The liver manufactures about half of the body's cholesterol; the rest comes from food. Cholesterol is used to make bile and is also needed to make certain hormones, including oestrogen, testosterone, and the adrenal hormones. The liver is the major site for converting excess carbohydrates and proteins into fatty acids and triglycerides, which are then exported and stored in adipose tissue. Sugars are also stored in the liver as glycogen and then broken down and released into the bloodstream as glucose when needed.
- The metabolism and excretion of bilirubin and bile acids (necessary for digestion and absorption of dietary fat).

In most western countries alcohol and hepatitis C are the major causes of liver disease. Elsewhere infection with hepatitis B virus is a common cause but the incidence is decreasing with vaccination.

## Symptoms of liver disease

Acute liver disease, e.g. viral hepatitis, may be asymptomatic or it presents with generalized symptoms of lethargy, anorexia and malaise in the early stages, with jaundice developing later (p. 116).

Chronic liver disease may also be asymptomatic and discovered from an incidental finding of abnormal liver biochemistry. Some patients with chronic liver disease may present at a late stage with complications of cirrhosis, causing:

- Ascites with abdominal swelling and discomfort (p. 138)
- Haematemesis and melaena due to bleeding oesophageal varices (p. 136)
- Confusion and drowsiness due to hepatic encephalopathy (p. 140).

Patients presenting in this way are often extremely unwell and a detailed history may not be obtained. However, physical examination will often reveal the signs of chronic liver disease (p. 128) and thus point to liver disease as the cause of the presenting illness.

Pruritus (itching) occurs in cholestatic jaundice from any cause (p. 116), but is particularly common in primary biliary cirrhosis, when it may be the only symptom (without jaundice) at presentation. Pruritus may occur in association with other systemic diseases (e.g. hyperthyroidism, polycythaemia, renal failure, malignant disease) and skin diseases (e.g. scabies, eczema), but in these cases there are usually additional symptoms or signs that suggest the diagnosis.

## Interpreting liver biochemistry and liver function tests (K&C p. 340)

A routine blood sample sent to the laboratory for liver biochemistry will be processed by an automated multichannel analyser to produce serum levels of bilirubin, aminotransferases, alkaline phosphatase, γ-glutamyl transpeptidase (γ-GT) and total proteins. Liver synthetic function is determined by measuring the serum albumin and the prothrombin time (clotting factors are synthesized in the liver). A prolonged prothrombin time may also occur as a result of vitamin K deficiency in biliary obstruction (low concentration of intestinal bile salts results in poor absorption of vitamin K); however, unlike liver disease, clotting is corrected by giving 10 mg of vitamin K intravenously.

- *Bilirubin* (normal range < 17 μmol/L, 1.00 mg/dL). A small or moderate rise in the serum bilirubin without accompanying abnormalities of liver enzymes is usually the result of Gilbert's syndrome, haemolysis or ineffective erythropoiesis (premature death of the red cell in the bone marrow). Hyperbilirubinaemia caused by hepatobiliary disease is almost always accompanied by other abnormalities of liver biochemistry; very high levels occur most frequently in biliary tract obstruction. Serial measurements are useful in following the progress of some diseases, e.g. primary biliary cirrhosis, or the response to treatment, e.g. after placement of a stent in cancer of the head of the pancreas.
- *Aminotransferases*. These enzymes are present in hepatocytes and leak into the blood with liver cell damage. Very high levels may occur with acute hepatitis (20–50 times normal). Aspartate aminotransferase (AST) (normal range 10–40 U/L) is also present in heart and skeletal muscle, and raised serum concentrations are seen with myocardial infarction and skeletal muscle damage. Alanine aminotransferase (ALT) (normal range 5–40 U/L) is more specific to the liver than AST.
- *Alkaline phosphatase* (normal range 25–115 U/L) is situated in the canalicular and sinusoidal membranes of the liver. Raised serum alkaline phosphatase concentrations are seen in cholestasis from any cause, whether intra- or extrahepatic disease. Circulating alkaline phosphatase is also derived from bone, and raised serum levels occur in Paget's disease, osteomalacia, growing children, and bony metastases. In these cases differentiation from cholestasis is made by the absence of a rise in serum γ-glutamyl transpeptidase (γ-GT) (see below). The placenta secretes its own isoenzyme and the serum level is raised in pregnancy.
- *γ-Glutamyl transpeptidase* (normal range, male < 50 U/L, female < 32 U/L) is a liver microsomal

enzyme which may be induced by alcohol and enzyme-inducing drugs, e.g. phenytoin. A raised serum concentration is a useful screen for alcohol abuse. In cholestasis the γ-GT rises in parallel with the serum alkaline phosphatase because it has a similar pathway of excretion.

## Imaging and liver biopsy (K&C p. 342)

The initial imaging tests used in the investigation of patients with suspected liver, biliary and pancreatic disease are all non-invasive and include transabdominal ultrasound, computed tomography (CT) examination and magnetic resonance cholangiopancreatography (MRCP). Endoscopic retrograde cholangiopancreatography (ERCP) is performed under intravenous sedation and usually without general anaesthesia. The pancreatic and bile ducts are imaged after the injection of radiographic contrast medium. Stones in the ducts can be removed and stents placed to relieve obstruction caused by strictures. Complications of ERCP include bleeding (after cutting of the sphincter to aid bile duct cannulation or stone removal) and acute pancreatitis. Percutaneous transhepatic cholangiopancreatography (PTC) involves injection of contrast into the biliary system by injection through a percutaneously placed needle inserted into an intrahepatic duct; ERCP is the preferred first-line investigation. Liver biopsy for histological examination is usually performed via a percutaneous approach under local anaesthesia. Contraindications include a prolonged prothrombin time (by more than 3 s), platelet count $< 80 \times 10^9/L$, ascites, extrahepatic cholestasis and renal transplant.

## Jaundice (K&C p. 346)

Jaundice (icterus) is a yellow discoloration of the sclerae and skin as a result of a raised serum bilirubin, and is usually detectable clinically when the bilirubin is greater than 50 μmol/L (3 mg/dL).

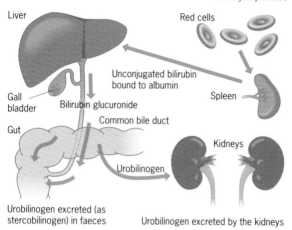

Fig. 4.1 **Pathways in bilirubin metabolism.**

Bilirubin is derived predominantly from the breakdown of haemoglobin in the spleen, and is carried in the blood bound to albumin. Unconjugated bilirubin is conjugated in the liver by glucuronyl transferase to bilirubin glucuronide, and this is excreted into the small intestine in bile. In the terminal ileum conjugated bilirubin is converted to urobilinogen and excreted in the faeces (as stercobilinogen) or reabsorbed and excreted by the kidneys (Fig. 4.1).

The usual division of jaundice into prehepatic, hepatocellular and obstructive is an oversimplification, because in hepatocellular jaundice there is invariably cholestasis and the clinical problem is whether the cholestasis is intrahepatic or extrahepatic. Jaundice is therefore considered under the following headings:

- Haemolytic jaundice
- Congenital hyperbilirubinaemias
- Cholestatic jaundice.

## Haemolytic jaundice

Increased breakdown of red cells leads to increased production of bilirubin, which usually results in mild jaundice only, as the liver can usually handle the increased bilirubin derived from haemolysis. The unconjugated bilirubin is not water soluble and therefore does not pass into the urine,

117

unlike the conjugated hyperbilirubinaemia of cholestatic jaundice. The urinary urobilinogen is increased. The causes are those of haemolytic anaemia (p. 178), with the clinical features dependent on the cause (e.g. anaemia, splenomegaly, jaundice). Investigations show features of haemolysis (p. 180), with raised serum unconjugated bilirubin and normal alkaline phosphatase and transferases.

## Congenital hyperbilirubinaemia (K&C p. 347)

The most common is Gilbert's syndrome, which affects 2–7% of the population. It is asymptomatic and is usually picked up as an incidental finding of a slightly raised serum bilirubin (17–102 μmol/L) which is caused by an increase in unconjugated bilirubin. Mutations in the gene coding for UDP-glucuronyl transferase lead to reduced enzyme activity and reduced conjugation of bilirubin with glucuronic acid. The diagnosis is based on the findings of unconjugated hyperbilirubinaemia with otherwise normal liver biochemistry, normal full blood count, smear and reticulocyte count (thus excluding haemolysis) and absence of signs of liver disease. No treatment is necessary.

The other congenital abnormalities of bilirubin metabolism (Crigler–Najar, Dubin–Johnson, and Rotor syndromes) are rare.

## Cholestatic jaundice

This can be divided into the following (Table 4.1):

- Intrahepatic cholestasis, caused by hepatocellular swelling in parenchymal liver disease or abnormalities at a cellular level of bile excretion
- Extrahepatic cholestasis resulting from obstruction of bile flow at any point distal to the bile canaliculi.

### Investigations

An outline of the approach to the investigation of jaundice is shown in Figure 4.2.

- Serum liver biochemistry will confirm the jaundice. The AST tends to be high early in the course of hepatitis, with a smaller rise in alkaline phosphatase. Conversely, in extrahepatic obstruction the alkaline

**Table 4.1**
Causes of cholestatic jaundice

**Intrahepatic**
Hepatitis – acute and chronic
Drugs
Cirrhosis
Pregnancy

**Extrahepatic**
Common bile duct stone
Carcinoma of head of pancreas/ampulla/bile duct
Iatrogenic biliary stricture following surgery
Pancreatitis
Sclerosing cholangitis

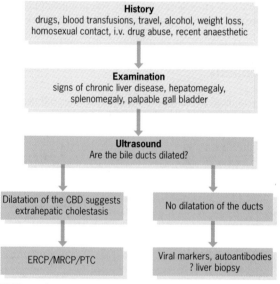

**History**
drugs, blood transfusions, travel, alcohol, weight loss,
homosexual contact, i.v. drug abuse, recent anaesthetic

**Examination**
signs of chronic liver disease, hepatomegaly,
splenomegaly, palpable gall bladder

**Ultrasound**
Are the bile ducts dilated?

Dilatation of the CBD suggests
extrahepatic cholestasis

No dilatation of the ducts

ERCP/MRCP/PTC

Viral markers, autoantibodies
? liver biopsy

ERCP = endoscopic retrograde cholangiopancreatography
MRCP = magnetic resonance cholangiopancreatography
PTC = percutaneous transhepatic cholangiogram

**Fig. 4.2 Approach to the investigation of cholestatic jaundice.** The
order of investigation is influenced by the age of the patient and hence the
likely cause of jaundice. A young person is most likely to have intrinsic liver
disease, e.g. viral hepatitis, and it may be more appropriate to organize
tests to exclude these conditions before proceeding to ultrasound. See
page 163 for clinical features.

119

phosphatase is elevated, with a smaller rise in the AST.

- Ultrasound examination will show dilated bile ducts in extrahepatic cholestasis and identify the level of obstruction.
- Serum viral markers for hepatitis A and hepatitis B may be present. Antibodies to hepatitis C virus develop late in the course of acute infection.
- Other tests. Cholestasis impairs the absorption of fat-soluble vitamins. Malabsorption of vitamin K often results in a prolonged prothrombin time, which is reversed by intravenous administration of vitamin K. Impairment of liver synthetic function in advanced liver disease also results in a prolonged prothrombin time and a low serum albumin. Serum autoantibodies are present in autoimmune liver disease (see later).

## Hepatitis

The pathological features of hepatitis are liver cell necrosis and inflammatory cell infiltration. Clinically the liver may be enlarged and tender, jaundice may be evident, and laboratory evidence of hepatocellular damage is invariably found in the form of elevated serum transferase levels. Hepatitis is divided into acute and chronic types (Table 4.2) on the basis of clinical and pathological criteria. Acute hepatitis is most commonly caused by one of the hepatitis viruses. Usually there is complete resolution of the liver cell damage, with a return to normal structure and function. Occasionally there is progression to massive liver cell necrosis, which may result in death. Chronic hepatitis is defined as sustained inflammatory disease of the liver lasting for more than 6 months.

### Viral hepatitis ND

The most common causes of viral hepatitis are hepatitis A, B and C. Hepatitis D and E are infrequent causes in the UK. Features of these viruses are summarized in Table 4.3. All cases of viral hepatitis must be notified to the appropriate public health authority. This allows contacts to be traced and provides data on disease incidence.

**Table 4.2**
The causes of acute and chronic hepatitis

| Acute | Chronic |
| --- | --- |
| Viruses | Viruses |
| Hepatitis A, B, C, D and E | Hepatitis B, C and D |
| Epstein–Barr virus | |
| Cytomegalovirus | |
| Non-viral infections | Autoimmune hepatitis |
| *Leptospira icterohaemorrhagica* | |
| *Toxoplasma gondii* | |
| *Coxiella burnetii* (Q fever) | |
| Alcohol | Alcohol |
| Drugs | Drugs |
| Anti-TB, e.g. isoniazid | Methyldopa |
| Halogenated anaesthetics | Nitrofurantoin |
| Paracetamol poisoning | |
| Others | Metabolic disorders |
| Pregnancy | Wilson's disease |
| Poisons, e.g. carbon tetrachloride | $\alpha_1$-Antitrypsin deficiency |
| Wilson's disease | |

## Hepatitis A ND (*K&C* p. 351)

### *Epidemiology*

Hepatitis A is the most common type of acute viral hepatitis. It occurs world-wide and affects particularly children and young adults. Spread is mainly faecal–oral and arises from the ingestion of contaminated food (e.g. shellfish, clams) or water. The virus is excreted in the faeces of infected individuals for about 2 weeks before, and 7 days after, the onset of the illness. It is most infectious just before the onset of the jaundice.

### *Clinical features*

Hepatitis A virus (HAV) infection varies from subclinical to fulminant hepatitis. The incubation period averages 30 days after which the illness in symptomatic patients begins with non-specific prodromal symptoms of nausea, vomiting, diarrhoea, malaise, abdominal discomfort and mild fever. After 1 or 2 weeks some patients become jaundiced with dark urine and pale stools and the prodromal symptoms improve. There is moderate hepatomegaly and the

Table 4.3
Some features of the hepatitis viruses

| Feature | A | B | C | D | E |
|---|---|---|---|---|---|
| | | | **Hepatitis** | | |
| **Virus** | RNA | DNA | RNA | RNA | RNA |
| Transmission | Faecal–oral | Parenteral Sexual Vertical | Parenteral | Parenteral | Faecal–oral |
| Incubation | Short (2–3 weeks) | Long (1–5 months) | Long | Intermediate | Short |
| **Chronicity** | No | Yes | Yes | Yes | No |
| **Mortality rate (%) in acute infection** | < 0.5 | < 1 | < 1 | (only with B) | 1–2 (20% in pregnancy) |

spleen is palpable in 10% of cases. Occasionally lympha-denopathy and a skin rash are present. The illness is self-limiting and usually over in 3–6 weeks. Rarely there is fulminant hepatitis (p. 130), coma and death.

### Investigations
- Liver biochemistry shows a raised serum AST and ALT and raised bilirubin when jaundice develops.
- The blood count may show a leucopenia with relative lymphocytosis and a high ESR.
- Serum antibodies to HAV are present, with anti-HAV IgM indicating an acute infection.

### Management
No specific treatment is required. Hospital admission is not usually necessary and avoidance of alcohol advised only when the patient is ill.

### Prophylaxis
Active immunization with an inactivated strain of the virus is recommended for people travelling to areas of high prevalence (Africa, Asia, South America, Eastern Europe and the Middle East), for individuals such as homosexuals who engage in high-risk behaviour, and in patients with chronic liver disease in whom the disease may be more severe. Control of hepatitis also depends on good hygiene. Travellers to high-risk areas should drink only boiled or bottled water and avoid risky foods.

## Hepatitis B ND (K&C p. 353)

### Epidemiology
Hepatitis B virus (HBV) is present world-wide and is particu-larly prevalent in parts of Africa, the Middle and Far East. It is spread through the intravenous route (infected blood products, contaminated needles of intravenous drug abusers and tattooists) and through sexual intercourse, particularly in male homosexuals. Vertical transmission from mother to child during parturition is the most common means of trans-mission world-wide. Hepatitis B is becoming rare in countries such as Taiwan where universal vaccination is per-formed. This approach has not been adopted in the UK.

## Viral structure

The whole virus is the Dane particle (Fig. 4.3) which consists of an inner core and an outer surface coat, the hepatitis B surface antigen (HBsAg). The inner core contains double-stranded DNA, DNA polymerase/reverse transcriptase, the core antigen (HBcAg) and e antigen (HBeAg). HBeAg is produced in excess during active viral replication, and its detection in the serum indicates a high degree of infectivity. Mutations in all regions of the HBV genome have been

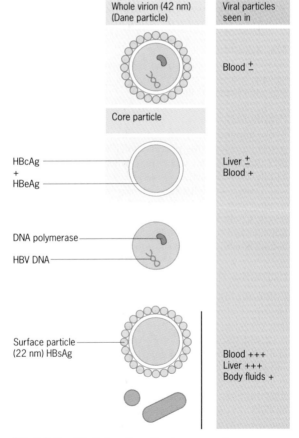

| | Whole virion (42 nm) (Dane particle) | Viral particles seen in |
| --- | --- | --- |
| | | Blood ± |
| | Core particle | |
| HBcAg + HBeAg | | Liver ± Blood + |
| DNA polymerase HBV DNA | | |
| Surface particle (22 nm) HBsAg | | Blood +++ Liver +++ Body fluids + |

**Fig. 4.3 Hepatitis B virus: the antigenic components.**

found in patients with chronic HBV infection. HBV mutations can potentially modulate the severity of liver disease by altering the level of HBV replication or the expression of immunogenic epitopes (the site against which T cells respond). Some variants such as that produced by the precore stop codon mutation, do not make HBeAg but the virus can continue to replicate with the presence of HBV DNA in the serum and elevated liver enzymes. HBV DNA must therefore always be measured in an HbsAg-positive patient to determine the level of viral replication.

## Acute infection

Acute infection with HBV may be asymptomatic or produce symptoms and signs similar to those seen in hepatitis A.

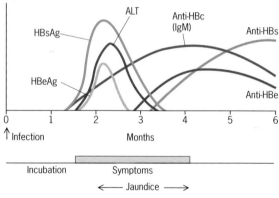

- **HBsAg**
    is found in acute hepatitis and persists in chronic carriers
- **HBsAg with HBeAg**
    is present in acute hepatitis
    its presence in chronic HBV infection is correlated with increased infectivity and development of chronic liver disease
- **HBsAg with anti-HBe**
    occurs in recovery from acute infection. In chronic infection it indicates decreased infectivity
- **Anti-HBs appears late and indicates immunity**
- **HBV DNA suggests continued viral replication**

**Fig. 4.4** Time course of the events and serological changes seen following infection with hepatitis B virus.

Occasionally it is associated with a rash or polyarthritis affecting the small joints. The sequence of events following acute infection is depicted in Figure 4.4.

Investigation is generally the same as for hepatitis A. The viral markers for HBV are shown in Figure 4.4. If HBsAg is present, a full viral profile is performed. There is no specific therapy for *acute* HBV infection and management is supportive.

Most patients recover completely. This is marked by the disappearance of HBsAg from the serum, the development of antibodies to surface antigen (anti-HBs) and immunity to subsequent infection (Fig. 4.4). One per cent of patients with acute hepatitis develop fulminant liver failure.

A minority of patients do not clear HBsAg from the serum and become chronic carriers. The risk of developing chronic HBV infection is inversely related to age at the time of infection. Ninety per cent of infants infected at birth will become chronically infected with HBV, but only about 5% of adults (Fig. 4.5).

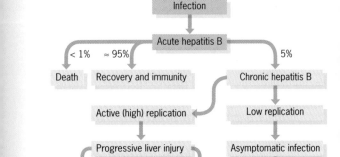

**Fig. 4.5 The natural history of hepatitis B infection in adults.**

## *Chronic carriers*

The persistence of HBsAg in the serum for more than 6 months after acute infection defines the carrier status. Carriers who, in addition, have HBeAg or viral DNA in the serum (i.e. have active viral replication) are highly infectious and are at greatest risk of developing chronic hepatitis (see below) and cirrhosis, with the attendant increased risk of hepatocellular carcinoma. These patients should be considered for treatment (see below). Patients with only HBsAg (low replication) are usually asymptomatic with normal liver biochemistry, and are of relatively low infective risk. Treatment is not indicated for this group of patients but they should be followed up since some will develop progressive disease and require treatment.

## *Chronic hepatitis* (*K&C* p. 360)

Approximately 3% of patients with acute viral hepatitis B progress to chronic hepatitis. The condition may be asymptomatic, or present with established liver disease and the signs of chronic liver disease on physical examination (see Fig. 4.6). Serum liver biochemistry, particularly the transferases, is usually abnormal. Liver biopsy and histological examination will show the severity of the disease varying from mild inflammatory changes to established cirrhosis.

## *Treatment of chronic hepatitis B*

Treatment is indicated for patients with HBsAg and HBV DNA in the serum with abnormal serum aminotransferases and chronic hepatitis on liver biopsy. Most of these patients will also have HBeAg in the serum unless they have a mutant virus (see above). The aim of treatment is to eliminate HBeAg and HBV DNA from the serum and reduce inflammatory necrosis of the hepatocyte; this is accomplished in 25–40% of patients. Treatment is with alpha-interferon (IFN-α) and/or lamivudine, both of which inhibit HBV replication. IFN-α is administered subcutaneously (by the patient) three times weekly for 4–6 months. It is expensive and associated with unpleasant side-effects (malaise, depression, bone marrow suppression). Pegylated IFN (p. 225) given once weekly is replacing IFN-α. Lamivudine is given by mouth.

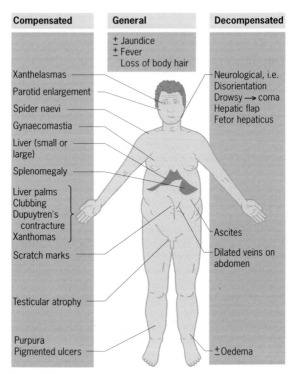

| Compensated | General | Decompensated |
| --- | --- | --- |

General:
± Jaundice
± Fever
Loss of body hair

Compensated:
Xanthelasmas
Parotid enlargement
Spider naevi
Gynaecomastia
Liver (small or large)
Splenomegaly
Liver palms
Clubbing
Dupuytren's contracture
Xanthomas
Scratch marks
Testicular atrophy
Purpura
Pigmented ulcers

Decompensated:
Neurological, i.e. Disorientation
Drowsy → coma
Hepatic flap
Fetor hepaticus
Ascites
Dilated veins on abdomen
± Oedema

**Fig. 4.6 Physical signs in chronic liver disease.**

## Prophylaxis (K&C p. 355)

The avoidance of high-risk factors (needle sharing, prostitutes and multiple male homosexual partners) and counselling patients who are potentially infective are important aspects of prevention. Active immunization with a recombinant yeast vaccine is universal in most developed countries. In the UK it is only recommended for those at increased risk, e.g. healthcare workers, homosexuals, intravenous drug abusers and haemodialysis patients. Combined prophylaxis (i.e. active immunization and passive immunization with specific antihepatitis B immunoglobulin) is given to non-immune individuals after high-risk exposure, e.g. a needle-stick injury from a carrier, newborn babies of HBsAg-positive mothers and HBV-negative sexual partners of HBsAg-positive patients.

## Hepatitis D (delta or δ agent) ND (*K&C* p. 356 & p. 362)

Hepatitis D virus is an incomplete RNA virus enclosed in a shell of HBsAg. It is unable to replicate on its own, but is activated by the presence of HBV. It can affect all risk groups for HBV infection, but is seen particularly in intravenous drug abusers. HDV infection can occur as a co-infection with HBV or as a superinfection in an already HBsAg-positive patient, and thus presents as an illness indistinguishable from acute HBV infection or as a flare-up of previously quiescent chronic HBV infection. Diagnosis is by finding IgM anti-D in the serum.

## Hepatitis C ND (*K&C* p. 356)

### Epidemiology

Hepatitis C virus (HCV) is an RNA virus. It is present world-wide, but is more common in southern Europe, Africa and Egypt. The virus is transmitted by blood and blood products. In about 20% of patients the exact mode of infection is not known.

129

### Clinical features

Acute infection is usually mild, with jaundice developing in less than 10% of cases. Most patients infected with HCV go on to develop chronic liver disease and will not be diagnosed until they present, years later, with elevated serum aminotransferase levels found on routine biochemistry (e.g. at health checks) or with symptoms and signs of chronic liver disease and cirrhosis. Patients with cirrhosis secondary to chronic HCV are at increased risk for the development of hepatocellular carcinoma. Extrahepatic manifestations of chronic HCV infection include essential mixed cryoglobulinaemia, membranoproliferative glomerulonephritis and lichen planus.

### Diagnosis

This is made by finding HCV antibody in the serum. Antibodies may take 6 weeks to appear after acute infection, and thus an early negative result does not exclude acute HCV infection. Patients with antibodies to hepatitis C should undergo further tests to look for the presence of HCV RNA in the serum. A positive result indicates ongoing infection, and a liver biopsy is usually then performed to assess the histological activity of disease and to detect the presence or absence of fibrosis and cirrhosis.

### Management (K&C p. 362)

Combination treatment with IFN-$\alpha$ (see HBV treatment) and ribavirin, both of which inhibit viral replication, is indicated for 6–12 months (depending on viral RNA load and genotype) in patients who have HCV RNA in the serum with raised serum aminotransferases and chronic hepatitis on liver biopsy. The aim of treatment is to eliminate HCV RNA from the serum and decrease serum aminotransferases in order to stop the progression of active liver disease and prevent the development of hepatocellular carcinoma. Success of treatment depends on the genotype and the viral load. Overall, a sustained loss of HCV RNA from the serum is achieved in 30–40% of treated patients. The prognosis is adversely affected by alcohol consumption, which should be discouraged.

## Hepatitis E ND

This is due to an RNA virus which causes enteral (epidemic or waterborne) hepatitis, particularly in developing countries. There is no chronic carrier state and it does not progress to chronic liver disease, but the mortality rate from fulminant hepatic failure is about 1–2%, rising to 20% in pregnant women.

## Fulminant hepatic failure (K&C p. 357)

Fulminant hepatic failure is defined as hepatic failure with encephalopathy developing in less than 2 weeks in a patient with a previously normal liver, or in patients with an acute exacerbation of underlying liver disease. It is an infrequent complication of acute hepatitis (from any cause) and occurs as a result of massive liver cell necrosis. In the UK, viral hepatitis and paracetamol overdose are the most common causes. Presentation is with hepatic encephalopathy of

**Table 4.4**
Grading of hepatic encephalopathy

| | |
|---|---|
| Grade I | Daytime somnolence, asterixis (flapping tremor of outstretched hands) |
| Grade II | Confusion, disorientation, agitation and impaired coordination |
| Grade III | Increasing drowsiness, stupor, no communication possible |
| Grade IV | Coma, increased rigidity, extensor plantar response |

varying severity (Table 4.4), accompanied by severe jaundice and a marked coagulopathy. The complications include cerebral oedema, hypoglycaemia, severe bacterial and fungal infections, hypotension and renal failure (hepatorenal syndrome). Fulminant hepatic failure is managed with supportive treatment in a specialist liver unit. Emergency liver transplantation has become a useful treatment for the very severe cases (grade IV encephalopathy), of which 80% might otherwise die.

13T

## Autoimmune hepatitis (K&C p. 362)

Autoimmune hepatitis is usually a progressive liver disease which is often associated with other autoimmune diseases, e.g. pernicious anaemia, thyroiditis. It is most common in young and middle-aged women but can occur in any age in either sex.

### Aetiology

The aetiology is unknown but there are many immunological abnormalities present. These include hypergammaglobulinaemia, with the most pronounced rise in IgG levels, circulating antibodies such as nuclear, smooth muscle and liver/kidney microsomal antibodies, and an increased helper/suppressor T cell ratio.

### Clinical features

The onset is often insidious, with anorexia, malaise, nausea and fatigue. Twenty-five per cent present as an acute hepatitis with rapidly progressive liver disease. The signs of chronic liver disease are often present, with palmar erythema, spider naevae, hepatosplenomegaly and jaundice. Features of other autoimmune diseases may be present.

### Investigations

Circulating autoantibodies (antinuclear and anti-smooth muscle antibodies) are the hallmarks of the disease. There is hypergammaglobulinaemia (particularly IgG), and the serum bilirubin and aminotransferases are elevated. Liver biopsy will show the non-specific changes of chronic hepatitis, with interface hepatitis and often cirrhosis.

### Treatment

Prednisolone 30 mg daily is given for 2–3 weeks. A subsequent reduction in the dose depends on clinical response, but maintenance doses of 10–15 mg are usually required. Azathioprine is used as a steroid-sparing agent and is usually continued lifelong.

### Prognosis

In treated patients the 5-year survival rate is 90%.

## Cirrhosis (K&C p. 363)

Cirrhosis is a histological diagnosis. It is a diffuse process that results from necrosis of liver cells followed by fibrosis and nodule formation. The end result is impairment of liver cell function and gross distortion of the liver architecture, leading to portal hypertension.

### Aetiology

The causes of cirrhosis are shown in Table 4.5. Alcohol is the most common cause in the western world, but viral hepatitis is the most common cause world-wide.

### Pathology

Histologically two types of cirrhosis have been described: micronodular and macronodular.

- Micronodular cirrhosis is characterized by uniform, small nodules up to 3 mm in diameter. This type is often caused by alcohol damage.

| **Table 4.5** |
|---|
| Causes of cirrhosis |

**Common**
Alcohol
Chronic hepatitis B
Chronic hepatitis C

**Others**
Haemochromatosis
Biliary cirrhosis: primary and secondary
Autoimmune hepatitis
Cystic fibrosis
Budd–Chiari syndrome
Wilson's disease
Drugs, e.g. methotrexate
$\alpha_1$-Antitrypsin deficiency
Fatty liver

- In macronodular cirrhosis large nodules up to several centimetres in diameter are present. This type is often seen following hepatitis B infection.
- There is also a mixed picture, with both small and large nodules.

### Clinical features

These are secondary to portal hypertension and liver cell failure (Fig. 4.6). Cirrhosis with the complications of encephalopathy, ascites or variceal haemorrhage is designated decompensated cirrhosis. Cirrhosis without any of these complications is termed compensated cirrhosis.

### Investigations

These are performed to identify the aetiology and assess the severity of liver disease.

#### Severity

- Liver biochemistry may be normal. In most cases there is at least a slight elevation of the serum alkaline phosphatase and aminotransferase.
- Liver function. Serum albumin and prothrombin time are the best indicators of liver function, both reflecting reduced hepatic synthesis.

- Serum electrolytes. A low sodium concentration indicates severe liver disease secondary to either impaired free water clearance or excess diuretic therapy.
- Serum α-fetoprotein (AFP). This is usually undetectable after fetal life, but raised levels may be found in chronic liver disease. A very high level (> 400 ng/mL) suggests the complication of hepatocellular carcinoma.

## Aetiology

This is determined by the following:

- Hepatitis B and C serology
- Serum autoantibodies and immunoglobulins
- Miscellaneous: serum iron, total iron-binding capacity and ferritin should be measured to exclude haemochromatosis. Serum copper, caeruloplasmin and $\alpha_1$-antitrypsin should be measured in young cirrhotic individuals to exclude Wilson's disease and $\alpha_1$-antitrypsin deficiency respectively.

## Further investigations

A liver biopsy is performed to confirm the severity and type of liver disease. Oesophageal varices are sought with endoscopy. An ultrasound is useful for detection of hepatocellular carcinoma, and to assess the patency of the portal vein.

## Management

Cirrhosis is irreversible and frequently progresses. Management is that of the complications seen in decompensated cirrhosis as they arise. Correcting the underlying cause, e.g. venesection for haemochromatosis, abstinence from alcohol for alcoholic cirrhosis, may halt the progression of liver disease. Liver transplantation should be considered in patients with end-stage cirrhosis.

## Prognosis

This is very variable and depends on the aetiology and the presence of complications. The severity and prognosis of

---

**Table 4.6**
Complications of cirrhosis

Portal hypertension and variceal haemorrhage
Ascites
Portosystemic encephalopathy
Acute renal failure
Hepatocellular carcinoma (HCC)

---

liver disease can be graded according to five variables: encephalopathy, ascites, prothrombin time, serum bilirubin and albumin (Child's grading, or modifications thereof). Overall the 5-year survival rate is approximately 50%.

## Complications
The complications of cirrhosis are shown in Table 4.6.

## Portal hypertension (K&C p. 367)
The portal vein carries blood from the gut and spleen to the liver and accounts for 85% of hepatic vascular inflow (15% is via the hepatic artery). The inflow of portal blood to the liver can be partially or completely obstructed at a number of sites, leading to high pressure proximal to the obstruction and the diversion of blood into portosystemic collaterals. The most important site for collateral formation is at the gastro-oesophageal junction (varices), where they are superficial and liable to rupture, causing massive gastrointestinal haemorrhage.

The main sites of obstruction are:

- Prehepatic, caused by blockage of the portal vein before the liver
- Intrahepatic, resulting from distortion of the liver architecture
- Posthepatic, as a result of obstruction of the hepatic veins.

## Aetiology
The causes of portal hypertension are outlined in Table 4.7. In the UK 90% of cases are caused by cirrhosis.

**Table 4.7**
Causes of portal hypertension

| Prehepatic | Portal vein thrombosis |
|---|---|
| Intrahepatic | Cirrhosis<br>Alcoholic hepatitis<br>Idiopathic non-cirrhotic portal hypertension<br>Schistosomiasis |
| Posthepatic | Budd–Chiari syndrome<br>Veno-occlusive disease<br>Right heart failure – rare<br>Constrictive pericarditis |

## Clinical features

The characteristic clinical manifestations of portal hypertension are:

- Gastrointestinal bleeding from oesophageal or less commonly gastric varices
- Ascites
- Hepatic encephalopathy.

Only 30% of patients with varices ever bleed from them, and bleeding is most common in those with large varices. Bleeding is often massive and mortality is as high as 50%.

## Management

The general management of GI bleeding is discussed on page 72.

**Acute bleeding** Patients should be resuscitated and undergo urgent gastroscopy to confirm the diagnosis and exclude bleeding from other sites.

- Endoscopic therapy is the treatment of choice for active variceal haemorrhage and will stop bleeding in 80% of cases. Two forms are available: sclerotherapy or variceal band ligation. Sclerotherapy involves injection of a sclerosant solution (e.g. ethanolamine) into the varices. Variceal band ligation is similar to haemorrhoidal banding and involves placing small elastic bands around the varices.
- Pharmacological treatment is used as a holding measure if sclerotherapy or banding is not available or

unsuccessful. The alternatives are intravenous terlipressin (1–2 mg bolus 6-hourly, contraindicated in patients with ischaemic heart disease) or octreotide infusion (50 µg/h), both of which restrict portal inflow by splanchnic arterial constriction.

- Balloon tamponade with a Sengstaken–Blakemore tube is used if bleeding continues (p. 749). It can have serious complications, such as aspiration pneumonia, oesophageal rupture and mucosal ulceration. To reduce complications, the airway should be protected, and the tube left in situ for no longer than 12 hours.

- TIPS (transjugular intrahepatic portosystemic shunting) is used if the above measures fail. A metal stent is passed over a guidewire in the internal jugular vein. The stent is then pushed into the liver substance, under radiological guidance, to form a shunt between the portal and hepatic veins, thus lowering portal pressure.

- Surgery (oesophageal transection and ligation of varices) is occasionally necessary if bleeding continues in spite of all the above measures.

- Additional treatment. Patients require high dependency/ITU nursing. Bacterial infection is common after upper gastrointestinal bleeding in cirrhotic patients and all patients should have antibiotic prophylaxis with ciprofloxacin. Lactulose should be given to prevent portosystemic encephalopathy and sucralfate to reduce oesophageal ulceration, a complication of endoscopic therapy.

**Prophylaxis** Following an episode of variceal bleeding there is a high risk of recurrence (60–80% over a 2-year period), and therefore treatment is given to prevent further bleeds (secondary prophylaxis). The main options are:

- Oral propranolol, which decreases portal pressure, but some patients are intolerant of treatment because of side-effects. Propranolol is also given to patients with varices who have never bled (primary prophylaxis).

- Repeated courses (every 1–2 weeks) of endoscopic therapy until the varices are obliterated; banding is preferred to sclerotherapy.

- TIPS or occasionally a surgical portosystemic shunt (portal vein to vena cava – or splenorenal) which is performed if endoscopic or medical therapy fails. Liver transplantation should always be considered when there is poor liver function.

## Ascites (K&C p. 370)

This is the presence of fluid in the peritoneal cavity and is a common complication of cirrhosis of the liver.

### Aetiology

In cirrhosis, peripheral arterial vasodilatation (mediated by nitric oxide and other vasodilators) leads to a reduction in effective blood volume, with activation of the sympathetic nervous system and renin–angiotensin system, thus promoting renal salt and water retention. The formation of oedema is encouraged by hypoalbuminaemia and mainly localized to the peritoneal cavity as a result of the portal hypertension.

### Clinical features

There is fullness in the flanks, with shifting dullness. Tense ascites is uncomfortable and may produce respiratory distress. A pleural effusion (usually right-sided) and peripheral oedema may be present.

### Investigations

A diagnostic aspiration (paracentesis, p. 748) of 10–20 ml of fluid should be carried out in all patients and the following performed:

- Cell count. A neutrophil count > 250 cells/mm$^3$ indicates underlying (usually spontaneous) bacterial peritonitis
- Gram stain and culture for bacteria and acid-fast bacilli
- Protein. An ascitic protein of 11 g/L or more below the serum albumin level suggests a transudate (exudate < 11 g/L)
- Cytology for malignant cells
- Amylase to exclude pancreatic ascites.

The causes of ascites are listed in Table 4.8; the commonest cause is cirrhosis.

**Table 4.8**
Causes of ascites

| Transudate | Exudate |
| --- | --- |
| Cirrhosis | Malignancy |
| Constrictive pericarditis | Infection, e.g. pyogenic, tuberculous |
| Cardiac failure | Pancreatitis |
| Hypoalbuminaemia, | Budd–Chiari syndrome |
| e.g. nephrotic syndrome | Myxoedema |
| Meig's syndrome* | Lymphatic obstruction |
| | (chylous ascites) |

* Meig's syndrome is the combination of an ovarian tumour, ascites and hydrothorax

## Management
Most patients with ascites secondary to cirrhosis are managed with diuretics.

**Diuretics** The management of ascites resulting from cirrhosis is based on a stepwise approach, starting with dietary sodium restriction (40 mmol/day) and spironolactone 100 mg daily, increasing gradually to 500 mg daily if necessary. Furosemide (frusemide) 20–40 mg daily is added if the response is poor. The rate of fluid loss is best assessed by changes in bodyweight. The aim of diuretic therapy is to produce weight loss of about 0.5 kg/day, because the maximum rate of transfer of fluid from the ascitic to the vascular compartment is only about 700 mL/day. Too rapid a diuresis causes volume depletion and hypokalaemia, and precipitates encephalopathy. In combination with dietary sodium restriction this medical approach is effective in over 90% of patients.

**Paracentesis** This is used in patients with tense ascites or who are resistant to standard medical therapy. All the ascites can be removed over several hours. There is therefore rapid symptom relief and reduced hospital stay compared to treatment with diuretics. The major danger of this approach is the production of hypovolaemia because the ascites reaccumulates at the expense of the circulating volume. This is largely overcome by the intravenous infusion of albumin administered immediately after para-centesis (p. 749).

*Transjugular intrahepatic portosystemic shunt* (TIPS, p. 137) is occasionally used for resistant ascites.

## Complications

Spontaneous bacterial peritonitis occurs in 8% of cirrhotic patients with ascites and has a mortality rate of 25%. The most common infecting organism is *Escherichia coli*. Clinical features may be minimal, but include abdominal pain and fever. Diagnosis is made on the ascitic fluid white cell count, and Gram stain and culture (p. 138). Empirical therapy, e.g. intravenous ceftazidine or cefotaxime, should be started before the results of culture are available. Spontaneous bacterial peritonitis frequently recurs and indicates a poor prognosis; it is an indication for liver trans-plantation.

## Portosystemic encephalopathy (K&C p. 372)

The term 'portosystemic encephalopathy' (PSE) refers to a chronic neuropsychiatric syndrome which occurs with advanced hepatocellular disease, either chronic (cirrhosis) or acute (fulminant hepatic failure). It is also seen in patients following TIPS.

### Pathophysiology

The mechanisms are unclear but are believed to involve 'toxic' substances, normally detoxified by the liver, bypass-ing the liver via the collaterals and gaining access to the brain. A putative toxin is ammonia produced from the breakdown of dietary protein by gut bacteria. In chronic liver disease there is an acute-on-chronic course, with acute episodes precipitated by a number of possible factors (Table 4.9).

### Clinical features

The earliest features are lethargy, mild confusion, anorexia and a reversal of the sleep pattern, with the patient sleep-ing during the day and restless at night. Later there is dis-orientation, a decreased conscious level and eventually coma (see Table 4.4). The signs are fetor hepaticus (a sweet

**Table 4.9**
Factors precipitating portosystemic encephalopathy

Gastrointestinal haemorrhage (i.e. a high protein load)
Infection
Fluid and electrolyte disturbance (spontaneous or diuretic-induced)
Sedative drugs, e.g. opiates, diazepam
Development of a hepatoma
Portosystemic shunt operations and TIPS
Constipation
High dietary protein

smell to the breath), a flapping tremor of the outstretched hand (asterixis), inability to draw a five-pointed star (constructional apraxia) and a prolonged trail-making test (the ability to join numbers and letters within a certain time). Serial attempts are easily compared and used to monitor patient progress.

## Differential diagnosis

None of the manifestations of hepatic encephalopathy are specific to this disorder. Alternative diagnoses such as other metabolic or toxic encephalopathies or intracranial mass lesions may present similarly and should be considered.

## Investigations

The diagnosis is clinical. An EEG (showing δ waves) and visual evoked potentials may aid diagnosis in difficult cases.

## Management

The aims of management are to identify and treat any precipitating factors (Table 4.9) and to minimize the absorption of nitrogenous material, particularly ammonia, from the gut. This is achieved by the following:

- Laxatives. Oral lactulose (10–30 mL three times daily) is an osmotic purgative that reduces colonic pH and increases transit. It may be given via a nasogastric tube if the patient is comatose. The dose should be titrated to result in 2–4 soft stools daily.
- Antibiotics are given to reduce the number of bowel organisms and hence production of ammonia.

141

Rifaximin is mainly unabsorbed and well tolerated. Oral metronidazole (200 mg four times daily) is also used.
- Maintenance of nutrition with a high-carbohydrate, low-protein diet.

Once the patient recovers the protein content of the diet may be increased and lactulose continued, to produce soft stools but not diarrhoea.

### Prognosis
The prognosis is that of the underlying liver disease.

## Types of cirrhosis

## Alcoholic
This is discussed in the section on alcoholic liver disease (p. 148).

## Primary biliary cirrhosis (K&C p. 373)
Primary biliary cirrhosis (PBC) is a chronic disorder in which there is progressive destruction of intrahepatic bile ducts causing cholestasis, eventually leading to cirrhosis.

### Epidemiology
It affects predominantly women in the age range 40–50 years.

### Aetiology
The cause of PBC is unknown but most data suggest that it is due to an inherited abnormality of immunoregulation, leading to immune-mediated damage to bile duct epithelial cells. It is thought that disease expression results from an environmental trigger, possibly infective, in a genetically susceptible individual. Antimitochondrial antibodies (AMAs) are present in almost all (> 95%) patients, but their role in the pathogenesis of this disorder is unclear.

### Clinical features
Pruritus, with or without jaundice, is the single most common presenting complaint. In advanced disease there

is, in addition, hepatosplenomegaly and xanthelasma (PBC is a cause of secondary hypercholesterolaemia). Asymptomatic patients may be discovered on routine examination or screening to have hepatomegaly, a raised serum alkaline phosphatase or autoantibodies. Patients with advanced disease may have steatorrhoea and mal-absorption of fat-soluble vitamins owing to decreased biliary secretion of bile acids and the resulting low concentrations of bile acids in the small intestine. Autoimmune disorders, e.g. Sjögren's syndrome, scleroderma and rheumatoid arthritis, occur with increased frequency.

## Investigations
- Liver biochemistry may show only a raised serum alkaline phosphatase, often very high (> 1000 U/L).
- Serum AMAs are found in more than 95% of patients and a titre of 1:160 or greater makes the diagnosis very likely. M2 antibody is specific. Other non-specific antibodies, e.g. antinuclear factor, may also be present.
- Serum IgM may be very high.
- Liver biopsy shows loss of bile ducts, lymphocyte infiltration of the portal tracts, granuloma formation and, at a later stage, fibrosis and eventually cirrhosis.
- An ultrasound scan is sometimes performed in the jaundiced patient to exclude extrahepatic biliary obstruction.

143

## Management
Ursodeoxycholic acid (ursodiol, 10–15 mg/kg by mouth) is a naturally occurring dihydroxy bile acid. It improves biochemistry, though it is unclear whether prognosis is altered. The mechanism of benefit of ursodiol in PBC is incompletely understood. Pruritus may be helped by colestyramine, and malabsorption of fat-soluble vitamins (A, D, K) is treated by supplementation. Liver transplantation is indicated for patients with advanced disease (bilirubin > 100 μmol/L).

## Prognosis
Asymptomatic patients may show a near-normal life expectancy. In symptomatic patients with jaundice there is a steady downhill course, with death in approximately 5 years without transplantation.

# Secondary biliary cirrhosis

Cirrhosis can result from prolonged (for months) large duct biliary obstruction. Causes include bile duct strictures, common bile duct stones and sclerosing cholangitis. Ultrasonography examination followed by MRCP is performed to outline the ducts. ERCP or PTC may then be necessary to treat the cause, e.g. stone removal.

# Hereditary haemochromatosis (K&C p. 375)

Hereditary haemochromatosis (HH) is an inherited disease characterized by excess iron deposition in various organs, leading to eventual fibrosis and functional organ failure. It is one of the most common inherited diseases in those of European descent, occurring in about 1 in 400 people, with approximately 10% of the population being carriers.

## Aetiology

Inappropriate and excessive iron absorption from the small bowel leads to overload, with deposition in, and damage to, the cells of the liver, heart, pancreas and pituitary gland. It is inherited as an autosomal recessive, with only homozygotes manifesting the clinical features of the disease. HH is due to a mutation in the gene *HFE* on the short arm of chromosome 6. The normal HFE protein is expressed in the small intestine and is thought to play a role in the regulation of iron absorption. HLA-A3, -B7 and -B14 occur with increased frequency compared to the general population.

## Clinical features

Most patients are currently diagnosed when elevated serum iron or ferritin levels are noted on routine biochemistry or screening is performed because a relative is diagnosed with HH. Presentation may also be with symptoms and signs of liver disease. Other features include gonadal atrophy and loss of libido secondary to pituitary dysfunction. There may be a cardiomyopathy and arthritis resulting from calcium pyrophosphate deposition in both large and small joints. There is a reduced incidence of overt disease in women, presumably because of iron lost in blood during menstruation.

The classic triad of bronze skin pigmentation (caused by melanin deposition), hepatomegaly and diabetes mellitus is only present in cases of gross iron overload.

## Investigations

- Serum liver biochemistry is often normal even with cirrhosis.
- Serum iron is elevated and total iron-binding capacity (TIBC) reduced. The transferrin saturation (serum iron/TIBC) is > 60%, normally < 33%.
- Serum ferritin reflects iron stores and is usually greatly elevated (often > 500 µg/L).
- Genotyping (by PCR reaction using whole blood samples) for mutation analysis of the *HFE* gene is performed in patients with elevated ferritin and transferrin saturation.
- Liver biopsy to document the degree of fibrosis is performed in patients who are likely to have significant hepatic injury or if the diagnosis is in doubt. Other patients with abnormal iron studies and mutations of the *HFE* gene may be treated by phlebotomy without the need for biopsy.

Causes of secondary iron overload, such as multiple transfusions, must be excluded. In addition, in alcoholic liver disease hepatic iron stores may increase. The precise reason is unknown, but the hepatic iron concentration does not reach the very high levels seen in haemochromatosis.

## Management

The aim of treatment is to remove excess tissue iron and render the patient iron deficient while maintaining a haemoglobin of greater than 11 g/dL. This is best achieved by venesection: 500 mL of blood are removed twice-weekly, and this may need to be continued for up to 2 years. Three or four venesections per year are then required to prevent the reaccumulation of iron.

Genotyping to detect *HFE* mutations and iron studies should be performed on first-degree relatives of affected individuals.

## Prognosis

The major complication is the development of hepato-cellular carcinoma in patients with cirrhosis. This can be prevented by venesection before cirrhosis develops, and life expectancy is then much the same as for the normal population.

# Wilson's disease (hepatolenticular degeneration) (K&C p. 376)

This is a rare, recessively inherited disorder in which there is failure of biliary excretion of copper, resulting in accumulation of copper and deposition in the liver, basal ganglia of the brain and the cornea. Although this is a rare disease it is potentially treatable and therefore all young patients with liver disease must be screened for this condition.

## Clinical features

Children usually present with hepatic problems ranging from fulminant hepatic failure to cirrhosis. Young adults have more neurological problems, which start with a mild tremor and speech problems and progress to involuntary movements and eventual dementia. A specific sign is the Kayser–Fleisher ring, which is caused by copper deposition in the cornea. It appears as a greenish-brown pigment at the periphery of the cornea, best seen with a slit-lamp. Additional features are haemolytic anaemia and renal tubular defects.

## Investigations

The diagnosis is usually made by demonstrating the following:

- Total serum copper and caeruloplasmin (the copper-carrying protein) are usually low but can be normal
- Urinary copper is usually increased on a 24-hour collection
- Increased hepatic copper concentration in a liver biopsy specimen.

## Management

Lifelong treatment with penicillamine is effective in chelating copper, which is then excreted in the urine. Liver transplantation may be offered to those with end-stage liver disease. First-degree relatives are screened by slit-lamp examination and serum caeruloplasmin measurements. Asymptomatic homozygotes should be treated.

## $\alpha_1$-Antitrypsin deficiency (K&C p. 377)

This is a rare cause of cirrhosis. Mutations in the $\alpha_1$-antitrypsin ($\alpha_1$-AT) gene on chromosome 14 lead to reduced production of $\alpha_1$-AT which normally inhibits the proteolytic enzyme elastase. The genetic variants of $\alpha_1$-AT are characterized by their electrophoretic mobilities as medium (M), slow (S) or very slow (Z). The normal genotype is PiMM, the homozygote for Z is PiZZ and the heterozygotes are PiMZ and PiSZ. S and Z variants are caused by single amino acid substitutions in the polypeptide chain that favours the formation of polymers which are retained within hepatocytes as inclusion bodies leading to hepatocellular damage. In the lung, deficiency of $\alpha_1$-AT leads to proteolytic lung damage and predisposes to emphysema.

147

### Clinical features

The majority of patients with clinical disease are homozygous with a PiZZ phenotype. They have very low circulating levels of $\alpha_1$-AT, associated with chronic liver disease and pulmonary emphysema (especially in smokers). The risk of liver disease is much smaller in heterozygotes, e.g. PiSZ or PiMZ.

### Investigations

The serum $\alpha_1$-AT is low. Liver biopsy demonstrates cirrhosis and $\alpha_1$-AT-containing globules in the hepatocytes.

### Management

There is no specific treatment. Patients should be advised to stop smoking.

# Alcohol and the liver (K&C p. 378)

Alcohol is the most common cause of chronic liver disease in the western world. Alcoholic liver disease occurs more commonly in men, usually in the fourth and fifth decades, although subjects can present in their 20s with advanced disease. Although alcohol acts as a hepatotoxin, the exact mechanism leading to hepatitis and cirrhosis is unknown. As only 10–20% of people who drink excessively develop cirrhosis, genetic predisposition and immunological mechanisms have been proposed.

There are three major pathological lesions and clinical illnesses associated with excessive alcohol intake: fatty liver, alcoholic hepatitis and cirrhosis.

## Fatty liver

This is the most common biopsy finding in alcoholic individuals. Metabolism of alcohol within the liver produces fat, which accumulates within the hepatocyte (steatosis). Symptoms are usually absent, and on examination there may be hepatomegaly. Laboratory tests are often normal, although an elevated mean corpuscular volume (MCV) often indicates heavy drinking. The $\gamma$-GT level is usually elevated. The fat disappears on cessation of alcohol intake but with continued drinking may progress to fibrosis and cirrhosis. Fat deposition is also seen in obesity, diabetes, hyperlipidaemia, and starvation when it is referred to as non-alcoholic fatty liver disease (NAFLD).

## Alcoholic hepatitis

There is necrosis of the liver cells and infiltration of polymorphonuclear leucocytes, with accumulation of dense cytoplasmic material called a Mallory body in the hepatocytes. It may progress to cirrhosis, particularly with continued alcohol consumption. Presentation encompasses a broad spectrum of patients, from those who are asymptomatic to those who are very ill with hepatic failure. Investigations show a leucocytosis with elevated bilirubin and transferases. The albumin may be low and prothrombin time prolonged. Treatment is supportive and adequate nutritional intake must be maintained. Corticosteroids are of benefit in severe disease.

## Alcoholic cirrhosis

This represents the final stage of liver disease from alcohol abuse. There is destruction and fibrosis, with regenerating nodules producing a classic micronodular cirrhosis. Patients may be asymptomatic, although they often present with one of the complications of cirrhosis and there are usually signs of chronic liver disease. Investigation is as for cirrhosis in general. Management is directed at the complications of cirrhosis, and patients are advised to stop drinking for life. Abstinence from alcohol improves the 5-year survival rate.

## Liver transplantation (K&C p. 378)

This is now an established treatment for end-stage chronic liver disease and, in some circumstances, for acute hepatic failure. Careful selection of patients is crucial. Psychological assessment and education of patients and their families is essential before transplantation. In adults primary biliary cirrhosis is the most common indication and, in these patients where the natural history is well defined, transplantation is offered when the serum bilirubin reaches 100 μmol/L. Absolute contraindications to transplantation are active sepsis outside the liver and biliary tree, HIV positivity and metastatic malignancy. With rare exceptions, patients over 65 years are not transplanted. Graft rejection is reduced by immunosuppression with a ciclosporin- or tacrolimus-(FK506)-based regimen. Early complications include haemorrhage, sepsis and acute rejection (< 6 weeks), which is reversible with intensive immunosuppression. Late complications include recurrence of disease (hepatitis B and C) and chronic rejection, which is not reversible and requires retransplantation. The outcome of liver transplantation is good, with an overall 5-year survival rate of 70–85%.

## Budd–Chiari syndrome (K&C p. 379)

Budd–Chiari syndrome is caused by occlusion of the hepatic vein, thereby obstructing venous outflow from the liver.

### Aetiology

Budd–Chiari syndrome may occur as a result of obstruction of the hepatic vein by malignancy, radiotherapy, trauma, or hypercoagulability states such as polycythaemia vera, taking the contraceptive pill or leukaemia. The cause is unknown in one-third of cases.

### Clinical features

The syndrome presents acutely with abdominal pain, nausea, vomiting, hepatomegaly and ascites, or more insidiously with enlargement of the caudate lobe, splenomegaly, ascites and jaundice. Chronic Budd–Chiari syndrome should be considered in the differential diagnosis of otherwise unexplained liver dysfunction particularly in association with ascites.

### Investigations

The ascitic fluid shows a high protein content. Ultrasonography or CT scanning will show an enlarged caudate lobe, and Doppler studies will demonstrate abnormalities in the direction of blood flow.

### Treatment

Treatment of Budd–Chiari syndrome can be divided into medical treatment (diuretics for ascites, anticoagulation) radiologic procedures (TIPS, angioplasty) and surgical intervention (including shunting procedures and liver transplantation). The choice of treatment depends on the clinical and anatomical features.

## Liver abscess (K&C p. 381)

## Pyogenic liver abscess

### Aetiology

The cause of pyogenic liver abscess is often unknown, although biliary sepsis or portal pyaemia from intra-abdominal sepsis may be responsible. Other causes include trauma, bacteraemia or direct extension from, for example, a perinephric abscess. The organism found most commonly is *Escherichia coli. Streptococcus milleri* and anaerobic organisms such as *Bacteroides* are often seen.

## Clinical features

Symptoms can be mild, although abdominal pain, fever, rigors, nausea and vomiting may occur. The patient may be jaundiced and the liver enlarged and tender.

## Investigations

- Blood count usually shows a normochromic/ normocytic anaemia and the ESR is elevated.
- Liver biochemistry shows a rise in serum alkaline phosphatase and an elevated bilirubin in 25% of cases.
- Ultrasonography and CT are useful for detecting fluid-filled lesions.

## Management

Treatment is with broad-spectrum antibiotics. Drainage of the abscess may be required under ultrasound guidance.

# Amoebic abscess

## Aetiology

An amoebic abscess results from spread of the organism *Entamoeba histolytica* from the bowel to the liver via the portal venous system (p. 27). Multiple microabscesses develop which coalesce to form single or multiple large abscesses.

## Clinical features

The onset is usually gradual with fever, weight loss and malaise, often with no history of dysentery. The patient looks ill, with tender hepatomegaly and sometimes consolidation or an effusion in the right side of the chest.

## Investigations

This is as for pyogenic abscess. Serological tests for amoebae, e.g. complement-fixation test or enzyme-linked immunosorbent assay (ELISA), are almost always positive. Aspiration of the abscess yields fluid 'like anchovy sauce'.

## Management

Metronidazole 800 mg three times daily is given by mouth for 10 days. Aspiration is used for large abscesses or those failing to respond to medical treatment.

## Hydatid disease (K&C p. 119 & p. 382)

For details of hydatid disease see page 38.

## Jaundice in pregnancy (K&C p. 382)

Viral hepatitis is the single most common cause of jaundice in pregnancy. Three types of liver disease are specific to pregnancy: acute fatty liver of pregnancy (a severe fulminating illness with jaundice, vomiting and hepatic coma); recurrent intrahepatic cholestasis (presenting with jaundice and pruritus); and haemolysis (occasionally producing jaundice), which occurs in pre-eclamptic toxaemia. The three conditions present most commonly in the third trimester and resolve with delivery of the baby.

# Liver tumours (K&C p. 383)

The most common malignant liver tumours are metastatic, particularly those from the gastrointestinal tract, breast or bronchus. Primary liver tumours may be either benign or malignant.

## Hepatocellular carcinoma (hepatoma)

Hepatocellular carcinoma (HCC) is one of the most common cancers world-wide, although it is uncommon in the West.

### Aetiology

Several risk factors have been identified, including cirrhosis, hepatitis B infection and hepatitis C infection. Other suggested aetiological factors include aflatoxin (a metabolite of a fungus found in groundnuts), androgenic steroids and, possibly the contraceptive pill.

### Clinical features

Weight loss, anorexia, fever, ascites and abdominal pain occur. The rapid development of these features in a patient with cirrhosis is suggestive of HCC. Because of surveillance, by measurement of serum α-fetoprotein and liver ultrasound, asymptomatic HCC is being found increasingly in cirrhotic patients.

### Investigations
- Serum α-fetoprotein may be raised but is normal in at least a third of patients.
- Ultrasound or CT scanning show large filling defects in 90% of cases.
- Liver biopsy under ultrasound control provides histological confirmation.

### Management
Surgical resection or transplantation is occasionally possible, but chemotherapy and radiotherapy are unhelpful.

### Prognosis
Survival is seldom for more than 6 months.

## Benign liver tumours

153

The most common are haemangiomas, usually found incidentally on a liver ultrasound or CT scan. They require no treatment. Hepatic adenomas are less common and associated with use of oral contraceptives. Resection is required if there are symptoms (e.g. pain, intraperitoneal bleeding).

## Gallstones (K&C p. 387)

Gallstones are present in 10–20% of the population. They are most common in women and the prevalence increases with age.

### Pathophysiology
Gallstones are of two types:

- *Cholesterol gallstones* are composed mainly of cholesterol and account for 80% of all gallstones in the western world. Cholesterol, insoluble in water, is held in solution by the detergent action of bile salts and phospholipids, with which it forms micelles and

**Table 4.10**
Risk factors for cholesterol gallstones

| Risk factor | Mechanism |
| --- | --- |
| Increased age | |
| Sex (F > M) | Increased cholesterol in bile |
| Obesity | Gall bladder stasis |
| Rapid weight loss | |
| Contraceptive pill | |
| Terminal ileal disease | Decreased bile salts in bile caused by |
| Terminal ileal resection | interruption of enterohepatic circulation |

vesicles. Cholesterol gallstones only form in bile which has an excess of cholesterol relative to bile salts and phospholipids (supersaturated or lithogenic bile), thus allowing cholesterol crystals to form and grow as stones (Table 4.10).

- *Pigment stones*, consisting of bilirubin polymers and calcium bilirubinate. They are seen in patients with chronic haemolysis, e.g. hereditary spherocytosis and sickle cell disease, in which bilirubin production is increased, and also in cirrhosis. Pigment stones may also form in the bile ducts after cholecystectomy and with duct strictures.

### Clinical presentation
Most gallstones never cause symptoms and cholecystectomy is not indicated in asymptomatic cases. The complications are summarized in Figure 4.7.

## Biliary pain
Biliary pain (colic) is the term used for the pain associated with the temporary obstruction of the cystic or common bile duct by a stone.

### Clinical features
There are recurrent episodes of severe constant pain in the upper abdomen which subsides after several hours. The pain may radiate to the right shoulder and right subscapular region and is often associated with vomiting. Examination is usually normal.

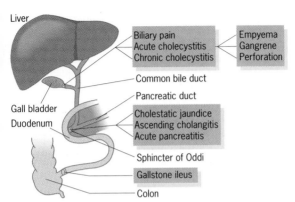

Fig. 4.7 The complications of gallstones.

## Investigations

The diagnosis is usually made on the basis of a typical history and an ultrasound showing gallstones. Increases of serum alkaline phosphatase and bilirubin during an attack support the diagnosis of biliary pain. The absence of inflammatory features (fever, white cell count and local peritonism) differentiates this from acute cholecystitis.

155

## Management

The treatment is analgesia and elective cholecystectomy. Abnormal liver biochemistry or a dilated CBD or stone in the CBD on ultrasonography, is an indication for preoperative MRCP and/or ERCP.

## Acute cholecystitis

Acute cholecystitis follows the impaction of a stone in the cystic duct or neck of the gall bladder. Very occasionally acute cholecystitis may occur without stones (acalculous cholecystitis).

### Clinical features

The initial clinical features are similar to those of biliary colic. However, over a number of hours there is progression to severe pain localized in the right upper quadrant which is associated with a fever and tenderness and muscle guarding on examination. The tenderness is worse on inspiration

(Murphy's sign). Complications include an empyema (pus) and perforation with peritonitis. The diagnosis of acute cholecystitis is usually straightforward. The differential diagnosis includes acute pancreatitis, perforated peptic ulcer, intrahepatic abscess and basal pneumonia.

### Investigations
- White cell count shows a leucocytosis.
- Serum liver biochemistry may be mildly abnormal.
- Radiology. The diagnosis is made by ultrasonography showing gallstones and a distended gall bladder with a thickened wall. There is focal tenderness directly over the visualized gall bladder (sonographic Murphy's sign).

### Management
The initial treatment is conservative, with nil by mouth, intravenous fluids, pain relief and intravenous antibiotics, e.g. cefotaxime. Cholecystectomy is usually performed within 48 hours of the acute attack, and always if complications (see above) develop.

## Chronic cholecystitis
Chronic inflammation of the gall bladder is often found in association with gallstones. There is no evidence that this produces any symptoms, and cholecystectomy is not indicated. Chronic right hypochondrial pain and fatty food intolerance are likely to be functional in origin and gallstones an incidental finding.

## Common bile duct stones (cholelithiasis)
### Clinical features
CBD stones may be asymptomatic. Usually one or more of the symptoms of pain, jaundice and fever are present. The jaundice is cholestatic in type, and therefore the urine is dark, the stools pale and the skin may itch. High fever and rigors indicate biliary tract infection (cholangitis). Charcot's triad is the three symptoms occurring together, and indicates cholangitis.

## Investigations

- White cell count shows a leucocytosis if infection is present.
- Blood cultures are often positive (*E. coli*, *E. faecalis*) in the presence of cholangitis.
- Liver biochemistry shows a cholestatic picture with a raised serum bilirubin and alkaline phosphatase.
- Ultrasound may show a dilated common bile duct containing a stone. Endoscopic ultrasound is more sensitive than transabdominal ultrasonography and is sometimes performed if there is a high index of suspicion and the latter is negative.
- MRCP is an alternative non-invasive technique for imaging the biliary system.
- ERCP confirms the diagnosis and allows stone removal. This must be performed urgently if there is cholangitis.

## Management *(K&C p. 392)*

Treatment depends on the clinical situation, but includes analgesia for pain, and intravenous antibiotics, e.g. cefotaxime, if infection is present. The stone must be removed from the duct either by ERCP followed by sphincterotomy and stone extraction with a Dormia basket or balloon, or by exploration of the CBD at the time of cholecystectomy.

## Management of gall bladder stones *(K&C p. 389)*

Cholecystectomy is the treatment of choice for symptomatic gallstones, and is now almost always done laparoscopically. Non-surgical treatment of gallstones by dissolution therapy or lithotripsy is occasionally performed in patients who are not fit for or refuse cholecystectomy.

## Primary sclerosing cholangitis

*(K&C p. 393)*

Primary sclerosing cholangitis (PSC) is a chronic cholestatic liver disease characterized by a progressive obliterating fibrosis of the intra- and extrahepatic ducts. Episodes of ascending cholangitis and jaundice are common. PSC is a progressive disease which may eventually lead to secondary biliary cirrhosis and, often, premature death from cholangiocarcinoma (bile duct cancer). It is of unknown cause; 75% or more cases have ulcerative colitis which may be asymptomatic. Eighty per cent of patients have myeloperoxidase ANCA antibodies (p. 800), liver biopsy shows fibrosis around the bile ducts (onion skin lesion) and ERCP shows multiple strictures. Extrahepatic strictures may be amenable to dilatation. Treatment is limited to management of the general complications of the disease, such as pruritus, fat malabsorption and complications arising from chronic liver disease. No specific treatment has been shown to retard the rate of disease progression and the only option is eventual liver transplantation. Patients with AIDS have been found to have sclerosing cholangitis that is believed to be infectious in origin.

# Pancreatitis

The classification of pancreatitis is difficult because of the inability to separate acute and chronic forms clearly. By definition, acute pancreatitis, which can occur as isolated or recurrent attacks, is distinguished from chronic pancreatitis in that the process occurs on the background of a previously normal pancreas and the pancreas returns functionally and structurally to normal after the episode. The causes are shown in Table 4.11.

## Acute pancreatitis (K&C p. 397)

This is an acute condition presenting with abdominal pain and raised pancreatic enzymes in the blood or urine, resulting from inflammatory disease of the pancreas.

### Pathogenesis

The exact pathophysiology is not well understood. Whatever the initiating event, there is acinar cell injury and release of activated proteases into the pancreatic interstitium. Disruption of acinar cells promotes migration of inflammatory cells from the microcirculation into the interstitium. Release of a variety of mediators and cytokines leads to a local inflammatory response, and sometimes a

**Table 4.11**
Causes of pancreatitis

| Acute | Chronic |
| --- | --- |
| Gallstones* | Alcohol* |
| Alcohol* | Idiopathic |
| Idiopathic (unknown cause) | Protein–energy malnutrition |
| Metabolic: hypercalcaemia, hyperlipidaemia | Hereditary |
| Iatrogenic: post-surgical, ERCP | Cystic fibrosis |
| Drugs: e.g. azathioprine, corticosteroids | |

ERCP, endoscopic retrograde cholangiopancreatography
* Commonest causes in the western world

systemic inflammatory response that can result in single or multiple organ failure.

## Clinical features

Epigastric or upper abdominal pain radiating through to the back is the cardinal symptom. There is often nausea and vomiting, and in severe cases multiorgan failure may develop. On examination there is epigastric tenderness, guarding and rigidity. Ecchymoses around the umbilicus (Cullen's sign) or in the flanks (Grey Turner's sign) indicate severe necrotizing pancreatitis.

## Diagnosis

- *Blood tests.* A raised serum amylase, in conjunction with an appropriate history and clinical signs, strongly suggests a diagnosis of acute pancreatitis. Normal levels occur if the patient presents late when urinary amylase or serum lipase levels may still be raised. Serum amylase may also be moderately raised in other abdominal conditions, such as acute cholecystitis and perforated duodenal ulcer, although very high amylase levels (> 3 times normal) strongly suggest pancreatitis. Full blood count, CRP, urea and electrolytes, liver biochemistry, plasma calcium, and arterial blood gases are also measured as a guide to the severity of pancreatitis.

- *Radiology*. An erect chest X-ray is performed to exclude perforated peptic ulcer as the cause of the pain and raised amylase. Abdominal ultrasound is performed as a screening test to look for gallstones as a cause of pancreatitis and may show swelling of the inflamed pancreas. Contrast-enhanced spiral CT scanning or MRI is performed in all but the mildest attack of pancreatitis to look for evidence of pancreatic necrosis (indicating a severe attack) and peripancreatic fluid collections.

## Management

The patient should be kept fasting and intravenous hydration is instituted. Nasogastric suction prevents abdominal distension and vomiting. Analgesics with opiates (other than morphine) are usually required. The majority of cases are mild without systemic complications and associated only with interstitial inflammation; these patients usually recover within 5–7 days. Less commonly, acute pancreatitis is associated with failure of one or more organ systems, such as renal or respiratory failure and impaired coagulation with disseminated intravascular coagulation. These severe attacks are usually associated with pancreatic necrosis, which is identified on CT scanning as focal areas of reduced tissue perfusion. Several scoring systems have been developed in order to identify those patients with severe pancreatitis; of these, the acute physiology and chronic health inquiry score (APACHE) is the most commonly used because it can be used continuously and may be the most accurate. In severe cases oral nutrition may not be possible for weeks. In this situation, enteral nutrition via a nasojejunal tube is now preferred over total parenteral nutrition as it is well tolerated and associated with fewer complications. Imipenem and cefuroxime reduce the number of septic complications and improve mortality in some patients with acute necrotizing pancreatitis. Surgical treatment is sometimes required for very severe necrotizing pancreatitis, particularly if it is infected, or if complications such as pancreatic abscesses or pseudocysts occur. Patients with biliary pancreatitis and evidence of cholangitis or progressive jaundice (both of which suggest a stone impacted in the common bile duct) may require urgent ERCP and stone removal.

## Complications
Acute complications include hyperglycaemia, hypocalcaemia, renal failure and shock.

## Prognosis
The mortality rate varies from 1% in mild cases to 50% in severe cases. Patients who recover may have recurrent attacks, depending on the aetiology.

# Chronic pancreatitis (*K&C* p. 400)
Chronic pancreatitis is defined as continuing inflammatory disease of the pancreas, characterized by irreversible morphological change and/or permanent impairment of function. Chronic calcifying pancreatitis is the commonest form in most developed countries, and is usually caused by alcohol. The disease is not reversible but it is possible to arrest the disease process, if the patient stops drinking alcohol.

## Clinical features

There is central abdominal pain which is located in the epigastrium and characteristically radiates to the back. The pain may be intermittent or constant, and exacerbations are precipitated by an alcoholic binge. The abdominal pain is accompanied by severe weight loss as a result of anorexia, and may be difficult to distinguish from the pain of pancreatic cancer.

Diabetes may develop and steatorrhoea (p. 54) occurs when the secretion of pancreatic lipase is reduced by 90%. Occasionally the patient presents with biliary obstruction, jaundice and cholangitis. The differential diagnosis is from pancreatic carcinoma which may also develop on a background of chronic pancreatitis. Carcinoma should be considered when there is a short history and localized ductular abnormalities on imaging.

## Investigations
The diagnosis of chronic pancreatitis is made by radiological techniques which demonstrate structural changes in the gland, and metabolic studies which demonstrate functional abnormalities.

- *Radiology.* A plain abdominal X-ray will show pancreatic calcification in some cases. Ultrasonography and CT scanning will show the dilated duct and demonstrate irregular consistency and outline of the gland. ERCP demonstrates dilatation of the pancreatic duct, with stenotic segments. MRCP and endoscopic ultrasound are sometimes used if the diagnosis is not confirmed with other imaging tests.
- *Functional assessment.* The pancreolauryl test involves the ingestion of fluorescein dilaurate, which is hydrolysed by pancreatic esterases to release fluorescein. Fluorescein is rapidly absorbed, conjugated in the liver and excreted in the urine. The various stages of the test require 3 days to perform and prolonged urine collection. Nevertheless, the test is simple, easily reproducible and has a high negative predictive value for pancreatic exocrine insufficiency. A faecal elastase level will be abnormal in patients with moderate to severe disease. The serum amylase is of no use in the diagnosis of chronic pancreatitis, but may be raised during an acute episode of pain. A raised blood sugar indicates diabetes mellitus.

### Treatment

The patient should be told to stop drinking alcohol. The pain may require opiates for control, with the attendant risk of addiction. Surgical resection combined with drainage of the pancreatic duct into the small bowel (pancreaticojejunostomy) is of value for severe disease with intractable pain. Pancreatic strictures or stones are sometimes amenable to endoscopic treatment with ERCP. Pancreatic supplements are useful for those with steatorrhoea and may reduce the frequency of attacks of pain in those with recurrent symptoms. Diabetes requires appropriate treatment with diet, oral hypoglycaemics or insulin.

## Carcinoma of the pancreas (K&C p. 402)

### Epidemiology

Pancreatic cancer is the fifth most common cause of cancer death in the western world. Men are affected more commonly than women, and the incidence increases with age (peak in the seventh decade).

## Aetiology
The aetiology is unknown but smoking, alcohol, coffee and dietary fat ingestion have all been implicated.

## Clinical features
Cancer affecting the head of the pancreas presents with painless jaundice as a result of obstruction of the common duct, and weight loss. Cancer of the body or tail presents with abdominal pain, weight loss and anorexia. Diabetes may occur and there is an increased risk of thrombophlebitis. In cancer of the head of the pancreas, examination may reveal jaundice and a distended palpable gall bladder (Courvoisier's law: if, in a case of painless jaundice, the gall bladder is palpable the cause will not be gallstones). In gallstone disease chronic inflammation and fibrosis prevent distension of the gall bladder.

## Investigations
The diagnosis is made with ultrasonography and/or CT. Duodenoscopy and ERCP may detect tumour in the head of the pancreas or at the ampulla. Endoscopic ultrasound is used for staging and in difficult cases for diagnosis.

## Management
Curative resection is not usually possible and treatment is therefore almost always palliative. Bypass of the obstructed common bile duct will relieve jaundice and this is usually performed with endoscopic placement of a stent, surgery being reserved for cases where the duodenum is obstructed. Chemotherapy and radiotherapy are of little value.

## Prognosis
The prognosis is appalling: overall the 5-year survival rate is 2%, most patients being dead within a year of diagnosis.

# Endocrine tumours (K&C p. 404)

These tumours arise in the pancreas from APUD (amine precursor uptake and decarboxylation) cells, and are sometimes called apudomas. They usually secrete one hormone that produces the clinical effect, although other hormones are often also synthesized. Circulating hormone concentrations can be measured and high levels provide the diagnosis. Most neuroendocrine tumours express large numbers of somatostatin receptors. Intravenous injection of $^{111}$In-labelled octreotide is therefore taken up readily by these tumours, and this test is the investigation of choice to localize the tumour and demonstrate the presence of metastases in patients suspected of having a neuroendocrine tumour. Endoscopic ultrasonography is also used in some patients to localize the tumour.

## Gastrinomas (Zollinger–Ellison syndrome)

Gastrinomas arise from the G cells of the pancreas and secrete large amounts of gastrin. This stimulates maximal gastric acid secretion, resulting in the development of peptic ulcers, which are often multiple, large and may be resistant to conventional treatment. Diarrhoea may also occur as a result of inhibition of digestive enzymes at low pH in the intestine. High-dose proton pump inhibitors are used to suppress symptoms but surgical resection is the only curative treatment.

## Vipomas

These rare tumours produce vasoactive intestinal polypeptide (VIP), which stimulates intestinal water and electrolyte secretion, causing severe watery diarrhoea, hypokalaemia and dehydration. Treatment is with surgical resection or octreotide.

## Glucagonomas

Glucagonomas arise from the α-cells of the pancreas and produce pancreatic glucagon. Patients present with diabetes mellitus and a unique necrolytic migratory erythematous rash.

# 5

# Diseases of the blood and haematological malignancies

## Introduction

Blood consists of red cells, white cells, platelets, and plasma in which the other components are suspended. Plasma is the liquid component of blood which contains soluble fibrinogen. Serum is what remains after the formation of the fibrin clot.

Haemopoiesis is the formation of blood cells (*K&C* p. 405). The bone marrow is the only source of blood cells during normal childhood and adult life. Pluripotential stem cells, under the influence of a number of haemopoietic growth factors, give rise to lymphoid and myeloid stem cells. The former gives rise to T and B cells. The myeloid stem cell gives rise to CFU-GEMM (colony-forming unit, committed to the production of granulocytes, erythroid cells, monocytes and megakaryocytes). The growth factor erythropoietin controls the production of red blood cells. Reticulocytes are young red cells recently released from the bone marrow and still contain RNA. Reticulocytes normally represent < 2% of total circulating red blood cells. The reticulocyte count gives a guide to the erythroid activity in the bone marrow and increases with haemorrhage, haemolysis and after treatment with specific haematinics in deficiency states.

## Anaemia (*K&C* p. 410)

### Introduction

The principal physiological function of haemoglobin (Hb) is to carry and deliver oxygen to the tissues from the lungs. Hb is a tetramer consisting of two pairs of globin polypeptide chains: one pair of alpha-like chains and one pair of non-alpha chains. A haem group, consisting of a single molecule of protoporphyrin IX bound to a single ferrous ion ($Fe^{2+}$) is linked covalently at a specific site to each globin

**Table 5.1**
Normal values for adult peripheral blood

|  | Men | Women |
|---|---|---|
| Hb (g/dL) | 13–18 | 11.5–15.5 |
| PCV (haematocrit, L/L) | 0.42–0.53 | 0.36–0.45 |
| RCC (10$^{12}$/L) | 4.5–6.0 | 3.9–5.1 |
| MCV (fL) | 80–96 | |
| MCH (pg) | 27–33 | |
| MCHC (g/dL) | 32–35 | |
| WCC (10$^9$/L) | 4.0–11.0 | |
| Platelets (10$^9$/L) | 150–400 | |
| ESR (mm/h) | < 20 | |
| Reticulocytes (% of total RCC) | 0.2–2.0 | |

ESR, erythrocyte sedimentation rate; Hb, haemoglobin; MCH, mean corpuscular haemoglobin; MCHC, mean corpuscular haemoglobin concentration; MCV, mean corpuscular volume of red cells; PCV, packed cell volume; RCC, red cell count; WCC, white cell count

chain. Oxygenation and deoxygenation of haemoglobin occur at the haem iron (*K&C* p. 408)

Anaemia is present when there is a decrease in the level of Hb in the blood below the reference range for the age and sex of the individual. Reduction of Hb is usually accompanied by a fall in red cell count (RCC) and packed cell volume (PCV, haematocrit), although an increase in plasma volume (as with massive splenomegaly) may cause anaemia with a normal RCC and PCV ('dilutional anaemia'). The normal values for these indices are given in Table 5.1, all of which are measured using automated cell counters as part of a routine full blood count (FBC).

## Clinical features

Symptoms depend on the severity and speed of onset of anaemia. A very slowly falling level of Hb allows for haemodynamic compensation and enhancement of the oxygen-carrying capacity of the blood. In general elderly people tolerate anaemia less well than young people. The symptoms are non-specific and include fatigue, faintness and breathlessness. Angina pectoris and intermittent claudication may occur in those with coexistent atheromatous arterial disease. On examination the skin and mucous membranes are pale; there may be a tachycardia and a systolic flow murmur. Cardiac failure may occur in elderly people or those with compromised cardiac function.

### Classification of anaemia (Table 5.2)

The causes of anaemia are classified according to the measurement of red blood cell size. The normal red blood cell has a volume of 80–96 femtoliters (fL). Automatic cell counters provide a value for the mean of the red blood cell volume based on counting millions of cells (the mean corpuscular volume, MCV). This classification is useful because the type of anaemia then indicates the underlying causes and necessary investigations. Irrespective of the cause, most patients with chronic anaemia do not require blood transfusion and the appropriate management, unless severely anaemic, is treatment of the underlying cause.

## Microcytic anaemia

Microcytosis usually reflects a decreased Hb content within the red blood cell and is then often associated with a re-duction in the mean corpuscular haemoglobin (MCH) and mean corpuscular haemoglobin concentration (MCHC) producing a hypochromic appearance on the blood film.

### Iron deficiency

Iron is necessary for the formation of haem, and iron deficiency is the most common cause of anaemia world-wide. Absorption of dietary iron occurs primarily in the duodenum at a rate of about 1–2 mg per day, which represents about 10% of dietary iron (*K&C* p. 412). Factors that promote intestinal absorption include gastric acid, iron deficiency and increased erythropoietic activity. Iron is transported in the plasma bound to the protein transferrin, which is synthesized in the liver and normally about one-third saturated with iron (Fig. 5.1). Most of the body's iron content is incorporated into haemoglobin in developing erythroid precursors and mature red cells. Most of the remaining body iron is stored as ferritin and haemosiderin in hepatocytes, skeletal muscle and reticuloendothelial macrophages. A fixed amount of iron, about 1 mg each day, is lost in sloughed skin and mucosal cells through sweat, urine and faeces. In women there is an additional loss during menses, and premenopausal women may often border on iron deficiency.

**Table 5.2**
Classification of the anaemias based on the MCV

| Microcytic | Normocytic | Macrocytic |
|---|---|---|
| **Small red cells, MCV < 80 fL** | **Normal-sized red cells, normal MCV** | **Large red cells, MCV > 96 fL** |
| Iron deficiency | Acute blood loss | Megaloblastic |
| Anaemia of chronic disease | Anaemia of chronic disease | Vitamin $B_{12}$ deficiency |
| Thalassaemia | Aplastic anaemia | Folate deficiency |
| Sideroblastic anaemia | Combined deficiency, e.g. iron and folate | Normoblastic |
| | Haemolytic anaemia | Myelodysplasia |
| | Endocrine disorders, e.g. hypothyroidism | Haemolysis |
| | | Other defects of DNA synthesis, e.g. chemotherapy |

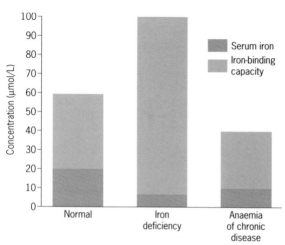

Fig. 5.1 **Serum iron and total iron-binding capacity (transferrin) in normal subjects and iron deficiency anaemia and anaemia of chronic disease.**

## Aetiology

The most common cause of iron deficiency is blood loss from the uterus or gastrointestinal tract. Other causes are:

- Increased demands, e.g. during growth and pregnancy
- Decreased absorption in small bowel disease or after gastrectomy
- Poor intake; this is rare in developed countries.

## Clinical features

Symptoms and signs are the result of anaemia (see earlier) and of decreased epithelial cell iron, which causes brittle hair and nails, atrophic glossitis, angular stomatitis and koilonychia (spoon-shaped nails). Rarely, pharyngeal webs occur which may cause dysphagia (Paterson–Brown–Kelly syndrome).

## Investigations

- Blood count shows a low Hb with a low MCV.
- Blood film. The red cells are microcytic and hypochromic, with anisocytosis (variation in size) and poikilocytosis (variation in shape).

169

- Serum ferritin reflects iron stores and is low.
- Serum iron is low and the total iron-binding capacity (TIBC) is high resulting in a transferrin saturation (serum iron divided by TIBC) < 19% (Fig. 5.1).
- Serum soluble transferrin receptor: the number of transferrin receptors increases in iron deficiency.
- Bone marrow examination is only necessary in complicated cases, and shows erythroid hyperplasia and absence of iron.

Iron deficiency is almost always the result of chronic, often occult, gastrointestinal blood loss in men and in post-menopausal women, and further investigation of the gastrointestinal tract is required to determine the cause of the blood loss (see p. 75). Mild anaemia in premenopausal women is usually the result of menstrual blood loss.

### Differential diagnosis
This is from other causes of a microcytic/hypochromic anaemia (see Table 5.2).

### Management
- Find and treat the underlying cause.
- Oral iron, e.g. ferrous sulphate 200 mg three times daily, is given for about 6 months to correct the anaemia and replace iron stores. A response to iron treatment is characterized by an increase in the reticulocyte count followed by an increase in Hb at a rate of about 1 g/dL every week until the Hb concentration is normal.
- Parenteral iron is rarely necessary and used only when patients are intolerant or there is a poor response to oral iron, e.g. severe malabsorption.

### Anaemia of chronic disease (K&C p. 416)
This occurs in patients with a variety of chronic diseases, including chronic renal failure, chronic inflammatory diseases such as Crohn's disease and polymyalgia rheumatica, and chronic infections such as tuberculosis and infective endocarditis. Anaemia of chronic disease presents with a normochromic, normocytic or microcytic anaemia.

Characteristic laboratory findings include low serum iron levels, low serum iron-binding capacity (Fig. 5.1) and increased or normal serum ferritin. The anaemia of chronic disease is the result of decreased release of iron from bone marrow to developing erythroblasts, inadequate erythropoietin response to the anaemia, and decreased red cell survival. Treatment is of the underlying cause.

### Sideroblastic anaemia (*K&C* p. 416)

Sideroblastic anaemia is a rare disorder of haem synthesis characterized by a refractory anaemia with hypochromic cells in the peripheral blood and ring sideroblasts in the bone marrow. Ring sideroblasts are erythroblasts with iron deposited in mitochondria and reflect impaired utilization of iron delivered to the developing erythroblast. It may be inherited or acquired (secondary to myelodysplasia, alcohol, lead or isoniazid, or idiopathic). Treatment is to withdraw the causative agents. Some cases respond to pyridoxine (vitamin $B_6$). In many cases anaemia is transfusion dependent and iron overload becomes a problem.

## Macrocytic anaemia

Macrocytosis is a rise in mean cell volume of the red cells above the normal range. Macrocytic anaemia can be divided into megaloblastic and non-megaloblastic types, depending on the bone marrow findings. In practice, macrocytosis is usually investigated without performing a bone marrow examination. The initial investigation is measurement of serum $B_{12}$ and red cell folate.

### Megaloblastic anaemia (*K&C* p. 417)

Megaloblastic anaemia is characterized by the presence in the bone marrow of developing red blood cells with delayed nuclear maturation relative to that of the cytoplasm (*megaloblasts*). The underlying mechanism is defective DNA synthesis, which may also affect the white cells (causing hypersegmented neutrophil nuclei with six lobes, and sometimes leucopenia) and platelets (causing thrombocytopenia). The most common cause (see Table 5.2) of megaloblastic anaemia is deficiency of vitamin $B_{12}$ or folate, which are both necessary to synthesize DNA.

## Vitamin B₁₂ deficiency

Animal products (meat and dairy products) provide the only dietary source of vitamin $B_{12}$ for humans. The daily requirement is 1 µg, which is easily supplied by a balanced western diet (containing 5–30 µg daily). Vitamin $B_{12}$ is liberated from protein complexes in food by gastric enzymes and binds to a vitamin $B_{12}$-binding protein 'R' binder derived from saliva. Free $B_{12}$ is then released by pancreatic enzymes and becomes bound to intrinsic factor, which, along with $H^+$ ions, is secreted from gastric parietal cells. This complex is delivered to the terminal ileum, where vitamin $B_{12}$ is absorbed and transported to the tissues by the carrier protein transcobalamin II. Vitamin $B_{12}$ is stored in the liver, where there is sufficient supply for 2 or more years. The causes of vitamin $B_{12}$ deficiency are listed in Table 5.3.

## Pernicious anaemia

Pernicious anaemia is an autoimmune condition in which there is atrophy of the gastric mucosa with failure of intrinsic factor production and consequent vitamin $B_{12}$ malabsorption. It is the most common cause of vitamin $B_{12}$ deficiency in adults in western countries.

## Epidemiology

This is a disease of elderly people (1–2% over the age of 60 years affected); most cases are undiagnosed. It is more

---

**Table 5.3**
Vitamin $B_{12}$ deficiency – causes

**Low dietary intake**
Vegans

**Impaired absorption**
Stomach
    Pernicious anaemia
    Gastrectomy
Small bowel
    Ileal disease or resection
    Coeliac disease
    Tropical sprue
    Bacterial overgrowth

**Congenital transcobalamin II deficiency (rare)**

---

common in women and in people with fair hair and blue eyes. There is an association with other autoimmune diseases, particularly thyroid disease and vitiligo.

## Pathology
There is glandular atrophy of the gastric mucosa causing absent acid and intrinsic factor secretion.

## Clinical features
The onset of pernicious anaemia is insidious, with progressively increasing symptoms of anaemia. There may be glossitis (a red sore tongue), angular stomatitis and mild jaundice. Neurological features can occur with very low levels of serum $B_{12}$ and include a polyneuropathy caused by symmetrical damage to the peripheral nerves and posterior and lateral columns of the spinal cord (subacute combined degeneration of the cord). The latter presents with progressive weakness, ataxia and eventually paraplegia if untreated. Dementia and visual disturbances due to optic atrophy may also occur.

173

## Investigations
- Blood count and film. A macrocytic anaemia (MCV often > 110 fL) is often seen with hypersegmented neutrophil nuclei and, in severe cases, leucopenia and thrombocytopenia.
- Serum vitamin $B_{12}$ is low, frequently < 50 ng/L (normal > 160 ng/L).
- Red cell folate may be reduced because vitamin $B_{12}$ is necessary to convert serum folate to the active intracellular form.
- Serum autoantibodies. Parietal cell antibodies are present in 90% and antibodies to intrinsic factor in 50%.
- Serum bilirubin is raised as a result of excess breakdown of haemoglobin, owing to ineffective erythropoiesis in the bone marrow.
- The Schilling test (Table 5.4) will differentiate pernicious anaemia from small bowel malabsorption as the cause of vitamin $B_{12}$ deficiency. Defective vitamin $B_{12}$ absorption is corrected by intrinsic factor

**Table 5.4**
Schilling test

**Part I**
- Give 1 μg radiolabelled vitamin $B_{12}$ orally to the fasting patient
- Give 1000 μg $B_{12}$ (non-radioactive) by intramuscular injection to saturate vitamin $B_{12}$-binding proteins and to flush out radiolabelled vitamin $B_{12}$
- Collect urine for 24 h. Normal subjects excrete more than 10% of the radioactive dose

*If abnormal:*
**Part II**
- Repeat part I after giving oral intrinsic factor capsules

*Result*
- If excretion still abnormal, lesion is in the terminal ileum or there is bacterial overgrowth
- If excretion now normal, diagnosis is pernicious anaemia or gastrectomy

in the former. In practice, the cause is often apparent from the history and autoantibody screen, and the Schilling test is rarely performed.

- Bone marrow examination shows a hypercellular bone marrow with megaloblastic changes. This is not necessary in straightforward cases.

## Differential diagnosis
Vitamin $B_{12}$ deficiency must be differentiated from other causes of megaloblastic anaemia, principally folate deficiency, but this is usually clear from the blood levels of these two vitamins. Pernicious anaemia should be distinguished from other causes of vitamin $B_{12}$ deficiency (Table 5.3).

## Management
Traditionally, treatment is with intramuscular hydroxocobalamin (vitamin $B_{12}$). Injections (1 mg) are given twice weekly for 3 weeks to replenish body stores, and then 3-monthly injections continued for life. However, gastrointestinal absorption of vitamin $B_{12}$ is not entirely dependent on the presence of intrinsic factor and there has been renewed interest in treatment with high-dose (2 mg daily) oral cobalamin.

## Complications

There is an increased incidence of gastric carcinoma. However, screening is not routinely recommended and endoscopy or barium meal examination of the stomach is performed only if there are gastric symptoms.

## Folate deficiency

Folate is found in green vegetables and offal, and absorbed in the upper small intestine. The daily requirement for folate is 100–200 µg and a normal mixed diet contains 200–300 µg. Body stores are sufficient for about 4 months, but folate deficiency may develop much more rapidly in patients who have a poor intake and excess utilization of folate, for example patients in intensive care. The causes of folate deficiency are shown in Table 5.5. The main cause is poor intake, which may occur alone or in combination with excessive utilization or malabsorption.

## Clinical features

Symptoms and signs are the result of anaemia.

## Investigations

Red cell folate is low (normal range 160–640 µg/mL) and is a more accurate guide of tissue folate than serum folate, which is also low (normal range 4.0–18 µg/L). If the history does not suggest dietary deficiency as the cause, further investigations such as a jejunal biopsy should be performed to look for small bowel disease.

175

**Table 5.5**
Causes of folate deficiency

| | |
|---|---|
| Poor intake | Old age, poverty, alcohol excess (also impaired utilization), anorexia |
| Malabsorption | Coeliac disease, tropical sprue |
| Excess utilization | |
|   Physiological | Pregnancy, lactation, prematurity |
|   Pathological | Chronic haemolytic anaemia, malignant and inflammatory diseases, dialysis |
| Drugs | Phenytoin, trimethoprim, sulfasalazine |

## Management

The underlying cause must be treated and folate deficiency corrected by giving oral folic acid 5 mg daily for 4 months; higher daily doses may be necessary with malabsorption. In megaloblastic anaemia of undetermined cause, folic acid alone must not be given, as this will aggravate the neuropathy of vitamin $B_{12}$ deficiency. Prophylactic folic acid is given to patients with chronic haemolysis (5 mg weekly) and pregnant women.

**Prevention of neural tube defects with folic acid** To prevent first occurrence of neural tube defects, women who are planning a pregnancy should be advised to take folate supplements (at least 400 µg/day) before conception and during the first 12 weeks of pregnancy. Larger doses (5 mg daily) are recommended for mothers who already have an infant with a neural tube defect.

## Differential diagnosis of megaloblastic anaemias

A raised MCV with macrocytosis on the peripheral blood film can occur with a normoblastic rather than a megaloblastic bone marrow (Table 5.6). The most common cause of macrocytosis in the UK is alcohol excess. The exact mechanism for the large red cells in each of these conditions is uncertain, but in some it is thought to be due to altered or excessive lipid deposition on red cell membranes.

**Table 5.6**
Causes of macrocytosis other than megaloblastic anaemia

**Physiological**
Pregnancy
Newborn

**Pathological**
Alcohol excess
Liver disease
Reticulocytosis
Hypothyroidism
Haematological disorders
Myelodysplastic syndrome (a frequent cause in the elderly)
Sideroblastic anaemia
Aplastic anaemia
Drugs: hydroxycarbamide (hydroxyurea) and azathioprine
Cold agglutinins

# Anaemia caused by marrow failure (aplastic anaemia) *(K&C p. 422)*

Aplastic anaemia is defined as pancytopenia (deficiency of all cell elements of the blood) with *hypocellularity* (aplasia) of the bone marrow. It is an uncommon but serious condition which may be inherited but is more commonly acquired.

## Aetiology

A list of the main causes of pancytopenia and aplasia is given in Table 5.7. Suppression of bone marrow pluripotential stem cells by cytotoxic T cells is responsible for many cases of idiopathic acquired aplastic anaemia. Many drugs have been associated with the development of aplastic anaemia, and this occurs as a predictable dose-related effect (e.g. chemotherapeutic agents) or as an idiosyncratic reaction (e.g. chloramphenicol).

## Clinical features

Symptoms are the result of the deficiency of red blood cells, white blood cells and platelets, and include anaemia, increased susceptibility to infection, and bleeding. Physical findings include bruising, bleeding gums and epistaxis. Mouth infections are common.

177

**Table 5.7**
Causes of pancytopenia

| Hypocellular bone marrow | Cellular bone marrow |
| --- | --- |
| Aplastic anaemia | Megaloblastic anaemia |
|   Congenital | Bone marrow infiltration or |
|   Idiopathic acquired |   replacement |
|     (50% of cases) |     Lymphoma |
|   Chemicals, e.g. benzene |     Acute leukaemia |
|   Drugs: cytotoxics, |     Myeloma |
|     chloramphenicol, gold |     Secondary carcinoma |
|   Insecticides |     Myelofibrosis |
|   Ionizing radiation | Myelodysplastic syndrome |
|   Infections, e.g. viral hepatitis, | Hypersplenism |
|     measles, HIV | Systemic lupus erythematosus |
| Paroxysmal nocturnal | |
|   haemoglobinuria | |
| Overwhelming sepsis | |

## Investigations

- Blood count shows pancytopenia with low or absent reticulocytes.
- Bone marrow examination shows a hypocellular marrow with increased fat spaces.

## Differential diagnosis

This is from other causes of pancytopenia (Table 5.7). A bone marrow trephine biopsy is essential for assessment of the bone marrow cellularity.

## Management

The cause of the aplastic anaemia must be eliminated if possible. Supportive care, including transfusions of red cells and platelets and antibiotic therapy, should be given as necessary. The course of aplastic anaemia is very variable, ranging from a rapid spontaneous remission to a persistent, increasingly severe pancytopenia, which may lead to death through haemorrhage or infection. Bad prognostic features are the following:

- A peripheral blood neutrophil count < $0.5 \times 10^9$/L
- A peripheral blood platelet count < $20 \times 10^9$/L
- A reticulocyte count of < $40 \times 10^9$/L (0.1% of total circulating red blood cells).

In those patients who do not undergo spontaneous recovery the options for treatment are as follows:

- Bone marrow transplantation (BMT) from a histocompatible sibling donor is the treatment of choice for patients under 50 years of age.
- Immunosuppressive therapy with antilymphocyte globulin and ciclosporin is used for patients over the age of 50 years in whom BMT is not indicated because of the high risk of graft-versus-host disease.

# Haemolytic anaemia (K&C p. 424)

Haemolytic anaemia results from increased destruction of red cells with a reduction of the circulating life-span (normally 120 days). Red cell destruction may be extravascular

**Table 5.8**
Causes of haemolytic anaemia

| Inherited | Acquired |
|---|---|
| Red cell membrane defect<br>  Hereditary spherocytosis<br>  Hereditary elliptocytosis | Immune<br>  Autoimmune haemolytic<br>    anaemia<br>  Haemolytic transfusion<br>    reactions<br>  Drug-induced |
| Haemoglobin abnormalities<br>  Thalassaemia<br>  Sickle cell disease | Non-immune<br>  Paroxysmal nocturnal<br>    haemoglobinuria<br>  Microangiopathic haemolytic<br>    anaemia<br>  March haemoglobinuria |
| Red cell metabolic defects<br>  Glucose-6-phosphate<br>    dehydrogenase deficiency<br>  Pyruvate kinase deficiency | Miscellaneous<br>  Infections (e.g. malaria)<br>  Drugs/chemicals<br>  Hypersplenism |

**179**

(within the reticuloendothelial system) or intravascular (within the blood vessels). The causes of haemolytic anaemia in adults are listed in Table 5.8.

In most haemolytic conditions, red cell destruction is extravascular and cells are removed from the circulation by macrophages in the reticuloendothelial system, particularly the spleen.

When red cells are broken down within the circulation, haemoglobin appears in the plasma as the oxidized form, methaemoglobin, which dissociates into ferrihaem and globin. Binding of ferrihaem to albumin, forms *methaem-albumin* and this can be detected in the plasma (Schumm's test). Free haemoglobin binds to plasma *haptoglobins*; the haemoglobin–haptoglobin is rapidly removed by the liver, leading to a reduction in plasma haptoglobin. Haemoglobin that is unbound to haptoglobin is filtered by the glomerulus and appears in the urine as *haemoglobinuria*. Some Hb is broken down in the renal tubular cells and appears as *haemosiderin* in the urine. Figure 5.2 shows an approach to investigating the patient with suspected haemolytic anaemia.

| Evidence for haemolysis | |
|---|---|
| **Increased red cell breakdown** | **Increased red cell production** |
| • Increased unconjugated serum bilirubin<br>• Increased serum lactate dehydrogenase (released from haemolysed RBC)<br>• Spherocytes on the blood film<br>• With intravascular haemolysis<br>  – increased free plasma Hb<br>  – haemosiderinuria<br>  – very low or absent plasma haptoglobins<br>  – presence of methaemalbumin (positive Schumm's test) | • Increased MCV (as a result of increased reticulocytes)<br>• Increased reticulocyte count<br>• Erythroid hyperplasia on the bone marrow |

| History | Examination |
|---|---|
| e.g. family history, systemic illness, drugs, race | e.g. jaundice, hepatosplenomegaly |

| Inherited defect suspected | Acquired defect suspected |
|---|---|
| Investigations<br>  Spherocytes or elliptocytes on blood film<br>  Haemoglobin electrophoresis<br>  Red cell enzyme assays | Investigations<br>  Coombs' test |

Fig. 5.2 An algorithm for investigation of suspected haemolytic anaemia.

# Inherited haemolytic anaemias

Inherited haemolytic anaemias are due to defects in one or more components of the mature red blood cell:

- Cell membrane
- Haemoglobin
- Metabolic machinery of the red blood cell.

## Membrane defects
### Hereditary spherocytosis (K&C p. 425)

Hereditary spherocytosis is the most common inherited haemolytic anaemia in northern Europeans, and is inherited in an autosomal dominant manner. It is the result of a defect in the red cell membrane of which the commonest cause is a deficiency of the structural membrane protein *spectrin*. Red cells become spherical in shape, are more rigid and less deformable than normal red cells, and are thus destroyed prematurely in the spleen.

## Clinical features

Hereditary spherocytosis may present with jaundice or be asymptomatic. Patients may develop anaemia, spleno-megaly and leg ulcers. As in many haemolytic anaemias, the course of the disease may be interrupted by aplastic, haemolytic and megaloblastic crises. Aplastic anaemia usually occurs after infections, particularly with parvovirus B19, whereas megaloblastic anaemia is the result of folate depletion caused by hyperactivity of the bone marrow. Chronic haemolysis may lead to the development of pigment gallstones.

## Investigations

- Blood count demonstrates reticulocytosis and anaemia, which is usually mild.
- The blood film shows spherocytes (also seen in autoimmune haemolytic anaemia) and reticulocytes.

The diagnosis is made by demonstration of increased red cell osmotic fragility when placed in hypotonic solutions.

## Management

Splenectomy should be performed in all but the mildest of cases. This is usually postponed until after childhood, to minimize the risk of overwhelming pneumococcal infec-tion. Prior to and following splenectomy, all patients should receive pneumococcal vaccine and long-term pro-phylactic penicillin.

### Hereditary elliptocytosis

Hereditary elliptocytosis is similar to spherocytosis but the red cells are elliptical in shape. It is milder clinically and usually does not require treatment.

## Haemoglobin abnormalities (*K&C* p. 426)

Normal adult Hb is made up of haem and two poly-peptide globin chains, $\alpha$ and $\beta$. The haemoglobinopathies can be classified into two subgroups: *abnormal chain production* or *abnormal chain structure* of the polypeptide chains (Table 5.9).

## Thalassaemia (*K&C* p. 427)

In normal Hb there is a balance (1:1) in the production of α and β chains. The thalassaemias are a group of disorders arising from one or multiple gene defects, resulting in a reduced rate of production of one or more globin chains. The imbalanced globin chain production leads to precipitation of globin chains within red cells or precursors. This results in cell damage, death of red cell precursors in the bone marrow (ineffective erythropoiesis), and haemolysis. The thalassaemias affect people throughout the world.

There are two main types:

- α-Thalassaemia: reduced α chain synthesis
- β-Thalassaemia: reduced β chain synthesis.

**β-Thalassaemia** In homozygous β-thalassaemia there is little or no β chain production, resulting in excess α chains. These combine with whatever δ and γ chains are produced, leading to increased Hb $A_2$ and Hb F. There are three main clinical forms of β-thalassaemia:

- *β-thalassaemia minor (trait)*. This is the asymptomatic heterozygous carrier state. Anaemia is mild or absent, with a low MCV and MCH. Iron stores and serum ferritin levels are normal.
- *β-Thalassaemia intermedia*. This includes patients with moderate anaemia (Hb 7–10 g/dL) that does not require regular blood transfusions. Splenomegaly, bone deformities, recurrent leg ulcers and gallstones are other features. This may be caused by a combination of homozygous β- and α-thalassaemias.
- *β-Thalassaemia major* (homozygous β-thalassaemia). This presents in the first year of life with severe anaemia (*Cooley's anaemia*), failure to thrive and recurrent infections. Hypertrophy of the ineffective bone marrow leads to bony abnormalities: the thalassaemic facies, with an enlarged maxilla and prominent frontal and parietal bones. Resumption of haemopoiesis in the spleen and liver (extramedullary

**Table 5.9**
Types of haemoglobin

| | Haemoglobin | Structure | Comment |
|---|---|---|---|
| Normal | A | $\alpha_2\beta_2$ | 97% of adult haemoglobin |
| | $A_{1c}$ | $\alpha_2\beta_2$ | $\leq 5\%$ of HbA (glycosylated Hb) |
| | $A_2$ | $\alpha_2\delta_2$ | 2% of adult haemoglobin; elevated in $\beta$-thalassaemia |
| | F | $\alpha_2\gamma_2$ | Normal haemoglobin in fetus from 3rd to 9th month; increased in $\beta$-thalassaemia |
| Abnormal chain production | H | $\beta_4$ | Found in $\alpha$-thalassaemia |
| | Barts | $\gamma_4$ | Found in homozygous $\alpha$-thalassaemia, biologically useless |
| Abnormal chain structure | S | $\alpha_2\beta_2$ | Substitution of valine for glutamic acid in position 6 of the $\beta$ chain |
| | C | $\alpha_2\beta_2$ | Substitution of lysine for glutamic acid in position 6 of the $\beta$ chain |

183

haemopoiesis), the chief sites of red cell production in fetal life, leads to hepatosplenomegaly.

## Investigations

In homozygous disease, blood count and film show a hypochromic/microcytic anaemia, raised reticulocyte count and nucleated red cells in the peripheral circulation.

The diagnosis is made by haemoglobin electrophoresis, which shows an increase in Hb F and absent or markedly reduced Hb A.

## Management

In homozygous patients, the mainstay of treatment is blood transfusion, aiming to keep the haemoglobin above 10 g/dL, thus suppressing ineffective erythropoiesis, preventing bony abnormalities and allowing normal development. Iron overload caused by repeated blood transfusions may lead to damage to endocrine glands, liver, pancreas and heart, with death in the second decade from cardiac failure. Treatment with the iron-chelating agent desferrioxamine decreases iron loading. Bone marrow transplantation has been used in some cases of thalassaemia.

*α*-**Thalassaemia**  The clinical manifestations of this disorder vary from a mild anaemia with microcytosis to a severe condition incompatible with life. There are four α-globin genes per cell. The manifestations depend on whether one, two, three or all four of the genes are deleted, and thus whether α chain synthesis is partial or completely absent. In the most severe form, where there is complete absence of α-globin (Hb Barts), infants are stillborn (hydrops fetalis).

# Antenatal diagnosis of haemoglobin abnormalities

It is possible to identify a fetus with severe haemoglobin abnormalities by DNA analysis of chorionic villous samples taken in the first trimester, or by testing umbilical cord blood in the second trimester. Abortion is offered if the fetus is found to be affected. This examination is appropriate if the mother is found to have a haemoglobin defect during antenatal testing and if on subsequent screening, her partner is also affected.

## Sickle cell disease (K&C p. 430)

Sickle cell disease is a family of haemoglobin disorders in which the sickle β-globin gene is inherited. The gene for sickle haemoglobin (haemoglobin S) results in the substitution of the amino acid valine for glutamic acid normally present in position 6 of the β chain of haemoglobin. In the homozygous state (*sickle cell anaemia*) both genes are abnormal (Hb SS), whereas in the heterozygous state (*sickle cell trait*, Hb AS) only one chromosome carries the abnormal gene. Inheritance of the HbS gene from one parent and HbC from the other parent gives rises to Hb SC disease, which tends to run a milder clinical course than sickle cell disease but with more thromboses.

The sickle β gene is spread widely throughout Africa (25% carry the gene), the Middle East and Mediterranean countries. One of the main factors in this distribution is that patients with sickle cell trait have a relative resistance to malaria, so are more likely to survive, breed and pass on their genes.

In the deoxygenated state Hb S molecules link to form chains, and this results in increased rigidity of the red cells, causing the classic sickle appearance. Sickling results in premature destruction of red cells (haemolysis) and obstruction of the microcirculation (vaso-occlusion), leading to tissue infarction. As the production of Hb F is normal, the disease is usually not manifest until Hb F decreases to adult levels at about 6 months of age.

## Clinical features

In the heterozygous state, Hb AS (sickle cell trait), there are usually no symptoms unless the patient is exposed to extreme hypoxia, e.g. very poor anaesthesia.

Symptoms of the homozygous state, Hb SS (sickle cell anaemia), are due to haemolysis and vaso-occlusion.

**Haemolysis** Symptoms vary from mild anaemia to severe haemolysis with recurrent sickle cell crises. Chronic haemolysis is associated with increased formation of pigment gallstones. Most patients with sickle cell anaemia have a steady-state Hb of 6–8 g/dL with a high reticulocyte count (10–20%). Most patients do not have symptoms of anaemia because tissue oxygen delivery is normal owing to a hyperdynamic circulation and the lower oxygen affinity of Hb S, which releases oxygen to the tissues more easily than normal Hb. A rapid fall in the Hb may be due to:

- Aplastic crisis. This is often due to parvovirus B19 infection, which destroys erythrocyte precursors
- Acute sequestration crisis. The liver and spleen become engorged with red cells, leading to a fall in Hb and rapid enlargement of these organs
- Haemolysis due to drugs or infection.

***Vaso-occlusion*** Avascular necrosis of bone marrow results in the bone pain crisis, which may be precipitated by hypoxia, dehydration or infection. In adults, bone pain most commonly affects the juxta-articular parts of the long bones, the ribs, spine and pelvis. In early childhood the small bones of the hands and feet are affected (dactylitis), which may result in shortened deformed bones. Most patients with a painful crisis are managed in the community, but hospital admission is necessary when the pain is not controlled by non-opiate analgesia such as paracetamol and non-steroidal anti-inflammatory drugs, or if there are complications listed in Table 5.10. The management of a painful sickle crisis is summarized in Emergency Box 5.1. Other complications of vaso-occlusion include:

- Splenic atrophy, which results in susceptibility to infection with pneumococcus, *Salmonella* species and haemophilus
- Cerebral infarction, causing fits and hemiplegia
- Retinal ischaemia, which may precipitate proliferative sickle retinopathy and visual loss.

Other complications of sickle cell disease include renal papillary necrosis and chronic renal failure, leg ulcers, and the acute chest syndrome. The latter is the commonest cause of death of adults with sickle cell disease. It is a medical emergency and characterized by fever, cough, dyspnoea and pulmonary infiltrates on the chest X-ray. It is caused by infection, fat embolism from necrotic bone marrow or pulmonary infarction due to sequestration of sickle cells. Sequestration of red cells within the corpora cavernosa causes priapism (prolonged erections) and eventual impotence.

**Table 5.10**
Complications of sickle cell disease requiring inpatient management

Pain uncontrolled by non-opiate analgesia
Swollen painful joints
Central nervous system deficit
Acute sickle chest syndrome or pneumonia
Mesenteric sickling and bowel ischaemia
Splenic or hepatic sequestration
Cholecystitis
Renal papillary necrosis resulting in colic or severe haematuria
Hyphema (a layer of red cells in anterior chamber of eye) or
    retinal detachment

 **Emergency Box 5.1**

**Management of a painful sickle cell crisis in hospital**

- **Analgesia**
  $\Rightarrow$ diclofenac 1 mg/kg every 8 hours orally
  $\Rightarrow$ morphine 10–40 $\mu$g/kg/h by intravenous or
  subcutaneous infusion if no response to diclofenac.
  Side-effects of morphine include nausea, respiratory
  depression and hypotension.
- **Oxygen**, 60% by face mask if arterial oxygen saturation
  < 95%.
- **Rehydrate** with intravenous fluids.
- **Immediate investigations:**
  – full blood count and reticulocyte count
  – urea and electrolytes
  – blood cultures
  – urine microscopy and culture
  – oxygen saturation by pulse oximetry
  – chest X-ray
  – arterial blood gases (if oxygen saturation < 90%
    breathing air, chest X-ray shadowing or respiratory
    symptoms).
- Search for and treat any source of infection.
- Check Hb and reticulocyte count at least once daily.
- Examine daily: the respiratory system for the acute chest
  syndrome, and the abdomen for increase in liver or spleen
  size which may indicate a sequestration crisis.

## Investigations

- Blood count. In sickle cell disease there is a low haemoglobin (6–8 g/dL) with a high reticulocyte count. Patients with sickle cell trait are not anaemic.
- Blood film shows sickled erythrocytes.

Diagnosis is made with Hb electrophoresis showing 80–90% Hb SS and absent Hb A. In addition, sickling can be induced in vitro with sodium metabisulphite.

## Treatment and screening

Asymptomatic anaemia requires no treatment. Folic acid is given to patients with severe haemolysis, and to women before conception and during pregnancy. The risk of pneumococcal infection is reduced by prophylaxis with pneumococcal vaccine and daily oral penicillin. Routine vaccination against *Haemophilus influenzae* is given to all children in the UK. Exchange transfusions may be used to reduce the frequency of crises, or as prophylaxis in pregnancy or before surgery.

In clinical trials hydroxycarbamide (hydroxyurea) has been shown to raise the concentration of fetal Hb and ameliorate the clinical course, but concerns remain over its myelosuppressive side-effects. Bone marrow transplantation from an HLA-matched sibling has been used in some patients with severe disease.

People from areas with a high prevalence of sickle cell disease should be screened before general anaesthesia, and before or during pregnancy.

## Prognosis

The median survival is 40–50 years; the commonest cause of death in adult sickle cell disease is the acute sickle chest syndrome.

# Metabolic red cell disorders (*K&C* p. 432)

A number of red cell enzyme deficiencies may produce haemolytic anaemia, the most common of which is glucose-6-phosphate dehydrogenase (G6PD) deficiency.

### Glucose-6-phosphate dehydrogenase deficiency

G6PD is a vital enzyme in the hexose monophosphate shunt, which maintains glutathione in the reduced state. Glutathione protects against oxidant injury in the red cell. G6PD deficiency is a common heterogeneous X-linked trait found predominantly in African, Mediterranean and Middle Eastern populations.

G6PD deficiency causes neonatal jaundice, chronic haemolytic anaemia, and acute haemolysis precipitated by the ingestion of fava beans and oxidizing drugs such as quinine, sulphonamides and nitrofurantoin. Diagnosis is by direct measurement of enzyme levels in the red cell. Treatment is the avoidance of precipitating factors, and transfusion if necessary.

## Acquired haemolytic anaemia

### Autoimmune haemolytic anaemia (K&C p. 435)

Acquired haemolytic anaemia is due to immunological destruction of red blood cells mediated by autoantibodies directed against antigens on the patient's red blood cells. Autoimmune haemolytic anaemia is classified according to whether the antibody reacts best at body temperature (*warm antibodies*) or at lower temperatures (*cold antibodies*) (Table 5.11). IgG or IgM antibodies attach to the red cell, resulting in extravascular haemolysis through sequestration in the spleen, or in intravascular haemolysis through activation of complement. The autoimmune haemolytic anaemias are diagnosed on the basis of a positive direct antiglobulin test (direct Coombs' test, Fig. 5.3).

#### Warm antibody haemolysis

##### Clinical features

This anaemia occurs at all ages in both sexes, with a variable clinical picture ranging from mild haemolysis to life-threatening anaemia. About 50% are associated with other autoimmune disorders or lymphoma.

**Table 5.11**
Features of autoimmune haemolytic anaemia

| | Warm antibody | Cold antibody |
| --- | --- | --- |
| Temperature at which antibody attaches best to red cell | 37°C | Lower than 37°C |
| Type of antibodies | IgG | IgM |
| Direct Coombs' test | Strongly positive | Positive |
| Cause of primary condition | Idiopathic | Idiopathic |
| Cause of secondary condition | Autoimmune disorders, e.g. SLE<br>Lymphomas<br>Drugs, e.g. methyldopa | Infections<br>  *Mycoplasma* sp.<br>  Infectious mononucleosis<br>  Viruses<br>Lymphomas<br>Paroxysmal cold haemoglobinuria (rare) |

### Direct antiglobulin test

Patient's cells sensitized in vivo
e.g. Autoimmune haemolytic anaemia
   Haemolytic transfusion reaction
   HDN
   Drug-induced immune haemolytic
   Anaemia

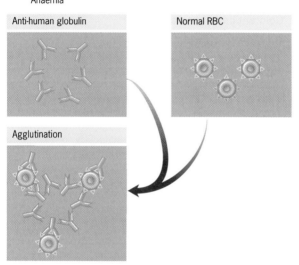

Anti-human globulin

Normal RBC

Agglutination

**Fig. 5.3 Antiglobulin (Coombs' test).** The red blood cells of the patient are washed free of adherent proteins and reacted with antiserum or monoclonal antibodies against various immunoglobulins and complement. The anti-human globulin forms bridges between the sensitized cells causing visible agglutinations. The direct test detects patients' cells sensitized in vivo. HDN, haemolytic disease of newborn; RBC, red blood cell.

### Investigation

There is evidence of haemolysis (p. 180) and the direct Coombs' test is positive. A Coombs' test is a test for antibodies or complement (another protein/enzyme that works with antibodies) attached to the surface of red blood cells. The red blood cells of the patient are reacted with antiserum or monoclonal antibodies prepared against the various immunoglobulins and the third component of complement (C3d). If either or both of these are present on the red cell surface, agglutination of red cells will be detected.

## Management

High-dose steroids (e.g. prednisolone 1 mg/kg daily) induce remission in 80% of cases. Splenectomy is useful in those failing to respond to steroids. Occasionally immunosuppressive drugs such as azathioprine and cyclophosphamide are beneficial.

### Cold antibody haemolysis

## Clinical features

IgM antibodies (cold agglutinins) attach to red cells in the cold peripheral parts of the body and cause agglutination and complement-mediated intravascular haemolysis. Infection with mycoplasma or Epstein–Barr virus may lead to increased synthesis of cold agglutinins (normally produced in insignificant amounts) and produce transient haemolysis. A chronic idiopathic form occurs in elderly people, with recurrent haemolysis and peripheral cyanosis.

## Investigation

There is evidence of haemolysis and the direct Coombs' test is positive. Examination of a peripheral blood film at room temperature shows red cell agglutination.

## Management

This does not usually require treatment other than for the underlying condition and avoiding exposure to cold.

### Drug-induced haemolysis

Two types of mechanisms have been identified:

- In the commonest form, the drug may associate with structures on the red cell membrane and thus be part of the antigen in a haptenic reaction. There is severe complement-mediated intravascular haemolysis which resolves quickly after drug withdrawal.
- The drug may induce a subtle alteration of one component of the red cell membrane, rendering it antigenic. There is extravascular haemolysis and a protracted clinical course.

The mechanisms for drug-induced haemolytic anaemia probably also apply to drug-induced thrombocytopenia and neutropenia.

# Non-immune haemolytic anaemia

**Paroxysmal nocturnal haemoglobinuria** (*K&C* p. 439)

The pathogenic defect in paroxysmal nocturnal haemo-globinuria (PNH) is an inability to produce the glycosyl-phosphatidylinositol (GPI) anchor which tethers several proteins to the cell membrane. Deficiency of two of these proteins, CD59 and delay accelerating factor, renders the red cell exquisitely sensitive to the haemolytic action of complement. The clinical manifestations of this rare disease are related to abnormalities in haemopoietic function including intravascular haemolysis, venous thrombosis and bone marrow aplasia. Progression to myelodysplasia and acute leukaemia can also occur. PNH should be considered in any patient with chronic or episodic haemolysis. Diagnosis is made by demonstrating deficiency of the GPI-anchored proteins on haematopoietic cells by flow cytometry. There is no specific treatment for PNH and management is supportive. Bone marrow transplantation has been successful in selected patients.

**Mechanical haemolytic anaemia** (*K&C* p. 440)

Red cells may be injured by physical trauma in the circulation. Examples of this form of haemolysis include the following:

- Prosthetic heart valves: damage to red cells in their passage through heart
- March haemoglobinuria: damage to red cells in the feet from prolonged marching
- Microangiopathic haemolysis: fragmentation of red cells in abnormal microcirculation caused by malignant hypertension, haemolytic uraemic syndrome or disseminated intravascular coagulation.

# Myeloproliferative and myelodysplastic disorders

Myeloproliferative and myelodysplastic syndromes are both clonal haemopoietic stem cell disorders which arise from a single abnormal multipotential cell in the bone marrow. Both have the potential to transform into acute leukaemia.

*Myelodysplastic syndromes* are characterized by ineffective erythropoiesis and peripheral blood cytopenias (see p. 198). *Myeloproliferative disorders* are characterized by the overproduction of one or more cell lines (myeloid, erythroid or megakaryocyte), and comprise chronic myeloid leukaemia (CML), polycythaemia vera, essential thrombocythaemia and myelofibrosis. These disorders differ from the acute leukaemias (also clonal proliferation of a single cell line), where the cells also do not differentiate normally but where there is progressive accumulation of immature cells.

## Polycythaemia

Polycythaemia is defined as an increase in Hb, packed cell volume (PCV) and red cell count (RCC). These measurements are all concentrations and are therefore directly dependent upon plasma volume as well as red blood cell mass. The production of red cells by the bone marrow is normally regulated by the hormone erythropoietin, which is produced in the kidney. The stimulus for erythropoietin production is tissue hypoxia. *Absolute polycythaemia* (Fig. 5.4) is therefore the result of an appropriate increase in erythropoietin secondary to hypoxia, an inappropriate increase in ery-

194

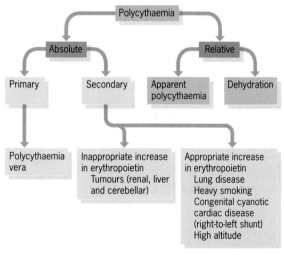

**Fig. 5.4 The causes of polycythaemia.**

thropoietin resulting from abnormal production by certain tumours, or escape by marrow stem cells from erythropoietin control (polycythaemia vera). Absolute polycythaemia must be differentiated from *apparent polycythaemia* (Gaisböck's syndrome), where PCV is normal but plasma volume is decreased. Apparent polycythaemia usually affects middle-aged obese men and is associated with smoking, increased alcohol intake and hypertension. The causes of polycythaemia are shown in Figure 5.4. The most common cause is hypoxia secondary to cardiopulmonary disease. Apparent polycythaemia is uncommon.

## Primary polycythaemia: polycythaemia vera
(*K&C* p. 440)

### Clinical features
Polycythaemia vera, like the other myeloproliferative disorders, occurs principally in middle-aged and elderly people. It is characterized by an excessive proliferation of erythroid, myeloid and megakaryocytic progenitor cells due to a failure of apoptosis. Symptoms and signs are the result of hypervolaemia and hyperviscosity. Typical symptoms include headache, dizziness, tinnitus, visual disturbance, angina pectoris, intermittent claudication, pruritus and venous thrombosis. Physical signs include a plethoric complexion and hepatosplenomegaly as a result of extramedullary haemopoiesis. Splenomegaly, if present, reliably distinguishes primary polycythaemia from the other polycythaemias. There is an increased risk of haemorrhage as a result of friable haemostatic plugs, and gout caused by increased cell turnover and uric acid production.

### Investigations
- Blood count shows a high Hb and PCV. The WCC is raised in 70% and the platelet count in 50% of patients; such abnormalities are rarely present in polycythaemia from other causes.
- Red cell volume, measured with $^{51}$Cr-labelled red cells, is increased.
- Plasma volume, measured using $^{131}$I-labelled albumin dilution, is normal or increased (compare with relative polycythaemia).

- Bone marrow shows erythroid hyperplasia with increased numbers of megakaryocytes.

## Differential diagnosis

This is from secondary and relative polycythaemia. An abdominal ultrasound, arterial $Po_2$ and carboxyhaemoglobin (increased in heavy smokers) and measurement of serum erythropoietin may be necessary to differentiate. Erythropoietin is low or normal in polycythaemia vera, and usually high in secondary polycythaemia.

## Management

There is no cure and treatment is given to maintain a normal blood count and to prevent the complications of the disease, particularly thrombosis and haemorrhage.

- Venesection to maintain PCV < 0.45 L/L. Regular venesection (e.g. 3-monthly) may be all that is needed in many patients.
- Chemotherapy. Hydroxycarbamide (hydroxyurea) and busulfan are particularly useful to reduce the platelet count.
- Radioactive phosphorus ($^{32}$P) is sometimes used in patients over 70 years of age. Its use is restricted in younger patients because of the increased incidence of leukaemic conversion in patients treated with $^{32}$P.
- Allopurinol is given to decrease uric acid levels.

## Prognosis

Median survival in untreated patients is 1–2 years and may be increased to approximately 14 years with treatment. Thirty per cent will develop myelofibrosis and 5% acute leukaemia. The risk of acute myeloid leukaemia is marginally increased by treatment with busulfan or $^{32}$P.

## Secondary polycythaemia *(K&C p. 441)*

Secondary polycythaemia presents with similar clinical features to primary polycythaemia, although the white cell and platelet counts are normal and the spleen is not enlarged. In patients with tumours the primary disease must be treated to lower the level of erythropoietin. In hypoxic patients, oxygen therapy (p. 455) may reduce the Hb, and a small-volume phlebotomy (400 mL) may help those with severe symptoms. Smokers should be advised to stop.

## Primary (essential) thrombocythaemia

(*K&C* p. 442)

Essential thrombocythaemia is characterized by very high platelet counts (usually $> 1000 \times 10^9$/L). Platelet size and function are abnormal, and presentation may be with bleeding or thrombosis. Busulfan, hydroxycarbamide (hydroxyurea) or α-interferon are used to reduce platelet production. Differential diagnosis is from secondary causes of a raised platelet count and other myeloproliferative disorders (Table 5.12).

## Primary myelofibrosis (myelosclerosis)

(*K&C* p. 442)

Myelofibrosis is characterized by haemopoietic stem-cell proliferation associated with marrow fibrosis (abnormal megakaryocyte precursors release fibroblast-stimulating factors such as platelet-derived growth factor).

### Clinical features

There are constitutional symptoms of fever, weight loss and lethargy. Bleeding occurs in the thrombocytopenic patient. There is hepatomegaly and massive splenomegaly caused by extramedullary haemopoiesis.

---

**Table 5.12**
Differential diagnosis of a raised platelet count

Reactive thrombocytosis
    Connective tissue disorders
    Chronic infections
    Inflammatory bowel disease
    Malignancy
    Haemorrhage
    Surgery
    Splenectomy and functional hyposplenism

Primary thrombocythaemia

Primary polycythaemia

Myelofibrosis

Myelodysplasia

### Investigations

- Blood count shows anaemia. The white cell and platelet counts are high initially, but fall with disease progression as a result of marrow fibrosis.
- Blood film examination shows a leucoerythroblastic picture (immature red cells caused by marrow infiltration) and 'teardrop'-shaped red cells.
- Bone marrow is usually unobtainable by aspiration ('dry tap'); trephine biopsy shows increased fibrosis.
- The Philadelphia chromosome is absent; this helps to distinguish myelofibrosis from most cases of CML which may present similarly.

### Management

- Supportive treatment including transfusions for anaemia and allopurinol to decrease serum uric acid levels.
- Hydroxycarbamide (hydroxyurea) or busulfan are used to reduce the raised white cell and platelet count.
- Splenic irradiation may be useful to reduce a large painful spleen.
- Splenectomy is performed if the spleen is very large and painful and the transfusion requirements are high.

### Prognosis

The median survival is 3 years. Transformation to acute myeloid leukaemia occurs in 10–20%.

## Myelodysplasia (K&C p. 443)

Myelodysplasia is a group of acquired bone marrow disorders caused by a defect in stem cells. There is progressive bone marrow failure, which tends to evolve into acute myeloid leukaemia. The myelodysplastic syndromes are predominantly diseases of the elderly, and are increasingly being diagnosed when a routine full blood count shows an unexplained macrocytosis, anaemia, thrombocytopenia or neutropenia. The diagnosis is made on the basis of characteristic blood film and bone marrow appearances. The paradox of peripheral pancytopenia and a hypercellular bone marrow reflects premature cell loss by apoptosis.

For most elderly patients with symptomatic disease treatment is supportive, with red cell and platelet transfusions.

198

Allogeneic bone marrow transplantation offers the hope of cure in the minority of patients who are under the age of 50 years. Overall median survival is 20 months.

## The spleen (K&C p. 443)

The spleen, situated in the left hypochondrium, is the largest lymphoid organ in the body. Its main functions are phagocytosis of old red blood cells, immunological defence, and to act as a 'pool' of blood from which cells may be rapidly mobilized. Pluripotential stem cells are present in the spleen and proliferate in severe haematological stress (*extramedullary haemopoiesis*), e.g. haemolytic anaemia.

## Hypersplenism

Hypersplenism can result from splenomegaly of any cause (Table 5.13). It results in pancytopenia, increased plasma

**Table 5.13**
Causes of splenomegaly

| **Sometimes massive** (extending into the right iliac fossa) | **Moderate** |
|---|---|
| Haematological<br>  Chronic myeloid<br>    leukaemia<br>  Myelofibrosis | Haematological<br>  Lymphomas<br>  Leukaemias<br>  Myeloproliferative disorders<br>  Haemolytic anaemia |
| Infections<br>  Chronic malaria<br>  Schistosomiasis<br>  Kala-azar | Infections<br>  Acute, e.g. endocarditis, typhoid<br>  Chronic, e.g. tuberculosis,<br>    brucellosis<br>  Parasitic, e.g. malaria |
| Other<br>  Tropical splenomegaly<br>  Gaucher's disease (rarely) | Inflammation<br>  Rheumatoid arthritis<br>  Sarcoidosis<br>  Systemic lupus erythematosus |
| | Others<br>  Portal hypertension, e.g. cirrhosis<br>  Amyloidosis<br>  Gaucher's disease |

volume and haemolysis caused by increased destruction of red cells.

## Splenectomy

This is performed mainly for:

- Trauma
- Idiopathic thrombocytopenic purpura
- Haemolytic anaemias
- Hypersplenism.

The main complications are an increased platelet count (thrombophilia) in the short term and overwhelming infection in the longer term. The main infecting organisms are *Streptococcus pneumoniae*, *Haemophilus influenzae* and the meningococci. Vaccination against *S. pneumoniae* and *H. influenzae* should be given to patients about to undergo splenectomy. Immunization with meningococcal group C vaccine is given to all hyposplenic patients; group A vaccine is given to travellers going to areas where there is an increased risk of group A infection. In addition, lifelong antibiotic prophylaxis (e.g. penicillin V 500 mg twice daily) is recommended (*K&C* p. 444)

## Blood products and transfusion

The components of whole blood are prepared by differential centrifugation of blood collected from volunteer donors.

- Blood components, such as red cell and platelet concentrates, fresh frozen plasma (FFP) and cryoprecipitate, are prepared from single donors.
- Plasma derivatives, such as coagulation factor concentrates, albumin and immunoglobulin are prepared using plasma from many donors as the starting material.

*Whole blood* itself is rarely used even for acute blood loss. Use of the required component is a more effective use of a scarce resource.

*Packed red cells and red cell concentrates* are used for acute bleeds (in combination with crystalloid or colloid) and correction of anaemia.

*Platelet concentrates* are used to treat or prevent bleeding in patients with severe thrombocytopenia.

*Fresh frozen plasma* (FFP) is separated from blood cells and frozen for storage. It contains all the coagulation factors and is used in acquired coagulation factor deficiencies.

*Cryoprecipitate* is the supernatant obtained after thawing of FFP at 4°C. It contains fibrinogen, antihaemophilic factor (factor VIII), fibrin stabilizing factor (factor XIII), and von Willebrand factor (vWf). It is used for the replacement of fibrinogen and von Willebrand factor.

*Albumin* is sometimes given to patients with acute severe hypoalbuminaemia.

*Immunoglobulins* are used in patients with hypogamma-globulinaemia to prevent infection and in patients with idiopathic thrombocytopenic purpura. Specific immuno-globulin, e.g. anti-hepatitis B, is used after exposure of a non-immune patient to infections.

## Blood groups (K&C p. 445)

The blood groups are determined by antigens on the surface of red cells; more than 400 blood groups have been found. The ABO (Table 5.14) and rhesus (Rh) systems are the two most important blood groups, but incompatibilities involving many other blood groups (such as Kell and Duffy) may cause haemolytic transfusion reactions and/or haemolytic disease of the newborn. Compatibility testing is performed

**Table 5.14**
Antigens and antibodies in the ABO system

| Blood group | Serum antibody | UK frequency (%) | Comment |
|---|---|---|---|
| O | Anti-A and anti-B | 44 | 'Universal donors' are O Rh negative |
| A | Anti-B | 45 | |
| B | Anti-A | 8 | |
| AB | None | 3 | Universal recipients |

by the transfusion service in order to select donor blood of the same ABO and Rh group as the recipient and to screen the patient's serum or plasma for antibodies against other red cell antigens that may cause a reduction in the survival of the transfused red cells. Many hospitals have guidelines for the ordering of blood for elective surgery. Many operations in which blood is required only occasionally can be classified as 'group and save' in order to conserve blood usage. In this case ABO and Rh testing is performed along with the antibody screen. Should blood unexpectedly be required during the course of the procedure, compatible units can be released within a matter of minutes after an immediate spin crossmatch whereby the patient's serum or plasma is incubated with the donor red cells to confirm ABO compatibility. The procedure for checking blood before transfusion is illustrated in Table 5.15.

Table 5.15
Blood transfusion checking procedure

**Blood must be checked by two nurses, one of whom is a registered nurse, before transfusion**

**Check the blood bag is not leaking or wet and has a compatibility label attached**

**Check the patient's surname, first names, sex, date of birth, hospital number on:**
Patient's name band which the patient must be wearing
Blood transfusion request form
Compatibility label
Medical case notes
Intravenous fluid prescription chart

**Check the expiry date of the unit of blood on:**
Compatibility label
Blood bag

**Check the blood group and unit number on:**
Blood transfusion request form
Compatibility label

**Record the unit number of the blood on:**
Intravenous fluid prescription chart

**Date and time and signature of both nurses on:**
Blood transfusion request form
Compatibility label
Intravenous fluid prescription chart

# Complications of transfusing red blood cells *(K&C p. 447)*

- ABO incompatibility is the most serious complication and often results from simple clerical errors, leading to the incorrect labelling and identification of blood and patient's blood sample for crossmatching. There is an immediate reaction, starting within minutes of the transfusion, leading to intravascular haemolysis, rigors, lumbar pain, dyspnoea and hypotension. The transfusion must be stopped and the donor units returned to the blood transfusion laboratory for testing with a new blood sample from the patient. Emergency treatment may be needed to maintain the blood pressure (p. 508). Autoimmune haemolysis may develop about a week after transfusion in patients alloimmunized by previous transfusions in whom the antibody level is too low to be detected during compatibility testing.

- Febrile reactions are usually the result of antileucocyte antibodies in the recipient acting against transfused leucocytes, leading to the release of pyrogens. The introduction of leucocyte-depleted blood in the UK in 1999, to minimize the risk of transmission of variant Creutzfeldt–Jakob disease by blood transfusion, is expected to reduce the incidence of febrile reactions.

- Anaphylactic reactions are seen in patients lacking IgA but who produce anti-IgA that reacts with IgA in the transfused blood. This is a medical emergency (p. 514). Urticarial reactions are treated by slowing of the infusion and giving intravenous antihistamines, e.g. chlorphenamine (chlorpheniramine) 10 mg i.v.

- Transmission of infection has decreased now that donated blood is tested for hepatitis B surface antigen and antibodies to hepatitis C and HIV. Other viruses that may cause post-transfusion hepatitis include cytomegalovirus and Epstein–Barr virus.

- Heart failure may occur, particularly in elderly people and those having large transfusions.

- Complications of massive transfusion (> 10 units within 24 hours) include hypocalcaemia, hyperkalaemia and hypothermia. Bleeding may occur

as a result of depletion of platelets and clotting factors in stored blood.
- Post-transfusion purpura, in which severe thrombocytopenia develops 7–10 days after the transfusion. Antibodies develop against the human platelet antigen 1a, leading to immune destruction of the patient's own platelets.

Concerns about the safety of blood transfusion have led to increased interest in strategies for avoiding or reducing the use of donor blood. These include artificial haemoglobin solutions and autologous blood transfusion. The latter is more popular in developing countries and involves collection of blood from the donor/patient either preoperatively or by intraoperative blood salvage.

## Bleeding disorders

A bleeding disorder is suggested when the patient has unexplained (i.e. no history of trauma) bruising or bleeding, or prolonged bleeding in response to injury or surgery, e.g. after tooth extraction.

## Reactions involved in haemostasis

(*K&C* p. 453)

Haemostasis is the process of blood clot formation at the site of vessel injury. When a blood vessel wall breaks, the haemostatic response must be quick, localized to the site of injury, and carefully regulated. Abnormal bleeding or a propensity to non-physiologic thrombosis (i.e. thrombosis not required for haemostatic regulation) may occur when specific elements of these processes are missing or dysfunctional.

Haemostasis is a complex process and depends on interactions between the vessel wall, platelets and coagulation and fibrinolytic mechanisms.

- *Blood vessel damage* leads to immediate vasoconstriction, reducing blood flow to the injured area and allowing contact activation of platelets and coagulation factors.

- *Formation of the platelet plug.* The intact vascular endothelium prevents the adherence of platelets. Intimal injury and exposure of subendothelial elements such as collagen lead to the adherence of platelets on the subendothelial matrix. Platelet *adhesion* to collagen is dependent on platelet membrane receptors, glycoprotein Ia (GPIa), which binds directly to collagen, and glycoprotein Ib (GPIb), which binds to von Willebrand factor (vWF) in the plasma; vWF in turn adheres to collagen. Deficiency of GPIb or vWF leads to congenital bleeding disorders: Bernard–Soulier disease and von Willebrand's disease, respectively. Following adhesion, platelets spread along the subendothelium and *release* the contents of their cytoplasmic granules containing ADP, serotonin, thromboxane $A_2$, fibrinogen and other factors. Release of ADP results in both exposure of, and a conformational change in the GP IIb/IIIa receptor on the platelet surface, leading to binding of the divalent molecule, fibrinogen, that bridges the activated platelets (*aggregation*). The importance of GP IIb/IIIa is illustrated by the clinical utility of GP IIb/IIIa antagonists in the treatment of coronary disease (p. 402). During aggregation, platelet membrane receptors are exposed, providing a surface for the interaction of coagulation factors and ultimately the formation of a stable haemostatic plug.

- *Clotting cascade and propagation of the clot.* The clotting cascade involves a series of enzymatic reactions leading to the conversion of soluble plasma fibrinogen to fibrin clot (Fig. 5.5). The local generation of fibrin enmeshes and reinforces the platelet plug. All of these proteins are synthesized in the liver except vWf, which is synthesized in megakaryocytes and endothelial cells. The vitamin K-dependent enzymes are prothrombin, factors VII, IX and X. Traditionally, the clotting cascade is depicted as consisting of an intrinsic and extrinsic pathway. Both pathways converge on the activation of factor X, which then activates prothrombin to thrombin, the final enzyme of the clotting cascade. It is now established that the generation or exposure of tissue factor (TF) at the wound site is the primary

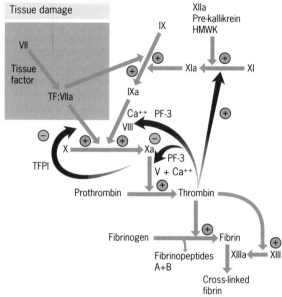

**Fig. 5.5 Coagulation cascade.** The pathway in vivo begins with activation of factor IX by factor VIIa. The factor XII and pre-kallikrein reactions are probably only relevant in vitro. Factor XI is activated by thrombin in vivo. HMWK, high-molecular-weight kininogen.

physiological event in initiating clotting. Deficiencies in the major proteins involved in the initiation of the intrinsic pathway, such as factor XII, are not associated with excessive bleeding.

## Limitation of coagulation

Coagulation would lead to dangerous occlusion of blood vessels if it were not limited to the site of injury by protective mechanisms:

**Rapid blood flow** Rapid blood flow at the periphery of the damaged area dilutes and removes coagulation factors.

### Circulating inhibitors of the coagulation factors

- Antithrombin binds to and forms stable complexes with coagulation factors. Activity is increased by heparin.

- Active protein C inactivates factors V and VIII.
- Protein S is a cofactor for protein C.

Inherited deficiency or abnormality of these natural anti-coagulant proteins is termed *thrombophilia* and places the patient at increased risk of both arterial and venous thrombosis.

***The fibrinolytic system*** The plasma protein plasminogen is converted to plasmin by activators present in the tissue and endothelial cells. Plasmin induces lysis of cross-linked (X-linked) fibrin, resulting in the formation of various X-linked fibrin degradation products (FDPs), which include D-dimers which can easily be measured using monoclonal antibodies.

Bleeding disorders are therefore the result of a defect in vessels, platelets or the coagulation pathway (Table 5.16).

## Investigation of bleeding disorders

The nature of the defect and therefore the most appropriate initial investigations may be suggested by the history and examination, e.g. family history, intercurrent disease, alcohol consumption, drugs. Vascular/platelet bleeding is

---

**Table 5.16**
Classification of bleeding disorders

**Blood vessel defect**
Hereditary
    Hereditary haemorrhagic telangiectasia (rare)
    Connective tissue disorders: Marfan's and Ehlers–Danlos
        syndromes
Acquired
    Severe infections: meningococcal, typhoid
    Drugs: steroids
    Allergic: Henoch–Schönlein purpura (mainly children)
    Others: scurvy, senile purpura
    Easy bruising syndrome

**Platelet defect**
Decreased platelet number or decreased function

**Coagulation defect**
Hereditary
    Haemophilia A or B, von Willebrand's disease
Acquired
    Anticoagulant treatment, liver disease, disseminated
        intravascular coagulation

---

characterized by bruising of the skin and bleeding from mucosal membranes. Bleeding into the skin is manifest as petechiae (small capillary haemorrhages of a few mm diameter) and superficial ecchymoses (larger areas of bleeding). The inherited coagulation disorders are typically associated with haemarthroses (bleeding into joints) and muscle haematomas. The most common cause of abnormal bleeding is thrombocytopenia.

- Platelet count and blood film will show the number and morphology of platelets and any blood disorder such as leukaemia.
- Coagulation tests are abnormal with deficiencies or inhibitors of the clotting factors. If the abnormal result is corrected by the addition of normal plasma to the patient's plasma in the assay, then the result is abnormal as a result of deficiency and not of inhibitors.
  - The prothrombin time (PT) is prolonged with abnormalities of factors VII, X, V, II or I, liver disease, or if the patient is on warfarin. The international normalized ratio (INR) is the ratio of the patient's PT to a normal control when using the international reference preparation. The advantage of the INR over the PT, is that it uses international standards and thus anticoagulant control can be compared in different hospitals across the world.
  - The activated partial thromboplastin time (APTT) is prolonged with deficiencies or inhibitors of one or more of the following factors: XII, XI, IX, VIII, X, V or I (but not factor VII).
  - Thrombin time (TT) is prolonged with fibrinogen deficiency, dysfibrinogenaemia (normal levels but abnormal function), heparin treatment or disseminated intravascular coagulation.
  The normal ranges of these tests vary from laboratory to laboratory and patient results must be compared with that laboratory reference range.
- The bleeding time is a measure of the interaction of platelets with the blood vessel wall and is abnormal with von Willebrand's disease, with blood vessel defects, and when there is a decrease in the number or function of platelets.

These tests will localize the site of the problem. Further specialized investigations, e.g. platelet aggregation studies and measurement of fibrinogen, FDPs and individual clotting factors, will be necessary to identify the exact haemostatic defect correctly.

## Platelet defects

Platelet defects are the result of thrombocytopenia (platelet count $< 150 \times 10^9$/L; Table 5.17) or disorders of platelet function, e.g. those occurring with aspirin treatment and uraemia. Congenital abnormalities of platelet number (e.g. Fanconi's anaemia, Wiskott–Aldrich syndrome) or function (e.g. Bernard–Soulier syndrome) are all extremely rare.

Mild thrombocytopenia can be artefactual and due to platelet clumping or a blood clot in the sample. This is excluded by asking the haematologist to confirm an unexpectedly low count by manual differentiation. Spontaneous bleeding from skin and mucous membranes is unlikely to

**Table 5.17**
Causes of thrombocytopenia

| Impaired production | Excessive destruction |
|---|---|
| **Bone marrow failure** | **Immune** |
| Megaloblastic anaemia | Autoimmune thrombocytopenia |
| Leukaemia | Secondary immune (SLE, CLL, |
| Myeloma | viruses, drugs, e.g. heparin) |
| Myelofibrosis | Post-transfusion purpura |
| Myelodysplasia | |
| Solid tumour infiltration | **Sequestration** |
| Aplastic anaemia | Hypersplenism |
|    drugs | |
|    chemicals | **Dilutional** |
|    viruses | Massive transfusion |
|    paroxysmal nocturnal | |
|      haemoglobinuria | **Other** |
| | Disseminated intravascular |
| |   coagulation |
| | Thrombotic thrombocytopenic |
| |   purpura |
| | Haemolytic uraemic syndrome |

SLE, systemic lupus erythematosus; CLL, chronic lymphocytic leukaemia
Thrombocytopenia due to impaired production is usually also associated with failure of red and white cell production

occur with platelet counts above $20 \times 10^9/L$. Increased destruction or decreased production can be differentiated by bone marrow examination, which will show respectively increased or decreased numbers of megakaryocytes (platelet precursors). When the platelet count is very low or the risk of bleeding is high, then platelet concentrate administration is indicated.

# Autoimmune thrombocytopenic purpura

(K&C p. 458)

Thrombocytopenia results from immune destruction of platelets. Acute autoimmune thrombocytopenic purpura (AITP) is seen in children, often following a viral infection. There is rapid onset of purpura, which is usually self-limiting and becomes chronic in only about 5% of cases. Chronic AITP is more commonly seen in adults and platelet autoantibodies are detected in 60–70% of patients.

## Aetiology

Chronic AITP is usually idiopathic, but may occur with autoimmune disorders, e.g. systemic lupus erythematosus, thyroid disease, chronic lymphatic leukaemia and some viral infections, e.g. HIV. The same drugs that cause autoimmune haemolytic anaemia may also cause thrombocytopenia (and neutropenia).

## Clinical features

The condition is characteristically seen in young women. There is a fluctuating course, with easy bruising, epistaxis and menorrhagia. Major haemorrhage is rare.

## Investigation

There is thrombocytopenia with normal or increased megakaryocytes on bone marrow examination. The detection of antiplatelet autoantibodies is unnecessary in a straightforward case.

## Management

Platelet transfusion and/or high-dose intravenous immunoglobulin produce a rapid but transient rise in the platelet count and may be useful in severe haemorrhage.

Prednisolone (60 mg/day) is the initial treatment of choice, and 20% will have a complete and sustained response. Splenectomy, which has a 60% cure rate, is indicated in those with moderate to severe thrombocytopenia who fail medical treatment. Immunosuppressive drugs (e.g. azathioprine) are indicated in refractory cases.

## Inherited coagulation disorders

Inherited disorders usually involve a deficiency of only one coagulation factor, whereas acquired disorders involve a deficiency of several factors.

### Haemophilia A (K&C p. 460)

This is the result of a deficiency of factor VIII:C, which is one part of the factor VIII molecule. It is inherited as an X-linked recessive, affecting 1 in 5000 males.

### *Clinical features*

Clinical features depend on the plasma levels of factor VIII:C. If more than 5% of the normal level is present the disease is mild, with post-traumatic bleeding only. Levels of less than 1% are associated with frequent spontaneous bleeding into muscles and joints that can lead to a crippling arthropathy. The joints most frequently involved are the knees, elbows, ankles, shoulders and hips.

### *Investigations*

The APTT is prolonged and plasma factor VIII:C levels are reduced. The PT and bleeding time are normal.

### *Management*

- Intravenous injection of factor VIII concentrates is the mainstay of treatment. They are given as prophylaxis, e.g. before and after surgery, or to treat an acute bleeding episode. Most severely affected patients are now given prophylaxis three times weekly from early childhood to try to prevent permanent joint damage. Many patients also have a supply of factor VIII concentrates at home to inject at the first sign of bleeding. Recombinant factor VIII is now well established as the treatment of choice, though cost constraints have resulted in some patients still being offered treatment with plasma-derived concentrates.

- Synthetic vasopressin (DDAVP) – intravenous, subcutaneous or intranasal administration – raises the level of factor VIII and may be used to treat patients with mild haemophilia.
- The cloning of the factor VIII gene, and progress in the development of gene-delivery systems, have led to considerable interest in the possibility that haemophilia A could be 'cured' by gene therapy.

## Complications

Recurrent bleeding into joints may lead to deformity and arthritis. In the past, multiple transfusions were associated with an increased risk of acquiring hepatitis C and HIV. This risk has been virtually eliminated because of the exclusion of high-risk blood donors, screening of donors and heat treatment of factor VIII concentrates. Ten per cent of people with haemophilia develop antibodies to factor VIII, and may need massive doses to overcome this. Recombinant factor VIIa is used to 'bypass' the inhibitor and shows promise in treating these patients.

### Haemophilia B (Christmas disease) (*K&C* p. 462)
This is the result of a deficiency of factor IX, and affects 1 in 30 000 males. Inheritance and clinical features are the same as for haemophilia A. Treatment is with factor IX concentrates.

### Von Willebrand's disease (vWD) (*K&C* p. 463)
vWD is the most common inherited bleeding disorder and is caused by an inherited deficiency of von Willebrand factor, an essential cofactor for normal platelet adhesion to damaged subendothelium. This factor also serves as a carrier for factor VIII:C to form the whole VIII complex.

## Clinical features

Types 1 and 2 are mild forms, with autosomal dominant inheritance and characterized by mucosal bleeding (nose bleeds and gastrointestinal bleeding) and prolonged bleeding after dental treatment or surgery.

Type 3 patients have more severe bleeding, but rarely experience the joint and muscle bleeds seen in haemophilia A.

## Investigations
Prolonged bleeding time reflects a defect in platelet adhesion. There is a prolonged APTT, normal PT and decreased plasma levels of VIII:C and VIII:vWF.

## Management
This depends on the severity of the bleeding, and includes treatment with factor VIII concentrates and synthetic vasopressin (DDAVP).

# Acquired coagulation disorders
**Disseminated intravascular coagulation** (*K&C* p. 463)
There is widespread generation of fibrin within blood vessels, caused by initiation of the coagulation pathway. There is consumption of platelets and coagulation factors, and secondary activation of fibrinolysis leading to production of fibrin degradation products (FDPs), which contribute to coagulation by inhibiting fibrin polymerization.

213

## Aetiology
Intravascular coagulation is initiated by:

- Release of procoagulant substances into the blood (malignancy, amniotic fluid embolism, abruptio placentae and snake bites)
- Contact of blood with an abnormal surface (septicaemia, burns and grafts)
- Generation of procoagulant substances in the blood (promyelocytic leukaemia, haemolytic transfusion reaction).

## Clinical features
The presentation varies from no bleeding at all to complete haemostatic failure, with bleeding from venepuncture sites and the nose and mouth. Thrombotic events may occur as a result of vessel occlusion by platelets and fibrin.

## Investigations

There is thrombocytopenia, prolonged PT, APTT and TT, decreased fibrinogen and elevated FDPs. The blood film shows fragmented red cells. In mild cases with compensatory increase of coagulation factors the only abnormality may be an increase in the FDPs, or in the D-dimer fragment.

## Management

- Treat the underlying condition.
- Platelets, fresh frozen plasma, cryoprecipitate and red cell concentrates are indicated in patients who are bleeding.

### Vitamin K deficiency (*K&C* p. 463)

Vitamin K is needed for the formation of active factors II, VII, IX and X. Deficiency, which occurs in malabsorption of vitamin K and with warfarin treatment (an inhibitor of vitamin K synthesis), leads to an increase in PT and APTT. Treatment, if required, is with parenteral phytomenadione (vitamin K).

### Liver disease (*K&C* p. 463)

Liver disease results in a number of defects of haemostasis: vitamin K deficiency in cholestasis, reduced synthesis of clotting factors, thrombocytopenia and functional abnormalities of platelets. DIC may occur in acute liver failure.

## Thrombosis

A thrombus is defined as a solid mass formed in the circulation from the constituents of the blood during life. Fragments of thrombi (emboli) may break off and block vessels downstream.

### Arterial thrombosis (*K&C* p. 465)

Arterial thrombosis is usually the result of atheroma, which forms particularly in areas of turbulent blood flow, such as the bifurcation of arteries. Platelets adhere to the damaged vascular endothelium and aggregate in response to ADP and thromboxane $A_2$. This may stimulate blood coagulation, leading to complete occlusion of the vessel, or embolization resulting in distal obstruction.

## Prevention and treatment of arterial thrombosis

### Prevention of thrombosis is with antiplatelet drugs

- Aspirin inhibits cyclo-oxygenase reducing production of thromboxane $A_2$ (p. 500). It is the most commonly used antiplatelet drug.
- Dipyridamole inhibits phosphodiesterase-mediated breakdown of cyclic AMP, which prevents platelet activation.
- Clopidogrel and ticlopidine block platelet aggregation and prolong platelet survival by inhibiting the binding of ADP to its platelet receptor. Ticlopidine has been associated with granulocytopenia and thrombotic thrombocytopenic purpura.
- Antibodies (e.g. abciximab), peptides (e.g. eptifibatide), and non-peptide antagonists (e.g. tirofiban) block the receptor of glycoprotein IIb/IIIa, inhibiting the final common pathway of platelet aggregation. Excessive bleeding has been a problem and research continues to identify their clinical role.

### Treatment of thrombosis (thrombolytic therapy)

- Streptokinase is a purified fraction of the filtrate obtained from cultures of haemolytic streptococci. It forms a complex with plasminogen which activates other plasminogen molecules to form plasmin. The dose in myocardial infarction is 1.5 million units given by infusion over 1 hour. The main disadvantage of streptokinase is the indiscriminate activation of plasminogen both in clots and in the circulation, leading to an increased risk of haemorrhage. Nevertheless, this is currently the thrombolytic agent of choice.
- Tissue-type plasminogen activator (tPA, alteplase, reteplase) is produced using recombinant gene technology, and was claimed to be more specific for clot-bound plasminogen. However, it has not been shown to produce fewer bleeding episodes than streptokinase.

Thrombosis

The use of thrombolytic therapy in myocardial infarction is discussed on page 406. The main risk of thrombolysis is bleeding. Contraindications are a recent major bleed, stroke (within 2 months), uncontrolled hypertension, surgery or other invasive procedure (within 10 days), and bleeding disorders.

## Venous thrombosis

Unlike arterial thrombosis, venous thrombosis usually occurs in normal vessels, often in the deep veins of the leg. It originates around the valves as red thrombi consisting of red cells and fibrin. Propagation occurs, inducing a risk of embolization to the pulmonary vessels. Chronic venous obstruction in the leg results in a permanently swollen leg which is prone to ulceration (post-phlebitic syndrome). Factors predisposing to venous thromboembolism are listed in Table 5.18. The clinical features and investigation of deep venous thrombosis and pulmonary embolism are discussed on pages 441 and 426.

**Table 5.18**
Risk factors for venous thromboembolism

| Patient factors | Disease or surgical procedure |
| --- | --- |
| Age | Trauma or surgery, especially pelvis, hip or lower limb |
| Obesity | Malignancy |
| Varicose veins | Cardiac failure |
| Long air travel | Recent myocardial infarction |
| Immobility (bed rest > 4 days) | Infection |
| Pregnancy and puerperium | Inflammatory bowel disease |
| Previous deep vein thrombosis or pulmonary embolism | Nephrotic syndrome |
| Thrombophilia | High doses of oestrogens |
| Antithrombin deficiency | Polycythaemia |
| Protein C or S deficiency | Thrombocythaemia |
| Resistance to activated protein C (factor V Leiden mutation) | Paroxysmal nocturnal haemoglobinuria |
| Prothrombin gene variant | Sickle cell anaemia |
| Homocysteinaemia | |
| Antiphospholipid antibody | |

### *Prevention and treatment of venous thromboembolism* (*K&C* p. 468)

Heparin and warfarin are the two drugs used most frequently in the prevention and treatment of thromboembolism (Table 5.19). In general, prophylaxis of venous thromboembolism relies on measures that prevent stasis, such as early mobilization, elevation of the legs and compression stockings, with heparin reserved for higher-risk patients. Low-molecular-weight heparins (e.g. enoxaparin 20–40 mg s.c. daily depending on risk), produced by the enzymatic or chemical breakdown of the heparin molecule, are now preferred to conventional heparin for venous prophylaxis in most cases. These can be administered on a once-daily basis, have greater efficacy than conventional heparin in high-risk patients, and do not require monitoring of clotting times.

Treatment of established thromboembolism:

- Obtain objective evidence of thrombosis as soon as possible; heparin treatment is often started on the basis of clinical suspicion.
- Perform a coagulation screen and platelet count before starting treatment to exclude a pre-existing haemostatic effect.
- Heparin treatment:
  - Low-molecular-weight heparin, e.g. enoxaparin 1.0 mg/kg s.c. every 12 hours. Where feasible, selected patients with DVT can be safely treated with LMW heparin as outpatients.

  OR
  - Give 5000 units of standard (unfractionated) heparin intravenously (10 000 units in severe pulmonary embolism) as a loading dose and continue with an intravenous infusion of 1000–2000 units per hour, or subcutaneous injections of 15 000 units every 12 hours. Check the APPT daily 4–6 hours after dose of heparin. Adjust the heparin dose to maintain an APPT of 1.5 to 2.5 times control.
- Warfarin 5–10 mg orally is started at the same time as the heparin.
- The dose of warfarin is adjusted to maintain the INR usually at two to three times the control value.

**Table 5.19**
Anticoagulant treatment

| | Heparin | Warfarin |
|---|---|---|
| Route of administration | s.c./i.v. | Oral |
| Half-life | 2 hours, longer for LMW | 2 days |
| Mode of action | Potentiates antithrombotic effects of antithrombin | Inhibits vitamin K-dependent gamma carboxylation of factors II, VII, IX and X |
| Monitoring | APPT | PT/INR |
| Reversal of anticoagulation (usually only if patient is bleeding) | Stop heparin Intravenous protamine sulphate 20–50 mg over 10 min FFP if life-threatening bleed | Stop warfarin Vitamin K, 1 mg by slow intravenous injection |

**Table 5.20**
Indications for oral anticoagulation and target INR

Target INR

| | |
|---|---|
| 2.5 | Pulmonary embolism, deep vein thrombosis, symptomatic inherited thrombophilia, atrial fibrillation, cardioversion, mural thrombus, cardiomyopathy |
| 3.5 | Recurrence of venous thromboembolism while on warfarin therapy, antiphospholipid syndrome, mechanical prosthetic heart valve, coronary artery graft thrombosis |

- Heparin can be discontinued when the INR is in the therapeutic range (Table 5.20).
- Major side-effects of heparin therapy are bleeding and thrombocytopenia. The platelet count should be measured in all patients receiving heparin for more than 5 days.

Anticoagulation for 6 weeks is sufficient for patients after their first thrombosis with a precipitating cause, provided there are no persisting risk factors. Long-term anticoagulation is required for those with repeated episodes or continuing risk factors.

219

# The haematological malignancies

## The leukaemias (*K&C* p. 489)

The leukaemias are malignant neoplasms of the haemopoietic stem cells, characterized by diffuse replacement of the bone marrow by neoplastic cells. In most cases, the leukaemic cells spill over into the blood, where they may be seen in large numbers. The cells may also infiltrate the liver, spleen, lymph nodes and other tissues throughout the body. They are rare diseases with an annual overall incidence of 5 per 100 000.

Leukaemias are classified on the basis of the cell type involved and the state of maturity of the leukaemic cells. Thus acute leukaemias are characterized by the presence of very immature cells (blast cells) and by a rapidly fatal course in untreated patients. Chronic leukaemias are associated, at least initially, with more mature leucocytes and a relatively indolent course. Acute and chronic leukaemias are further subdivided into the cell type involved:

- Acute myelogenous leukaemia (AML)
- Acute lymphoblastic leukaemia (ALL)
- Chronic myeloid leukaemia (CML)
- Chronic lymphocytic leukaemia (CLL).

## Aetiology
In most cases the aetiology is unknown.

**Genetic factors** Genetic factors are suggested by the increased incidence in patients with chromosomal disorders (e.g. Down's syndrome) and in identical twins of affected patients. Chromosomal abnormalities have been described in patients with leukaemia. The earliest described was the Philadelphia (Ph) chromosome, found in 95% of cases with CML and some patients with ALL. In the Ph chromosome the long arm of chromosome 22 is shortened by reciprocal translocation to the long arm of chromosome 9 (t9;22). Bcr-abl, a chimeric protein with tyrosine kinase activity, results from the formation of the Ph chromosome. This enzyme is central to the signalling machinery that controls the proliferation of cells and its incessant activity results in altered cell growth, stromal attachment and apoptosis. Inhibitors of the Bcr-abl tyrosine kinase activity may offer new opportunities for cancer-specific therapy. The leukaemic cells of most patients with acute promyelocytic leukaemia have the translocation t(15;17) involving the retinoic acid receptor alpha (*RARa*) on chromosome 17 and the promyelocytic leukaemia gene (*PML*) on chromosome 15. The resulting PML-RARa fusion protein shows reduced sensitivity to retinoic acid and prevents differentiation of myeloid cells.

## Environmental factors
- Chemicals, e.g. benzene compounds used in industry
- Drugs, e.g. chemotherapy using chlorambucil and procarbazine
- Radiation exposure, e.g. nuclear generators and treatment for Hodgkin's disease.

# Treatment of haematological malignancies

The treatment of the haematological malignancies is based on the use of chemotherapy and radiotherapy. Surgery and other treatments (e.g. steroids and interferon) are used less often.

## *Chemotherapeutic agents* (K&C p. 481)

There are many chemotherapy drugs in common use. They directly damage DNA and RNA and kill cells by promoting apoptosis and sometimes cell necrosis. They therefore affect not only tumour cells, but also the rapidly dividing normal cells of the bone marrow, gastrointestinal tract and germinal epithelium. The principal side-effects are:

- Bone marrow suppression, leading to anaemia, thrombocytopenia and infection
- Mucositis, causing mouth ulceration
- Loss of hair (alopecia)
- Sterility, which can be irreversible.

To minimize these side-effects, chemotherapy is given at intervals to allow some recovery of normal cell function between cycles. Nausea and vomiting may be severe with some drugs, such as cisplatin, and is related to the direct actions of cytotoxic agents on the brainstem chemoreceptor trigger zone. Antiemetics such as metoclopramide and domperidone are used initially, but the serotonin 5-HT$_3$ antagonists (ondansetron and granisetron) combined with dexamethasone are used for severe vomiting. Chemotherapy drugs may themselves cause cancer, particularly acute leukaemia presenting years after treatment. Finally there are additional side-effects that are specific to one class of drug, e.g. cardiotoxicity with the anthracyclines such as doxorubicin.

## *Radiotherapy* (K&C p. 487)

Radiation induces strand breaks in DNA and induces apoptosis. The complications of radiotherapy depend on the radiosensitivity of normal tissue in the path of the radiation field. General side-effects are lethargy and loss of energy. There may be damage to the skin (erythema and

221

desquamation), gut (nausea, mucosal ulceration and diarrhoea), testes (sterility) and bone marrow (anaemia, leucopenia).

## Acute leukaemia (K&C p. 490)

The acute leukaemias are characterized by a clonal proliferation of myeloid or lymphoid precursors with reduced capacity to differentiate into more mature cellular elements. There is accumulation of leukaemic cells in the bone marrow, peripheral blood and other tissues with a reduction in red cells, platelets and neutrophils.

### Epidemiology

Both types of acute leukaemia can occur in all age groups, but ALL is predominantly a disease of childhood, whereas AML is seen most frequently in older adults (middle-aged and elderly).

### Clinical features

These are the result of marrow failure: anaemia, bleeding and infection, e.g. sore throat and pneumonia. Sometimes there is peripheral lymphadenopathy and hepatosplenomegaly.

### Investigations

A definitive diagnosis is made on the peripheral blood film and a bone marrow aspirate. The various subtypes (Table 5.21) are classified on the basis of morphology and immunophenotyping, and cytogenetic studies of blast cells. However, the presence of Auer rods (a rod-like conglomeration of granules in the cytoplasm) within blast cells is pathognomonic of AML. If the patient has a fever, blood cultures and chest radiograph are essential.

- The full blood count shows anaemia and thrombocytopenia. The white cell count is usually raised, but may be normal or low.
- The peripheral blood film shows characteristic leukaemic blast cells.
- Bone marrow aspirate usually shows increased cellularity, with a high percentage of abnormal lymphoid or myeloid blast cells.

**Table 5.21**
The World Health Organization classification of acute leukaemia

**a. AML (acute myeloid leukaemia)**
1. AML with recurrent cytogenetic abnormalities (including acute promyelocytic leukaemia with t(15;17) or variants
2. AML with multi-lineage dysplasia (usually secondary to a pre-existing myelodysplastic syndrome)
3. Therapy-related AML, i.e. occurring after chemotherapy or radiotherapy
4. AML – other (including minimally differentiated AML)
5. Acute biphenotypic leukaemia (acute leukaemia expressing both lymphoid and myeloid phenotype)

**b. ALL (acute lymphoblastic leukaemia)**
1. Precursor B acute lymphoblastic leukaemia
2. Burkitt cell leukaemia
3. Precursor T acute lymphoblastic leukaemia

## Management

The aim of treatment is to achieve complete remission (defined as a normal full blood count and less than 5% of blasts in the bone marrow) and restore the patient to a normal state of health.

223

*General* Before starting treatment the following need to be considered:

- Correction of anaemia and thrombocytopenia by administration of blood and platelets
- Treatment of infection with intravenous antibiotics
- Prevention of the acute tumour lysis syndrome (ATLS) with adequate hydration and allopurinol. ATLS results from a massive release of cellular breakdown products consequent upon tumour cell death following effective therapy. The biochemical disturbances include hyperkalaemia, hyperuricaemia, hyperphosphataemia and hypocalcaemia (due to precipitation of calcium phosphate).

## Treatment of AML (K&C p. 492)

This is in two parts: induction of remission and post-remission/consolidation. This is due to the fact that when complete remission is achieved, there are still $10^8$ or $10^9$ leukaemic blast cells detectable using molecular techniques.

- Induction of remission is achieved with an aggressive combination of intravenous chemotherapy, e.g. cytosine arabinoside (cytarabine) and daunorubicin given at intervals to allow marrow recovery in between.
- Post-remission therapy. The options are further courses of chemotherapy or myeloablative therapy with allogeneic/autologous bone marrow transplantation (BMT) (see p. 231).

Chemotherapy achieves an initial remission rate of 70%, although long-term cure is only around 35% with chemotherapy alone. BMT improves long-term remission to 50%.

### Prognosis
Patients under 55 years with AML have a 40% chance of cure. The prognosis for older patients is poor.

### Treatment of acute promyelocytic leukaemia (APML) (K&C p. 492)
Acute promyelocytic leukaemia is specifically associated with disseminated intravascular coagulation (DIC) which may worsen when treatment is started. Management of DIC is discussed on page 213. Pharmacological doses of retinoic acid induce differentiation of the malignant promyelocytic clone into mature granulocytes and all-*trans*-retinoic acid (ATRA) is used to induce remission in APML. Remission induction therapy as in other forms of AML is also necessary for long-term survival.

### Treatment of acute lymphoblastic leukaemia (ALL) (K&C p. 493)
The principles of treatment are similar to those for AML; cyclical combination chemotherapy (vincristine, prednisolone and daunorubicin) is given to induce a remission and for post-remission therapy. However, ALL has a propensity to involve the CNS, so treatment also includes prophylactic intrathecal drugs, methotrexate or cytosine arabinoside (cytarabine) with or without prophylactic cranial radiotherapy. Most patients also receive oral maintenance chemotherapy for 2–3 years. Relapse may occur in the blood, testes and CNS.

Overall 90% of children with ALL respond to treatment and 50–60% are cured. The results in adults are not so good, with only about 30% being cured.

# Chronic myeloid leukaemia (K&C p. 493)

## Clinical features

Chronic myeloid leukaemia (CML) occurs most commonly in middle age. There is an insidious onset, with fever, weight loss, sweating and symptoms of anaemia. Massive splenomegaly is characteristic.

## Investigations

- Blood count usually shows anaemia and a raised white cell count (often $> 100 \times 10^9$/L). The platelet count may be low, normal or raised.
- Bone marrow aspirate shows a hypercellular marrow with an increase in myeloid progenitors. On cytogenetic analysis the Ph chromosome (p. 220) is present in all patients. The *BCR-ABL* oncogene can be detected by reverse transcriptase polymerase chain reaction (RT-PCR) in all patients.

225

## Management

Alpha-interferon has antiproliferative actions and stimulates cell-mediated and humoral responses to the malignant cells. It induces haematological remission in the majority of patients with CML and cytogenetic remissions in a minority. Side-effects such as anorexia and fatigue are common with the doses required. Preparations of interferon conjugated to polyethylene glycol (pegylated interferon) reduce the need for daily injections and hence toxicity. The mainstay of treatment for younger patients (< 50 years old) is allogeneic bone marrow transplantation, which may be curative. Palliative chemotherapy in the form of oral hydroxycarbamide (hydroxyurea) induces a haematological remission and is used in elderly patients who are intolerant of interferon. Preliminary results with STI571 (blocks the dysregulated tyrosine kinase activity of Bcr-abl fusion protein) are encouraging.

## Prognosis

The chronic phase described above lasts 3–4 years. This is followed by blast transformation, with the development of acute leukaemia (usually acute myeloid) and, commonly, rapid death. Less frequently, CML transforms into myelo-fibrosis, death ensuing from bone marrow failure.

# Chronic lymphocytic leukaemia (K&C p. 494)

CLL is an incurable disease of older people, characterized by an uncontrolled proliferation and accumulation of mature B lymphocytes (although T cell CLL does occur).

## Clinical features

CLL usually follows an indolent course. Early CLL is generally asymptomatic and isolated peripheral blood lymphocytosis is frequent. Symptoms are a consequence of bone marrow failure: anaemia, infections and bleeding. An autoimmune haemolysis contributes to the anaemia. Some patients may be asymptomatic, the diagnosis being a chance finding on the basis of a blood count done for a different reason. There may be lymphadenopathy and, in advanced disease, hepatosplenomegaly.

## Investigations

- Blood count shows a raised white cell count $> 15 \times 10^9/L$, of which at least 40% are lymphocytes. There may be anaemia and thrombocytopenia.
- The peripheral blood film shows small lymphocytes of mature appearance with 'smear cells', an artefactual finding due to cell rupture while the film is being made.
- Phenotyping of cells from blood or bone marrow is essential to exclude reactive lymphocytosis and other lymphoid neoplasms.

## Management

Treatment, usually with intermittent oral chlorambucil with or without prednisolone, is indicated only for those with symptomatic disease.

## Prognosis

The median survival is 8 years for those with lymphocytosis only. The prognosis is much worse (median survival 2 years) for those patients with marrow failure at presentation.

# The lymphomas

The lymphomas are neoplastic transformations of normal B or T cells which reside predominantly in lymphoid tissues. They are classified on the basis of histological appearance into Hodgkin's disease and non-Hodgkin's lymphoma (NHL).

## Hodgkin's disease (K&C p. 496)

### Clinical features

Hodgkin's disease is primarily a disease of young adults. The most common presentation is painless lymph node enlargement (most often cervical nodes). Systemic symptoms, known as 'B' symptoms, are fever, night sweats and weight loss. Other constitutional symptoms may occur, such as pruritus, fatigue, anorexia and alcohol-induced pain at the site of the enlarged lymph nodes.

227

On examination enlarged nodes are typically non-tender, discrete and with a rubbery consistency. There may be hepatosplenomegaly.

### Investigations

- Blood count may be normal or show a normochromic, normocytic anaemia.
- The ESR is usually raised.
- Liver biochemistry may be abnormal, with liver involvement.
- Radiology. Chest X-ray and CT are necessary for staging and may show mediastinal, intrathoracic or abdominal lymphadenopathy.
- Lymph node biopsy and histological examination are required for a definitive diagnosis. Classically, Sternberg–Reed (binucleate or multinucleate malignant B lymphocytes) cells are present, with a characteristic admixture of lymphocytes and histiocytes.

**Table 5.22**
Differential diagnosis of lymphadenopathy

| Localized | Generalized |
| --- | --- |
| Local infection<br>    Pyogenic infection,<br>    e.g. tonsillitis<br>    Tuberculosis | Infection<br>    Epstein–Barr virus<br>    Cytomegalovirus<br>    *Toxoplasma* sp.<br>    Tuberculosis<br>    HIV infection |
| Lymphoma | Lymphoma |
| Secondary carcinoma | Leukaemia |
| | Systemic disease<br>    Systemic lupus erythematosus<br>    Sarcoidosis<br>    Rheumatoid arthritis |
| | Drug reaction, e.g. phenytoin |

- Bone marrow aspirate and trephine biopsy may show involvement in patients with advanced disease.

### Differential diagnosis

This includes any other cause of lymphadenopathy (Table 5.22). The management of persistently enlarged lymph nodes includes surgical excision for histological and micro-biological examination for diagnostic purposes.

### Management

Treatment is always given with a curative intent and consists of radiotherapy, cyclical combination chemotherapy or both. The choice of treatment depends on:

- Stage (Table 5.23)
- Involved sites
- 'Bulk' of lymph nodes involved
- Presence or absence of 'B' symptoms.

Stage IA and stage IIA disease are treated with radiotherapy. All other stages are usually treated with combination chemotherapy. The prognosis is related to the stage of the disease, with a 5-year survival rate of approximately 90% in stage I. The presence of B symptoms indicates more severe disease with a worse prognosis.

**Table 5.23**
Staging classification of Hodgkin's disease*

| Stage | Definition |
|-------|------------|
| I | Involvement of a single lymph node region or a single extralymphatic organ or site |
| II | Involvement of two or more lymph node regions on the same side of the diaphragm, or localized involvement of an extralymphatic organ or site and of one or more lymph node regions on the same side of the diaphragm |
| III | Involvement of lymph node regions on both sides of the diaphragm, which may also be accompanied by involvement of the spleen or by localized involvement of an extralymphatic organ or site or both |
| IV | Diffuse or disseminated involvement of one or more extralymphatic organs or tissues, with or without associated lymph node involvement |

* Each stage is subdivided into A (no systemic symptoms) and B (unexplained fever, night sweats and weight loss >10% of bodyweight)

229

## Non-Hodgkin's lymphoma (K&C p. 498)

This is a heterogeneous group of disorders which encompasses many different histological subtypes. Subdivisions of the lymphomas into 'low grade' and 'high grade' reflects the rate at which the cells are dividing and thus the clinical progression of the disease. Paradoxically, high-grade lymphomas (rapidly dividing cells) are potentially curable, whereas low-grade lymphomas are generally considered to be incurable with conventional chemotherapy (Table 5.24). The classification of non-Hodgkin's lymphoma is currently

**Table 5.24**
Non-Hodgkin's lymphoma: low grade and high grade

| Low grade | High grade |
|-----------|------------|
| Middle-aged/older people | Any age group |
| Bone marrow infiltration common | Bone marrow infiltration unusual |
| Incurable with conventional chemotherapy | Potentially curable |

based on histological, cytogenetic and immunochemical information.

## Clinical features

Non-Hodgkin's lymphoma (NHL) is rare before the age of 40. The presentation can be very varied and almost any organ in the body can be involved. Peripheral lymph node enlargement is the most common clinical presentation. Systemic symptoms as in Hodgkin's disease may occur. Bone marrow infiltration, leading to anaemia, recurrent infections and bleeding, is often seen in low-grade lymphoma.

## Investigations

- Blood count may show anaemia. An elevated white cell count or thrombocytopenia suggests bone marrow involvement.
- Liver biochemistry may be abnormal if the liver is involved.
- Radiology, such as a chest radiograph and CT, will show involvement of mediastinal, intrathoracic or intra-abdominal lymph nodes.
- Lymph node biopsy is required for definitive diagnosis and subtype classification.
- Bone marrow aspiration and trephine biopsy will confirm marrow involvement.

## Management

Treatment depends on the grade and histological subtype.

- Low-grade disease in general is not curable. However, patients may survive for many years and usually experience several remissions with relatively simple treatment such as chlorambucil, or radiotherapy in localized disease.
- High-grade disease requires combination chemotherapy. Modern regimens, e.g. doxorubicin, cyclophosphamide, vincristine and prednisolone (CHOP), achieve a 60–70% response rate, and cure in about 40%. Some patients with localized disease can be cured with local radiotherapy.

## MALT lymphoma

MALT (mucosa-associated lymphoid tissue) lymphoma is an unusual lymphoma affecting the gastrointestinal tract, most commonly the stomach. It has gained increasing recognition because of the close association in the stomach with *Helicobacter pylori* infection. In certain cases, eradication of this organism alone has led to resolution of the lymphoma.

## Mycosis fungoides and Sézary syndrome

(*K&C* p. 1307)

These are rare cutaneous T cell lymphomas that may spread in the later stages to involve lymph nodes and other organs.

## Burkitt's lymphoma (*K&C* p. 500)

This is a form of NHL occurring mainly in African children, and is associated with Epstein–Barr virus infection. Jaw tumours are common, usually with gastrointestinal involvement. Treatment is with radiotherapy and chemotherapy.

231

## Myeloablative therapy with bone marrow transplantation

Myeloablative therapy is a term used for treatment that employs high-dose chemotherapy or chemotherapy plus radiation, with the aim of clearing the bone marrow completely of both benign and malignant cells. Without bone marrow replacement or 'transplantation', the patient would die of bone marrow failure. Approaches to restore bone marrow function include the following:

- *Allogeneic* bone marrow transplantation: bone marrow or peripheral blood stem cells *from another individual*, usually an HLA-identical sibling, are infused intravenously following myeloablative therapy. Immunosuppression is required to prevent host rejection and graft-versus-host disease (GVHD). The latter is a syndrome in which donor T lymphocytes infiltrate the skin, gut and liver, causing a maculopapular rash, diarrhoea and liver necrosis. Following allogeneic BMT the blood count usually recovers within 3–4 weeks. The mortality rate is 20–40%, depending on the person's age, and is often a result of infection or GVHD.

- *Autologous* (the patient acts as his or her own source of stem cells) peripheral blood progenitor cells (PBPCs) have virtually replaced autologous BMT as support for myeloablative therapy. With this technique it is possible, by using chemotherapy followed by the growth factor, colony-stimulating factor (G-CSF), to stimulate haemopoietic progenitor cells in the marrow to proliferate so that they can be collected from the peripheral blood. They are stored and re-infused after myeloablative therapy. The main advantage is the short time for blood count recovery because PBPCs are more differentiated. This technique has been used predominantly in patients with Hodgkin's disease, NHL, myeloma and breast cancer.
- *Syngeneic*: donor cells are from an identical twin.

# The paraproteinaemias

## Multiple myeloma *(K&C p. 501)*

Multiple myeloma is a neoplastic clonal proliferation of bone marrow plasma cells usually capable of producing monoclonal immunoglobulins (M proteins or paraproteins), which in most cases are IgG or IgA. The paraprotein may be associated with excretion of light chains in the urine, which are either κ or λ; the excess light chains are known as Bence Jones protein.

### Clinical features

The peak age of presentation is 60 years. The neoplastic clone of cells induces excess osteoclastic activity, which results in osteoporosis, osteolytic lesions, pathological fractures and hypercalcaemia. Bone pain is the most common presenting symptom. Progressive marrow infiltration results in anaemia, infections and bleeding. Renal failure has multiple causes: deposition of light chains in the tubules, hypercalcaemia, hyperuricaemia and amyloid deposition in the kidneys. Paraproteins may form aggregates in the blood, which greatly increase the viscosity, leading to blurred vision, gangrene and bleeding.

## Investigations

The diagnosis is made by demonstrating the following:

- Plasma cell infiltration on bone marrow aspirate or trephine biopsy
- Osteolytic bone lesions (often in the skull) on skeletal survey
- Monoclonal ('M') bands on serum protein electrophoresis, or Bence Jones protein in the urine. There is also a reduction in the normal polyclonal immunoglobulins (immune paresis).

Other essential investigations are as follows:

- Blood count, which may show anaemia, thrombocytopenia and leucopenia. The ESR is almost always high.
- Serum biochemistry may show evidence of renal failure and hypercalcaemia. The alkaline phosphatase is usually normal.

## Management

Combination chemotherapy with alkylating agents (melphalan or cyclophosphamide) given in conjunction with prednisolone has improved the median survival of patients with myeloma from 7 months to 2.5 years. Selected patients are treated with high-dose melphalan supported by autologous BMT or PBPC. Adjuvant interferon therapy following chemotherapy has been shown to prolong remission. Localized bone pain can be helped by radiotherapy, and pathological fractures prevented by pinning of lytic bone lesions. Renal failure (p. 340) and hypercalcaemia (p. 585) may be corrected by adequate hydration alone. In addition bony complications may be reduced in patients in 'plateau phase' by long-term administration of bisphosphonates. Hyperviscosity is treated by plasmapheresis together with systemic therapy.

### Prognosis
The median survival with treatment is about 2 years.

## Waldenström's macroglobulinaemia
(*K&C* p. 502)
As in myeloma the neoplastic B cells secrete a monoclonal immunoglobulin. However, unlike myeloma, but similar to lymphoma, the tumour infiltrates the lymphoid tissues, including bone marrow, spleen and lymph nodes.

### Clinical features
The most common features are malaise, weight loss, lymph node enlargement and symptoms of hyperviscosity.

### Investigations
- Blood count may show a normal or low Hb and WCC, although the ESR is almost always high.
- Protein electrophoresis shows an IgM paraprotein.
- Bone marrow aspirate shows infiltration with lymphoplasmacytoid cells.

### Management
Treatment is with alkylating agents or doxorubicin-containing regimens. Hyperviscosity is treated with plasmapheresis.

## Monoclonal gammopathy of undetermined significance (*K&C* p. 503)
This is usually seen in older patients, where a raised level of paraprotein (usually IgA) is found in the blood, but without other features of myeloma. Patients are often asymptomatic and no treatment is required. Regular follow-up is usually indicated in case they later develop lymphoma or myeloma.

# 6

# Rheumatology

Musculoskeletal problems are common and account for about one in six GP consultations. Most of these are non-articular problems (see below). Osteoarthritis and rheumatoid arthritis are more commonly seen in hospital clinics. Pain, stiffness, and swelling are the most common presenting symptoms of joint disease and may be localized to a single joint or affect many joints.

*Arthralgia* is the term used to describe joint pains when the joint appears normal on examination. *Arthritis* is the term used when there is objective evidence of joint inflammation (swelling, deformity or an effusion). In a patient presenting with joint pains, the history and examination must assess the distribution of joints affected (symmetrical?, axial or peripheral?), the presence of morning stiffness (common in inflammatory arthropathies), aggravating and relieving factors, past medical history and family history. Table 6.1 lists the likely causes of joint pains based on the age and sex of the patient and the presence of associated features.

Pain in or around a single joint may arise from the joint itself (articular problem) or from structures surrounding the joint (periarticular problem). Enthesitis (inflammation at the site of attachment of ligaments, tendons and joint capsules), bursitis and tendinitis are all causes of periarticular pain. Pain arising from the joint may be the result of a mechanical problem (e.g. torn meniscus) or an inflammatory problem.

The causes of a large joint monoarthritis include osteoarthritis, gout, pseudogout, trauma and septic arthritis (p. 250). Disseminated gonococcal infection is a common cause of acute non-traumatic monoarthritis or oligoarthritis in young adults. Less common causes are rheumatoid arthritis, the spondyloarthropathies, tuberculous infection and haemarthrosis (e.g. in haemophilia, or on warfarin). Acute monoarthritis requires urgent investigation and treatment (p. 251). The key investigation is synovial fluid aspiration with Gram stain and culture and analysis for crystals in gout and pseudogout.

**Table 6.1**
Differential diagnosis of polyarticular disease in adults in the UK

| Age | Predominantly males | | Predominantly females |
|---|---|---|---|
| Young | Reiter's syndrome<br>Reactive arthritis<br>Ankylosing spondylitis | Psoriatic arthropathy<br>Enteropathic arthropathy | Systemic lupus erythematosus<br>Rheumatoid arthritis<br>Sjögren's syndrome |
| Middle age | Gout | Sjögren's syndrome<br>Generalized osteoarthritis | Rheumatoid arthritis |
| Elderly | | Polymyalgia rheumatica<br>Pseudogout | |

**Uncommon arthropathies:** Malignancy (hypertrophic pulmonary osteoarthropathy), Lyme disease, rheumatic fever, Henoch–Schönlein purpura, Behçet's syndrome

# Arthritis

## Osteoarthritis (K&C p. 533)

Osteoarthritis (OA) is the most common form of arthritis. It is a disease of synovial joints characterized by articular cartilage loss with an accompanying periarticular bone response. Radiological changes of OA are seen in about 10% of the population as a whole, and in 50% of those aged over 60, although only a proportion of these have symptoms.

### Epidemiology

Osteoarthritis occurs world-wide, although it is uncommon in the black population. It is twice as common in women as in men, and there is a marked familial tendency.

### Pathology and pathogenesis

Osteoarthritis is the result of active, sometimes inflammatory but potentially reparative processes, rather than the inevitable result of trauma and ageing. It is characterized by a progressive destruction and loss of articular cartilage. The exposed subchondral bone becomes sclerotic, with increased vascularity and cyst formation. Attempts at repair produce cartilaginous growths at the margins of the joint which later become calcified (osteophytes).

Several mechanisms have been suggested for the pathogenesis:

- Metalloproteinases, such as stromelysin and collagenase, degrade the cartilage components, collagen and proteoglycans
- Inflammatory mediators such as interleukin-1 and tumour necrosis factor-$\alpha$ stimulate metalloproteinase production and inhibit collagen production
- Deficiency of growth factors such as insulin-like growth factor and transforming growth factor impairs matrix repair
- Genetic factors (35–65% influence).

Most OA is primary. Secondary OA occurs in joints that have been damaged in some way (e.g. intra-articular fractures, avascular necrosis) or are congenitally abnormal (e.g. slipped femoral epiphysis).

## Clinical features

The main symptom is pain, which is made worse by movement and relieved by rest. Stiffness occurs after sitting down and for a short period (< $^1/_2$ h) on waking in the morning. The joints most commonly involved are the distal interphalangeal joints (DIPJ) and first carpometacarpal joint of the hands, first metatarsophalangeal joint of the foot and the weight-bearing joints – vertebrae, hips and knees. On examination there is deformity and bony enlargement of the joints, limited joint movement and muscle wasting of surrounding muscle groups. There may occasionally be a joint effusion. Heberden's nodes are bony swellings at the DIPJ. Bouchard's nodes are similar but occur at the proximal interphalangeal joint.

## Differential diagnosis

Osteoarthritis is differentiated from rheumatoid arthritis by the pattern of joint involvement (Fig. 6.1) and the absence

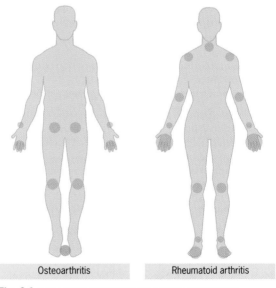

Osteoarthritis                    Rheumatoid arthritis

**Fig. 6.1 The pattern of joint involvement in osteoarthritis compared with rheumatoid arthritis.** Joint involvement in RA is usually symmetrical, whereas asymmetry is frequent in OA, especially of the large joints.

of the systemic features that occur in rheumatoid arthritis. Pyrophosphate arthropathy (p. 268) affects a similar age group as OA but the wrists are usually involved. Chronic tophaceous gout (p. 265) and psoriatic arthritis affecting the DIPJ (p. 249) may mimic OA.

## Investigations

- FBC and ESR are both normal. Rheumatoid factor is negative, but positive low-titre tests may occur incidentally in elderly people.
- X-rays are only abnormal in advanced diseased and show narrowing of the joint space (resulting from loss of cartilage), osteophytes, subchondral sclerosis and cyst formation.
- MRI demonstrates early cartilage changes.

## Management

Treatment should focus on the symptoms and disability, not the radiological appearances. There are three main types of treatment: physical measures, drugs and surgery. Obese patients should be encouraged to lose weight, particularly if weight-bearing joints are affected.

239

- Physical therapy. Heat applied to an affected joint may provide pain relief. Exercises maintain muscle power and improve the mobility of weight-bearing joints. Hydrotherapy may be helpful.
- Drugs. Paracetamol and non-steroidal anti-inflammatory drugs (NSAIDs), e.g. ibuprofen, are used to control symptoms, and should ideally be used on an intermittent rather than a continuous basis. The primary effect of NSAIDs is to inhibit cyclo-oxygenase (COX, prostaglandin synthase) with impaired production of prostaglandins, thromboxane and prostacyclin. NSAIDs inhibit both isoforms of the enzyme, COX-1 (expressed in most tissues) and COX-2 (expression increased at sites of inflammation). Inhibition of COX-1 in the gastroduodenal mucosa leads to reduced production of protective prostaglandins and an increased rate of mucosal damage. The specific COX-2 inhibitors (rofecoxib and celecoxib) are similarly efficacious to the traditional

non-specific NSAIDs but are associated with reduced rates of peptic ulceration. Side-effects of both drugs include fluid retention and chronic tubulointerstitial nephritis. Indications for COX-2 specific inhibitors include previous peptic ulceration, age > 65 years and associated co-morbidity such as cardiac or respiratory failure. Intra-articular steroids can be used for inflammatory exacerbations, but systemic corticosteroid therapy is not used.

- Surgery. Replacement of the joint is indicated if pain and loss of function have failed to respond to drugs and physical therapy.

## Rheumatoid arthritis (K&C p. 537)

Rheumatoid arthritis (RA) is a chronic symmetrical poly-arthritis of unknown cause. It is a systemic disorder associated with extra-articular involvement, e.g. the lungs and many other organs.

### Epidemiology

Rheumatoid arthritis affects 1–3% of the population worldwide, with a peak prevalence between the ages of 30 and 50 years. Women are affected three times more often than men. There is an increased incidence in those with a family history of rheumatoid arthritis and an association with HLA-DR4 in most ethnic groups.

### Aetiology

The cause of RA is unknown. The most widely held view is that an interplay of genetic factors, sex hormones and an unknown antigen triggers activation of T cells and initiates an autoimmune mechanism with inflammatory and destructive features.

### Pathology

Rheumatoid arthritis is a disease of the synovium. There is infiltration by chronic inflammatory cells: lymphocytes, plasma cells and macrophages with secretion of pro-inflammatory cytokines (e.g. TNF-$\alpha$, IL-8) and autoantibody production. Generation of new synovial blood vessels is induced by angiogenic cytokines, and activated endothelial cells produce adhesion molecules such as vascular cell adhesion molecule-1 (VCAM-1) which expedite extravasation of leucocytes into the synovium. The synovium proliferates and grows out over the surface of cartilage, producing a tumour-like mass called 'pannus'. Pannus destroys the articular cartilage and subchondral bone, producing bony erosions. Rheumatoid factors (RhF) are antibodies directed against the Fc portion of immunoglobulin. Their role in the pathogenesis of RA is not known but they are associated with nodules and more aggressive disease.

Subcutaneous nodules (rheumatoid nodules) have a characteristic microscopic appearance with a central area of necrosis surrounded by macrophages and fibrous tissue. Similar lesions occur in the pleura, pericardium and lung.

## Clinical features

The typical presentation is with an insidious onset of pain, stiffness and swelling in the small joints of the hands and feet, which is most marked on waking in the mornings. There is spindling of the fingers caused by swelling of the proximal but not the distal interphalangeal joints. The metacarpophalangeal and wrist joints are also swollen. As the disease progresses there is weakening of joint capsules, causing joint instability, subluxation (partial dislocation) and deformity. The characteristic deformities of the rheumatoid hand are shown in Figure 6.2. Most patients eventually have many joints involved, including the wrists, elbows, shoulders, cervical spine, knees, ankles and feet. The dorsal and lumbar spine are not involved. Joint effusions and wasting of muscles around the affected joints are early features. Later there is joint deformity, subluxation and instability. Less common presentations are 'explosive' (sudden onset of widespread arthritis), palindromic (relapsing and remitting monoarthritis of different large joints), or with a systemic illness with few joint symptoms initially.

## Extra-articular manifestations

Periarticular features of RA include bursitis, tenosynovitis, muscle wasting and nodule formation. Rheumatoid nodules are found in about 20% of cases, usually on the ulnar surface of the forearm just below the elbow. Patients with nodules are usually seropositive, i.e. they have circulating RhF.

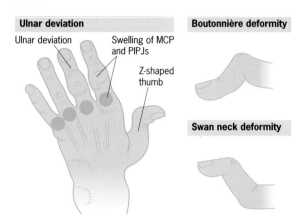

**Fig. 6.2 Characteristic hand deformities in rheumatoid arthritis.**
MCP, metacarpophalanges; PIPJs, proximal interphalangeal joints. (Adapted from Read et al (1992) Essential Medicine. Churchill Livingstone, Edinburgh.)

Other extra-articular disease manifestations are summarized in Table 6.2. The most common manifestations are highlighted; these may be present but cause few symptoms, e.g. atlantoaxial subluxation is commonly seen on a cervical spine X-ray, but much less commonly causes problems.

### Investigations

The diagnosis is usually clinical, but appropriate investigations include:

- Blood count. There is a normochromic, normocytic anaemia and thrombocytosis which correlates with disease activity. Other forms of anaemia may also occur (Table 6.2). The ESR and CRP are raised in proportion to the activity of the inflammatory process.
- Serum autoantibodies. RhF (p. 241) is positive in 70% of cases and antinuclear factor in 30% (p. 800).
- Radiology. X-ray of the affected joints may show joint narrowing, erosions at the joint margins, porosis of periarticular bone and cysts.
- Synovial fluid is sterile with a high neutrophil count in uncomplicated disease.

242

**Table 6.2**
Extra-articular manifestations of rheumatoid arthritis

| | |
|---|---|
| Systemic | **Fever** |
| | **Fatigue** |
| | Weight loss |
| Eyes | **Secondary Sjögren's syndrome** |
| | Scleritis |
| | Scleromalacia perforans |
| | (perforation of the eye) |
| Neurological | **Carpal tunnel syndrome** |
| | **Atlanto-axial subluxation** |
| | Cord compression |
| | Polyneuropathy, predominantly sensory |
| | Mononeuritis multiplex |
| Reticuloendothelial | **Lymphadenopathy** |
| | Felty's syndrome (rheumatoid |
| | arthritis, splenomegaly, neutropenia) |
| Blood | **Anaemia caused by:** |
| |     Chronic disease |
| |     NSAID-induced gastrointestinal blood loss |
| |     Haemolysis |
| |     Hypersplenism |
| | **Thrombocytosis** |
| Pulmonary | Pleural effusion |
| | Diffuse fibrosing alveolitis |
| | Rheumatoid nodules |
| | Rheumatoid pneumoconiosis |
| | (Caplan's syndrome) |
| | Small airway disease |
| Heart | **Pericarditis (rarely clinically apparent)** |
| | Pericardial effusion |
| Kidneys | Amyloidosis |
| | Analgesic nephropathy |
| Vasculitis | Leg ulcers |
| | Nail fold infarcts |
| | Gangrene of fingers and toes |

The most common manifestations are in bold

## Differential diagnosis

In the patient with symmetrical peripheral arthritis, nodules and positive RhF the diagnosis is straightforward. RA must be distinguished from the symmetrical seronegative arthropathy occurring in psoriasis. Severe RA can also mimic a form of psoriatic arthritis known as 'arthritis mutilans' (p. 249). In a young woman presenting with joint pains SLE must be considered, but characteristically the joints look normal on examination in this condition.

## Management

Effective management of RA requires a multidisciplinary approach, with input from rheumatologists, orthopaedic surgeons (joint replacement, arthroplasty), occupational therapists (aids to reduce disability) and physiotherapists (improvement of muscle power and maintenance of mobility to prevent flexion deformities).

*NSAIDs* and *COX-2 specific inhibitors* (p. 239) are effective in relieving the joint pain and stiffness of RA, but they do not slow disease progression. Individual response to NSAIDs varies considerably and it is reasonable to try several drugs in a particular patient to find the best. Slow-release preparations (e.g. slow-release diclofenac) taken at night may produce dramatic relief of symptoms on the following day.

*Disease-modifying drugs* (DMARDs) should be used early (within 3–6 months) in disease onset to prevent the irreversible effects of long-term inflammation of the joints. These drugs, which act mainly through inhibition of inflammatory cytokines, reduce inflammation and slow the development of joint erosions, though they may take up to 6 months to achieve maximum effect. The most effective drugs are methotrexate, penicillamine and azathioprine. Hydroxychloroquine, sulfasalazine and auranofin are a little less effective but safer. Methotrexate is considered to be the drug of first choice for most patients, though all drugs can have serious side-effects (Table 6.3) so careful monitoring with blood tests is necessary. The antimalarial drug hydroxychloroquine may produce corneal deposits (which disappear when treatment is stopped) and rarely retinopathy, which may be permanent. Visual acuity must be checked and ophthalmoscopy performed 6 monthly.

Leflunomide is a newer immunomodulatory agent which acts by blocking T cell proliferation. It has a similar initial response rate to sulfasalazine but improvement continues and it is better sustained at 2 years. Tumour necrosis factor-$\alpha$ blockers such as etanercept, a soluble TNF-$\alpha$ receptor fusion protein that binds TNF-$\alpha$, or infliximab a chimeric (human/mouse) antibody to TNF-$\alpha$, have had a

**Table 6.3**
Side-effects of drugs used in long-term suppressive therapy for rheumatoid arthritis. Rash is an additional side-effect of most of the drugs listed

| Drug | Side-effects |
| --- | --- |
| Methotrexate | Neutropenia<br>Liver fibrosis |
| Penicillamine | Thrombocytopenia<br>Proteinuria |
| Azathioprine | Neutropenia<br>Nausea and vomiting |
| Intramuscular gold (sodium aurothiomalate) | Thrombocytopenia |
| Oral gold (auranofin) | Diarrhoea |
| Hydroxychloroquine | Retinopathy |
| Sulfasalazine | Nausea<br>Leucopenia and thrombocytopenia<br>Male infertility (reversible) |

major impact in the treatment of RA. Both products slow or halt erosion formation in up to 70% of patients. TNF blocking therapy should be considered for patients who have active disease despite adequate treatment with one or more DMARDs. The cost of these agents and the lack of long-term data remain barriers to their more widespread use.

*Corticosteroids* suppress disease activity but the dose required is often large, with the considerable risk of long-term toxicity (p. 577). They are seldom used except in the elderly patient with explosive RA or in patients with severe extra-articular manifestations. Local injection of a troublesome joint (see below) with a long-acting corticosteroid improves pain, synovitis and effusion. Repeated injections into an individual joint are possible, but usually limited to four a year because too-frequent injections may accelerate joint damage.

In patients presenting with disproportionate involvement of a single joint, septic arthritis (p. 250) must be excluded before the symptoms are attributed to a disease flare-up.

### Prognosis

The prognosis is variable. After 10 years 10% of patients will be severely disabled and 25% will have minimal if any symptoms. Other patients lie between these two extremes.

## The seronegative spondarthritides
(*K&C* p. 547)

This title describes a group of conditions affecting the spine and peripheral joints which cluster in families and are linked to certain type I HLA antigens (Table 6.4). The joint involvement is more limited than that seen in RA and its distribution is different. The synovitis itself is difficult to distinguish from that of RA histologically, but there is no production of rheumatoid factors, hence 'seronegative'. All are associated with an increased frequency of sacroiliitis and an increased frequency of HLA-B27 or structurally associated class I antigens which cross-react with HLA-B27. The explanation for the association with HLA-B27 is unknown.

## Ankylosing spondylitis (*K&C* p. 548)
This is an inflammatory disorder of the back, affecting mainly young adults. Men are affected more severely than women and so more likely to present with symptoms of the disease.

### Clinical features
The typical patient with ankylosing spondylitis is a young man (late teens, early 20s) who presents with increasing pain and morning stiffness in the lower back. There is a

---

**Table 6.4**
Seronegative spondarthritides

Ankylosing spondylitis (AS)
Psoriatic arthritis
Reactive arthritis
    Sexually acquired (Reiter's disease)
    Post-dysenteric reactive arthritis
Ulcerative colitis/Crohn's (enteropathic) arthritis

progressive loss of spinal movement. Inspection of the spine reveals two characteristic abnormalities:

- Loss of lumbar lordosis and increased kyphosis (Fig. 6.3)
- Variable limitation of spinal flexion and a reduction in chest expansion.

Other features include Achilles tendinitis and plantar fasciitis (enthesitis) and tenderness around the pelvis and chest wall.

Non-articular features include iritis (in 25%) and, rarely, aortic incompetence, cardiac conduction defects and apical lung fibrosis.

## Investigations

- The ESR and CRP are often raised.
- X-rays may be normal or show erosion and sclerosis of the margins of the sacroiliac joints, proceeding to ankylosis (immobility and consolidation of the joint). In

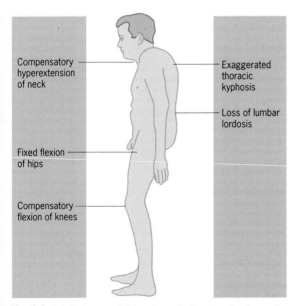

Compensatory hyperextension of neck

Exaggerated thoracic kyphosis

Loss of lumbar lordosis

Fixed flexion of hips

Compensatory flexion of knees

**Fig. 6.3 Ankylosing spondylitis – the typical posture in advanced cases.** (Adapted from Calin A. Seronegative spondylarthrities. *Medicine* 1994 22.4: 145–151 by kind permission of The Medicine Publishing Company.)

the spinal column, squaring of the vertebrae (caused by erosion of the corners) and progressive calcification of the interspinous ligaments produce the 'bamboo spine'.

## Management

- Twice-daily exercises are essential to maintain posture and mobility.
- Slow-release NSAIDs taken at night are particularly effective in relieving night pain and morning stiffness. Sulfasalazine or methotrexate may help the peripheral arthritis but there is little evidence that they control the spinal disease.

## Prognosis

Most patients are able to lead a normal active life and remain at work. In severe cases the spine becomes completely fused and brittle, with a risk of fracture (on minimal trauma) and cord compression. The fixed kyphosis of the cervical and thoracic spine may impair ventilation.

## Reiter's syndrome (K&C p. 550)

Reiter's syndrome consists of the triad of a seronegative reactive arthritis, non-specific urethritis and conjunctivitis. Two types are recognized:

- Following a gastrointestinal infection with *Shigella, Salmonella, Yersinia* or *Campylobacter* (enteric)
- Following non-specific urethritis.

### Clinical features

**Arthritis** The typical case is a young man who presents with an acute arthritis shortly (within 4 weeks) after an enteric or venereal infection, which may have been mild or asymptomatic. The joints of the lower limbs are particularly affected in an asymmetrical pattern; the knees, ankles and feet are the most common sites.

**Urethritis** is associated with a sterile urethral discharge and dysuria.

**Conjunctivitis** occurs in one-third of patients and is usually mild and bilateral.

Occasional additional features are iritis, enthesiopathy (plantar fasciitis, Achilles tendinitis), circinate balanitis (superficial ulceration around the penile meatus) and keratoderma blenorrhagica, an intense scaling of the soles of the feet resembling pustular psoriasis.

## Investigations
The diagnosis is clinical. The ESR is raised in the acute stage. Aspirated synovial fluid is sterile, with a high neutrophil count.

## Management
Three types of therapy are used in the management of Reiter's syndrome: the acute inflammation is treated with NSAIDs together with local joint aspiration and injection of corticosteroid; the infection with antibiotics; and chronic disease with sulfasalazine or azathioprine.

## Prognosis
The acute arthritis resolves within a few months. However, 50% of patients develop recurrent arthritis, iritis or ankylosing spondylitis.

# Reactive arthritis (K&C p. 550)
The full triad of Reiter's syndrome is rare, but a large joint arthritis following enteric or venereal infection is common and is the most common cause of arthritis in young men.

# Psoriatic arthritis (K&C p. 549)
This is a seronegative arthritis occurring in 5–8% of patients with psoriasis, particularly in those with nail disease (p. 725). Arthritis may precede the skin disease.

## Clinical features
There are several types:

- *Asymmetrical involvement* of the small joints of the hand, including the distal interphalangeal joints
- *Symmetrical polyarthritis* resembling rheumatoid arthritis
- *Arthritis mutilans*, a severe form with destruction of the small bones in the hands and feet

- *Ankylosing spondylitis* occurs with increased frequency in patients with psoriasis.

### Investigations
- Blood count. Routine blood tests are unhelpful in the diagnosis. The ESR is often normal.
- Radiology. X-rays may show erosions and periarticular osteoporosis in the terminal interphalangeal joints.

### Treatment
This is with analgesia and NSAIDs. Local synovitis responds to intra-articular corticosteroid injections. In severe cases methotrexate or ciclosporin are used, as they control both the arthritis and the skin lesions.

## Enteropathic arthritis *(K&C p. 551)*
Enteropathic arthritis is a large joint mono- or asymmetrical oligoarthritis occurring in 10–15% of patients with ulcerative colitis and Crohn's disease. It usually parallels the activity of the inflammatory bowel disease and consequently improves as bowel symptoms improve. Ankylosing spondylitis occurs in 5% of patients with inflammatory bowel disease but is not related to disease activity.

## Infective arthritis

Joint infection is uncommon but is important because it can lead to considerable joint destruction. Infection of the joints may be caused by the following:

- Bacteria (see below)
- Viruses. Rubella, mumps and hepatitis B virus infections are associated with a mild self-limiting arthritis. HIV infection is associated with an intermittent arthritis
- Spirochaetes and fungi (rare).

## Septic arthritis *(K&C p. 554)*
Septic arthritis results from infection of the joint with pyogenic organisms, most commonly *Staphylococcus aureus*. The organism reaches the joint through the bloodstream from a

distant site of infection, from local spread of adjacent osteomyelitis, or through direct injury or trauma.

### Clinical features

Classically there is a hot painful red joint, often the knee, which has developed acutely. There may be fever and evidence of infection elsewhere. Fever and systemic reactions may be absent in those with rheumatoid arthritis or in patients taking corticosteroids.

### Management

This is summarized in Emergency Box 6.1.

---

 **Emergency Box 6.1**

#### Acute monoarthritis

**Investigations**

- **Joint aspiration** and synovial fluid analysis: white cell count and differential (normal < 180/mm$^3$), Gram stain and culture, polarized light microscopy for crystals (in gout and pseudogout). Purulent fluid (white cell count > 50 000/mm$^3$, mostly neutrophils) and/or positive Gram stain indicates bacterial infection.
- **Bloods:** FBC, ESR, C-reactive protein, blood cultures.
- **X-rays of the affected joint** play little part in the diagnosis because these only become abnormal when joint destruction has occurred. However, a baseline X-ray may be useful for later comparison.
- **Swab** of urethra, cervix and anorectum if gonococcal infection a possibility.

**Treatment of acute non-gonococcal bacterial arthritis**

- Antibiotics for 6 weeks, initial 2 weeks i.v. Treatment depends on the organism concerned, but a suitable 'blind' regimen would be flucloxacillin 1–2 g 6-hourly i.v. (erythromycin if penicillin allergic), together with oral fusidic acid 500 mg 8-hourly. Modify treatment depending on culture and sensitivity.
- Adequate joint drainage: by needle aspiration, arthroscopy or open drainage. Consider orthopaedic referral.
- Immobilize joint in acute stages, mobilize early to avoid contractures.
- NSAIDs or specific COX-2 inhibitor for pain relief.

# Tuberculous arthritis (K&C p. 555)

Approximately 1% of patients with TB have skeletal involvement, which is usually caused by haematogenous spread from pulmonary or renal disease.

## Clinical features

Spinal involvement is particularly common (50%) but the knee, hip, sacroiliac and other joints may be involved. There is an insidious onset of pain, swelling and dysfunction, often associated with general symptoms of malaise, anorexia and night sweats.

## Diagnosis

Culture of the synovial fluid may give the diagnosis. Occasionally, synovial biopsy is required.

## Treatment

Treatment is as for tuberculosis elsewhere (see p. 481), in addition to joint rest and immobilization.

# Meningococcal arthritis (K&C p. 555)

Meningococcal arthritis usually occurs as part of a meningococcal septicaemia and results from the deposition of circulating immune complexes containing meningococcal antigens. It is a migratory polyarthritis, not associated with joint destruction. Treatment is with penicillin.

# Gonococcal arthritis (K&C p. 555)

Gonococcal arthritis occurs secondary to genital or oral infection (often asymptomatic) and presents with a mild inflammatory polyarthritis. Concomitant skin involvement is common (maculopapular pustules). It affects particularly young women and homosexual men. The organism can usually be cultured from the bloodstream, and from the joints. Treatment is with penicillin.

# Salmonella arthritis

Salmonella arthritis presents as a mild polyarthritis and occurs with types of salmonellae that invade the bloodstream rather than staying within the gastrointestinal tract.

Gastrointestinal symptoms may be minor or absent. Treatment is with amoxicillin.

## Connective tissue disease

The term 'connective tissue disease' is used for three diseases:

- Systemic lupus erythematosus (SLE)
- Systemic sclerosis (scleroderma)
- Polymyositis and dermatomyositis.

Their relationship is illustrated in Figure 6.4.

These diseases have a number of features in common, including arthritis, immune complex deposition and vasculitis. Features of all three occur in overlap syndrome.

### Systemic lupus erythematosus (*K&C* p. 557)

SLE is the most common of the connective tissue disorders and is characterized by the presence of serum antibodies against nuclear components. It is a multisystem disease and has a varied clinical presentation.

### *Epidemiology*

253

SLE is mainly a disease of young women, with a peak age of onset between 20 and 40 years. It affects about 0.1% of the population but is more common in Africans.

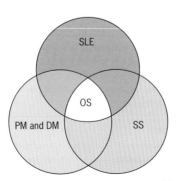

**Fig. 6.4 The family of connective tissue diseases.** OS, overlap syndrome; PM, DM, poly- and dermatomyositis; SLE, systemic lupus erythematosus; SS, systemic sclerosis.

Connective tissue disease

## Aetiology

The cause of the disease is unknown but is probably multi-factorial. Factors that are thought to play a role include the following:

- *Genetic factors.* There is a 25% concordance for SLE between identical twins and an increased incidence of HLA-B8 and -DR3.
- *Immunological factors.* Antinuclear antibodies are present which are thought to result from polyclonal activation of B cells by an antigenic stimulus, possible viral antigens. This may be associated with impaired T cell regulation and deficiencies in complement. Most of the visceral lesions are mediated by vascular immune complex (DNA–anti-DNA) deposition.
- *Drugs.* Hydralazine and procainamide may cause a mild lupus-like syndrome, which often resolves after the drug is withdrawn.
- *Infection.* Viral infections may be responsible.
- *Hormonal factors.* The high incidence in women suggests that female hormones may modify the immune response.

254

## Clinical features

Clinical manifestations are varied (Fig. 6.5) and most are due to the consequences of vasculitis. A migratory asymmetrical arthralgia is one of the most common presenting features. Synovitis and joint effusions are uncommon and joint destruction is very rare. Non-specific features such as fever, malaise and depression may dominate the clinical picture.

Discoid lupus is a benign variant of the disease, in which skin involvement may be the only feature. There is a characteristic facial rash with erythematous plaques which progress to scarring and pigmentation. Sunlight is an exacerbating factor in most patients.

## Investigations

- Blood count usually shows a normochromic, normocytic anaemia, often with neutropenia and thrombocytopenia. The ESR is raised but the CRP is usually normal.

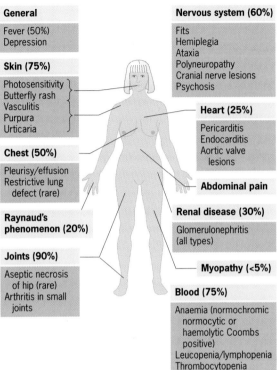

**General**

Fever (50%)
Depression

**Skin (75%)**

Photosensitivity
Butterfly rash
Vasculitis
Purpura
Urticaria

**Chest (50%)**

Pleurisy/effusion
Restrictive lung
defect (rare)

**Raynaud's
phenomenon (20%)**

**Joints (90%)**

Aseptic necrosis
of hip (rare)
Arthritis in small
joints

**Nervous system (60%)**

Fits
Hemiplegia
Ataxia
Polyneuropathy
Cranial nerve lesions
Psychosis

**Heart (25%)**

Pericarditis
Endocarditis
Aortic valve
lesions

**Abdominal pain**

**Renal disease (30%)**

Glomerulonephritis
(all types)

**Myopathy (<5%)**

**Blood (75%)**

Anaemia (normochromic
normocytic or
haemolytic Coombs
positive)
Leucopenia/lymphopenia
Thrombocytopenia

**Fig. 6.5 Clinical features of SLE.** The frequency of organ involvement is indicated as a percentage.

- Serum autoantibodies: antinuclear antibodies are positive in almost all cases. Double-stranded DNA (dsDNA) binding is specific for SLE but is positive in only 50% of cases. Rheumatoid factor is positive in 25% of cases.
- Serum complement levels are reduced in active disease.
- Anticardiolipin antibodies are present in 35–45%.
- Histological examination, for example of a renal biopsy, shows a vasculitis.

## Management

Treatment depends on the symptoms and severity of disease.

- NSAIDs or specific COX-2 inhibitors are useful for patients with mild disease and with arthralgia.
- Hydroxychloroquine is used for mild disease when symptoms cannot be controlled with NSAIDs, or for cutaneous disease.
- Corticosteroids form the mainstay of treatment, particularly in moderate to severe disease. The aim is to control disease activity (e.g. prednisolone 30 mg/day for 4 weeks) before gradually reducing the dose.
- Immunosuppressives (e.g. azathioprine, cyclophosphamide), usually in combination with corticosteroids, are used for patients with severe manifestations, e.g. renal or cerebral disease.
- Topical steroids are used for discoid lupus. These patients should also avoid excessive sunlight.

## Prognosis

The disease is characterized by relapses and remissions even in severe disease. The 10-year survival is about 90%. Infection has replaced renal failure as the most common cause of death in SLE.

## Antiphospholipid syndrome (K&C p. 560)

This syndrome is characterized by autoantibodies directed against either phospholipids or plasma proteins bound to anionic phospholipids. Three types of antibodies have been described: lupus anticoagulant, anticardiolipin and $\beta_2$-glycoprotein I antibodies. The antibodies are thought to play a role in thrombosis by reacting with plasma proteins and phospholipids with an effect on platelet membranes, endothelial cells and clotting compounds such as pro-thrombin, protein C and protein S (p. 206). Although first described in patients with SLE, it is more common than SLE and most patients (often young women) with the syndrome do not have SLE.

## Clinical features

The major clinical features are the result of thrombosis:

- In arteries: stroke, transient ischaemic attacks, myocardial infarction
- In veins: deep vein thrombosis, Budd–Chiari syndrome (p. 149)
- In the placenta: recurrent abortions.

Other features include valvular heart disease, migraine, epilepsy and thrombocytopenia.

## Investigations

The diagnosis is made on finding one or more of the specific serum antibodies (see above) in a patient with thrombosis or recurrent abortion.

## Management

Aspirin is given in mild cases; warfarin is used in more severe cases.

# Systemic sclerosis (K&C p. 561)

Systemic sclerosis (scleroderma) is a chronic multisystem disease which predominantly affects the skin and is usually accompanied by Raynaud's phenomenon (p. 440). It is three to five times more common in women than men, and presents before the age of 50 years.

257

## Aetiology

The cause of systemic sclerosis is unknown, although many abnormalities in both cellular and humoral immunity have been documented. There is an increase in dermal collagen and a decrease in elastic tissue which leads to the typical thickening and immobility.

## Clinical features

*Limited cutaneous scleroderma (60% of cases)* This starts initially with Raynaud's phenomenon, often prior to the development of cutaneous manifestations. The skin changes that dominate this disease are usually limited to the hands, face and feet. Typically the skin is thickened, bound down to underlying structures, and the fingers taper (sclerodactyly). There is often a characteristic facial appearance, with beaking of the nose, a fixed expression, radial furrowing of the lips and limitation of mouth movements. There may be telangiectasia and palpable subcutaneous nodules of calcium deposition in the fingers (calcinosis). The CREST syndrome (Calcinosis, Raynaud's phenomenon, oEsophageal involvement, Sclerodactyly, Telangiectasia) was the term previously used to describe this syndrome.

**Diffuse cutaneous scleroderma (40% of cases)** The skin changes develop more rapidly after the development of Raynaud's phenomenon and are more widespread than in limited cutaneous scleroderma. There is early involvement of other organs (Table 6.5).

## Investigations

The diagnosis of scleroderma is primarily based upon the presence of characteristic skin changes.

- Blood count shows a normochromic, normocytic anaemia and the ESR may be raised.
- Serum autoantibodies. Antinuclear antibodies are often positive. Specific types are antinucleolar and antitopoisomerase (Scl 70). Anticentromere antibodies occur in the CREST syndrome.
- Radiology. An X-ray of the hands may show deposits of calcium around the fingers, and there may be erosion and resorption of the tufts of the distal phalanges. High-resolution CT demonstrates fibrotic lung involvement.
- Oesophageal manometry demonstrates failure of peristalsis in the distal oesophagus, with reduced oesophageal sphincter pressure.

## Management

Management is symptomatic. There is no specific treatment. Control of hypertension is necessary to prevent further kidney damage.

## Prognosis

The 10-year survival is 70% and 55% in limited cutaneous and diffuse cutaneous disease respectively. Lung disease is

**Table 6.5**
Major clinical features of scleroderma

| Organ | Clinical manifestation | Involved in (%) |
|---|---|---|
| Skin | Thickened skin, sclerodactyly, telangiectasia, calcinosis | 90 |
| Vascular | Raynaud's phenomenon | 80 |
| Oesophagus | Impaired peristalsis causing reflux with eventual stricture formation | 80 |
| Lungs | Fibrosis, pulmonary hypertension | 45 |
| Heart | Myocardial fibrosis with arrhythmias and conduction defects | 40 |
| Kidney | Obliterative endarteritis of renal vessels with renal failure and hypertension | 35 |
| Eyes | Sjögren's syndrome | 15 |
| Joints/muscle | Joint deformity, myopathy, myositis | 20–25 |

now the major cause of death (previously accelerated hypertension and renal failure).

# Polymyositis and dermatomyositis

(*K&C* p. 563)

Polymyositis is a rare muscle disorder of unknown aetiology in which there is inflammation and necrosis of skeletal muscle fibres. When accompanied by a rash it is called dermatomyositis.

## Clinical features

Peak ages of onset are in childhood and in the fifth and sixth decades. Muscle weakness affecting the proximal muscles of the shoulder and pelvic girdle is the chief symptom. Patients have difficulty squatting, going upstairs, rising from a chair and raising their hands above the head. This may be accompanied by pain, tenderness and muscle wasting. The skin changes of dermatomyositis are characteristic: a heliotrope (purple) periorbital skin rash, a photosensitive scaling rash on the face, and erythematous plaques over the dorsal aspects of the fingers and knuckles. Other features include arthralgia or arthritis, dysphagia resulting from oesophageal muscle involvement, and Raynaud's phenomenon. Dermatomyositis is associated with an increased incidence of underlying malignancy, particularly in the older age groups.

## Investigations

- Muscle biopsy is the definitive test in establishing the diagnosis and in excluding other causes of myopathy. There is inflammatory cell infiltration and necrosis of muscle cells.
- Muscle enzymes (aldolase or creatine phosphokinase) are elevated in the serum.
- Anti-Jo-1 antibodies (anti-histidyl-tRNA synthetase) are positive.
- ESR is elevated in 5% of cases.
- Electromyography (EMG) shows characteristic changes.
- MRI can demonstrate areas of muscle inflammation.

## Management
Oral prednisolone is the treatment of choice. Sometimes immunosuppressive therapy with azathioprine or methotrexate is required.

## Prognosis
Fifty per cent of affected children die within 2 years. In adults the prognosis is better, except in association with malignancy.

# Overlap syndrome (K&C p. 564)
This rare disorder combines features of more than one of the connective tissue diseases. Cerebral and renal disease is unusual and the prognosis is good. High titres of antibodies to extractable nuclear antigens (p. 807) such as ribonucleo-protein (RNP) are commonly found.

# Sjögren's syndrome (K&C p. 564)
Sjögren's syndrome is a chronic autoimmune disorder predominantly affecting middle-aged women. It is characterized by immunologically mediated destruction of epithelial exocrine glands, especially the lacrimal and salivary glands.

## Clinical features
The main features are dry eyes (keratoconjunctivitis sicca) and dry mouth (xerostomia). It occurs as an isolated disorder (primary Sjögren's syndrome), also known as the sicca syndrome, or in association with another systemic disease (secondary Sjögren's syndrome), commonly rheumatoid arthritis, SLE, and primary biliary cirrhosis. Other features of primary Sjögren's syndrome are arthritis, Raynaud's phenomenon and interstitial nephritis. Six per cent develop lymphomas.

## Investigations
- Antinuclear antibodies are found in 60–70% of patients. Anti-Ro and anti-La antibodies are present in 70% of patients with primary Sjögren's syndrome.
- Labial gland biopsy shows characteristic changes of lymphocyte infiltration and destruction of acinar tissue.
- A positive Schirmer test (a standard strip of filter paper is placed on the inside of the lower eyelid;

wetting of less than 10 mm in 5 min is positive)
confirms defective tear production.

## Management

Treatment is symptomatic with artificial tears for dry eyes.

## Vasculitis (K&C p. 564)

Vasculitis is inflammation of the blood vessel walls and
may be associated with SLE, rheumatoid arthritis,
polymyositis and some allergic drug reactions. The term
'systemic vasculitides' describes a group of multisystem
disorders in which vasculitis is the principal feature. These
disorders are all rare except for giant cell (temporal) arteritis. Classification of the systemic vasculitides is based on
the size of the vessels affected (Table 6.6).

## Polymyalgia and giant cell arteritis (temporal arteritis) (K&C p. 565)

Polymyalgia and giant cell arteritis are clinical syndromes
affecting elderly people. Both are associated with the
finding of a giant cell arteritis on temporal artery biopsy.

**Table 6.6**
Classification of vasculitis

**Large-vessel vasculitis** (aorta and its major branches)
Giant-cell arteritis
Takayasu's arteritis (affects young women, causing coronary and
CNS ischaemia)

**Medium-sized-vessel vasculitis** (main visceral vessels, e.g.
renal, coronary)
Classic polyarteritis nodosa
Kawasaki's disease (affects young children)

**Small-vessel vasculitis** (small arteries, arterioles, venules and
capillaries)
ANCA positive
    Microscopic polyangiitis
    Wegener's granulomatosis (p. 486)
    Churg–Strauss syndrome
ANCA negative
    Henoch–Schönlein purpura
    Cutaneous leucocytoclastic angiitis
    Essential cryoglobulinaemia

ANCA, antineutrophil cytoplasmic antibodies (p. 800)

Patients may have symptoms and signs limited to polymyalgia or to giant cell arteritis throughout the course of their illness while others have manifestations of both.

## Clinical features

Polymyalgia is characterized by an abrupt onset of stiffness and intense pain in the proximal muscles of the shoulder and pelvic girdle. Significant objective weakness is uncommon. There may be constitutional symptoms, with malaise, fever, weight loss and anorexia. Arteritic involvement by inflammation is most frequently noticed in the superficial temporal arteries and causes localized headache, temporal artery tenderness and loss of pulsation (p. 702). Giant cell arteritis affecting the vertebrobasilar, and sometimes the carotid, circulation may result in stroke.

## Investigations

The diagnosis is usually based on clinical findings.

- Blood count usually shows a very high ESR (around 100 mm/h) and a normochromic, normocytic anaemia.
- Temporal artery biopsy may be performed if arteritis is suspected and should be performed before or within a week of starting corticosteroids.

## Management

Treatment of polymyalgia rheumatica and giant cell arteritis is with corticosteroids. The usual starting dose is 15 mg/day for polymyalgia and 60 mg/day for temporal arteritis. The dose is gradually reduced by weekly decrements of 5 mg. Once 10 mg is reached a reduction of 1 mg every 2–4 weeks is usually sufficient. The dose is titrated against symptoms and the ESR. Prophylaxis against steroid-induced osteoporosis should be given (p. 279). The disease may relapse when steroid treatment is stopped.

## Polyarteritis nodosa (classic polyarteritis nodosa) (K&C p. 566)

Polyarteritis nodosa (PAN) predominantly affects middle-aged men. Hepatitis B surface antigen is detected in some patients and may be involved in the pathogenesis. There is a necrotizing arteritis associated with microaneurysm formation, thrombosis and infarction. Clinical features include fever, malaise, weight loss, mononeuritis multiplex, abdominal pain (resulting from visceral infarcts), renal impairment and hypertension. The diagnosis is made by biopsy of a clinically affected organ, often the kidney, which shows focal necrotizing glomerulonephritis and inflammation of medium-sized arteries. Mesenteric or renal arteriography shows microaneurysms.

## Microscopic polyangiitis (K&C p. 901)

A necrotizing focal segmental glomerulonephritis causes haematuria, proteinuria and sometimes progressive renal failure. Other features include arthralgia and purpuric rashes. Diagnosis is by renal biopsy and measurement of serum perinuclear antineutrophil cytoplasmic antibodies (pANCA, present in 70%; see p. 800). Treatment is similar to Churg–Strauss syndrome (see below).

## Churg–Strauss syndrome (K&C p. 901)

This is rare and characterized by a triad of asthma, eosinophilia and a systemic vasculitis. The treatments for Churg–Strauss syndrome, PAN and microscopic polyangiitis are similar, using prednisolone, azathioprine and cyclophosphamide.

## Henoch–Schönlein purpura (K&C p. 570 & p. 605)

This condition is most commonly seen in children and presents as a purpuric rash, mainly on the legs and buttocks. The rash is caused by a vasculitis with intradermal bleeding. Abdominal pain, arthritis, haematuria and nephritis also occur. It is characterized by vascular deposition of IgA-dominant immune complexes, and the onset is often preceded by an acute upper respiratory tract infection. Recovery is usually spontaneous.

## Behçet's disease (K&C p. 568)

This is a rare multisystem chronic disease of unknown cause, characterized by recurrent oral ulceration. Diagnosis is clinical and requires the presence of oral ulceration and any two of the following:

- Genital ulcers
- Eye lesions (uveitis, retinal vascular lesions)
- Skin lesions (erythema nodosum, papulopustular lesions)
- Positive skin pathergy test (skin injury, e.g. needle prick, leads to pustule formation in 48 h).

Other features include arthritis, gastrointestinal ulceration with pain and diarrhoea, pulmonary and renal lesions, meningoencephalitis, and organic confusional states. Treatment is with immunosuppressive therapy (steroids, azathioprine, ciclosporin).

## Arthritis in children

There are three main types: juvenile chronic arthritis, juvenile rheumatoid arthritis and juvenile ankylosing spondylitis discussed in detail in *Clinical Medicine* (*K&C* p. 569).

## Crystal deposition diseases

Two main types of crystal account for the majority of crystal-induced arthritis: sodium urate and calcium pyrophosphate. Neutrophils ingest the crystals and initiate a pro-inflammatory reaction. Crystals may be found in asymptomatic joints.

### Gout (*K&C* p. 552)

Gout is an abnormality of uric acid metabolism resulting in the deposition of sodium urate crystals in:

- Joints, causing arthritis
- Soft tissue, causing tophi and tenosynovitis
- Urinary tract, causing urate stones and renal failure.

### *Epidemiology*

The prevalence of gout is about 0.2% in Europeans. The disease is 10 times more common in men, rarely occurs before puberty and is more prevalent in the upper social classes. One-third have a positive family history.

## Pathogenesis

The biochemical abnormality is hyperuricaemia resulting from overproduction or renal underexcretion of uric acid. Urate is derived from the breakdown of purines (adenine and guanine in DNA and RNA), which are synthesized in the body or ingested (a minor component). In idiopathic (primary) gout, the most common form, impaired renal excretion is the most common cause of hyperuricaemia. The causes of hyperuricaemia are shown in Table 6.7.

## Clinical features

The typical patient is an obese middle-aged man who presents with acute gout, characterized by the sudden onset of severe pain and swelling, most frequently in the first metatarsophalangeal joint of the big toe. The joint becomes red, hot, swollen and exquisitely tender. The attack may be precipitated by a surgical operation, dietary or alcoholic excess, starvation or drugs, particularly thiazide diuretics. With persisting hyperuricaemia there is recurrent acute arthritis affecting more joints, associated with the permanent deposition of urate in and around joints (chronic tophaceous gout). Tophaceous urate deposits may also occur in cartilage, particularly the pinna of the ear. Acute attacks must be differentiated from other causes of monoarthritis, particularly septic arthritis.

## Investigations

- Serum uric acid is usually raised, but may be normal in acute gout. However, the diagnosis is excluded if the serum uric acid is in the lower half of the normal range. Conversely, asymptomatic hyperuricaemia is common.
- Serum urea and creatinine for signs of renal impairment.
- Joint fluid microscopy reveals long needle-shaped crystals which are negatively birefringent under polarized light.

## Management

Acute attacks are treated with anti-inflammatory drugs:

- NSAIDs, e.g. naproxen, or a COX-2 specific inhibitor (p. 239), are the treatment of choice.

**Table 6.7**
Causes of hyperuricaemia

| Impaired excretion of uric acid | Increased production of uric acid |
|---|---|
| Idiopathic (primary) gout | Idiopathic (primary) gout |
| Chronic renal disease (clinical gout unusual) | Increased turnover of purines |
| Drug therapy, e.g. thiazide diuretics, low-dose aspirin |   Myeloproliferative disorders, e.g. polycythaemia vera |
| Hypertension |   Lymphoproliferative disorders, e.g. leukaemia |
| Lead toxicity |   Others, e.g. carcinoma, severe psoriasis |
| Alcohol | Increased de novo purine synthesis (very rare) |
| Glucose-6-phosphatase deficiency |   HGPRT deficiency (Lesch–Nyhan syndrome) |
| |   PPS overactivity |

HGPRT, hypoxanthine-guanine phosphoribosyltransferase; PPS, phosphoribosyl-pyrophosphate synthetase

- Intra-articular corticosteroid injection after aspiration of effusion.
- Other treatments. Intramuscular ACTH is very effective for difficult cases. Oral colchicine may be useful if NSAIDs are contraindicated, e.g. active peptic ulceration.

Long-term therapy is considered when the acute attack subsides. Obese patients should lose weight, alcohol consumption should be reduced, and drugs such as thiazides and salicylates should be withdrawn. Drugs used to reduce serum uric acid include:

- Allopurinol inhibits xanthine oxidase (an enzyme in the purine breakdown pathway) and is the drug of choice. It may precipitate an acute attack and is used initially in conjunction with an NSAID.
- Probenecid, a uricosuric agent, is used in those allergic to allopurinol.

## Pyrophosphate arthropathy (pseudogout)

(*K&C* p. 554)

This condition is associated with the deposition of calcium pyrophosphate dihydrate in articular cartilage and peri-articular tissue. The acute attacks of synovitis that occur in 25% of patients are known as pseudogout. The aetiology is unknown and it occurs most commonly in elderly women. It may occur secondary to other diseases, including primary hyperparathyroidism, haemochromatosis, hypothyroidism and gout.

### Clinical features

The clinical picture is similar to primary osteoarthritis, with acute attacks most commonly involving the knee. There is often polyarticular involvement or involvement of unusual joints such as the wrist, and the patient may be pyrexial.

### Investigations

- Blood count may show a raised white cell count.
- Synovial fluid examination reveals small brick-shaped pyrophosphate crystals which are positively birefringent under polarized light (compare uric acid).

- X-ray of the knee may show linear calcification parallel to the articular surfaces (chondrocalcinosis).
- Serum calcium is normal.

### Management

Rest with joint aspiration and NSAIDs forms the mainstay of treatment. Injection of local corticosteroids may also be useful.

## Back pain

### Lumbar back pain (K&C p. 522)

Lumbar back pain is an extremely common symptom experienced by most people at some time in their lives. Mechanical back pain is a common cause in young people. It starts suddenly, is often unilateral, and may be helped by rest. It may arise from the facet joints, spinal ligaments or muscle. The history, physical examination and simple investigations will also often identify the minority of patients with other causes of back pain (Table 6.8).

The age of the patient is important in deciding the aetiology of back pain because certain causes are more common in particular age groups. These are illustrated in Table 6.9.

### Investigations

A detailed history and physical examination (see Table 6.8) will lead to the diagnosis in many cases. The key points are age, speed of onset, the presence of motor or sensory symptoms, involvement of the bladder or bowel, and the presence of stiffness and the effect of exercise. Young adults with a history suggestive of mechanical back pain and with no physical signs do not need further investigation.

- Blood count is usually normal. The ESR may be raised with inflammatory back pain and tumours.
- Serum biochemistry. A raised calcium and alkaline phosphatase suggest metastases. Typically with myeloma the calcium is raised, with a normal alkaline phosphatase. A raised alkaline phosphatase with a normal calcium occurs with metabolic bone disease.

**Table 6.8**
Causes of lumbar back pain

| | | Relevant points in the history and examination |
|---|---|---|
| Mechanical | Prolapsed intervertebral disc<br>Osteoarthritis<br>Fractures<br>Spondylolisthesis<br>Spinal stenosis | Often sudden onset<br>Pain worse in the evening<br>Morning stiffness is absent<br>Exercise aggravates pain |
| Inflammatory | Ankylosing spondylitis<br>Infection (see below) | Gradual onset<br>Pain worse in the morning<br>Morning stiffness is present<br>Exercise relieves pain |
| Serious cause | Metastatic carcinoma<br>Myeloma<br>Tuberculosis osteomyelitis<br>Bacterial osteomyelitis<br>Cord or cauda equina compression | Constant pain without relief<br>Systemically unwell: fever, weight loss<br>Localized bone tenderness<br>Bilateral signs in the legs<br>Neurological deficit involving more than one root level<br>Bladder, bowel or sexual function deficits |
| Others | Osteomalacia, Paget's disease, referred pain<br>from pelvic/abdominal disease | |

Table 6.9
Low back pain – disorders most commonly found in specific age groups

| 15–30 years | 30–50 years | 50 years and over |
|---|---|---|
| Mechanical | Mechanical | Degenerative joint disease |
| Prolapsed intervertebral disc | Prolapsed intervertebral disc | Osteoporosis |
| Ankylosing spondylitis | Degenerative joint disease | Paget's disease |
| Spondylolisthesis | Malignancy | Malignancy, myeloma |
| Fractures (all ages) | | |
| Infective lesions (all ages) | | |

Prostate-specific antigen should be measured if secondary prostatic disease is suspected.

- Radiology. X-rays may be useful for excluding serious disease, although they may be misleading, e.g. degenerative disease is virtually always present in older people.
- Technetium bone scan will show increased uptake with infection or malignancy.
- MRI is useful when neurological symptoms and signs are present. It is useful for the detection of disc and cord lesions, and has largely taken over from CT and myelography.

### Management

The treatment depends on the cause. Mechanical back pain is managed with analgesia, brief rest and physiotherapy. Exercise programmes reduce long-term problems.

## Intervertebral disc disease

272

### Acute disc disease (K&C p. 524)

Acute disc disease is a syndrome in which there is prolapse of the intervertebral disc resulting in acute back pain (lumbago), with or without radiation of the pain to areas supplied by the sciatic nerve (sciatica). It is a disease of younger people (20–40 years) because the disc degenerates with age and in elderly people is no longer capable of prolapse. In older patients sciatica is more likely to be the result of compression of the nerve root by osteophytes in the lateral recess of the spinal canal.

### Clinical features

There is a sudden onset of severe back pain, often following a strenuous activity. The pain is often clearly related to position and is aggravated by movement. Muscle spasm leads to a sideways tilt when standing. The radiation of the pain and the clinical findings depend on the disc affected (Table 6.10), the lowest three discs being those most commonly affected.

**Table 6.10**
Symptoms and signs of common root compression syndromes produced by lumbar disc prolapse

| Root lesion | Pain | Sensory loss | Motor weakness | Reflex lost | Other signs |
|---|---|---|---|---|---|
| S1 | From buttock down back of thigh and leg to ankle and foot | Sole of foot and posterior calf | Plantar flexion of ankle and toes | Ankle jerk | Diminished straight leg raising |
| L5 | From buttock to lateral aspect of leg and dorsum of foot | Dorsum of foot and anterolateral aspect of lower leg | Dorsiflexion of foot and toes | None | As above |
| L4 | Lateral aspect of thigh to medial side of calf | Medial aspect of calf and shin | Dorsiflexion and inversion of ankle; extension of knee | Knee jerk | Positive femoral stretch test |

273

## Investigations

Investigations are of very limited value in acute disc disease and X-rays are often normal. MRI or myelography are usually reserved for patients in whom surgery is being considered (see later).

## Management

Treatment is aimed at the relief of symptoms and has little effect on the duration of the disease. In the acute stage, treatment consists of bed rest on a firm mattress, analgesia, and occasionally epidural corticosteroid injection in severe disease. Surgery is only considered for severe or increasing neurological impairment, e.g. foot drop or bladder symptoms. Physiotherapy plays an important role in the recovery phase, helping to correct posture and restore movement.

# Chronic disc disease

This common syndrome is characterized by the presence of chronic lower back pain associated with 'degenerative' changes in the lower lumbar discs and apophyseal joints. Pain is usually of the mechanical type (see above). Sciatic radiation may occur and there may be a history of acute disc prolapse. Usually the pain is long-standing and the prospects for cure are limited. However, measures that have been found useful include NSAIDs, physiotherapy and weight reduction. Surgery can be considered when pain arises from a single identifiable level and has failed to respond to conservative measures. Fusion at this level, with decompression of the affected nerve roots, can be successful.

# Mechanical problems

### Spondylolisthesis (K&C p. 525)

Spondylolisthesis is characterized by a slipping forward of one vertebra on another, most commonly at L4/L5. It arises because of a defect in the pars interarticularis of the vertebra, and may be either congenital or acquired (e.g. trauma). The condition is associated with mechanical pain which worsens throughout the day. The pain may radiate to one or other leg and there may be signs of nerve root irritation. Small spondylolistheses, often associated with degenerative disease of the lumbar spine, may be treated conservatively with simple analgesics. A large spondylolisthesis causing severe symptoms should be treated with spinal fusion.

### Spinal stenosis (*K&C p. 525*)

Narrowing of the lower spinal canal compresses the cauda equina, resulting in back and buttock pain typically coming on after a period of walking and easing with rest. Accordingly it is sometimes called spinal claudication. Causes include disc prolapse, degenerative osteophyte formation, tumour and congenital narrowing of the spinal canal. CT and MRI will demonstrate cord compression and treatment is by surgical decompression.

## Neck pain (*K&C p. 518*)

Pain in the neck may be caused by rheumatoid arthritis, ankylosing spondylitis or fibrositis (chronic muscle pain in young women with no underlying cause; large psychological overlay in some patients). In addition, disc disease, both acute and chronic, the latter in association with osteoarthritis, may occur in the neck as well as in the lumbar spine. The three lowest cervical discs are most often affected, and there is pain and stiffness of the neck with or without root pain radiating to the arm. Chronic cervical disc disease is known as cervical spondylosis.

## Bone disease

Bone normally consists of 70% mineral and 30% organic matrix (mostly type 1 collagen fibres). The mineral component consists mostly of a complex crystalline salt of calcium and phosphate called hydroxyapatite. Although major skeletal growth occurs in childhood, adult bone is continuously being remodelled, with bone formation and resorption. Two major cell types are involved in bone remodelling:

- Osteoblasts produce type 1 collagen and growth factors, and also regulate osteoclast activity.
- Osteoclasts produce lysosomal enzymes which degrade collagen matrix (*K&C p. 574*)

# Control of calcium and bone metabolism

(*K&C* p. 576)

Vitamin D and parathyroid hormone (PTH) are the major factors that control plasma calcium concentration and bone turnover. Bone metabolism is also controlled by calcitonin, glucocorticoids, sex hormones, growth hormone and thyroid hormone.

## Vitamin D

The metabolism and actions of vitamin D are shown in Figure 6.6.

## Parathyroid hormone (PTH)

PTH levels rise as serum ionized calcium falls. The effects are several, all serving to increase plasma calcium and decrease plasma phosphate:

- Increased osteoclastic resorption of bone
- Increased intestinal absorption of calcium
- Increased synthesis of $1,25\text{-}(OH)_2D_3$
- Increased renal tubular reabsorption of calcium
- Increased renal excretion of phosphate.

# Osteomalacia (*K&C* p. 584)

Inadequate mineralization of the osteoid framework, leading to soft bones, produces rickets during bone growth in children and osteomalacia following epiphyseal closure in adults.

## Aetiology

- Deficiency of vitamin D as a result of a combination of poor diet and inadequate sunlight. This is seen in immobile elderly people and in female Asian immigrants in the UK.
- Malabsorption, e.g. coeliac disease and small bowel resection.
- Renal disease leading to inadequate conversion of $25\text{-}(OH)D_3$ to $1,25\text{-}(OH)_2D_3$ (Fig. 6.6).
- Other causes include liver failure, renal phosphate loss and anticonvulsant therapy (caused by increased vitamin D inactivation).

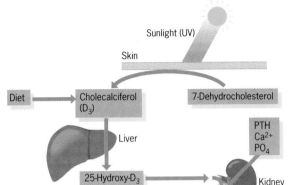

**Fig. 6.6 The metabolism and actions of vitamin D.** Cholecalciferol is predominantly formed from photoactivation of 7-dehydrocholesterol in the skin. In the liver, cholecalciferol is converted to 25-hydroxycholecalciferol, which is then converted to the much more active form, 1,25-dihydroxycholecalciferol, in the kidney. PTH, parathyroid hormone.

## Clinical features

In the adult osteomalacia produces muscle and bone pain and fractures. In addition, a proximal myopathy leads to a 'waddling' gait and difficulty in rising from a chair. The principal differential diagnosis in a patient presenting with bone pain, bone fractures and osteopenia on the X-ray is osteoporosis versus osteomalacia. The distinction can usually be made from the history, physical examination and a combination of laboratory and radiological studies.

## Investigations

- Serum biochemistry shows a low phosphate, low or low–normal calcium and increased alkaline phosphatase.
- Serum 25-hydroxyvitamin $D_3$ is usually low.

- Radiology. X-ray appearance is characteristic, showing defective mineralization and Looser's zones (low-density bands extending from the cortex inwards in the shafts of the long bones).
- Bone biopsy is the definitive investigation and shows increased non-mineralized bone. However, this procedure is uncomfortable and rarely necessary.

## Management

The treatment is with oral vitamin D; the dose and formulation depend on the cause (Table 6.11). Treatment is monitored by measurement of serum alkaline phosphatase and calcium.

## Osteoporosis (K&C p. 578)

Osteoporosis means thin bone and the term implies a reduction in bone mass, including all components of bone, not just calcium. The bone is fragile, with an increased risk of fracture.

## Aetiology

Bone resorption is part of the normal ageing process, occurring more in women than in men, largely as a result of postmenopausal oestrogen deficiency. The risk factors for osteoporosis are those that cause a reduction in peak bone mass attained in adult life or those that cause increased bone loss (Table 6.12).

## Clinical features

Symptoms of osteoporosis are the result of fractures, which typically occur at three sites: the thoracic and lumbar

**Table 6.11**
Treatment of osteomalacia

| | |
|---|---|
| Vitamin D deficiency | Vitamin D$_2$ 10 μg (400 U) daily |
| Malabsorption | Vitamin D$_2$ 1–2.5 mg (40 000–100 000 U) daily |
| Renal failure | 1α-Hydroxycholecalciferol (alfacalcidol or 1α-(OH)D$_3$) or 1,25-dihydroxycholecalciferol (calcitriol or 1,25-(OH)$_2$D$_3$) |

**Table 6.12**
Risk factors for osteoporosis

Increasing age
Female sex
Early menopause
Oophorectomy
Slender habitus
Smoking
Excess alcohol
Lack of exercise
Family history
White race
Drugs (corticosteroids, heparin, ciclosporin)
Endocrine disease (Cushing's syndrome, hyperparathyroidism, acromegaly)
Other chronic disease (Crohn's disease, coeliac disease, primary biliary cirrhosis)

vertebrae, neck of the femur and the distal radius (Colles' fracture). Vertebral fractures may lead to kyphosis and loss of height.

### Investigations

- Bone densitometry. Dual-energy X-ray absorptiometry (DXA) measures real bone density, usually of the lumbar spine and proximal femur. It is the gold standard in osteoporosis diagnosis and reflects fracture risk which may influence treatment decisions.
- Radiology. X-rays may show reduced bone density (osteopenia) and will demonstrate fractures.
- Serum biochemistry. Calcium, phosphate and alkaline phosphatase are normal.

### Management

Prevention is better than treatment of established disease. Predisposing factors should be addressed and those at risk (Table 6.12) identified for DXA.

Non-drug therapy of osteoporosis includes regular exercise, adequate intake of calcium (1500 mg/day) and vitamin D (400–800 IU/day) and, cessation of smoking.

Selected patients with osteoporosis or at high risk for osteoporosis should also be given drug treatment.

- Bisphosphonates (e.g. etidronate, alendronate and risedronate) inhibit bone resorption through inhibition of osteoclast activity, increase bone mass at the hip and spine and most have been shown to reduce fracture incidence. Optimal duration of therapy is unknown.

- Oestrogen therapy as hormone replacement therapy (HRT) should be considered for women at high risk (see Table 6.12) to reduce bone loss during the postmenopausal years. Oestrogens are combined with progestogens in women with an intact uterus because oestrogens alone increase the risk of developing endometrial cancer.

- Raloxifene, a selective oestrogen-receptor modulator (SERM), activates oestrogen receptors on bone while having no stimulatory effect on endometrium. It has been shown to reduce bone mineral density loss at spine and hip, though fracture rates are reduced only in the spine.

## Paget's disease (K&C p. 582)

Paget's disease is characterized by excessive osteoclastic bone resorption followed by disordered osteoblastic activity, leading to abundant new bone formation which is structurally abnormal and weak.

### Aetiology

A gene predisposing to Paget's disease has been identified on chromosome 18q. Osteoclasts contain viral inclusion bodies, suggesting a possible 'slow viral' aetiology.

### Epidemiology

The incidence increases with age; it is rare in the under-40s and affects up to 10% of adults by the age of 90.

### Clinical features

The most common sites are the femur, pelvis, tibia, skull and lumbosacral spine, although any bone can be involved. Most cases are asymptomatic, but features include the following:

- Bone pain
- Apparent joint pain when the involved bone is close to a joint

- Deformities: enlargement of the skull, bowing of the tibia
- Complications: nerve compression (deafness, paraparesis), fractures, rarely cardiac failure and osteogenic sarcoma.

## Investigations

The diagnosis is often clinical and supported by:

- Serum biochemistry, shows a raised alkaline phosphatase concentration (reflects level of bone formation), often > 1000 U/L, with a normal calcium and phosphate.
- X-rays showing characteristic changes, most often in the pelvis, skull or spine. There is localized bony enlargement and distortion, sclerotic changes (increased density) and osteolytic areas (loss of bone and reduced density).
- Radionuclide bone scans showing increased uptake of bone-seeking radionuclides, which is due to increased bone formation. The appearances on bone scans and plain X-rays may be difficult to distinguish from metastatic carcinoma, especially sclerotic secondaries seen with breast and prostate cancer.
- Urinary hydroxyproline, though not commonly measured in practice, is usually increased and reflects the level of bone resorption.

## Treatment

Bisphosphonates inhibit bone resorption by decreasing osteoclastic activity, and form the mainstay of treatment. They are indicated for symptomatic patients and asymptomatic patients at risk of complications (e.g. fracture, nerve entrapment). Disease activity is monitored by symptoms and measurement of serum alkaline phosphatase.

# 7

# Water and electrolytes

## Body fluid compartments

A 70 kg man contains approximately 42 L of water (i.e. about 50–60% of total bodyweight is water) and 3000 mmol of osmotically active sodium (Table 7.1). Maintenance of the total amount depends on the balance between intake and loss. Water and electrolytes are taken in as food and water, and lost in urine, sweat and faeces (Table 7.2). In addition, about 500 mL of water are lost daily in expired air.

Body water is distributed between three major compartments:

- The intracellular fluid (28 L, about 35% of lean bodyweight)
- The interstitial fluid that bathes the cells (9.4 L, about 12%)
- Plasma (4.6 L, about 4–5%).

Water moves freely between compartments and the distribution is determined by the osmotic equilibrium between them. Osmolality is determined by the concentration of osmotically active particles. Thus 1 mole of sodium chloride dissolved in 1 kg of water has an osmolality of 2 mmol/kg, as sodium chloride freely dissociates into two particles, the sodium ion $Na^+$ and the chloride ion $Cl^-$. One mole of urea (which does not dissociate) in 1 kg of water has an osmolality of 1 mmol/kg. Sodium is the major extracellular ion and therefore the main determinant of plasma osmolality. The plasma osmolality can be calculated from the plasma concentrations of sodium, urea and glucose, as follows:

$$\text{Calculated plasma osmolality (mmol)} = (2 \times \text{plasma } Na^+) + [\text{urea}] + [\text{glucose}].$$

The factor of 2 applied to sodium concentration allows for associated anions (chloride and bicarbonate). The other extracellular solutes, e.g. calcium, potassium and

284

**Table 7.1**
Normal adult total body content and serum electrolyte concentrations

| Cation | Total body content (mmol) | Extracellular/intracellular distribution | Serum concentration (mmol/L) | Dietary intake/day (mmol) |
|---|---|---|---|---|
| Sodium | 3000 | 95% extracellular | 136–144 | 140 |
| Potassium | 3500 | 98% intracellular | 3.6–5.0 | 80–150 |
| Magnesium | 1000 | 99% intracellular | 0.7–1.1 | 15 |

**Table 7.2**
The normal daily water and sodium balance in a 75 kg man

| | Input | | | Output |
|---|---|---|---|---|
| **Water (mL)** | | | | |
| Drink | 1500 | Urine | | 1500 |
| Food | 800 | Insensible loss | | 800 |
| Metabolism | 200 | (skin, lungs) | | |
| | | Faeces | | 200 |
| Total | 2500 | | | 2500 |
| **Sodium (mmol)** | | | | |
| Food and drink | 140 | Urine | | 140 |
| | | Sweat | | Negligible |
| | | Faeces | | Negligible |

magnesium, and their associated anions exist in very low concentrations and contribute so little to osmolality that they can be ignored when calculating the osmolality. The normal plasma osmolality is 285–300 mmol/kg.

The *calculated* osmolality is the same as the osmolality *measured* by the laboratory, unless there is an unmeasured, osmotically active substance present. For instance, plasma alcohol or ethylene glycol concentration (substances sometimes taken in cases of poisoning) can be estimated by subtracting the calculated from the measured osmolality.

## Distribution of extracellular fluid (K&C p. 667)

The distribution of extracellular water between vascular and extravascular (interstitial) space is determined by the equilibrium between hydrostatic pressure (i.e. intracapillary blood pressure), which tends to force fluid out of the capillaries, and oncotic pressure (i.e. osmotic pressure exerted by plasma proteins), which acts to retain fluid within the vessel. The net flow of fluid outwards is balanced by 'suction' of fluid into the lymphatics which returns it to the bloodstream (Fig. 7.1).

Oedema is defined as an increase in interstitial fluid and results from:

- Increased hydrostatic pressure, e.g. sodium and water retention in cardiac failure

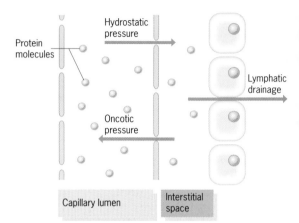

**Fig. 7.1 Distribution of water between the vascular and extravascular (interstitial) spaces.** This is determined by the equilibrium between hydrostatic pressure, which tends to force fluid out of the capillaries, and oncotic pressure, which acts to retain fluid within the vessel. The net flow of fluid outwards is balanced by 'suction' of fluid into the lymphatics, which returns it to the bloodstream. Similar principles govern the volume of the peritoneal and pleural spaces.

286

- Reduced oncotic pressure, e.g. as a result of nephrotic syndrome with hypoalbuminaemia
- Obstruction to lymphatic flow
- Increased permeability of the blood vessel wall, e.g. at a site of inflammation, cytokines lead to an increase in vascular permeability.

Inspection and palpation are usually sufficient to identify oedema. Compression of the skin of the affected area with a finger tip for 10 seconds results in 'pitting'. Localized oedema is most likely to result from a local alteration. The location of generalized oedema, e.g. with cardiac failure, is often most prominent in the lower legs and feet in ambulatory patients and in the sacral region in those who are confined to bed.

## Regulation of extracellular volume

The total body content of sodium controls extracellular volume. Regulation of body sodium is dependent on tight control over renal excretion. This is achieved by activation of 'volume' receptors (which respond to extracellular volume rather than changes in sodium concentration). There are two types of volume receptors:

- Extrarenal: in the large vessels near the heart
- Intrarenal: in the afferent renal arteriole, which controls the renin–angiotensin system via the juxtaglomerular apparatus.

A decreased effective circulating volume leads to activation of these volume receptors, which leads to an increase in sodium (and hence water) reabsorption by the kidney and expansion of the extracellular volume via stimulation of the sympathetic nervous system and activation of the renin–angiotensin system (p. 590). In contrast, atrial natriuretic peptide (ANP), produced by the atria of the heart in response to an increase in blood volume, increases sodium excretion.

## Regulation of body water content

Body water is controlled mainly by changes in the plasma osmolality. An increased plasma osmolality, sensed by osmoreceptors in the hypothalamus, causes thirst and the release of antidiuretic hormone (ADH, vasopressin) from the posterior pituitary, which increases water reabsorption from the renal collecting ducts. In addition, non-osmotic stimuli may cause the release of ADH even if serum osmolality is normal or low. These include hypovolaemia, stress (surgery and trauma) and nausea.

## Abnormalities of extracellular volume

### Increased extracellular volume (K&C p. 673)
Extracellular volume expansion is the result of increased sodium (and hence water) reabsorption or impaired excretion by the kidney.

### Aetiology
- *Cardiac failure* caused by impaired perfusion (therefore effective hypovolaemia) of the volume receptors.

- *Hypoalbuminaemia.* Loss of plasma oncotic pressure leads to loss of water from the vascular to the interstitial space, and therefore activation of intravascular volume receptors.
- *Cirrhosis.* This is through a complex mechanism, but there is vasodilatation and hence underperfusion of the volume receptors. There may also be hypoalbuminaemia.
- *Sodium retention.* This may be as a result of renal impairment, where there is a reduction in renal capacity to excrete sodium, or due to drugs such as mineralocorticoids, non-steroidal anti-inflammatory drugs (NSAIDs) and selective cyclo-oxygenase-2 (COX-2) inhibitors. NSAIDs and COX-2 inhibitors inhibit synthesis of vasodilatory prostaglandins in the kidney with an increase in renal vascular resistance and increase in water and sodium reabsorption.

### Clinical features

These depend on the distribution of extracellular water, e.g. with hypoalbuminaemia caused by loss of plasma oncotic pressure there is predominantly interstitial volume overload. Cardiac failure leads to expansion of both compartments:

- *Interstitial volume overload* – ankle oedema, pulmonary oedema, pleural effusion and ascites
- *Intravascular volume overload* – raised jugular venous pressure, cardiomegaly, and a raised arterial pressure in some cases.

This must be differentiated from local causes of oedema (e.g. ankle oedema as a result of venous damage following thrombosis) which do not reflect a disturbance in the control of extracellular volume.

### Management

The underlying cause must be treated. The cornerstone of treatment is diuretics, which increase sodium and water excretion in the kidney. There are a number of different classes of diuretic, of which the most potent are the loop diuretics, e.g. furosemide (frusemide) (Table 7.3).

**Table 7.3**
The main classes of diuretics in clinical use

| Class | Example | Mechanism of action | Relative potency |
|---|---|---|---|
| Loop diuretics | Furosemide (frusemide)<br>Bumetanide | Reduce $Na^+$ and $Cl^-$ reabsorption in ascending limb of loop of Henle | ++++ |
| Thiazides | Bendroflumethiazide (bendrofluazide) | Reduce sodium reabsorption in distal convoluted tubule | ++ |
| Potassium-sparing diuretics | Spironolactone<br>Amiloride | Aldosterone antagonist<br>Prevents potassium exchange for sodium in distal tubule | + |

# Decreased extracellular volume (K&C p. 676)

This may be the result of loss of sodium and water, plasma or blood.

## Aetiology

Volume depletion occurs in haemorrhage, plasma loss in extensive burns, or loss of salt and water from the kidneys, gastrointestinal tract or skin (Table 7.4.).

## Clinical features

Symptoms include thirst, nausea and postural dizziness. Interstitial fluid loss leads to loss of skin elasticity ('turgor'). Loss of circulating volume causes peripheral vasoconstriction and tachycardia, a low jugular venous pressure and postural hypotension. Severe depletion of circulating volume causes hypotension, which may impair cerebral perfusion, resulting in confusion and eventual coma.

## Investigations

The diagnosis is usually made clinically. A central venous line allows the measurement of central venous pressure (p. 740) which helps in assessing the response to treatment. Plasma urea may be raised because of increased urea reabsorption and, later, prerenal failure (when the creatinine rises as well). This is, however, very non-specific. Urinary sodium is low ($< 20$ mmol/L) if the kidneys are working normally, which can be misleading if the cause of the

**Table 7.4**
Causes of extracellular volume depletion

**Haemorrhage**
External
Concealed, e.g. leaking aortic aneurysm

**Burns**

**Gastrointestinal losses**
Vomiting, diarrhoea, ileostomy losses

**Renal losses**
Diuretic use, impaired tubular sodium conservation, e.g. reflux nephropathy, papillary necrosis

volume depletion involves the kidneys (e.g. diuretics or intrinsic renal disease).

## Management

The overriding aims of treatment are to replace what is missing:

- Haemorrhage involves the loss of whole blood. The rational treatment of acute haemorrhage is therefore whole blood, or a combination of red cells and a plasma substitute.
- Loss of plasma, as in burns or severe peritonitis, should be treated with human plasma or a plasma substitute (see p. 509).
- Loss of sodium and water, as in vomiting, diarrhoea or excessive renal losses, should be treated with replacement of water and electrolytes. This is best done orally if possible, with an increased intake of water and salt. Glucose–electrolyte solutions are often used to restore fluid balance in patients with diarrhoeal diseases. This is based on the fact that the presence of glucose stimulates intestinal absorption of salt and water (p. 29).
- In the acute situation if there have been large losses of sodium and water, patients are usually treated with intravenous physiological saline (Tables 7.5 and 7.6) and replacement is assessed clinically and by measurement of serum electrolytes.
- Loss of water alone, e.g. diabetes insipidus, only causes extracellular volume depletion in severe cases because the loss is spread evenly over all the compartments of body water. The correct treatment is to give water. If intravenous treatment is required, water is given as 5% dextrose (pure water is not given because it would cause osmotic lysis of blood cells).

## Disorders of sodium regulation

As discussed above, sodium content is regulated by volume receptors, with water content adjusted to maintain a normal

**Table 7.5**
Intravenous fluids in general use*

|  | Na+ | K+ | HCO₃⁻ | Cl- mmol/L |
|---|---|---|---|---|
| Normal plasma constituents | 142 | 4.5 | 26 | 103 |
| Sodium chloride 0.9% (isotonic physiological saline) | 150 | – | – | 150 |
| Glucose 5% | – | – | – | – |
| Sodium chloride (0.18%) + glucose 4% (1/5 physiological saline) | 30 | – | – | 30 |

* Accounting for 95% of the fluids used in clinical practice

Table 7.6
Guidelines for intravenous fluid administration in maintenance and replacement of losses

**For maintenance fluid balance**
Each day 2500 mL fluid containing about 140 mmol sodium and 60 mmol potassium are required to maintain balance in a 75 kg man. A good regimen is 1.5–2 L 5% dextrose and 1 L physiological saline every 24 h

**For hypovolaemic patients**
An estimate of the losses is made (e.g. in hospital patients from a review of the input/output charts) and these must be given in addition to the normal daily requirements

osmolality and a normal plasma sodium concentration. Disturbances of sodium concentration are usually caused by disturbances of water balance, rather than an increase or decrease in total body sodium.

## Hyponatraemia (K&C p. 679)

Hyponatraemia (serum sodium < 135 mmol/L) may be the result of the following:

- Relative water excess (dilutional hyponatraemia); this is the most common cause.
- Salt loss in excess of water, e.g. diarrhoea and renal diseases as described above.
- Pseudohyponatraemia, in which hyperlipidaemia or hyperproteinaemia results in a spuriously low measured sodium concentration. The sodium is confined to the aqueous phase but its concentration is expressed in terms of the total volume of plasma (i.e. water plus lipid). In this situation plasma osmolality is normal and therefore treatment of 'hyponatraemia' is unnecessary.
- True hyponatraemia must be differentiated from artefactual 'hyponatraemia' caused by taking blood from the drip arm into which a fluid of low sodium is being infused.

Once preliminary evaluation reveals that the hyponatraemia reflects hypo-osmolality (i.e. it is not pseudohyponatraemia or artefactual), assessment of the extracellular volume (pp. 288, 290) allows patients to be classified as hypovolaemic, normovolaemic or hypervolaemic (Fig. 7.2).

293

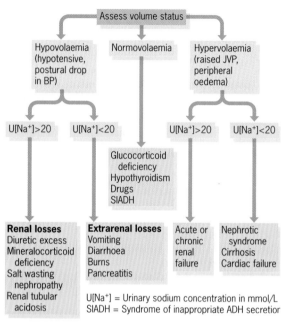

Fig. 7.2 **Diagnosis of hyponatraemia.**

U[Na+] = Urinary sodium concentration in mmol/L
SIADH = Syndrome of inappropriate ADH secretion

# Hyponatraemia resulting from salt loss (hypovolaemic hyponatraemia)

These patients have a deficit of both total body sodium and water, with the sodium deficit exceeding the water deficit. Measurement of urinary sodium will help to differentiate between renal and extrarenal sources of fluid loss (Fig. 7.2). For example, vomiting and diarrhoea are associated with avid sodium retention as the kidney responds to volume contraction by conserving NaCl.

Diuretics are the most common cause of hypovolaemic hyponatraemia with a high urinary [Na+].

## Clinical features

These are usually a result of the hypovolaemia and extra-cellular volume depletion (p. 290). Symptoms directly related to the hyponatraemia are rare, as the loss of both sodium and water limits osmotic shifts in the brain.

## Management

Restoration of extracellular volume with crystalloids or colloids interrupts non-osmotic release of ADH and normalizes serum sodium.

# Hyponatraemia resulting from water excess (dilutional hyponatraemia)

An excess of body water relative to sodium is differentiated from hyponatraemia caused by sodium loss, because there are none of the clinical features of extracellular volume depletion. This is the most common mechanism of hyponatraemia seen in hospital patients.

## Aetiology

Hyponatraemia is often seen in patients with severe cardiac failure, hepatic cirrhosis or the nephrotic syndrome, in which there is an inability of the kidney to excrete 'free water'. This is compounded by the use of diuretics. There is evidence of volume overload and the patient is usually oedematous. Where there is no evidence of extracellular volume overload, causes include the syndrome of inappropriate ADH secretion (SIADH) (p. 381), Addison's disease and hypothyroidism.

## Clinical features

Symptoms rarely occur until the serum sodium is less than 120 mmol/L and are more conspicuous when hyponatraemia has developed rapidly, i.e. over hours. They result from the movement of water into the brain cells (cerebral oedema) in response to the fall in extracellular osmolality, and include headache, confusion, convulsions and coma.

## Investigation

Hyponatraemia in association with cardiac failure, cirrhosis or nephrotic syndrome is usually clinically obvious and no further investigation is necessary. If there is no evidence of volume overload the most probable cause is SIADH or diuretic therapy.

## Management

The underlying cause must be corrected where possible. Most cases (those without severe symptoms) are simply managed by water restriction (to 1000 mL or even 500 mL/ day) with a review of diuretic treatment. Management of SIADH syndrome is described on page 582. Patients with hyponatraemia developing acutely, in less than 48 hours (often a hospital patient on intravenous dextrose), are at the greatest risk of developing cerebral oedema and should be treated more urgently (see Emergency Box 7.1).

## Central pontine myelinolysis

Over-rapid correction of the sodium concentration by whatever means must be avoided, as this can result in a severe, neurological syndrome due to local areas of demyelination, called central pontine myelinolysis or the osmotic demyelination syndrome. Features of this include quadriparesis, respiratory arrest, pseudobulbar palsy, mutism, and, rarely, fits. The distribution of the areas of demyelination include most often the pons, but also, in some cases, the basal ganglia, internal capsule, lateral geniculate body, and even the cerebral cortex.

## Hypernatraemia (K&C p. 681)

Hypernatraemia (serum sodium > 145 mmol/L) is almost always the result of reduced water intake or water loss in

### Emergency Box 7.1

**Management of hyponatraemia resulting from water excess**

**Treat the underlying cause**

**Restrict water intake to 500–1000 mL/day**

**With acute symptomatic hyponatraemia:**
- Hypertonic saline is indicated in patients who present with seizures or other severe neurological abnormalities
- Infuse 3% (hypertonic) NaCl at a rate of 1–2 mL/kg/h
- Aim to raise serum sodium by 2 mmol/L/h until symptoms resolve
- Give furosemide (frusemide) 40–80 mg i.v. to enhance free water excretion
- Subsequent correction should be very slow so that the total increase in serum sodium is less than 8 mmol/L in 24 h

excess of sodium. More rarely it is caused by excessive administration of sodium.

## Aetiology

Insufficient fluid intake is most often found in elderly people, neonates or unconscious patients when access to water is denied or confusion or coma eliminates the normal response to thirst. The situation is exacerbated by increased losses of fluid, e.g. sweating, diarrhoea.

Water loss relative to sodium occurs in pituitary diabetes insipidus, nephrogenic diabetes insipidus, osmotic diuresis and water loss from the lungs or skin.

## Clinical features

Symptoms are non-specific and include nausea, vomiting, fever and confusion.

## Investigations

Simultaneous urine and plasma osmolality and sodium should be measured.

The passage of urine with an osmolality lower than that of plasma in this situation is clearly abnormal and indicates diabetes insipidus (p. 582). If urine osmolality is high this suggests an osmotic diuresis or excessive extrarenal water loss (e.g. heat stroke).

## Management

Treatment is that of the underlying cause and replacement of water, either orally if possible or intravenously with 5% dextrose. The aim is to correct over 48 hours, as over-rapid correction may lead to cerebral oedema. In severe hypernatraemia (> 170 mmol/L), 0.9% saline (150 mmol/L) should be used to avoid too rapid a drop in serum sodium. In addition, if there is clinical evidence of volume depletion this implies that there is a sodium deficit as well as a water deficit, and intravenous 0.9% saline should be used.

# Disorders of potassium regulation

Dietary intake of potassium varies between 80 and 150 mmol daily. Potassium is predominantly an intracellular ion, only

2% of total body potassium being extracellular (Table 7.1). Serum levels are controlled by:

- Uptake of $K^+$ into cells – by altering activity of the $Na^+$–$K^+$-ATPase pump in the cell membrane
- Renal excretion – mainly controlled by aldosterone
- Extrarenal losses, e.g. gastrointestinal.

# Hypokalaemia (K&C p. 682)
This is a serum potassium concentration of < 3.5 mmol/L.

## Aetiology
The most common causes of hypokalaemia (Table 7.7) are diuretic treatment and hyperaldosteronism. Blood taken from a drip arm may produce a spurious result.

**Table 7.7**
Causes of hypokalaemia

| | |
|---|---|
| **Increased renal excretion** (spot urinary $K^+$ > 20 mmol/L) | Diuretics, e.g. thiazides, loop diuretics |
| | Solute diuresis, e.g. glycosuria |
| | Hypomagnesaemia |
| | Increased aldosterone secretion |
| | Liver failure |
| | Heart failure |
| | Nephrotic syndrome |
| | Cushing's syndrome |
| | Conn's syndrome |
| | Exogenous mineralocorticoid |
| | Corticosteroids |
| | Carbenoxolone |
| | Liquorice |
| | Renal disease |
| | Renal tubular acidosis: types 1 and 2 |
| | Renal tubular damage |
| **Gastrointestinal losses** | Vomiting, diarrhoea, villous adenoma, fistulae, ileostomies |
| **Redistribution into cells** (by increasing activity of $Na^+$–$K^+$-ATPase) | Alkalosis |
| | β-Agonists |
| | Insulin |
| **Reduced intake** | Severe dietary deficiency |
| | Inadequate replacement in i.v. fluids |

## Clinical features

Hypokalaemia is usually asymptomatic, although muscle weakness may occur if severe. It results in an increased risk of cardiac arrhythmias, particularly in patients with cardiac disease. Hypokalaemia also predisposes to digoxin toxicity.

## Management

The underlying cause should be identified and treated where possible. Usually withdrawal of purgatives, assessment of diuretic treatment, and replacement with oral potassium chloride supplements (20–80 mmol/day in divided doses with monitoring of serum $K^+$ every 1–2 days) is all that is required. Serum magnesium concentrations should be normalized, as hypomagnesaemia makes hypokalaemia difficult or impossible to correct. Indications for the intravenous infusion of potassium chloride include hypokalaemic diabetic ketoacidosis and severe hypokalaemia (< 2.5 mmol/L), which may be associated with cardiac arrhythmias. This should be performed slowly, and replacement at rates of greater than 20 mmol/h should only be done with ECG monitoring and hourly measurement of serum potassium. Concentrations over 60 mmol/L cannot be given via a peripheral vein because of pain and sclerosis.

## Hyperkalaemia (K&C p. 681)

This is defined as a serum potassium concentration of > 5.0 mmol/L. True hyperkalaemia must be differentiated from artefactual hyperkalaemia, which results from lysis of red cells during vigorous phlebotomy.

## Aetiology

The most common causes (Table 7.8) are renal impairment and drug interference with potassium excretion.

## Clinical features

Hyperkalaemia usually produces few symptoms or signs until it is high enough to cause cardiac arrest. Symptoms produced by hyperkalaemia are related to impaired neuromuscular transmission and include muscle weakness and paralysis. It may be associated with metabolic acidosis

> **Table 7.8**
> Causes of hyperkalaemia
>
> **Excessive intake**
>
> **Impaired renal excretion**
> Acute renal failure
> Potassium-sparing diuretics (amiloride)
>
> **Hypoaldosteronism**
> Addison's disease
> Hyporeninaemic hypoaldosteronism (type 4 renal tubular acidosis)
> Angiotensin-converting enzyme (ACE) inhibitors
>
> **Release from cells**
> Diabetic ketoacidosis
> Acidosis
> Crush injury
> Suxamethonium

causing Kussmaul's respiration (low deep sighing inspiration and expiration).

## Management

A serum potassium of more than 7 mmol/L is a medical emergency (Emergency Box 7.2) and may be associated with typical ECG changes (Fig. 7.3).

# Disorders of magnesium regulation

Disturbance of magnesium balance is uncommon and usually associated with more obvious fluid and electrolyte disturbance. Like potassium, magnesium is mainly an intracellular cation (Table 7.1) and balance is maintained mainly via the kidney.

## Hypomagnesaemia (K&C p. 687)

### Aetiology

A low serum magnesium is most often caused by loss of magnesium from the gut or kidney. Gastrointestinal causes include severe diarrhoea, malabsorption, extensive bowel resection and intestinal fistulae. Excessive renal loss of magnesium occurs with diuretics, alcohol abuse, and with an osmotic diuresis such as glycosuria in diabetes mellitus.

**Emergency Box 7.2**

## Management of hyperkalaemia

1. **Protect myocardium from hyperkalaemia (if K$^+$ > 7.0 mmol/L or ECG changes present)**

   10 mL of 10% calcium gluconate bolus i.v. over 2–3 min with ECG monitoring
   Repeat after 5 min if ECG changes persist
   NB: This treatment does not alter serum K$^+$

2. **Drive K$^+$ into cells**

   Soluble insulin 10 units + 50 mL 50% dextrose intravenously over 15–30 min and/or correction of severe acidosis with sodium bicarbonate (1.26%)
   Effect lasts 1–2 h; repeated doses may be necessary

3. **Deplete body K$^+$ (after emergency treatment)**

   Calcium or sodium resonium orally (15 g three times daily with laxatives) or rectally (30 g) binds potassium
   Treat the cause
   Stop any extra source of potassium intake or potentiating drugs, e.g. NSAIDs and ACE inhibitors
   Haemodialysis or peritoneal dialysis if conservative measures fail

4. **Monitor**

   Blood glucose (finger-prick Stix testing) hourly during and after insulin/dextrose infusion
   Serum K$^+$ every 2–4 hours acutely and daily thereafter

## Clinical features

Hypomagnesaemia increases renal excretion of potassium, inhibits secretion of parathyroid hormone and leads to parathyroid hormone resistance. Many of the symptoms of hypomagnesaemia are therefore due to hypokalaemia (p. 298) and hypocalcaemia (p. 588).

## Management

The underlying cause must be corrected where possible and oral supplements given (magnesium chloride 5–20 mmol daily). Symptomatic severe magnesium deficiency should be treated by intravenous infusion (50 mmol of MgCl in 1 L of 5% dextrose over 12–24 h), plus a loading dose (4 mmol over 10 min) if there are seizures or ventricular arrhythmias.

Disorders of acid–base balance

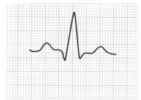

**(a)** Normal

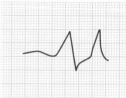

**(c)** Reduced P wave with increased QRS complex

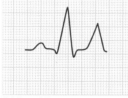

**(b)** Tented T wave

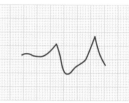

**(d)** 'Sine wave' pattern (pre-cardiac arrest)

**Fig. 7.3 Progressive ECG changes with increasing hyperkalaemia.**

## Hypermagnesaemia (K&C p. 687)

Hypermagnesaemia is rare and is usually iatrogenic, occurring in patients with renal failure who have been given magnesium-containing laxatives or antacids. Symptoms include neurological and cardiovascular depression, with narcosis, respiratory depression and cardiac conduction defects. The only treatment usually necessary is to stop magnesium treatment. In severe cases intravenous calcium gluconate may be necessary to reverse the cellular toxic effects of magnesium and dextrose/insulin (as for hyperkalaemia) to lower the plasma magnesium level.

## Disorders of acid–base balance

(*K&C* p. 689)

The pH (the negative logarithm of $[H^+]$) is maintained at 7.4 (normal range 7.35–7.45). The metabolism of food and endogenous body tissues produces about 70–100 mmol of $H^+$ each day, which is excreted by the kidneys.

carbonic anhydrase

$$H^+ + HCO_3^- \rightleftharpoons H_2CO_3 \rightleftharpoons H_2O + CO_2$$

**Fig. 7.4** The carbonic anhydrase reaction.

Bicarbonate ($HCO_3^-$) is the main plasma and extracellular fluid buffer. It mops up free $H^+$ ions and prevents increases in the $H^+$ concentration (Fig. 7.4). Bicarbonate is filtered at the glomerulus but is then reabsorbed in the proximal and distal renal tubule. The lungs also constantly regulate acid–base balance through the excretion of $CO_2$. Between production and excretion of $H^+$ ions there is an extremely effective buffering system maintaining a constant $H^+$ ion concentration inside and outside the cell. Buffers include haemoglobin proteins, bicarbonate and phosphate.

Acid–base disturbances may be caused by:

- Abnormal carbon dioxide removal in the lungs ('respiratory' acidosis and alkalosis)
- Abnormalities in the regulation of bicarbonate and other buffers in the blood ('metabolic' acidosis and alkalosis).

In general, the body compensates to some extent for changes in pH by regulating renal bicarbonate excretion and altering the respiratory rate. For instance, metabolic acidosis causes hyperventilation (via medullary chemoreceptors), leading to increased removal of $CO_2$ in the lungs and partial compensation for the acidosis. Conversely, respiratory acidosis is accompanied by renal bicarbonate retention, which could be mistaken for primary metabolic alkalosis.

Measurement of pH, $P_{CO_2}$ and [$HCO_3^-$] will reveal which type of disturbance is present (Table 7.9). These measurements are made on an arterial blood sample (p. 738) using an automated blood gas analyser. Clinical history and examination usually point to the correct diagnosis.

## Respiratory acidosis

This is usually associated with ventilatory failure, with retention of carbon dioxide (p. 515). Treatment is of the underlying cause.

303

Table 7.9
Changes in arterial blood gases

| | pH | $P_a$co$_2$ | HCO$_3^-$ |
|---|---|---|---|
| **Acidosis** | | | |
| Metabolic | Normal or reduced | Normal or reduced | Reduced ++ |
| Respiratory | Normal or reduced | Increased ++ | Normal or increased |
| **Alkalosis** | | | |
| Metabolic | Normal or increased | Increased | Increased ++ |
| Respiratory | Normal or increased | Reduced ++ | Reduced |

The pH may be at the limits of the normal range if the acidosis or alkalosis is compensated, e.g. respiratory compensation (hyperventilation) of a metabolic acidosis. The clue to the abnormality from the blood gases will be the abnormal $P_a$co$_2$ and HCO$_3^-$

## Respiratory alkalosis

Hyperventilation results in increased removal of carbon dioxide, resulting in a fall in $P_aCO_2$ and $[H^+]$.

## Metabolic acidosis (K&C p. 692)

This is the result of the accumulation of any acid other than carbonic acid. The most common cause is lactic acidosis following shock or cardiac arrest.

### Clinical features

These include hyperventilation, hypotension caused by arteriolar vasodilatation and the negative inotropic effect of acidosis, and cerebral dysfunction associated with confusion and fits.

### Differential diagnosis (the anion gap)

The first step is to identify whether the acidosis is the result of retention of HCl or of another acid. This is achieved by measurement of the anion gap. The main electrolytes measured in plasma are sodium, potassium, chloride and bicarbonate. The sum of the cations, sodium and potassium, normally exceeds that of chloride and bicarbonate by 6–12 mmol/L. This anion gap is usually made up of negatively charged proteins, phosphate and organic acids. If the anion gap is normal in the presence of acidosis, it can be concluded that HCl is being retained or $NaHCO_3$ is being lost. The causes of a normal anion gap acidosis are given in Table 7.10.

If the anion gap is increased (i.e. > 12 mmol/L), the acidosis is the result of an exogenous acid, e.g. salicylates or one of the acids normally present in small unmeasured quantities, such as lactate. Causes of a high anion gap acidosis are given in Table 7.11.

### Lactic acidosis (K&C p. 695)

Increased production of lactic acid occurs when cellular respiration is abnormal, resulting from either lack of oxygen (type A) or a metabolic abnormality (type B). The most common form in clinical practice is type A lactic acidosis, occurring in septicaemic or cardiogenic shock.

> **Table 7.10**
> Causes of metabolic acidosis with a normal anion gap
>
> **Increased gastrointestinal HCO$_3$ loss**
> Diarrhoea
> Ileostomy
> Ureterosigmoidostomy
>
> **Increased HCO$_3^-$ renal loss**
> Acetazolamide ingestion
> Proximal (type 2) renal tubular acidosis
> Hyperparathyroidism
> Tubular damage, e.g. drugs, heavy metals
>
> **Decreased renal H$^+$ excretion**
> Distal (type 1) renal tubular acidosis
> Type 4 renal tubular acidosis
>
> **Increased HCl production**
> Ammonium chloride ingestion
> Increased catabolism of lysine, arginine

**Diabetic ketoacidosis** (*K&C* p. 695 & p. 1088)
This is a high anion gap acidosis caused by the accumulation of organic acids, acetoacetic acid and hydroxybutyric acid (see p. 609).

**Renal tubular acidosis** (*K&C* p. 693)
Renal tubular acidosis may occur in the absence of renal failure and is a normal anion gap acidosis. There is failure of the kidney to acidify the urine adequately. This group of disorders is uncommon and only rarely a cause of significant clinical disease.

*Type 4 renal tubular acidosis* This is the most common of these disorders and is also known as hyporeninaemic hypoaldosteronism. Typical features are acidosis and hyperkalaemia occurring in the setting of mild chronic renal failure, usually caused by tubulointerstitial disease or diabetes. Plasma aldosterone and renin are low and do not respond to stimulation. Treatment is with fludrocortisone, diuretics, sodium bicarbonate and ion exchange resins for the reduction of serum potassium.

*Proximal (type 2) renal tubular acidosis* This is failure to absorb bicarbonate in the proximal tubule. Typical features

**Table 7.11**
Causes of metabolic acidosis with a high anion gap

**Renal failure (sulphate, phosphate)**

**Ketoacidosis**
Diabetes
Starvation
Alcohol poisoning

**Lactic acidosis**
Type A
    Shock
    Severe hypoxia
    Methanol
    Ethylene glycol
    Strenuous exercise
Type B
    Acute liver failure
    Poisoning: ethanol, paracetamol
    Metformin accumulation
    Leukaemia, lymphoma

**Drug poisoning**
Salicylates

are hypokalaemia, an inability to produce an acid urine in spite of systemic acidosis, and the appearance of bicarbonate in the urine. This disorder normally occurs as part of a generalized tubular defect, together with other features such as glycosuria and aminoaciduria. Treatment is with oral sodium bicarbonate.

*Distal (type 1) renal tubular acidosis* There is failure of $H^+$ excretion in the distal tubule. Typical features include hypokalaemia and an inability to produce an acid urine in spite of systemic acidosis. Causes include autoimmune diseases, SLE and nephrocalcinosis. Presentation is often with renal stones as a result of hypercalciuria, low urinary citrate (citrate inhibits calcium phosphate precipitation) and alkaline urine (favours precipitation of calcium phosphate). Treatment is with sodium bicarbonate.

## Uraemic acidosis (K&C p. 695)
Reduction of the capacity to secrete $H^+$ and $NH_4^+$, in addition to bicarbonate wasting, contributes to the acidosis of chronic renal failure. Acidosis occurs particularly when

there is tubular damage, such as reflux and chronic obstructive nephropathy. It is associated with hypercalciuria and renal osteodystrophy because $H^+$ ions are buffered by bone in exchange for calcium. Treatment is with calcium or sodium bicarbonate, although acidosis in end-stage renal failure is only usually fully corrected by adequate dialysis.

# Metabolic alkalosis (K&C p. 696)

This is much less common than acidosis and is often associated with potassium or volume depletion. The main causes are persistent vomiting, diuretic therapy or hyperaldosteronism. Vomiting causes alkalosis both by causing volume depletion and through loss of gastric acid.

### Clinical features

Cerebral dysfunction is an early feature of alkalosis. Respiration may be depressed.

### Management

This includes fluid replacement, if necessary, with replacement of sodium, potassium and chloride. The bicarbonate excess will correct itself.

# 8

# Renal disease

## Renal physiology

The kidney's principal role is the elimination of waste material and the regulation of the volume and composition of body fluid. Urine is produced by glomerular filtration, which depends on the maintenance of a relatively high perfusion pressure within the glomerular capillary and an adequate renal blood flow. In health glomerular blood flow is autoregulated by the preglomerular arteriole and remains relatively constant within a range of mean arterial pressures. The proximal renal tubules reabsorb most of the filtered solute required to maintain fluid and electrolyte balance, but elimination of potassium, water and non-volatile hydrogen ions is regulated in the distal tubules. As renal perfusion and glomerular filtration fall, reabsorption of water and sodium by the proximal tubules increases so that minimal fluid reaches the distal tubule. Hence hypotensive or hypovolaemic patients cannot excrete potassium and hydrogen ions. Patients with distal tubular damage, e.g. caused by drugs, also cannot excrete potassium and hydrogen ions. The kidney also acts as an endocrine organ and produces erythropoietin, renin and vitamin D in its active form (*K&C* p. 588)

## Presenting features of renal disease

The most common diseases of the kidney and urinary tract are benign prostatic hypertrophy in men and urinary tract infection (UTI) in women. The symptoms suggesting renal tract disease are frequency of micturition, dysuria, haematuria, urinary retention and alteration of urine volume (either polyuria or oliguria). In addition there may be pain situated anywhere along the renal tract, from loin to groin. Non-specific symptoms, e.g. lethargy, anorexia and pruritus, may be the presenting features of chronic renal failure.

Renal disease may be asymptomatic and discovered by the incidental finding of hypertension, a raised serum urea, or proteinuria and haematuria on Stix testing. Once renal disease is suspected, the purpose of investigations is to determine the presence or degree of renal dysfunction and the cause of the renal disease. Estimation of the glomerular filtration rate (GFR, see below) is used clinically to determine the degree of renal dysfunction. Creatinine clearance is a reasonably accurate measure of GFR and is measured from a 24-hour urine collection and measurement of a single serum creatinine value during the 24-hour period (*K&C* p. 590). The clinical history and examination together with Stix testing and microscopy of urine are the starting points for determining the cause.

## Dysuria

Dysuria (pain on micturition) is caused by:

- Inflammation involving the urethra (urethritis) or bladder (cystitis). Dysuria is common in adult women and is usually due to lower urinary tract bacterial infection (p. 325) with inflammation of the urethra and bladder. Other causes of urethritis include infection with *Chlamydia trachomatis* or *Neisseria gonorrhoeae* (p. 39).
- Inflammation involving the vagina in women or glans penis in men. Causes include infection with *Candida albicans* and *Gardnerella vaginalis*.

## Polyuria and nocturia

Polyuria can be arbitrarily defined as a urine output exceeding 3 L in 24 hours. It must be differentiated from the more common complaints of urinary frequency and nocturia, which are not necessarily associated with an increase in the total urine output. The causes of polyuria include polydipsia, solute diuresis (e.g. hyperglycaemia with glycosuria), diabetes insipidus and chronic renal failure. Nocturia is most often due to drinking before bed or, in men over 50 years, prostatic enlargement (p. 359).

## Oliguria

Oliguria (low urine output) is defined as a urine output of less than 300 mL in 24 hours. It may be 'physiological', as in patients with hypotension and hypovolaemia, where urine is maximally concentrated in an attempt to conserve water. It may also be due to intrinsic renal disease or urinary tract obstruction. Anuria (no urine) suggests bilateral ureteric or bladder outflow obstruction. Management of the oliguric patient is in three steps:

1. *Exclude obstruction.* The patient with outflow obstruction (acute retention of urine) is typically in great discomfort with an intense desire to micturate. The bladder is palpable as a tender mass that is dull to percussion, arising out of the pelvis. The diagnosis is confirmed by passing a urethral catheter and releasing a large volume of urine. If the patient is already catheterized, the catheter should be flushed with sterile saline to relieve any blockage. Obstruction proximal to the bladder (e.g. ureteric obstruction) is often painless, and ultrasound examination is indicated to exclude pelvicalyceal dilatation.

2. *Assess for hypovolaemia.* Once obstruction has been excluded the patient must be assessed for evidence of hypovolaemia by measurement of blood pressure, pulse, JVP, and urinary electrolytes (p. 342). If the patient is hypovolaemic the urine output in response to a fluid challenge (500 mL saline intravenously over 30 minutes) should be assessed.

3. *Management of established acute renal failure* (p. 346) once obstruction and hypovolaemia have been excluded.

311

## Urine Stix testing *(K&C p. 94)*

Commercial reagent Stix detect the presence of protein, glucose, ketones, bilirubin, urobilinogen and blood in the urine. They also measure urine pH, which is useful in the investigation and management of renal tubular acidosis (p. 306). Each test is based on a colour change in a strip of absorbent cellulose impregnated with the appropriate reagent. The Stix is dipped briefly into a fresh specimen of urine collected in a clean container and the colour changes compared with the manufacturer's colour charts on the reagent strip container. The degree of colour change is a semiquantitative assessment of the amount of substance present. Haematuria or proteinuria suggests renal tract disease. Dipsticks are also available for testing for urinary nitrites, which if present indicate bacteriuria (p. 326).

## Proteinuria

The glomerular ultrafiltrate normally contains a small amount of protein, most of which is absorbed in the proximal renal tubule and only small amounts (up to 200 mg/24 h) appear in the urine. Most reagent Stix can detect a protein concentration of 150 mg/L or more in the urine. Pyrexia, exercise and adoption of the upright posture may all produce a mild increase in urinary protein output. 'Postural proteinuria' is the term used when proteinuria occurs in the upright posture but not when supine. It may be diagnosed by testing for protein in several early morning urine samples passed after overnight recumbency, and then testing several samples after being up and about. The condition is usually benign and the amount of protein excreted small.

Persistent proteinuria (Fig. 8.1) detected on Stix testing requires full investigation. The first step is to quantify protein excretion by a 24-hour urine collection. Proteinuria

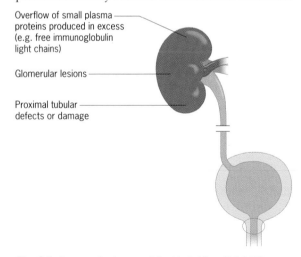

Overflow of small plasma proteins produced in excess (e.g. free immunoglobulin light chains)

Glomerular lesions

Proximal tubular defects or damage

**Fig. 8.1 Sources of urinary protein.** Adapted from Mallick N P. Presenting features of renal disease. *Medicine* 1995 23:3: 91–96 by kind permission of The Medicine Publishing Company.

greater than 2 g/24 h is usually the result of glomerular disease (p. 315) and greater than 3–5 g/24 h may result in the nephrotic syndrome (p. 322). Proteinuria caused by failure of proximal tubular reabsorption is uncommon and is seldom an isolated defect: there are usually multiple proximal tubular defects causing glycosuria, amino-aciduria, phosphaturia and renal tubular acidosis (Fanconi's syndrome). Bence Jones proteins (immunoglobulin light chains in patients with myeloma) are not detected by Stix and are identified by immunoelectrophoresis of urine.

Microalbuminuria is defined as an increase above the normal range in urinary albumin excretion (normal less than 43 mg/day) but undetectable by conventional dip-sticks. In patients with diabetes mellitus, microalbuminuria is the earliest indicator of glomerular damage which may, in turn, progress to intermittent albuminuria followed by persistent proteinuria, sometimes with a frank nephrotic syndrome. Microalbuminuria is detected by measurement of the albumin in a 24-hour urine collection.

## Haematuria

Haematuria arises from any site in the kidney or urinary tract (Fig. 8.2) and may be macroscopic, with bloody urine, or microscopic and found only on Stix testing. Vaginal bleeding is a common source of false positives. A positive Stix test must always be followed by careful microscopy of fresh urine to confirm the presence of red cells, to look for red cell casts and to exclude haemoglobinuria or myo-globinuria, which are uncommon but also result in a positive result on Stix testing. The presence of red cell casts on urine microscopy indicates bleeding of glomerular origin, i.e. glomerulonephritis (see later). In the absence of red cell casts, further investigations, such as urine cytology, ultrasonography, excretion urography and cystoscopy, are required to define the site of bleeding.

With macroscopic haematuria, the source of bleeding may be suggested by a careful history. Haematuria that is only apparent at the start of micturition is usually associated with urethral disease. Haematuria that occurs at the end of micturition suggests bleeding from the prostate or bladder base, whereas blood seen as an even discoloration

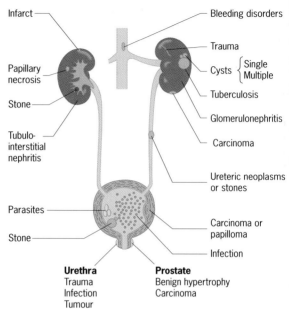

Fig. 8.2 Sites and causes of bleeding from the urinary tract.

throughout the urine suggests bleeding from a source in the bladder or above.

### Glycosuria

Diabetes mellitus must be excluded in any patients with a positive Stix test for glucose.

## Urine microscopy

Microscopy of urine is performed on all patients suspected of having renal disease. A fresh clean-catch mid-stream specimen of urine is essential to make a valid interpretation of the results (*K&C* p. 595)

### White cells

A value of $> 10/mm^3$ of urine is abnormal and indicates an inflammatory reaction within the urinary tract. Usually it is the result of a urinary tract infection (UTI). The causes of sterile pyuria (i.e. pus cells without bacterial infection) are a partially treated UTI, urinary tract tuberculosis, calculi, bladder tumour, papillary necrosis and tubulointerstitial nephritis.

### Red cells
A value of $> 1/mm^3$ is abnormal and must be investigated (see above).

### Casts
Mucoprotein precipitated in the renal tubules results in the formation of hyaline casts, which on their own are a normal finding. The incorporation of red cells results in red cell casts, a finding pathognomonic of glomerulonephritis. White cell casts may be seen in acute pyelonephritis. Granular casts result from the disintegration of cellular debris and indicate renal disease.

### Bacteria
A bacterial count over 100 000 organisms per mL of urine in a fresh mid-stream specimen is a reliable indicator of a UTI (p. 325).

## Glomerulonephritis (K&C p. 600)

### Normal glomerular structure

315

A renal glomerulus (there are about 1 million glomeruli in each kidney) consists of a capillary plexus invaginating the blind end of the proximal renal tubule (Fig. 8.3). The glomerular capillaries are lined by a fenestrated endothelium, which rests on the glomerular basement membrane (GBM). External to the GBM are the visceral epithelial cells (podocytes). These cells only make contact with the GBM by finger-like projections, called foot processes, which are separated from one another by 'slit pores'. This unique structure of the glomerular membrane accounts for its tremendous permeability, allowing 125–200 mL of glomerular filtrate to be formed every minute (this is the glomerular filtration rate or GFR). The composition of the glomerular filtrate is similar to plasma but contains only small amounts of protein (all of low molecular weight), most of which is reabsorbed in the proximal tubule. Tubular reabsorption and secretion

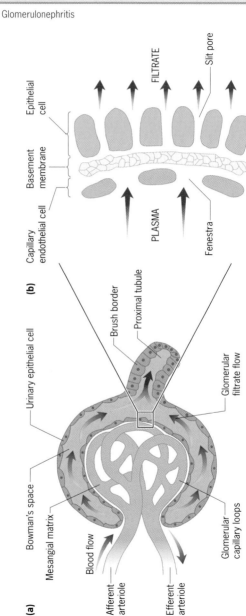

**Fig. 8.3 (a) Diagrammatic representation of the normal glomerulus. (b) Components of the glomerular membrane.** (Adapted from Read et al 1993 Essential Medicine. Churchill Livingstone, Edinburgh; Guyton (1987) Human Physiology and Mechanisms of Disease, 4th edn. WB Saunders, London.)

**(b)**

FILTRATE

Slit pore

Epithelial cell

Basement membrane

Capillary endothelial cell

PLASMA

Fenestra

Brush border

Proximal tubule

Urinary epithelial cell

Glomerular filtrate flow

Bowman's space

Mesangial matrix

Blood flow

Glomerular capillary loops

Afferent arteriole

Efferent arteriole

**(a)**

316

normally substantially alter the water and electrolyte composition of the glomerular filtrate until it reaches the renal pelvis as urine. The presence of some form of glomerular disease is usually suspected from the history and from one or more of the following urinary findings: haematuria, red cell casts, and proteinuria which may be in the nephrotic range (> 3 g/day).

Glomerulonephritis is a general term for a group of disorders in which there is bilateral, symmetrical immunologically mediated injury to the glomerulus. Pathogenetic mechanisms include:

- Deposition or in situ formation of immune complexes. Circulating antigen–antibody complexes are deposited in the kidney, or complexes are formed locally when antigen becomes trapped in the glomerulus. The antigen may be exogenous, e.g. β-haemolytic streptococci, or endogenous, e.g. DNA in systemic lupus erythematosus.
- Deposition of antiglomerular basement membrane antibody (anti-GBM, < 5% of glomerulonephritides). The principal target for the anti-GBM antibodies is the α-3 chain of type IV collagen. The antibody may also react with alveolar capillary basement membrane and can cause both lung haemorrhage and glomerulonephritis (Goodpasture's syndrome).
- Deposition of an immunoglobulin of atypical configuration in glomeruli. IgA nephropathy is the commonest type of glomerulonephritis and is an important cause of end-stage renal failure.

In some glomerulonephritides, e.g. associated with Wegener's granulomatosis and microscopic polyangiitis, there is no evidence of immune complex deposition. Injury is mediated by a vasculitis causing a focal segmental necrotizing glomerulonephritis with haematuria, proteinuria and deteriorating renal function.

## Pathogenesis

Deposition of immune complexes in the glomerulus leads to an inflammatory response, which triggers secondary mechanisms of glomerular injury. These include complement activation, fibrin deposition, platelet aggregation and activation of kinin systems. The histological response to immune complex deposition is very variable.

Renal tissue, obtained at transcutaneous renal biopsy, is examined by light microscopy, electron microscopy and immunofluorescence to determine the extent and type of disease and to assess the type of immunological injury. The main forms of histopathologically identified glomerulonephritis and the clinical features most often associated with each are listed in Table 8.1. The terms 'focal' and 'diffuse' refer to the kidney as a whole, and 'segmental' and 'global' refer to the glomeruli. Thus in focal segmental glomerulonephritis only some glomeruli are affected and only a part of the glomerulus.

## Aetiology

In most patients with immune complex-mediated glomerulonephritis the cause is unknown, i.e. the nature of the antigen is not determined. In a minority of cases antigens derived from viruses, bacteria, parasites, drugs and from the host may be involved (Table 8.2).

## Clinical features

Glomerulonephritis presents in one of four ways:

- Asymptomatic proteinuria and/or microscopic haematuria (p. 312)
- Acute nephritic syndrome
- Nephrotic syndrome
- Renal failure, acute and chronic (p. 340).

## Acute nephritic syndrome (K&C p. 606)

Diffuse proliferative glomerulonephritis underlies many of the cases of acute nephritic syndrome in adults and children. The prototype exogenous pattern is poststreptococcal glomerulonephritis, whereas that produced by an endogenous antigen is lupus nephritis, seen in systemic lupus erythematosus (SLE). The typical case of poststreptococcal glomerulonephritis develops in a child 1–3 weeks after a streptococcal infection (pharyngitis or cellulitis) with a Lancefield group A β-haemolytic streptococcus. The bacterial antigen becomes trapped in the glomerulus, leading to an acute diffuse proliferative glomerulonephritis.

**Table 8.1**
Categories of glomerulonephritis (GN) and associated clinical conditions*

| Histological type | Light microscopic appearances | Most common clinical presentation |
|---|---|---|
| Proliferative glomerulonephritis | | |
| Diffuse | Endothelial and mesangial cell proliferation | Acute nephritic syndrome |
| Focal segmental | As above but changes are focal | Haematuria, proteinuria |
| With crescent formation (rapidly progressive GN) | Crescent formation (aggregates of macrophages and epithelial cells in Bowman's space) | Acute renal failure |
| Mesangiocapillary (mesangioproliferative) | Thickening of GBM, mesangial cell proliferation | Haematuria, proteinuria, nephritic and nephrotic syndrome |
| IgA nephropathy | Mesangial cell proliferation | Haematuria in young men |
| Membranous GN | Thickening of GBM | Nephrotic syndrome in adults |
| Minimal change nephropathy | Normal (fusion of epithelial cell foot processes on EM) | Nephrotic syndrome in children |
| Focal glomerulosclerosis | Segmental scarring of glomeruli | Proteinuria or nephrotic syndrome |

* There is not a complete correlation between the histopathological types and the clinical features. GBM, glomerular basement membrane

> **Table 8.2**
> Some causes of immune complex-mediated glomerulonephritis
>
> **Infections**
> Lancefield group A β-haemolytic streptococci
> *Streptococcus viridans* (infective endocarditis)
> Mumps virus
> Hepatitis B and C virus
> Tropical infections: schistosomiasis, *Plasmodium malariae*, filariasis
>
> **Systemic disease**
> Systemic lupus erythematosus (SLE)
>
> **Malignant tumours**
>
> **Drugs**, e.g. penicillamine, gold

## Clinical features

The syndrome comprises:

- Haematuria (macroscopic or microscopic)
- Proteinuria (usually < 2 g in 24 hours)
- Hypertension caused by salt and water retention
- Oedema (periorbital, leg or sacral)
- Oliguria
- Uraemia.

## Investigations

A thorough history and examination are essential to assess the severity of the illness and to determine any associated underlying conditions. The investigations to consider in the nephritic syndrome are listed in Table 8.3. If the clinical diagnosis of a nephritic illness is clear-cut, e.g. in post-streptococcal glomerulonephritis, renal ultrasonography and renal biopsy are usually unnecessary.

## Management

Poststreptococcal glomerulonephritis usually has a good prognosis, and supportive measures are often all that is required until spontaneous recovery takes place. Hypertension is treated with salt restriction, loop diuretics and vasodilators. Fluid balance is monitored by daily weighing and daily recording of fluid input and output. In oliguric patients with evidence of fluid overload (e.g. oedema, pulmonary congestion and severe hypertension) fluid restriction is necessary. The management of life-threatening

**Table 8.3**

Investigations indicated in glomerular disease

| Investigations | Significance |
|---|---|
| **Baseline measurements** | |
| Creatinine clearance as a measure of GFR | To determine current status, monitor progress and response to treatment |
| 24-hour urinary protein excretion | |
| Serum urea and electrolytes | |
| Serum albumin | |
| **Diagnostically useful tests** | |
| Urine microscopy | Red cell casts indicate glomerulonephritis |
| Culture (swab from throat or infected skin) } | Diagnosis of recent streptococcal infection |
| Serum antistreptolysin-O titre | |
| Blood glucose | Diagnosis of diabetes mellitus |
| Serum tests: | |
| Antinuclear and anti-DNA antibodies | Systemic lupus erythematosus |
| Antineutrophil cytoplasmic antibodies (ANCA) | Wegener's granulomatosis and other types of vasculitis |
| Antiglomerular basement membrane antibody | Goodpasture's syndrome |
| Hepatitis B surface antigen | Hepatitis B infection |
| Hepatitis C antibody | Hepatitis C infection |
| HIV antibody | HIV infection |
| Cryoglobulins | Cryoglobulinaemia |
| Chest radiograph | Cavities in Wegener's granulomatosis, malignancy |
| Renal biopsy | Indicated in some adults with nephrotic or nephritic syndrome |

complications such as hypertensive encephalopathy (see p. 439), pulmonary oedema (p. 395) and severe uraemia (p. 347) is discussed in the appropriate chapters. In glomerulonephritis complicating SLE or the systemic vasculitides (see below), immunosuppression with prednisolone, cyclophosphamide or azathioprine improves renal function.

# Nephrotic syndrome *(K&C p. 611)*

Nephrotic syndrome consists of heavy proteinuria (> 3–5 g/24 h), hypoalbuminaemia and oedema. Hyperlipidaemia and thrombotic disease are also frequently observed. Structural damage to the glomerular basement membrane leads to loss of electrostatic and physical barriers, which normally prevent the passage of large molecular weight proteins into the glomerular filtrate. Increased protein loss, in addition to increased catabolism of protein in the kidney, leads to hypoalbuminaemia. The pathogenesis of oedema in the nephrotic syndrome is poorly understood. The classic explanation is that intravascular hypovolaemia (hypoalbuminaemia reduces plasma oncotic pressure, salt and water move into extravascular compartment) results in activation of the renin–angiotensin–aldosterone system, which promotes sodium and water reabsorption in the distal nephron. However, it seems probable that there is also a primary intrarenal defect in sodium excretion.

## Aetiology

All types of glomerulonephritis can cause the nephrotic syndrome, although in Europe and the USA membranous disease is the most common cause in adults and minimal change glomerulonephritis in children. Membranous glomerulonephritis is usually idiopathic but may occur in association with drugs, neoplasms or infections (Table 8.2). Focal glomerulosclerosis also presents with nephrotic syndrome and may be idiopathic or secondary to HIV infection.

Minimal change glomerulonephritis occurs most commonly in boys under 5 years of age. It accounts for 90% of cases of nephrotic syndrome in children and 20–25% in adults; however, it is rare in black African populations. The pathogenesis of this condition is not known; immune complexes are absent on immunofluorescence but the increase in glomerular permeability is thought to be immunologically mediated in some way.

Amyloid (p. 632) involving the kidneys and diabetes mellitus (p. 616) are also important causes of the nephrotic syndrome but, unlike minimal change and membranous glomerulonephritis, the mechanism is not immune mediated.

Other renal diseases, e.g. polycystic kidneys, reflux nephropathy, may cause proteinuria, but are rarely severe enough to cause the nephrotic syndrome.

## Clinical features

Oedema of the ankles, genitals and abdomen is the principal finding. The face (periorbital oedema) and arms may also be involved in severe cases.

## Differential diagnoses

Nephrotic syndrome must be differentiated from other causes of oedema and hypoalbuminaemia. In congestive cardiac failure (p. 389) there is oedema and a raised jugular venous pressure (JVP). In nephrotic syndrome the JVP is normal or low unless there is concomitant renal failure and oliguria. Hypoalbuminaemia and oedema occur in cirrhosis, but there are usually signs of chronic liver disease on examination (p. 128).

323

## Investigations

The diagnosis is established by demonstrating:

- Heavy proteinuria (> 3–5 g/24 h in adults)
- Hypoalbuminaemia (serum albumin < 30 g/L).

Hyperlipidaemia is common in the nephrotic syndrome and is the result of increased hepatic synthesis of cholesterol and triglycerides, which accompanies hepatic albumin synthesis. Further investigations to be considered are listed in Table 8.3.

In the UK most cases of childhood nephrotic syndrome are caused by minimal change glomerulonephritis, and therefore treatment is usually started with corticosteroids without recourse to a renal biopsy. In adults a renal biopsy is performed unless the diagnosis is clear-cut, e.g. nephrotic syndrome in a patient with long-standing diabetes mellitus must be advanced diabetic glomerulopathy. If a drug is implicated, e.g. penicillamine, the correct management is to stop the drug.

## Management

**General** Oedema is treated with bed rest, dietary salt restriction and diuretic therapy. Intravenous diuretics and occasionally intravenous salt-poor albumin is required to initiate a diuresis which, once established, can usually be maintained with oral diuretics alone. If diuresis is too vigorous it may precipitate circulatory collapse and acute renal failure.

**Specific treatment** Minimal change disease is almost always steroid responsive in children, although less commonly in adults. High-dose prednisolone therapy (40–60 mg daily) should be given over a period of 8 weeks and then reduced slowly. Of patients who enter remission 30–50% will have a relapse within 3 years, and this is treated with a further course of steroids. In patients with frequent relapses and in steroid-unresponsive patients, immunosuppressive therapy with cyclophosphamide or ciclosporin is used.

The benefits of immunosuppressive therapy in membranous glomerulonephritis remain contentious. In other types of glomerulonephritis remission may occur if the underlying disease can be treated, e.g. in patients with SLE, treatment with steroids or cyclophosphamide may induce long-term remission.

## Complications

- *Venous thrombosis.* Hypovolaemia and a hypercoagulable state predispose to thrombus formation in both renal (seen on ultrasonography) and peripheral veins. Prolonged bed rest should be avoided but, if necessary, patients should receive prophylactic anticoagulation with subcutaneous heparin (p. 217). Renal vein thrombosis presents with renal pain, haematuria and a deterioration in renal function.

- *Sepsis.* Loss of immunoglobulin in the urine increases the susceptibility to infection which is a cause of death in these patients.
- *Acute renal failure* is rarely the result of progression of the underlying renal disease. However, acute renal failure occurs as a result of hypovolaemia (particularly after diuretic therapy) or with renal vein thrombosis.

## Urinary tract infection *(K&C p. 615)*

Urinary tract infection (UTI) is common in women, with about 35% having symptoms of a UTI at some time in their lives. It is relatively uncommon in children and in men, when it usually indicates underlying disease.

### Pathogenesis

Infection of the urinary tract is most often via the ascending transurethral route, and this is facilitated by sexual intercourse and urethral catheterization. Women are more susceptible to infection because the short urethra and its proximity to the anus facilitates the transfer of bowel organisms to the bladder. Infection is most often caused by bacteria from the patient's own bowel flora (Table 8.4), but in 20–30% of young women it is caused by skin organisms: *Staphylococcus saprophyticus* or *Staph. epidermidis.*

**Table 8.4**
Organisms causing urinary tract infection in domiciliary practice

| Organism | Approximate frequency (%) |
|---|---|
| *Escherichia coli* and other coliforms | > 70 |
| Proteus mirabilis | 12 |
| *Klebsiella aerogenes**  | 4 |
| Enterococci* | 6 |
| *Staphylococcus saprophyticus* or *Staph. epidermidis†* | 8 |

* More common in hospital practice
† More common in women

Abnormalities that encourage bladder infection (*cystitis*) include:

- Urinary obstruction or stasis
- Previous damage to the bladder epithelium
- Bladder stones
- Poor bladder emptying.

Ascending infection of the ureters results in renal parenchymal infection (*acute pyelonephritis*). This is facilitated by vesicoureteric reflux and dilated hypotonic ureters. Reflux nephropathy arises from childhood UTIs in combination with vesicoureteric reflux, leading to progressive renal scarring. It presents as hypertension or chronic renal failure in childhood and adult life.

## Clinical features

The most common symptoms of lower urinary tract infection are frequency of micturition, dysuria, suprapubic pain and tenderness, haematuria and smelly urine. In acute pyelonephritis there may also be loin pain and tenderness, with fever and systemic upset. However, localization of infection on the basis of symptoms alone is unreliable. In elderly people the symptoms may be atypical, with incontinence, nocturia or just a vague change in well-being.

## Investigations

- Dipstick tests can be used to detect the presence of urinary nitrites (produced by reduction of urinary nitrates by bacteria) and elastase produced by neutrophils. Dipstick tests positive for both nitrite and elastase are highly predictive of acute infection.
- Urine microscopy and culture and antimicrobial susceptibility testing of pathogens. The diagnosis depends on finding more than 100 000 of the same organism per mL of urine in a clean-catch mid-stream urine specimen (MSU). Lower counts or mixed growths are of uncertain significance and the test should be repeated. Rarely and if in doubt, urine must be obtained by suprapubic bladder aspiration, where any growth of a uropathogenic organism is evidence of infection.

- Excretion urography (pp. 335, 807) is performed to look for physiological and anatomical abnormalities of the urinary tract that predispose to UTI. It is indicated in women with repeated infections and after a single infection in children and men.

## Management

A 3–5-day course of oral amoxicillin, nitrofurantion or trimethoprim is usually effective. The treatment regimen may be modified in light of the result of urine culture and sensitivity testing and the clinical response. A high fluid intake should be encouraged during treatment and for some weeks afterwards. In women with relapsing infection, low-dose prophylactic antibiotics are required for a period of 6–12 months. Patients with acute pyelonephritis are often acutely ill and usually require initial treatment with parenteral antibiotics, such as intravenous cefuroxime, ciprofloxacin or an aminoglycoside (e.g. gentamicin). In patients with an indwelling catheter, treatment is indicated only in the presence of symptoms.

## Complications

Acute cystitis in the otherwise healthy non-pregnant adult woman is generally considered to be uncomplicated and will rarely result in serious kidney damage. Patients with abnormal urinary tracts (e.g. stones) or systemic disease involving the kidney (e.g. diabetes mellitus), are considered to have complicated infection and are more likely to fail treatment and develop complications which include renal papillary necrosis (p. 329) and the development of a renal or perinephric abscess with the risk of Gram-negative septicaemia. Abscesses can be seen on ultrasonography and usually require surgical drainage as well as antibiotic therapy.

# Urinary tract infection in pregnancy

(*K&C* p. 620)

Approximately 6% of pregnant women have significant bacteriuria in pregnancy; if untreated, 20% of these will develop acute pyelonephritis with significant risk to both mother and fetus (e.g. septic shock, low birthweight and prematurity). Early detection and treatment of bacteriuria is thus indicated.

## Abacteriuric frequency or dysuria ('urethral syndrome') (*K&C* p. 618)

The urethral syndrome occurs in women and presents with dysuria and frequency but in the absence of bacteriuria. It may be associated with vaginitis in postmenopausal women, irritant chemicals (e.g. soaps) and sexual intercourse.

## Tuberculosis of the urinary tract (*K&C* p. 620)

Tuberculosis (TB) of the urinary tract may present with all the symptoms of a UTI, i.e. dysuria, frequency or haematuria, and should be considered particularly in the Asian immigrant population of the UK. Classically, there is sterile pyuria (p. 314). Diagnosis depends on culture of mycobacteria from early-morning urine samples. Treatment is as for pulmonary tuberculosis (p. 481).

## Tubulointerstitial nephritis (*K&C* p. 621)

Interstitial inflammation with tubular damage is a regular feature of bacterial pyelonephritis but it rarely, if ever, leads to chronic renal damage in the absence of reflux, obstruction or other complicating factors. The importance of other factors, particularly drugs, in the causation of this disorder has now been realized.

## Acute tubulointerstitial nephritis

Acute tubulointerstitial nephritis is most often the result of a hypersensitivity reaction to drugs (Table 8.5), most commonly drugs of the penicillin family and non-steroidal anti-inflammatory drugs (NSAIDs). Patients present with fever, eosinophilia and eosinophiluria, normal or only mildly increased urine protein excretion (< 1 g/day) and acute renal failure. Renal biopsy shows an intense interstitial cellular infiltrate, predominantly eosinophils, and variable tubular necrosis. Management involves withdrawal of the offending drug and treatment of acute renal failure (p. 346). High-dose

**Table 8.5**
Common causes of acute tubulointerstitial nephritis

Penicillins
NSAIDs
Sulfonamides
Allopurinol
Cephalosporins
Rifampicin
Diuretics – furosemide (frusemide), thiazides
Cimetidine
Phenytoin

NSAIDs, non-steroidal anti-inflammatory drugs

prednisolone therapy is often used, although its value has not been proven. The prognosis is generally good; patients should avoid further exposure to the offending drug.

## Chronic tubulointerstitial nephritis

The most common cause of chronic tubulointerstitial nephritis is prolonged consumption of large amounts of analgesic drugs, particularly NSAIDs ('analgesic nephropathy'). Some causes are shown in Table 8.6. Presentation is usually with polyuria, proteinuria (usually <1 g/day) or uraemia. Polyuria and nocturia are the result of tubular damage in the medullary area of the kidney, leading to defects in the renal concentrating ability. Necrosis of the papillae, which may subsequently slough off and be passed in the urine, sometimes causes ureteric colic or acute ureteral obstruction. Management is largely supportive. In cases of analgesic nephropathy the drug should be stopped and replaced if necessary with paracetamol or dihydrocodeine.

**Table 8.6**
Causes of chronic tubulointerstitial nephritis

Reflux nephropathy
NSAIDs
Diabetes mellitus
Sickle cell disease
Sjögren's syndrome
Hyperuricaemic nephropathy

NSAIDs, non-steroidal anti-inflammatory drugs

# Hypertension and the kidney (*K&C* p. 623)

Hypertension can be the cause or the result of renal disease, and it is often difficult to differentiate between the two on clinical grounds. Investigations, as described on page 437, should be performed on all patients, although excretion urography (p. 807) is usually unnecessary.

## Essential hypertension

Hypertension leads to characteristic histological changes in the renal vessels and intrarenal vasculature over time. These include intimal thickening with reduplication of the elastic lamina, reduction in kidney size, and an increase in the proportion of sclerotic glomeruli. The changes are usually accompanied by some deterioration in renal function.

Accelerated or malignant-phase hypertension is marked by the development of fibrinoid necrosis in afferent glomerular arterioles and fibrin deposition in arteriolar walls. A rapid rise in blood pressure may trigger these arteriolar lesions, and a vicious circle is then established whereby fibrin deposition leads to renal damage, increased renin release and a further increase in blood pressure.

Treatment of hypertension is described on page 437. The outlook is good if treatment is started before renal impairment has occurred.

## Renal hypertension

### Bilateral renal disease

Hypertension commonly complicates bilateral renal disease, such as chronic glomerulonephritis, reflux nephropathy or analgesic nephropathy. Two main mechanisms are responsible:

- Activation of the renin–angiotensin–aldosterone system
- Retention of salt and water, leading to an increase in blood volume and hence blood pressure.

Good control of blood pressure will prevent further deterioration in renal function, with angiotensin-converting enzyme (ACE) inhibitors being the drugs of choice.

## Unilateral renal disease

Hypertension may arise as a result of unilateral renal artery stenosis (caused by fibromuscular hyperplasia in young women, atheroma in elderly people) or unilateral reflux nephropathy. The mechanism of hypertension with renal artery stenosis is illustrated in Figure 8.4.

### Screening for unilateral renal disease

- *MR angiography* is a valuable non-invasive technique for visualizing the renal arteries, with close correlation with conventional angiography.
- *Helical (spiral) CT scanning* with intravenous contrast injection (CT angiography) also permits non-invasive imaging of the renal arteries, though it exposes the patient to ionizing radiation and to a large volume of contrast which may be harmful to patients with poor renal function.
- *Renal arteriography* remains the 'gold standard' for the diagnosis of renal artery disease, though the technique is invasive and requires cannulation of the femoral artery.
- *Radionuclide studies* using technetium-labelled diethylenetriaminepentaacetic acid ([$^{99m}$TC]DTPA).

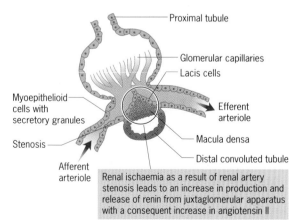

Fig. 8.4 **The mechanism of hypertension in unilateral renal artery stenosis.** (Adapted from Davidson (1991) Principles and Practice of Medicine. Churchill Livingstone, Edinburgh.)

With significant renal artery stenosis, a fall in uptake of isotope on the affected side follows administration of an angiotensin-converting enzyme (ACE) inhibitor, such as captopril. A completely normal result renders the diagnosis unlikely.

## Management

Most patients do well with hypotensive therapy without the need for surgery. ACE inhibitors are avoided because they can lead to acute renal failure in the presence of renal artery stenosis. Surgical options for renal artery stenosis include transluminal angioplasty to dilate the stenotic region, insertion of a stent across the stenosis, reconstructive vascular surgery and nephrectomy. With good patient selection more than 50% are cured or improved by intervention. In unilateral reflux nephropathy nephrectomy is advocated, particularly if the abnormal kidney is making an insignificant contribution to overall excretion function.

# Renal stone disease (K&C p. 625)

Renal and ureteral stones (urolithiasis) are a common problem affecting 2% of the UK population at some time in their life. There is a male:female ratio of 2:1. Bladder stones are common in developing countries.

## Aetiology

80% of patients with urolithiasis form calcium stones, most of which are composed primarily of calcium oxalate or, less often, calcium phosphate. The other main types include uric acid, struvite (magnesium ammonium phosphate), and cystine stones. Stone formation occurs when normally soluble material (e.g. calcium) supersaturates the urine and begins the process of crystal formation. In normal urine, inhibitors of crystal formation also prevent stone formation.

More than half of all patients with calcium oxalate stones have idiopathic hypercalciuria. People with this condition both absorb from the gut and excrete in the urine a higher fraction of dietary calcium than normal people. Serum calcium levels are normal. Less common causes of hypercalciuria are:

- Hypercalcaemia (p. 585): most patients with hypercalcaemia who form stones have primary hyperparathyroidism
- Excessive dietary intake of calcium
- Excessive resorption of calcium from the skeleton, as occurs with prolonged immobilization or weightlessness.

Increased oxalate excretion favours the formation of calcium oxalate, even if calcium excretion is normal:

- Dietary hyperoxaluria from excessive ingestion of high-oxalate-containing foods (e.g. spinach, rhubarb and tea), or from dietary calcium restriction with compensatory increased absorption of oxalate.
- Enteric hyperoxaluria: small bowel disease, e.g. Crohn's disease or resection, is associated with increased absorption of oxalate from the colon. Dehydration secondary to fluid loss from the gut also plays a part in stone formation.
- Primary hyperoxaluria is a rare autosomal recessive enzyme deficiency leading to increased oxalate production and corresponding oxalate excretion. There is widespread calcium oxalate crystal deposition in the kidneys, and later in other tissues (myocardium, tissues and bone). Renal failure typically develops in the late teens or early 20s.

Primary renal disease may lead to calcium stone formation. Medullary sponge kidney is associated with hypercalciuria and a tendency to develop stones (p. 357). The alkaline urine seen in the renal tubular acidoses favours the precipitation of calcium phosphate.

***Uric acid stones*** are sometimes associated with hyperuricaemia (p. 267) with or without clinical gout. Patients with ileostomies are also at risk of developing urate stones, as loss of bicarbonate from gastrointestinal secretions results in the production of an acid urine (uric acid is more soluble in an alkaline than an acid medium).

***Infection-induced stones*** Urinary tract infection with organisms that produce urease (*Proteus*, *Klebsiella* and

*Pseudomonas* spp.) is associated with stones containing ammonium, magnesium and calcium. Urease hydrolyses urea to ammonia and thus raises the urine pH. An alkaline urine and high ammonia concentration favour stone formation. These stones are often large and fill the pelvicalyceal system, producing the typical radio-opaque staghorn calculus.

**Cystine stones** may occur with cystinuria, an autosomal recessive condition affecting cystine and dibasic amino acid transport (lysine, ornithine and arginine) in the epithelial cells of renal tubules and the gastrointestinal tract. The excessive urinary excretion of cystine, which is the least soluble of the naturally occurring amino acids, leads to the formation of crystals and calculi.

### Clinical features (Table 8.7)

Most people with urinary tract calculi are asymptomatic; pain is the most common symptom. Large staghorn renal calculi may cause loin pain. *Ureteric stones* cause renal colic, a severe intermittent pain lasting for hours. The pain is felt anywhere between the loin and the groin, and may radiate into the scrotum or labium or into the tip of the penis. Nausea and vomiting are common. Microscopic haematuria is almost always present. The patient will be pyrexial only if there is a UTI associated with the stone. *Bladder stones* present with urinary frequency and haematuria. *Urethral stones* may cause bladder outflow obstruction, resulting in anuria and painful bladder distension.

### Differential diagnosis

Bleeding within the kidney, e.g. after renal biopsy, can produce clots that lodge temporarily in the ureter and

**Table 8.7**
Clinical features of urinary tract calculi

Asymptomatic
Pain
Haematuria
Urinary tract infection
Urinary tract obstruction

produce ureteric colic. Pain may also occur from sloughed necrotic renal papillae (p. 329). Pain from an ectopic pregnancy or leaking aortic aneurysm may be mistaken for renal colic.

## Investigations

In a patient presenting with renal colic the clinical diagnosis is confirmed by plain abdominal X-ray (KUB: kidney, ureters and bladder) and emergency excretion urography. Ninety per cent of renal stones are radio-opaque and calcification may be seen in the line of the renal tract. Excretion urography (intravenous urography, IVU) shows a delayed nephrogram (opacification of the renal parenchyma) on the side of the stone and may identify the site and degree of obstruction. An IVU is relatively safe despite the need for intravenous contrast (1% risk of 'allergic reaction, 1 in 200 000 mortality) and remains the diagnostic procedure of choice in most cases, although it may eventually be replaced by unenhanced spiral CT scan.

A detailed history may reveal possible aetiological factors for stone formation, e.g. vitamin D consumption, gouty arthritis, recurrent UTIs, intestinal resection. The subsequent work-up for a renal calculus is indicated in Table 8.8.

**Table 8.8**
Investigations in a patient with urinary calculi

| First line | Second line in recurrent stone formers |
|---|---|
| **Urine**<br>Chemical analysis of any stone passed<br>MSU for culture and sensitivity | 24-h urine collection for: calcium, oxalate, cystine and uric acid |
| **Blood**<br>Serum urea and electrolytes<br>Serum calcium<br>Serum uric acid<br>Serum bicarbonate | |
| **Radiography**<br>Plain film<br>Intravenous (excretion) urography<br>Helical CT scanning | |

## Management

**Initial treatment**  In the case of renal colic, a strong analgesic (e.g. an opiate or an NSAID) should be given to relieve the pain. Patients can be managed at home if there is no evidence of sepsis and they are able to take oral medications and fluids. Most ureteric stones that are 5 mm or less in diameter will pass spontaneously. Indications for intervention include persistent pain, infection above the site of obstruction, and failure of the stone to pass down the ureter. The options for stone removal include the following:

- Extracorporeal shock wave lithotripsy (ESWL) is the treatment of choice in 85% of patients and is particularly good for stones in the renal pelvis and upper ureter. Shock wave lithotripsy fragments the stones and allows them to pass spontaneously down the urethra.
- Endoscopy (ureteroscopy) and some form of in situ stone fragmentation are used for ureteric calculi. Bladder stones are removed at cystoscopy.
- Percutaneous nephrolithotomy for stones in the renal pelvis and calyces. Stones are removed by creating a percutaneous track followed by endoscopic removal of stones along this track.
- Open surgery for very large stones.

**Prevention of recurrence**  Further therapy depends on the type of stone and any underlying condition identified during screening investigations. For prevention of all stones whatever the cause, a high intake of fluid (to produce a urine volume of 2–2.5 L/day) must be maintained, particularly during the summer months. When no metabolic or renal abnormality has been identified ('idiopathic stone formers') adequate hydration is the mainstay of treatment.

- *Idiopathic hypercalciuria.* Reduction of dietary intake of calcium by avoiding milk, cheese and white bread is recommended, though its value has been questioned. A water softener may be helpful for patients who live in hard water areas. If hypercalciuria persists, a thiazide diuretic, e.g. bendroflumethiazide (bendrofluazide), will reduce urinary calcium excretion.

- *Mixed infective stones.* Recurrent stones should be prevented by maintenance of a high fluid intake and measures to stop bacteriuria. This will require long-term follow-up and may demand the use of long-term, low-dose, prophylactic antibiotics.

- *Uric acid stones* are prevented by the long-term use of the xanthine oxidase inhibitor, allopurinol, which allows the excretion of the soluble precursor compound, hypoxanthine, in preference to uric acid. Oral sodium bicarbonate supplements to maintain an alkaline urine, and hence increased solubility of uric acid, are an alternative approach in those patients unable to tolerate allopurinol.

- *Cystine stones.* Patients may be unable to tolerate the very high fluid intake (5 litres of water in 24 hours) needed to maintain solubility of cystine in the urine. An alternative is D-penicillamine, which chelates cystine, forming a more soluble complex.

## Nephrocalcinosis (Table 8.9) (*K&C* p. 631)

The term 'nephrocalcinosis' means diffuse renal parenchymal calcification that is detectable radiologically. The condition is typically painless. Hypertension and renal impairment commonly occur. The treatment is of the underlying cause.

337

**Table 8.9**
Common causes of nephrocalcinosis

**Mainly medullary**
Hypercalcaemia
Renal tubular acidosis
Primary hyperoxaluria
Medullary sponge kidney
Tuberculosis

**Mainly cortical (rare)**
Renal cortical necrosis

# Urinary tract obstruction (K&C p. 631)

The urinary tract may be obstructed at any point along its length between the kidney and the urethral meatus. This results in dilatation of the tract above the obstruction. Dilatation of the renal pelvis is known as *hydronephrosis*.

## Aetiology

The causes of obstruction may be classified into three groups (Table 8.10). In adults the most common causes are prostatic hypertrophy or tumour, gynaecological cancer and calculi.

## Clinical features

- *Upper urinary tract obstruction* results in a dull ache in the flank or loin, which may be provoked by an increase in urine volume, e.g. high fluid intake or diuretics. Complete anuria is strongly suggestive of complete bilateral obstruction or complete obstruction

**Table 8.10**
Causes of urinary tract obstruction

**Within the lumen**
Calculi
Tumour
Blood clots
Sloughed renal papillae (diabetes, NSAIDs, sickle cell disease or trait)

**Within the wall**
Stricture: ureteric or urethral
Neuropathic bladder
Pelviureteric junction obstruction (functional disturbance in peristalsis of collecting system)
Obstructive megaureter (defective peristalsis at lower end of ureter)

**Within the wall**
Prostatic hypertrophy/tumour
Pelvic tumours
Phimosis
Retroperitoneal fibrosis
Accidental surgical ligation of the ureter

NSAIDs, non-steroidal anti-inflammatory drugs

of a single functioning kidney. Partial obstruction causes polyuria as a result of tubular damage and impairment of concentrating mechanisms.

- *Bladder outlet obstruction* results in hesitancy, poor stream, terminal dribbling and a sense of incomplete emptying. Retention with overflow is characterized by the frequent passage of small quantities of urine. Infection commonly occurs and may precipitate acute retention of urine.

Depending on the site of obstruction an enlarged bladder or hydronephrotic kidney may be felt on examination. Pelvic and rectal examination is essential in determining the cause of obstruction.

### Investigations

Imaging studies are performed to identify the site and nature of the obstruction and, together with serum bio-chemistry, to assess function of the affected kidney.

- Ultrasonography and intravenous urography are the initial investigations. Ultrasonography confirms the diagnosis of obstruction and may show hydronephrosis. Excretion urography identifies the site of obstruction and shows a characteristic appearance (a delayed nephrogram, which eventually becomes denser than the non-obstructed side).

- Radionuclide studies (p. 812) are of no value in the investigation of acute obstruction but may help, in long-standing obstruction, to differentiate true obstructive uropathy from retention of tracer in a baggy low-pressure unobstructed pelvicalyceal system.

- Subsequent investigations may include helical (spiral) CT scanning, retrograde and anterograde uretography, cystoscopy and pressure–flow studies during bladder filling and voiding. Anterograde uretography is particularly useful in both the diagnosis and therapy of patients with urinary obstruction. A fine catheter is introduced into the renal pelvis under ultrasound guidance. This allows the introduction of dye to determine the site and cause of obstruction; in addition, urine may be temporarily drained from an obstructed system while definitive treatment is planned.

## Management

Surgery is the usual treatment for persistent urinary tract obstruction. Elimination of the obstruction may be associated with a massive postoperative diuresis, resulting partly from a solute diuresis from salt and urea retained during obstruction and partly from the renal concentrating defect. In some cases definitive relief of obstruction is not possible and urinary diversion may be required. This may be simply an indwelling urethral catheter, a stent placed across the obstructing lesion, or the formation of an ileal conduit.

# Renal failure

The term 'renal failure' means failure of renal excretory function as a result of the depression of the glomerular filtration rate (GFR). This is accompanied to a variable extent by failure of erythropoietin production, vitamin D hydroxylation, regulation of acid–base balance, regulation of salt and water balance and blood pressure control.

- *Acute renal failure* (ARF) is a sudden and rapid decline in renal function which lasts days to weeks. It is usually reversible or self-limiting.
- *Chronic renal failure* (CRF) develops over months or years. It is usually not reversible but treatment may slow progression.

## Acute renal failure (K&C p. 637)

Acute renal failure (ARF) can be defined as an abrupt sustained rise in serum urea and creatinine due to a rapid decline in glomerular filtration rate leading to loss of normal water and solute homeostasis. There is no universally accepted biochemical definition of ARF, but commonly used definitions include an increase in the serum creatinine of more than 44 µmol/L or more than 50% over the baseline value.

### Aetiology

ARF may be:

- Prerenal
- Renal
- Postrenal.

It may also result from a combination of these factors, e.g. in post-surgical ARF, fluid depletion (prerenal), systemic infection and nephrotoxic drugs (renal) may all play a role. ARF may also complicate chronic renal failure ('*acute-on-chronic*').

**Prerenal** Failure of perfusion of the kidneys with blood occurs in prerenal failure. The kidney is able to maintain glomerular filtration close to normal in spite of wide variations in the renal perfusion pressure and volume status – so-called 'autoregulation'. Maintenance of a normal GFR in the face of decreased systemic pressure depends on the intrarenal production of prostaglandins and angiotensin II. With severe or prolonged hypovolaemia there is eventually a drop in glomerular filtration, termed 'prerenal failure'. Drugs that impair renal autoregulation, such as angiotensin-converting enzyme (ACE) inhibitors, and non-steroidal anti-inflammatory drugs, increase the risk of prerenal failure in hypovolaemia. ACE inhibitors may also cause renal failure (ischaemic nephropathy) in patients with atherosclerotic renal artery stenosis (p. 331), who may have evidence of atherosclerosis elsewhere, e.g. ischaemic heart disease and peripheral vascular disease.

Prerenal failure is most commonly the result of hypovolaemia (Table 8.11), and is characterized in the early stages by lack of structural damage and rapid reversibility once normal renal perfusion has been restored. Hypovolaemia is identified from the clinical history and, on physical examination, by the presence of hypotension, a postural drop in blood pressure, a low jugular venous pressure (JVP) and reduced tissue turgor. Measurement of urinary electrolytes (Table 8.12) can help differentiate between prerenal ARF, in which the reabsorptive capacity of tubular cells and the concentrating ability of the kidney are preserved, and intrinsic renal failure, in which both these functions are impaired. However, the urinary indices do not completely segregate the two conditions and they are no substitute for a proper clinical assessment.

If, on the basis of the history and clinical examination, prerenal (hypovolaemia) failure is diagnosed or strongly suspected, the effect of volume repletion on renal function must be tested. Volume repletion should be with an

**Table 8.11**
Prenatal causes of acute renal failure

**Hypovolaemia**
Haemorrhage
Diarrhoea
Diuretics
Pancreatitis
Diabetic ketoacidosis
Sepsis
Burns

**Decreased cardiac output**
Myocardial infarction
Massive pulmonary embolism
Congestive cardiac failure

**Severe liver failure (hepatorenal syndrome)**

**Renal artery obstruction**
Stenosis
Thrombosis
Embolization

appropriate fluid: blood in the case of post-haemorrhagic shock and physiological saline if fluid depletion is caused by vomiting, diarrhoea or polyuria. In some cases, e.g. with a very sick patient, volume replacement is guided by measurement of the central venous pressure (p. 740). With pure prerenal failure, urine output should increase with volume replacement. If hypovolaemia is corrected (i.e. the JVP or CVP is normal) and urine output does not increase, the kidneys may respond to a strong diuretic stimulus (e.g.

**Table 8.12**
Criteria for distinction between prerenal and intrinsic causes of renal dysfunction

|  | Prerenal | Intrinsic |
|---|---|---|
| Urine specific gravity | > 1.020 | < 1.010 |
| Urine osmolality (mOsm/Kg) | > 500 | < 350 |
| Urine sodium (mmol/L) | < 20 | > 40 |
| Fractional excretion of sodium ($Na^+$) | < 1% | > 1% |

$$\text{Fractional excretion of } Na^+ = \frac{[\text{urine } Na^+ \times \text{plasma Cr}]}{[\text{plasma } Na^+ \times \text{urine Cr}]} \times 100\%$$

where Cr is creatinine

furosemide (frusemide) 120 mg i.v. over 10 minutes, which may be repeated once if there is no response). If urine output does not increase with these measures, then the patient has progressed to acute tubular necrosis (ATN) and the management is that of established intrinsic renal failure (see later).

**Postrenal** Postrenal ARF occurs when both urinary outflow tracts are obstructed or when one tract is obstructed in a patient with a single functional kidney (p. 338). It is usually quickly reversed if the obstruction is relieved. All patients with ARF must be examined for evidence of obstruction (enlarged palpable kidneys or bladder, large prostate on rectal examination, pelvic masses on vaginal examination in women) and undergo renal ultrasonography to look for hydronephrosis and dilated ureters. Bladder outflow obstruction is ruled out by flushing of an existing catheter or insertion of a urethral catheter, which should then be removed unless a large volume of urine is obtained. Treatment of obstruction is usually by a temporary measure, e.g. urethral/suprapubic catheterization or percutaneous nephrostomy, until definitive treatment of the obstructing lesion can be undertaken (p. 339).

**Intrinsic renal failure** Intrinsic renal diseases that result in ARF are categorized according to the primary site of injury: tubules, interstitium, renal vessels or glomerulus (Table 8.13). Injury to the tubules is most often ischaemic or toxic in origin. Prerenal ARF and ischaemic tubular necrosis represent a continuum, with the former leading to the latter when blood flow is sufficiently compromised to result in the death of tubular cells. In established renal failure the kidney loses its ability to concentrate the urine and conserve sodium. This may, in addition to clinical examination, be useful in differentiating renal from prerenal failure where the kidney is able to concentrate the urine and conserve sodium (see Table 8.12).

## Clinical features of established ARF

The early stages of renal failure are often completely asymptomatic. Symptoms are common when the plasma urea concentration is over 40 mmol/L, but many patients

> **Table 8.13**
> Causes of intrinsic renal failure
>
> **Acute tubular necrosis\***
> Ischaemia
> Exogenous nephrotoxins: gentamycin, cefaloridine, intravenous
>   contrast agents
> Endogenous nephrotoxins: Bence Jones protein, uric acid,
>   myoglobin (secondary to rhabdomyolysis)
>
> **Acute tubulointerstitial nephritis**
> Drug hypersensitivity
> Infections
>
> **Large renal vessels**
> Renal artery thrombosis
> Renal vein thrombosis
>
> **Small renal vessels**
> Vasculitis
> Malignant hypertension
> Haemolytic uraemic syndrome/thrombotic thrombocytopenic
> purpura
>
> **Acute glomerulonephritis**

\* Accounts for about 90% of intrinsic ARF

develop uraemic symptoms at lower levels of plasma urea. It is not the accumulation of urea itself that causes symptoms, but a combination of many different metabolic abnormalities.

- *Alteration of urine volume.* Oliguria (urinary output < 300 mL/day) usually occurs with acute renal failure, but there may be polyuria with the passage of large quantities of dilute urine.
- *Neurological.* Weakness, fatigue and lassitude occur. Mental confusion, seizures and coma may also occur with severe uraemia, but this is less commonly seen since the introduction of effective renal replacement therapy.
- *Skin.* Symptoms include pallor, pruritus, pigmentation and bruising.
- *Cardiopulmonary.* Breathlessness occurs from a combination of anaemia and pulmonary oedema secondary to volume overload. There may be deep sighing respiration (Kussmaul's respiration) resulting from systemic metabolic acidosis. Pericarditis occurs

with severe untreated uraemia and may be complicated by a pericardial effusion and tamponade.

- *Gastrointestinal.* Nausea, anorexia and vomiting are common.
- *Haematological.* Anaemia is most commonly seen in chronic renal failure but may occur in ARF. Impaired platelet function causes bruising and exacerbates gastrointestinal bleeding.

## Investigation of the uraemic emergency

The purpose of investigation, together with clinical examination, is threefold:

1. To differentiate acute from chronic renal failure (see p. 350).
2. To document the degree of renal impairment and obtain baseline values so that the response to treatment can be monitored. This is accomplished by measurement of serum urea and electrolytes, and a 24-hour creatinine clearance.
3. To establish whether ARF is prerenal, renal or postrenal, and to determine the underlying cause so that specific treatment (e.g. intensive immunosuppression in Wegener's granulomatosis) may be instituted as early as possible and thus prevent progression to irreversible renal failure.
   - Urinary electrolytes: measurement of urinary electrolytes (see Table 8.12) may help to exclude a significant prerenal element to ARF.
   - Urine Stix testing and microscopy: glomerulonephritis is suggested by haematuria and proteinuria on urine Stix testing and by the presence of red cell casts on urine microscopy (p. 315).
   - Serum calcium, phosphate and uric acid.
   - Blood count: anaemia, a very high ESR, or eosinophilia may suggest myeloma or a vasculitis.
   - Radiology: every patient should undergo renal ultrasonography (for renal size and to exclude obstruction); CT is useful for the diagnosis of retroperitoneal fibrosis and some other causes of urinary obstruction, and may also indicate cortical scarring.

- Histological investigations: renal biopsy should be considered in every patient with unexplained renal failure and normal-sized kidneys.
- Urine and blood cultures to exclude infection.
- Optional investigations (depending on the case):
  - Serum protein electrophoresis for myeloma
  - Serum autoantibodies, ANCAs (p. 800) and complement
  - Antibodies to hepatitis B and C may point to polyarteritis or cryoglobulinaemia
  - Antibodies to HIV may point to HIV-related renal disease.

## Management

The principles of management of established ARF are summarized in Emergency Box 8.1. In all patients with intrinsic renal failure, hypovolaemia and obstruction must be excluded as contributing factors.

Indications for dialysis include:

- Hyperkalaemia not controlled by conservative measures
- Severe metabolic acidosis
- Pulmonary oedema
- Progressive uraemia with encephalopathy or pericarditis.

Whether haemodialysis, haemofiltration or peritoneal dialysis (p. 352) is used depends on the facilities available and the clinical circumstances, e.g. haemodialysis requires anticoagulation and thus would be inappropriate in a patient with recent haemorrhage from peptic ulceration.

## Prognosis

The prognosis depends on the underlying cause. The most common cause of death is sepsis as a result of impaired immune defence (from uraemia and malnutrition) and instrumentation (dialysis and urinary catheters and vascular lines). In those who survive, renal function usually begins to recover within 2–3 weeks. ARF is irreversible in a few patients, probably because of cortical necrosis which, unlike tubules, which regenerate, heals with the formation of scar tissue.

**Emergency Box 8.1**

## Principles of management of a patient with acute renal failure

### Emergency resuscitation
To prevent death from hyperkalaemia (p. 301) or pulmonary oedema (p. 396)

### Establish the aetiology and treat the underlying cause
- History, including family history, systemic disease, use of nephrotoxic drugs
- Examination includes assessment of haemodynamic status, pelvic and rectal examination
- Investigations, including bladder catheterization or flush of existing catheter

### Prevention of further renal damage
Early detection of infection and prompt treatment with antibiotics. Avoid hypovolaemia, nephrotoxic drugs, NSAIDs and ACE inhibitors

### Management of established renal failure
- Seek advice from a nephrologist
- Once fluid balance has been corrected the daily fluid intake should equal fluid lost on the previous day plus insensible losses (approximately 500 mL)
- Adequate nutrition – enteral route preferred over parenteral
- Nursing care, e.g. prevention of pressure sores
- Adjust doses of drugs that are excreted by the kidney and monitoring of serum drug levels where appropriate (refer to BNF for guidance)
- Monitor daily: urine volume, serum biochemistry, bodyweight
- Frequent review regarding the need for dialysis

### Careful fluid and electrolyte balance during recovery phase
The patient may pass large volumes of dilute urine until the kidney recovers its concentrating ability

NSAIDs, non-steroidal anti-inflammatory drugs; ACE, angiotensin-converting enzyme; BNF, *British National Formulary*

## Chronic renal failure (K&C p. 642)

### Aetiology

The causes of chronic renal failure (CRF) are listed in Table 8.14. In European countries diabetes mellitus is the single most common cause of end-stage renal failure.

**Table 8.14**
Causes of end-stage renal failure

**Congenital and hereditary disease**
Polycystic kidneys

**Glomerular disease**
Primary glomerular disease
Secondary glomerular disease, e.g. diabetes mellitus,
    amyloidosis, systemic lupus

**Tubulointerstitial disease**
Reflux nephropathy
Tuberculosis
Nephrocalcinosis
Interstitial nephritis, e.g. drugs, idiopathic

**Vascular disease**
Atherosclerotic renal artery stenosis
Hypertensive nephropathy
Vasculitis

**Urinary tract obstruction**

**Other**
HIV-associated nephropathy

Hypertensive nephropathy and glomerulonephritis are other common causes. Regardless of the underlying cause, fibrosis of the remaining tubules, glomeruli and small blood vessels results in progressive renal scarring and eventually end-stage renal failure.

### Clinical features and investigations
Clinical features are summarized in Table 8.15. Investigations are similar to those in ARF (p. 345).

In addition there may be symptoms and signs resulting from the long-term complications of CRF.

***Anaemia*** This is present in the great majority of patients with CRF. The pathogenesis is multifactorial:

- Decreased erythropoietin production by the diseased kidney
- Depressed bone marrow activity
- Shortened red cell survival
- Increased blood loss (from the gut, during haemodialysis and as a result of repeated sampling)
- Dietary deficiency of haematinics (iron and folate).

**Table 8.15**
Symptoms and signs of chronic renal failure

**Anaemia**
Pallor, lethargy, breathlessness on exercise

**Platelet abnormality**
Epistaxis, bruising

**Skin**
Pigmentation
Pruritus

**Gastrointestinal tract**
Anorexia, nausea, vomiting, diarrhoea

**Endocrine/gonads**
Amenorrhoea, erectile impotence, infertility

**Central nervous system**
Confusion, coma, fits (in severe uraemia)

**Cardiovascular system**
Uraemic pericarditis, hypertension, peripheral vascular disease, heart failure

**Renal**
Nocturia, polyuria, salt and water retention causing oedema

**Renal osteodystrophy**
Osteomalacia, muscle weakness, bone pain, hyperparathyroidism, osteosclerosis

**Bone disease** The term 'renal osteodystrophy' embraces the various forms of bone disease that develop in CRF, i.e. osteomalacia, osteoporosis, secondary and tertiary hyperparathyroidism, and osteosclerosis. Renal phosphate retention and impaired production of 1,25-dihydroxyvitamin D (the active hormonal form of vitamin D) lead to a fall in serum calcium concentration and hence to a compensatory increase in parathyroid hormone (PTH) secretion. A sustained excess of PTH results in skeletal decalcification with the classic radiological features described in Figure 8.5. Osteosclerosis (hardening of bone) may be a result of hyperparathyroidism. Alternate bands of sclerotic and porotic bone in the vertebra produce the characteristic 'rugger jersey spine' radiographic appearance.

**Neurological** A motor and sensory neuropathy may occur in uraemia. Most commonly the sensory neuropathy may manifest as peripheral paraesthesiae. Median nerve

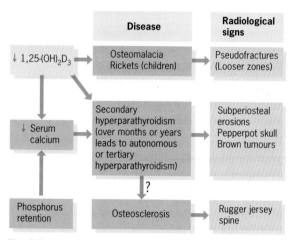

Fig. 8.5 **Pathogenesis and radiological features of renal osteodystrophy.**

compression in the carpal tunnel is common and is usually caused by $\beta_2$-microglobulin-related amyloidosis (see later). Autonomic dysfunction may present as postural hypotension and disturbed gastrointestinal motility. Dialysis produces an improvement in neuropathy.

**Cardiovascular disease** The highest mortality in CRF is from cardiovascular disease, which is increased as a result of the presence of hypertension, abnormalities of lipid metabolism and vascular calcification. Renal disease also results in a form of cardiomyopathy with both systolic and diastolic dysfunction.

**Other complications** include an increased risk of peptic ulceration, acute pancreatitis, hyperuricaemia, sexual dysfunction and, in children, failure to thrive.

### Differentiating ARF from CRF
Distinction between ARF and CRF depends on the history, duration of symptoms and previous urinalysis or measurement of renal function. A normochromic anaemia, small kidneys on ultrasonography and the presence of renal osteodystrophy (see below) favour a chronic process.

## Management

The underlying cause of renal disease should be treated aggressively wherever possible, e.g. tight metabolic control in diabetes.

**Dietary restrictions** Reduction of protein intake (0.8–1.0 g/kg/day) lessens the amount of nitrogenous waste products generated and this may delay the onset of symptomatic uraemia. Clinical trials have provided some evidence that a low-protein diet may benefit some patients with CRF, particularly patients with diabetes mellitus. Most patients will also require a diet restricted in sodium, potassium and phosphate.

**Good blood pressure control** may slow the decline in renal function. Of the antihypertensive agents, ACE inhibitors have particular protective effects on the glomeruli but must be used with caution in the presence of coexistent renal vascular disease.

**Calcium and phosphate** Hyperphosphataemia is treated by dietary restriction and oral calcium carbonate (a phosphate-binding agent). The serum calcium should be maintained in the normal range through the use of synthetic vitamin D analogues such as $1_\alpha$-colecalciferol or the vitamin D metabolite 1,25-dihydroxyvitamin $D_3$ (1,25-$(OH)_2D_3$).

**Anaemia** Recombinant human erythropoietin is a very effective but expensive treatment for the anaemia of CRF and has largely replaced repeated blood transfusions. It is administered subcutaneously or intravenously three times weekly. Failure to respond may be the result of haematinic deficiency, bleeding, malignancy or infection. The disadvantages of treatment are that erythropoietin may accelerate hypertension and, rarely, lead to encephalopathy with convulsions.

**Acidosis** Systemic acidosis accompanies the decline in renal function and may contribute to increased serum potassium levels as well as dyspnoea and lethargy. Treatment is with oral sodium bicarbonate; the increased

Renal replacement therapy

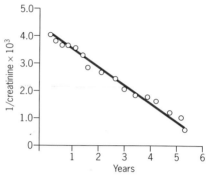

**Fig. 8.6 A reciprocal plot of serum creatinine against time.** Such a slope is particular to an individual patient. It may be used to predict the time of onset of end-stage renal failure and thus prepare the patient for dialysis, e.g. the formation of an arteriovenous fistula.

sodium load may exacerbate oedema and reduce blood pressure control.

**_Preparation_ for dialysis and transplantation** In most patients with CRF there is a progressive loss of renal function, which proceeds at a constant rate for that patient (Fig. 8.6). The graph of the reciprocal creatinine concentration plotted against time may be used to predict when the patient is likely to develop end-stage renal failure and thus require a form of renal replacement therapy. This may be haemodialysis, chronic ambulatory peritoneal dialysis or renal transplantation. Patients should be referred to a nephrologist by the time the serum creatinine reaches 350 mmol/L (250 mmol/L in diabetics), or earlier if the primary diagnosis is unknown.

## Renal replacement therapy (K&C p. 650)

### Dialysis

'Uraemic toxins' can be efficiently removed from the blood by the process of diffusion across a semipermeable membrane towards the low concentrations present in dialysis fluid (Fig. 8.7). The gradient is maintained by replacing

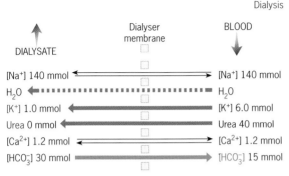

**Fig. 8.7 The principle of haemodialysis.**

used dialysis fluid with fresh solution. In haemodialysis, blood in an extracorporeal circulation is exposed to dialysis fluid separated by an artificial semipermeable membrane. In peritoneal dialysis the peritoneum is used as the semipermeable membrane and dialysis fluid is instilled into the peritoneal cavity.

## Haemodialysis

Adequate dialysis requires a blood flow of at least 200 mL/min and the most reliable way of achieving this is by surgical construction of an arteriovenous fistula, usually in the forearm. This provides a permanent and easily accessible site for the insertion of needles. An adult of average size usually requires 4–5 hours of haemodialysis three times a week, which may be performed in hospital; in the UK some patients have self-supervised home haemodialysis. All patients are anticoagulated during treatment (usually with heparin) because contact of blood with foreign surfaces activates the clotting cascade. The most common acute complication of haemodialysis is hypotension, caused in part by excessive removal of extracellular fluid.

## Haemofiltration

Haemofiltration involves the removal of plasma water and its dissolved constituents (e.g. $Na^+ K^+$, urea, phosphate) and replacing it with a solution of the desired biochemical composition. The procedure employs a highly permeable membrane, which allows large amounts of fluid and solute to be removed from the patient (Fig. 8.8). The procedure is costly

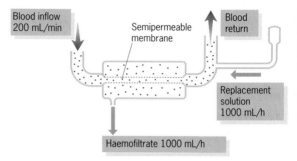

**Fig. 8.8 Principles of haemofiltration.**

and only a tiny minority of patients with end-stage renal failure are managed in this way. However, it is readily performed in intensive care units on very sick patients, as haemofiltration can be managed by ITU nursing staff rather than renal unit nurses.

### Peritoneal dialysis

- *Continuous ambulatory peritoneal dialysis* (CAPD) requires the insertion of a permanent catheter (Tenkoff catheter) into the peritoneal cavity via a subcutaneous tunnel. Up to 3 litres of dialysate are introduced and exchanged three to five times a day.
- *Intermittent peritoneal dialysis.* Dialysate is introduced into the peritoneal cavity via a catheter and exchanged every 60–120 minutes, requiring the patient to remain in bed during treatment. It is mainly used in ARF.

Peritonitis is the most common serious complication of peritoneal dialysis. Infection with *Staph. epidermidis* accounts for 50% of cases. Treatment is with appropriate antibiotics, which are often given intraperitoneally.

## Long-term complications of dialysis

(*K&C* p. 654)

Cardiovascular disease (as a result of atheroma) and sepsis are the leading causes of death in long-term dialysis patients. Causes of fatal sepsis include peritonitis complicating peritoneal dialysis and *Staph. aureus* infection (including endocarditis) complicating the use of indwelling access devices for haemodialysis. Amyloidosis is the result of the accumulation and polymerization of $\beta_2$-microglobulin. This molecule (a component of HLA proteins on most cell membranes) is normally excreted by the kidneys, but is not removed by dialysis membranes. Deposition results in the carpal tunnel syndrome and joint pains, particularly of the shoulders.

## Transplantation (K&C p. 656)

Successful renal transplantation offers the potential for complete rehabilitation in end-stage renal failure. It allows freedom from dietary and fluid restriction, anaemia and infertility are corrected and the need for parathyroidectomy reduced. In the best centres graft survival is 80% at 10 years. Kidneys are obtained from cadavers or, less frequently, from healthy close relatives. The donor must be ABO compatible and good HLA matching increases the chances of successful transplantation. The donor kidney is placed in the iliac fossa and anastomosed to the iliac vessels of the recipient; the donor ureter is placed into the recipient's bladder.

Long-term immunosuppressive treatment is employed in all cases (unless the donor is an identical twin, i.e. genetically identical) to reduce the incidence of graft rejection. This treatment comprises corticosteroids, azathioprine or mycophenolate mofetil and ciclosporin or tacrolimus. Antilymphocyte globulin is a potent immunosuppressive and is increasingly used in both the treatment and prevention of rejection. The complications of renal transplantation and immunosuppression include opportunistic infection (e.g. *Pneumocystis carinii*), hypertension, the development of tumours (skin malignancies and lymphomas) and, occasionally, recurrence of the renal disease (e.g. Goodpasture's syndrome).

## Cystic renal disease

### Solitary and multiple renal cysts

Renal cysts are common, particularly with advancing age. They are usually asymptomatic and discovered incidentally on ultrasonography or excretion urography performed for some other reason. Occasionally they may cause pain and/or haematuria.

# Adult polycystic disease (K&C p. 658)

Adult polycystic disease (APCD) is a common autosomal dominantly inherited condition in which multiple cysts develop throughout both kidneys. Cysts increase in size with advancing age and lead to renal enlargement and the progressive destruction of normal kidney tissue, with gradual loss of renal function. Most cases are due to a mutation in the *PKD1* gene (short arm of chromosome 16), which encodes for a protein, polycystin, an integral membrane protein thought to be involved in cell adhesion. The underlying mechanism by which cysts form remains unclear.

## Clinical features

The disease presents at any age after the second decade. Presenting symptoms include the following:

- Acute loin pain and/or haematuria as a result of haemorrhage into a cyst
- Abdominal discomfort caused by renal enlargement
- Development of hypertension or symptoms of uraemia.

About 30% of patients will develop hepatic cysts, which are usually clinically insignificant. More rarely cysts develop in the pancreas, spleen, ovary and other organs. Berry aneurysms of the cerebral vessels are found in 8% of patients; these may result in subarachnoid haemorrhage.

## Diagnosis

Clinical examination commonly reveals large irregular kidneys, hypertension and possibly hepatomegaly. A definitive diagnosis is established by ultrasonography.

## Management

Treatment involves careful control of blood pressure, and salt replacement if necessary. As the disease is always progressive, many patients will require renal replacement by dialysis and/or transplantation. Children and siblings of patients with the disease should be offered ultrasonographic screening. This is carried out in the second decade because diagnosis before this age is difficult and hypertension is rare in the very young.

## Medullary sponge kidney (K&C p. 660)

Medullary sponge kidney is an uncommon condition characterized by dilatation of the collecting ducts in the papillae with associated stasis of urine. In severe cases there are numerous cysts and the medullary area has a sponge-like appearance. In 20% of patients there is hypercalciuria or renal tubular acidosis (see p. 306). Most patients have intermittent colic, with the passage of small stones, or haematuria with well-preserved renal function. The diagnosis is made by excretion urography.

## Tumours of the kidney and genitourinary tract

### Renal cell carcinoma (K&C p. 661)

Renal cell carcinomas are the most common renal tumours in adults, presenting most commonly in the fifth decade, with a male:female ratio of 2:1. They arise from the proximal tubular epithelium and may be solitary, multiple and occasionally bilateral.

#### Clinical features

Haematuria, loin pain and a mass in the flank are the most common presenting features. Other features include malaise, weight loss, fever and occasionally polycythaemia (p. 194). Twenty-five per cent have metastases at presentation to bone, liver and the lung, where they are often solitary and large ('cannonball' metastases).

#### Investigations

- Excretion urography will reveal a space-occupying lesion in the kidney.
- Ultrasonography will demonstrate a solid lesion and can assess the patency of the renal vein and inferior vena cava.
- MRI and CT are useful for tumour staging.

#### Management

Surgery forms the mainstay of treatment. Nephrectomy is carried out unless there is bilateral involvement or the contralateral kidney functions poorly. Medroxyprogesterone may be of value in controlling metastatic disease. Treatment with interleukin-2 and alpha-interferon produces a remission in about 20% of cases.

### Prognosis

The 5-year survival rate is 60–70% when the tumour is confined to the renal parenchyma, but less than 5% in those with distant metastases.

## Urothelial tumours (K&C p. 662)

The calyces, renal pelvis, ureter, bladder and urethra are lined by transitional cell epithelium. Bladder tumours are the most common form of transitional cell malignancy. They occur most commonly after the age of 40 years and are four times more common in males. Predisposing factors for bladder cancer include:

- Cigarette smoking
- Industrial chemicals, e.g. β-naphthylamine, benzidine
- Drugs, e.g. phenacetin, cyclophosphamide
- Chronic inflammation, e.g. schistosomiasis.

### Clinical features

Painless haematuria is the most common symptom of bladder cancer, although pain sometimes occurs from clot retention. Transitional cell cancers of the kidney and ureters present with haematuria and flank pain.

### Investigations

- Cytology of the urine may show malignant cells.
- Excretion urography shows filling defects, but small tumours may not be seen.
- Cystoscopy if no evidence of upper urinary tract pathology has been found.

### Management

Pelvic and ureteric tumours are treated with surgical resection. Treatment of bladder tumours depends on the stage, but options include local diathermy or cystoscopic resection, bladder resection, radiotherapy, and local and systemic chemotherapy.

# Diseases of the prostate gland

## Benign enlargement of the prostate gland
(*K&C* p. 663)
Benign prostatic enlargement is extremely common, occurring most commonly after the age of 60 years. There is hyperplasia of both glandular and connective tissue elements of the gland, although the aetiology of the condition remains unknown.

### Clinical features
Frequency of micturition, nocturia, delay in initiation of micturition and post-void dribbling are common symptoms. Acute urinary retention or retention with overflow incontinence also occurs. An enlarged smooth prostate may be felt on rectal examination.

### Investigations
Serum electrolytes and renal ultrasonography are performed to exclude renal damage resulting from obstruction. Serum prostate-specific antigen (PSA) is markedly raised in patients with prostate cancer, which presents similarly (see below).

### Management
Patients with mild or moderate symptoms require no treatment or medical treatment only. Selective $\alpha_1$-adrenoceptor antagonists such as tamsulosin relax smooth muscle in the bladder neck and prostate. $5\alpha$-reductase inhibitors such as finasteride block the conversion of testosterone to dihydrotestosterone – the latter is thought to be responsible for the development of prostatic hypertrophy. $\alpha$-Blockers provide better symptom relief than finasteride. Patients with acute retention of urine or retention with overflow require urethral catheterization or if this is not possible, suprapubic catheter drainage. Patients with persistent severe symptoms or with dilatation of the upper urinary tract require surgery, most commonly with transurethral resection of the prostate (TURP).

Diseases of the prostate gland

# Prostatic carcinoma (K&C p. 506 & p. 664)

Prostatic adenocarcinoma is common, accounting for 7% of all cancers in men. Malignant change within the prostate is increasingly common with increasing age, being present in 80% of men aged 80 and over. In most cases these malignant foci remain dormant.

## Clinical features

In developed countries most patients now present as a result of screening for prostate cancer by measurement of prostate-specific antigen (PSA). Presentation is also with symptoms of bladder outflow obstruction identical to those of benign prostatic hypertrophy. Occasionally, presenting symptoms are due to metastases, particularly to bone. In some cases malignancy is unsuspected until histological investigation is carried out on the resected specimen after prostatectomy. Rectal examination may reveal a hard irregular gland.

## Investigation

Investigation is as for benign prostatic enlargement, with measurement of serum PSA. Supplemental tests include transrectal ultrasonography, which helps in tumour staging, and transrectal biopsy for histological confirmation.

## Management

Microscopic tumour is sometimes managed by watchful waiting. Treatment of disease confined to the gland is radical prostatectomy or radiotherapy, both resulting in 80–90% 5-year survival. The treatment of metastatic disease depends on removing androgenic drive to the tumour. This is achieved by bilateral orchidectomy, synthetic luteinizing hormone-releasing hormone analogues, e.g. goserelin, or antiandrogens, e.g. cyproterone acetate.

## Screening

The value or otherwise of screening for prostate cancer remains uncertain. Annual measurement of PSA in asymptomatic men does result in earlier diagnosis and large-scale trials are in progress to determine the potential benefits (i.e. increased survival) and drawbacks of screening (expense, side-effects of treatment, emotional impact of a positive result).

## Testicular tumours (K&C pp. 506 & 664)

Testicular cancer is the most common cancer in young men. More than 96% of testicular tumours arise from germ cells. There are two main types: seminomas and teratomas. The aetiology is unknown and the risk of malignant change is greater in undescended testes.

### Clinical features
Typically the man or his partner finds a painless lump in the testicle. Presentation may also be with metastases in the lungs causing cough and dyspnoea, or para-aortic lymph nodes causing back pain.

### Investigations
- Ultrasound scanning will help to differentiate between masses in the body of the testes and other intrascrotal swellings.
- Measurement of serum concentrations of tumour markers ($\alpha$-fetoprotein and human chorionic gonadotrophin) will help to make the diagnosis, to assess response to treatment and in following up patients.
- Tumour staging is assessed by chest X-ray and CT scanning of the chest, abdomen and pelvis.

### Treatment
Orchidectomy is performed to permit histological evaluation of the primary tumour and to provide local tumour control. Seminomas with metastases below the diaphragm only are treated by radiotherapy. More widespread tumours are treated with chemotherapy. Teratomas with metastases are also treated with chemotherapy. Sperm banking should be offered prior to therapy to men who wish to preserve fertility.

361

## Urinary incontinence

### Normal bladder physiology

As the bladder fills with urine, two factors act to ensure continence until it is next emptied:

- Intravesical pressure remains low as a result of stretching of the bladder wall and the stability of the bladder muscle (detrusor), which does not contract involuntarily.
- The sphincter mechanisms of the bladder neck and urethral muscles.

At the onset of voiding the sphincters relax (mediated by decreased sympathetic activity) and the detrusor muscle contracts (mediated by increased parasympathetic activity). Overall control and coordination of micturition is by higher brain centres, which include the cerebral cortex and the pons.

### Stress incontinence

Stress incontinence occurs as a result of sphincter weakness, which may be iatrogenic in men (post-prostatectomy) or the result of childbirth in women. There is a small leak of urine when intra-abdominal pressure rises, e.g. with coughing, laughing or standing up. In young women pelvic floor exercises may help. In postmenopausal women the contributing factor of urethral atrophy may be helped by oestrogen creams.

### Urge incontinence

In urge incontinence there is a strong desire to void and the patient may be unable to hold his or her urine. The usual cause is detrusor instability, which occurs most often in women, and the aetiology is not known. Mild cases may respond to bladder retraining (gradually increasing the time interval between voids). More severe cases are treated with anticholinergic agents, e.g. oxybutynin, which decrease detrusor excitability. Less commonly, urge incontinence is caused by bladder hypersensitivity from local pathology (e.g. UTI, bladder stones, tumours) and treatment is then of the underlying cause.

# Overflow incontinence

Overflow incontinence is most often seen in men with prostatic hypertrophy causing outflow obstruction. There is leakage of small amounts of urine, and on abdominal examination the distended bladder is felt rising out of the pelvis. If the obstruction is not relieved with urethral or suprapubic catheterization then renal damage will develop.

## Neurological causes (*K&C* p. 1153)

These are usually apparent from the history and examination, which reveal accompanying neurological deficits. Brainstem damage, e.g. trauma, may lead to incoordination of detrusor muscle activity and sphincter relaxation, so that the two contract together during voiding. This results in a high-pressure system with the risk of obstructive uropathy. The aim of treatment is to reduce outflow pressure, either with α-adrenergic blockers or by sphincterotomy. Autonomic neuropathy, e.g. in diabetic individuals, decreases detrusor excitability and results in a distended atonic bladder with a large residual urine which is liable to infection. Permanent catheterization may be necessary.

In elderly people incontinence may be the result of a combination of factors: diuretic treatment, dementia (antisocial incontinence) and difficulty in getting to the toilet because of immobility.

# 9

# Cardiovascular disease

## Common presenting symptoms of heart disease

The common symptoms of heart disease are chest pain, breathlessness, palpitations and syncope.

### Chest pain (K&C p. 707)

Acute chest pain or discomfort is a common presenting symptom of cardiovascular disease and must be differentiated from non-cardiac causes. The site of pain, its character, radiation and associated symptoms will often point to the cause (Table 9.1).

### Dyspnoea (K&C p. 706)

Dyspnoea is an awareness of the sensation of breathing. The causes are discussed on page 445. Left heart failure is the most common cardiac cause of exertional dyspnoea.

### Orthopnoea (K&C p. 707)

This is a form of breathlessness that occurs on lying flat as a result of gravitational redistribution of blood leading to increased pulmonary blood volume. Paroxysmal nocturnal dyspnoea occurs when there is an accumulation of fluid in the lungs at night causing the patient to awake suddenly from sleep.

### Palpitations (K&C p. 707)

A palpitation is an awareness of the heartbeat. The normal heartbeat is sensed when the patient is anxious, excited, exercising or lying on the left side. In other circumstances it usually indicates a cardiac arrhythmia, commonly ectopic beats or a paroxysmal tachycardia (p. 376).

**Table 9.1**
Common causes of chest pain

**Usually retrosternal**

| | |
|---|---|
| Angina pectoris | Crushing pain on exercise, relieved by rest. May radiate to jaw or arms |
| Myocardial infarction | Similar in character to angina but more severe, occurs at rest, lasts longer |
| Pericarditis | Sharp pain aggravated by movement, respiration and changes in posture |
| Aortic dissection | Severe tearing chest pain which radiates to the back |
| Reflux oesophagitis | Pain may occur at night and when bending or lying down. Pain may radiate into the neck |

**Other sites: usually lateral**

| | |
|---|---|
| Pulmonary infarct | |
| Pneumonia | } Typically pleuritic in nature, i.e. sharp, well-localized pain aggravated by inspiration, coughing and movement |
| Pneumothorax | |
| Costochondritis | } Musculoskeletal pain is usually a sharp, well-localized pain with a tender area on palpation |
| Fractured rib | |

## Syncope and dizziness (K&C p. 708)

Syncope means a temporary impairment of consciousness as a result of cerebral ischaemia. There are many causes, but the most common is a simple faint (p. 637). The cardiac causes of syncope are the result of either very fast (e.g. ventricular tachycardia) or very slow heart rates (e.g. complete heart block) which are unable to maintain an adequate cardiac output. Attacks occur suddenly and without warning. They last only 1 or 2 minutes, with complete recovery in seconds (compare with epilepsy, where complete recovery may be delayed for some hours). Obstruction to ventricular outflow also causes syncope (e.g. aortic stenosis, hypertrophic cardiomyopathy), which typically occurs on exercise when the requirements for increased cardiac output cannot be met.

## Other symptoms

Tiredness, lethargy and exertional fatigue occur with cardiac failure and result from poor perfusion of brain and skeletal muscle. Heart failure also causes salt and water retention, leading to oedema, which in ambulant patients is most prominent over the ankles. In severe cases it may involve the genitalia and thighs.

## The electrocardiogram (K&C p. 719)

367

The electrocardiogram (ECG) is a recording from the body surface of the electrical activity of the heart. The standard ECG has 12 leads:

- Chest leads, $V_1$–$V_6$, look at the heart in a *horizontal plane* (Fig. 9.1)
- Limb leads, look at the heart in a *vertical plane* (Fig. 9.2). Limb leads are unipolar (AVR, AVL and AVF) or bipolar (I, II, III).

The ECG machine is arranged so that when a depolarization wave spreads towards a lead the needle moves upwards on the trace, and when it spreads away from the lead the needle moves downwards.

**(a)**

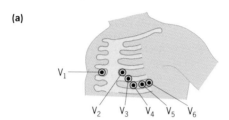

**(b)**

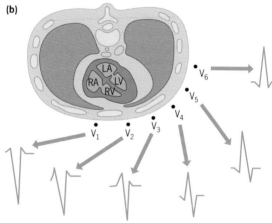

**Fig. 9.1 ECG chest leads. (a)** The V leads are attached to the chest wall overlying the intercostal spaces as shown: $V_4$ in the mid-clavicular line, $V_5$ in the anterior axillary line, $V_6$ in the mid-axillary line. **(b)** Leads $V_1$ and $V_2$ look at the right ventricle, $V_3$ and $V_4$ at the interventricular septum, and $V_5$ and $V_6$ at the left ventricle. The normal QRS complex in each lead is shown. The R wave in the chest (precordial) leads steadily increases in amplitude from lead $V_1$ to $V_6$ with a corresponding decrease in S wave depth, culminating in a predominantly positive complex in $V_6$.

## ECG waveform and definitions (Fig. 9.3)

The *heart rate*. At normal paper speed (usually 25 mm/s) each 'big square' measures 5 mm wide and is equivalent to 0.2 s. The heart rate (if the rhythm is regular) is calculated by counting the number of big squares between two consecutive R waves and dividing into 300.

The *P wave* is the first deflection and is caused by atrial depolarization. When abnormal it may be:

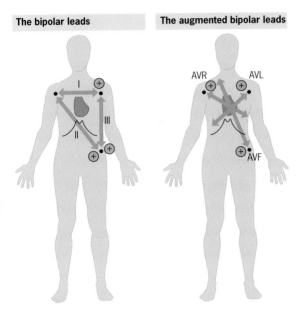

**The bipolar leads**

**The augmented bipolar leads**

**Fig. 9.2 ECG limb leads.** Lead I is derived from electrodes on the right arm (negative pole) and left arm (positive pole), lead II is derived from electrodes on the right arm (negative pole) and left leg (positive pole), and lead III from electrodes on the left arm (negative pole) and the left leg (positive pole).

**369**

- Broad and notched (> 0.12 s, i.e. 3 small squares) in left atrial enlargement ('P mitrale', e.g. mitral stenosis)
- Tall and peaked (> 2.5 mm) in right atrial enlargement ('P pulmonale', e.g. pulmonary hypertension)
- Replaced by flutter or fibrillation waves (p. 378)
- Absent in sinoatrial block (p. 374).

The *QRS complex* represents ventricular depolarization:

- A negative (downward) deflection preceding an R wave is called a Q wave. Normal Q waves are small and narrow; deep (> 2 mm), wide (> 1 mm) Q waves (except in AVR and $V_1$) indicate myocardial infarction (p. 403).
- A deflection upwards is called an R wave whether or not it is preceded by a Q wave.

The electrocardiogram

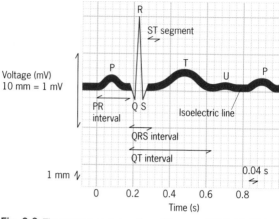

**Fig. 9.3 The waves and elaboration of the normal ECG.** (Modified from Goldman (1976) Principles of Clinical Electrocardiography, 9th edn. McGraw-Hill Companies.)

- A negative deflection following an R wave is termed an S wave.

Ventricular depolarization starts in the septum and spreads from left to right (Fig. 9.4). Subsequently the main free walls of the ventricles are depolarized. Thus, in the right ventricular leads ($V_1$ and $V_2$) the first deflection is upwards (R wave) as the septal depolarization wave spreads towards those leads. The second deflection is downwards (S wave) as the bigger left ventricle (in which depolarization is spreading away) outweighs the effect of the right ventricle (see Fig. 9.1). The opposite pattern is seen in the left ventricular leads ($V_5$ and $V_6$), with an initial downwards deflection (small Q wave reflecting septal depolarization) followed by a large R wave caused by left ventricular depolarization.

*Left ventricular hypertrophy.* The increased bulk of the left ventricular myocardium in left ventricular hypertrophy (e.g. with systemic hypertension) increases the voltage-induced depolarization of the free wall of the left ventricle. This gives rise to tall R waves (> 25 mm) in the left ventricular leads ($V_5$, $V_6$) and/or deep S waves (> 30 mm) in the right ventricular leads ($V_1$, $V_2$). The sum of the R wave in

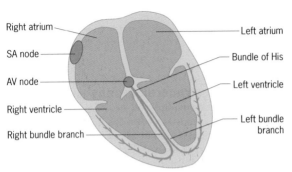

**Fig. 9.4 The normal cardiac conduction system.** In normal circumstances only the specialized conducting tissues of the heart undergo spontaneous depolarization (automaticity) which initiates an action potential. The sinus (SA) node discharges more rapidly than the other cells and is the normal pacemaker of the heart. The impulse generated by the sinus node spreads first through the atria, producing atrial systole, and then through the atrioventricular (AV) node to the His–Purkinje system, producing ventricular systole.

the left ventricular leads and the S wave in the right ventricular leads exceeds 40 mm. In addition to these changes there may also be ST-segment depression and T wave flattening or inversion in the left ventricular leads.

*Right ventricular hypertrophy* (e.g. in pulmonary hypertension) causes tall R waves in the right ventricular leads.

The QRS duration reflects the time that excitation takes to spread through the ventricle. A wide QRS complex (> 0.10 s, 2.5 small squares) occurs if conduction is delayed, e.g. with right or left bundle branch block, or if conduction is through abnormal pathways, e.g. ventricular ectopic.

*T waves* result from ventricular repolarization. In general the direction of the T wave is the same as that of the QRS complex. Inverted T waves occur in many conditions and, although usually abnormal, they are a non-specific finding.

The *PR interval* is measured from the start of the P wave to the start of the QRS complex whether this is a Q wave or an R wave. It is the time taken for excitation to pass from the sinus node, through the atrium, atrioventricular node and His–Purkinje system to the ventricle. A prolonged PR interval (> 0.22 s) indicates heart block (p. 374).

The *ST segment* is the period between the end of the QRS complex and the start of the T wave. ST elevation (> 1 mm above the isoelectric line) occurs in the early stages of myocardial infarction (p. 403) and with acute pericarditis. ST segment depression (> 0.5 mm below the isoelectric line) indicates myocardial ischaemia.

# Exercise electrocardiography (K&C p. 721)

Exercise eletrocardiography is an ECG recording made during standard graded exercise treadmill testing (e.g. the Bruce protocol) and is used in the investigation of patients with known or suspected ischaemic heart disease. Contraindications include recent myocardial infarction (within 6 days), unstable angina, severe hypertrophic cardiomyopathy, severe aortic stenosis and malignant hypertension. A positive test and indications for stopping the test are:

- Chest pain
- ST segment depression > 1 mm
- ST segment elevation > 1 mm
- Fall in systolic blood pressure > 20 mmHg, a sustained fall in blood pressure usually indicates severe coronary artery disease
- Fall in heart rate despite an increase in workload
- BP > 240/110
- Significant arrhythmias or increased frequency of ventricular ectopics.

# Cardiac arrhythmias (K&C p. 734)

An abnormality of the cardiac rhythm is called a cardiac arrhythmia. Such a disturbance may cause sudden death, syncope, dizziness, palpitations or no symptoms at all. Paroxysmal arrhythmias may not be detected on a single ECG recording. Twenty-four-hour ambulatory ECG monitoring (continuous recording for 24 hours) and event recorders (a portable device activated by the patient to record the ECG when symptoms occur) are outpatient investigations often used to detect arrhythmias causing intermittent symptoms.

There are two main types of arrhythmia:

- *Bradycardia*, where the heart rate is slow (< 60 beats/min). The slower the heart rate the more probable that the arrhythmia will be symptomatic.
- *Tachycardia*, where the heart rate is fast (> 100 beats/min). Tachycardias are more likely to be symptomatic when the arrhythmia is fast and sustained. They are subdivided into *supraventricular tachycardias*, which arise from the atrium or the atrioventricular junction, and *ventricular tachycardias*, which arise from the ventricles.

Arrhythmias and conduction disturbances complicating acute myocardial infarction are discussed on page 408.

## Sinus rhythms *(K&C p. 735)*

### Sinus arrhythmia
Fluctuations of autonomic tone result in phasic changes in the sinus discharge rate. Thus, during inspiration parasympathetic tone falls and the heart rate quickens, and on expiration the heart rate falls. This variation is normal, particularly in children and young adults.

### Sinus bradycardia
Sinus bradycardia is normal during sleep and in well-trained athletes. During the acute phase of a myocardial infarction it often reflects ischaemia of the sinus node. Other causes include hypothermia, hypothyroidism, cholestatic jaundice, raised intracranial pressure, and drug therapy with β-blockers, digitalis and other antiarrhythmic drugs. Patients with persistent symptomatic bradycardia are treated with a permanent cardiac pacemaker. Intravenous atropine is used in the acute situation.

### Sinus tachycardia
Sinus tachycardia is a physiological response during exercise and excitement. It may also occur with fever, anaemia, cardiac failure, thyrotoxicosis and drugs (e.g. catecholamines and atropine). Treatment is aimed at correction of the underlying cause. If necessary, β-blockers may be used to slow the sinus rate, but not in uncontrolled heart failure.

# Pathological bradycardias (K&C p. 736)

There are two main forms of severe bradycardia: sinus node dysfunction and atrioventricular block.

## Sinus node dysfunction (sick sinus syndrome)

Most cases of chronic sinus node dysfunction are the result of idiopathic fibrosis occurring in elderly people. Bradycardia is caused by intermittent failure of sinus node depolarization (sinus arrest) or failure of the sinus impulse to propagate through the perinodal tissue to the atria (sinoatrial block). This is seen on the ECG as intermittent long pauses between consecutive P waves (> 2 s). The slow heart rate predisposes to ectopic pacemaker activity and tachyarrhythmias are common (tachy–brady syndrome).

Insertion of a permanent pacemaker is only indicated in symptomatic patients to prevent dizzy spells and blackouts. Antiarrhythmic drugs are used to treat tachycardias. Thromboembolism is common in sinus node dysfunction and patients should be anticoagulated unless there is a contraindication.

## Atrioventricular block

There are three forms: first-degree heart block, second-degree (partial) block and third-degree (complete) block. The common causes are coronary artery disease, cardiomyopathy and, particularly in elderly people, fibrosis of the conducting tissue.

- *First-degree atrioventricular (AV) block* is the result of delayed atrioventricular conduction and reflected by a prolonged PR interval (> 0.22 s) on the ECG. No change in heart rate occurs and treatment is unnecessary.
- *Second-degree (partial) AV block* occurs when some atrial impulses fail to reach the ventricles. There are three forms (Fig. 9.5):
  - Mobitz type 1 block (Wenckebach's phenomenon), in which the PR interval gradually increases, culminating in a dropped beat, i.e. absent QRS after the P wave. The PR interval then returns to normal and the cycle repeats itself.

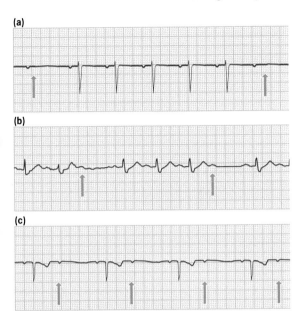

**Fig. 9.5 Three varieties of second-degree atrioventricular (AV) block. (a)** Wenckebach (Mobitz type I) AV block. The PR interval gradually prolongs until the P wave does not conduct to the ventricles (arrows). **(b)** Mobitz type II AV block. The P waves that do not conduct to the ventricles (arrows) are not preceded by gradual PR interval prolongation. **(c)** Two P waves to each QRS complex. The PR interval prior to the dropped P wave is always the same. It is not possible to define this type of AV block as type I or type II Mobitz block and it is, therefore, a third variety of second-degree AV block (arrows show P waves), not conducted to the ventricles.

- Mobitz type II block occurs when a dropped QRS complex is not preceded by progressive PR prolongation.
- A 2:1 or 3:1 block occurs when only every second or third P wave conducts to the ventricles. A 4:1 or 5:1 block can also occur.

Progression to complete heart block occurs more frequently following anterior myocardial infarction and in Mobitz type II block, and treatment with pacing is usually indicated. Patients with Wenckebach AV block or those with second-degree block following inferior infarction are usually monitored.

- *Third-degree AV block (complete heart block).* There is no association between atrial and ventricular activity and ventricular contractions are maintained by a spontaneous escape rhythm (usually about 40/min) from an automatic centre below the site of the block. The ECG shows regular P waves and QRS complexes which occur independently of one another. The usual symptoms are dizziness and blackouts (Stokes–Adams attacks). If the ventricular rate is very slow, cardiac failure may occur. Insertion of a permanent pacemaker is always required for sustained complete heart block. In the acute situation, e.g. myocardial infarction, recovery may be expected and intravenous atropine or a temporary pacemaker may be all that is necessary.

### Intraventricular conduction disturbances

The intraventricular conduction system consists of the His bundle, the right and left bundle branches and the antero-superior and posteroinferior divisions of the left bundle branch block (Fig. 9.4). Complete block of a bundle branch is associated with a wider QRS complex (0.12 s or more). The shape of the QRS depends on whether the right or the left bundle is blocked.

## Pathological tachycardias

### *Mechanisms of arrhythmia production*

The mechanisms responsible for most tachyarrhythmias are abnormal automaticity and re-entry mechanisms.

### Abnormal automaticity

Arrhythmias arise if there is enhanced automaticity of the normal conducting tissue or automaticity is acquired by damaged cells of the atria or ventricles; this causes ectopic beats and, if sustained, tachyarrhythmias.

**Re-entry** Re-entry may occur if there are two separate pathways for impulse conduction (Fig. 9.6).

### Atrial tachyarrhythmias (K&C p. 743)

Ectopic beats, tachycardia, flutter and fibrillation may all

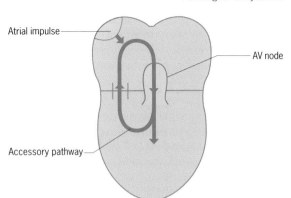

**Fig. 9.6 A re-entry circuit.** The impulse is conducted normally through the AV node and initiates ventricular depolarization. In certain circumstances the accessory pathway is able to transmit the impulse retrogradely back into the atria, thus completing a circuit and initiating a self-sustaining re-entry tachycardia.

arise from the atrial myocardium. They share common aetiologies, which are listed in Table 9.2.

### Atrial ectopic beats (K&C p. 746)

These are caused by premature discharge of an ectopic atrial focus. On the ECG this produces an early and abnormal P wave, usually followed by a normal QRS complex. Treatment is not usually required unless they

---

**Table 9.2**
Causes of atrial arrhythmias

Ischaemic heart disease
Rheumatic heart disease
Thyrotoxicosis
Cardiomyopathy
Lone atrial fibrillation (i.e. no cause discovered)
Wolff–Parkinson–White syndrome
Pneumonia
Atrial septal defect
Carcinoma of the bronchus
Pericarditis
Pulmonary embolus
Acute and chronic alcohol abuse
Cardiac surgery

cause troublesome palpitations or are responsible for provoking more significant arrhythmias when β-blockade may be effective.

### Atrial flutter (*K&C p. 745*)

Atrial flutter is almost always associated with organic disease of the heart. The atrial rate is usually about 300 beats/min. The AV node usually conducts every second flutter beat, giving a ventricular rate of 150 beats/min. The ECG (Fig. 9.7a) characteristically shows 'sawtooth' flutter waves (F waves), which are most clearly seen when AV conduction is transiently impaired by carotid sinus massage or drugs. Treatment of an acute paroxysm is electrical cardioversion (p. 741). Prophylaxis is achieved with class Ia, Ic or III drugs (Table 9.3). Rate control of a chronic arrhythmia is with AV nodal blocking drugs, e.g. digoxin. Recurrent atrial flutter is best treated with radiofrequency catheter ablation of focal arrhythmogenic sites.

**(a)**

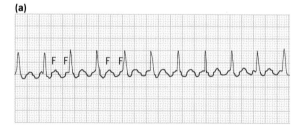

**(b)**

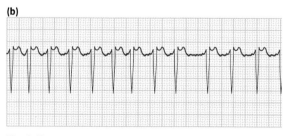

**Fig. 9.7 (a) Atrial flutter.** The flutter waves are marked with an F, only half of which are transmitted to the ventricles. **(b) Atrial fibrillation.** There are no P waves; the ventricular response is fast and irregular.

**Table 9.3**
Vaughan Williams' classification of antiarrhythmic drug therapy

| Class | Mechanism of action | Individual drugs |
|---|---|---|
| 1a | | Quinine, procainamide, disopyramide |
| 1b | Membrane stabilizing action | Lidocaine (lignocaine), mexiletine |
| 1c | | Flecainide, propafenone |
| II | β-Adrenergic blockers | Metoprolol, atenolol, propranolol |
| III | Increases refractory period of conducting system | Amiodarone, sotalol, bretylium |
| IV | Calcium-channel blocking agents | Verapamil, diltiazem |

Adenosine and digoxin are other antiarrhythmic drugs which do not fit into this classification

These drugs all have proarrhythmic side-effects (among others) and should be used with caution

All except amiodarone are negatively inotropic and may exacerbate heart failure

## Atrial fibrillation (AF) (K&C p. 743)

This is a common arrhythmia, occurring in 5–10% of patients over 65 years of age. It also occurs, particularly in a paroxysmal form, in younger patients. Atrial activity is chaotic and mechanically ineffective. The AV node conducts a proportion of the atrial impulses to produce an irregular ventricular response. Symptoms range from palpitations and fatigue to acute pulmonary oedema. There are no clear P waves on the ECG (Fig. 9.7b), only a fine oscillation of the baseline (so-called fibrillation or f waves).

When AF arises in an apparently normal heart it is sometimes possible to convert to sinus rhythm, either electrically (by cardioversion, p. 741) or chemically (with class Ia, Ic or III drugs – Table 9.3). When AF is caused by an acute precipitating event, such as alcohol toxicity, chest infection or thyrotoxicosis, the underlying cause should be treated initially.

Strategies for the long-term management of atrial fibrillation include:

- Maintenance of sinus rhythm with anti-arrhythmic drugs after DC cardioversion
- Rate control and consideration of anticoagulation (e.g. digoxin and warfarin).

Atrial fibrillation is associated with an increased risk of thromboembolism, and anticoagulation with warfarin should be given for at least 3 weeks before (with the exception of those who require emergency cardioversion) and 4 weeks after cardioversion. Most patients with chronic AF should also be anticoagulated (INR 2.0–3.0). The exception is young patients (< 65 years) with lone AF, i.e. in the absence of demonstrable cardiac disease, diabetes or hypertension. This group has a low incidence of thromboembolism and is treated with aspirin alone.

## Junctional tachycardia (K&C p. 742)

Junctional tachycardias are paroxysmal in nature and usually occur in the absence of structural heart disease. They are re-entrant arrhythmias caused by an abnormal pathway in the AV node or by an accessory pathway (bundle of Kent), as in the Wolff–Parkinson–White syndrome (Fig. 9.8). The usual history is of a sudden onset of fast (140–280/min) regular palpitations. On the ECG the P waves may be seen very close to the QRS complex, or are not seen at all. The QRS complex is usually of normal shape because, as with other supraventricular arrhythmias, the ventricles are activated in the normal way, down the bundle of His. Occasionally the QRS complex is wide, because of a rate-related bundle branch block, and it may be difficult to distinguish from ventricular tachycardia.

### Termination of an attack

- Manoeuvres that increase vagal stimulation of the sinus node: carotid sinus massage, ocular pressure or the Valsalva manoeuvre.
- Drug treatment: Adenosine is a very short-acting AV nodal blocking drug given as a 3 mg bolus dose intravenously. It will terminate most junctional tachycardias. If there is no response after 1–2 minutes a further bolus of 6 mg is given. A third bolus of 12 mg may be given if there is still no response. Transient side-effects include complete heart block, hypotension, nausea and bronchospasm. Asthma and second- or third-degree AV block are contraindications to adenosine.

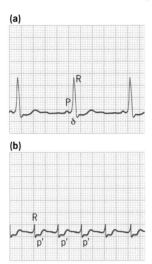

**Fig. 9.8 (a) An ECG showing Wolff–Parkinson–White syndrome.**
There is an abnormal connection, termed an accessory pathway, between
the atria and ventricles. The accessory pathway has a more rapid rate of
conduction from the atria to the ventricles than does the normal AV node
and ventricular depolarization occurs sooner than expected. Such pre-
excitation is apparent on the ECG during sinus rhythm as a short PR
interval and wide QRS complex with a 'slurred' upstroke (δ wave).
**(b) A trace demonstrating the paroxysmal tachycardia which may
result from this syndrome.** Note the tachycardia p wave visible between
QRS and T wave complexes.

381

An alternative treatment is intravenous verapamil
10 mg i.v. over 5–10 minutes (contraindicated if the
QRS complex is wide and therefore differentiation
from ventricular tachycardia difficult).
- Rapid atrial pacing or DC cardioversion is used if
  adenosine fails.

### Prophylaxis
- Radiofrequency ablation of the accessory pathway via
  a cardiac catheter
- Flecainide, disopyramide, amiodarone and β-blockers
  are the drugs most commonly used.

# Ventricular arrhythmias (K&C p. 746)

## Ventricular ectopic beats (extrasystoles, premature beats) (K&C p. 748)

Ventricular ectopic beats may be asymptomatic or patients may complain of extra beats, missed beats or heavy beats. The ectopic electrical activity is not conducted to the ventricles through the normal conducting tissue and thus the QRS complex on the ECG is widened, with a bizarre configuration (Fig. 9.9). In normal individuals ectopic beats are of no significance, but treatment is sometimes given for symptoms. In patients with heart disease they are associated with an increased risk of sudden death. Prophylaxis with amiodarone may reduce mortality by preventing arrhythmias and sudden death.

## Ventricular tachycardia (K&C p. 746)

Ventricular tachycardia and ventricular fibrillation are usually associated with underlying heart disease, e.g. ischaemia, cardiomyopathy and hypertensive heart disease. Ventricular tachycardia is defined as three or more consecutive ventricular beats occurring at a rate of 120/min or more. The ECG shows a rapid ventricular rhythm with broad abnormal QRS complexes which can sometimes be confused with a broad complex junctional tachycardia. Ventricular tachycardia may produce severe hypotension, when urgent DC cardioversion is necessary. If there is no haemodynamic compromise, treatment is usually with intravenous lidocaine (lignocaine) (50–100 mg i.v. over 5 min followed by an intravenous infusion of 2–4 mg/min).

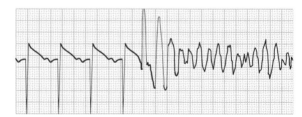

**Fig. 9.9 A rhythm strip demonstrating four beats of sinus rhythm followed by a ventricular ectopic beat that initiates ventricular fibrillation.** The ST segment is elevated owing to acute myocardial infarction.

Prophylaxis is with mexiletine, disopyramide, flecainide or amiodarone. Patients who are refractory to all medical treatment may need an implantable defibrillator. This is a small device implanted behind the rectus abdominis and connected to the heart; it recognizes ventricular tachycardia or ventricular fibrillation and automatically delivers a defibrillation shock to the heart.

## Ventricular fibrillation (K&C p. 746)

This is a very rapid and irregular ventricular activation (see Fig. 9.9) with no mechanical effect and hence no cardiac output. Ventricular fibrillation rarely reverts spontaneously and management is immediate cardioversion (Emergency Box 9.1).

## Torsades de pointes (K&C p. 747)

This uncommon arrhythmia is characterized by rapid irregular sharp QRS complexes that continuously change from an upright to an inverted position on the ECG. It arises when ventricular repolarization (QT interval) is greatly prolonged – the so-called long QT syndrome. Torsades de pointes causes palpitations and syncope and usually terminates spontaneously. It can, however, degenerate to ventricular fibrillation and cause sudden death. Causes include electrolyte abnormalities (hypokalaemia, hypomagnesaemia), drugs (quinidine, sotalol and chlorpromazine) and congenital syndromes.

383

## Cardiac arrest (K&C p. 730)

In cardiac arrest there is no effective cardiac output. The patient is unconscious and apnoeic with absent arterial pulses (best felt in the carotid artery in the neck). Irreversible brain damage occurs within 3 minutes if an adequate circulation is not established. Management of a cardiac arrest is described below (Emergency Box 9.1).

***Prognosis of cardiac arrest*** In many patients resuscitation is unsuccessful, particularly in those who collapse out of hospital and are brought into hospital in an arrested state. In patients who are successfully resuscitated the prognosis is often poor because they have severe underlying heart disease. The exception is those who are successfully resuscitated from a ventricular fibrillation arrest in the early stages of myocardial infarction, when the prognosis is much the same as for other patients with an infarct.

### Emergency Box 9.1

#### Basic life support
Call for help
Thump the chest firmly over the sternum; occasionally reverts VT/VF to sinus rhythm

**AIRWAY**

- Place patient on his or her back on a firm surface
- Remove obstructing material, e.g. blood and vomit
- Open the airway by flexing the neck and extending the head

**BREATHING**

- Give four breaths in quick succession of mouth-to-mouth resuscitation. Watch for the rise and fall of the patient's chest, indicating adequate ventilation

**CIRCULATION**

- Circulation is achieved by external chest compression
- The heel of one hand is placed over the lower half of the victim's sternum and the heel of the second hand is placed over the first with the fingers interlocked. With straight arms the sternum is depressed by 1–2 inches

Compressions : respiration in a ratio of 15 : 2 with 100 compressions per minute

#### Advanced life support

- Institute as soon as help arrives; continue cardiac massage throughout except during defibrillation
- Defibrillate immediately (ventricular fibrillation is the most common arrhythmia in cardiac arrest)
- Give 100% $O_2$ via Ambu-bag, intubate as soon as possible and initiate positive-pressure ventilation
- Establish intravenous access and connect ECG leads
- Drugs administered by the peripheral route should be followed by a flush of 20 mL of 0.9% saline
- If intravenous access not possible give drugs via endotracheal tube (3 × intravenous dose) diluted to 10 mL with 0.9% saline

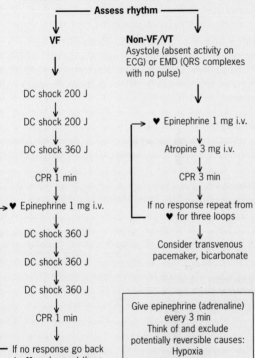

**Management of arrhythmias causing cardiac arrest**

─── **Assess rhythm** ───

**VF**

**Non-VF/VT**
Asystole (absent activity on
ECG) or EMD (QRS complexes
with no pulse)

DC shock 200 J

DC shock 200 J

DC shock 360 J

CPR 1 min

♥ Epinephrine 1 mg i.v.

DC shock 360 J

DC shock 360 J

DC shock 360 J

CPR 1 min

If no response go back
to ♥ and repeat three
loops. If no response
consider amiodarone **or**
lidocaine (lignocaine) **or**
procainamide

♥ Epinephrine 1 mg i.v.

Atropine 3 mg i.v.

CPR 3 min

If no response repeat from
♥ for three loops

Consider transvenous
pacemaker, bicarbonate

Give epinephrine (adrenaline)
every 3 min
Think of and exclude
potentially reversible causes:
Hypoxia
Hypovolaemia
Hypothermia
Hyper- or hypokalaemia
Tension pneumothorax
Tamponade (cardiac)
Toxicity (drug overdose)
Thromboembolic (PE)

EMD, electromechanical dissociation; VF, ventricular
fibrillation; VT ventricular tachycardia; PE, pulmonary embolus
http://www.resus.org.uk/pages/als.htm

385

# Cardiac failure (*K&C p. 754*)

Cardiac failure occurs when, in spite of normal venous pressures, the heart is unable to maintain sufficient cardiac output to meet the demands of the body. It is a common condition, with an estimated annual incidence of 10% in patients over 65 years. The long-term outcome is poor and approximately 50% of patients are dead within 5 years.

## *Aetiology*

The causes of heart failure are given in Table 9.4. Coronary artery disease is the commonest cause in western countries.

**Table 9.4**
Causes of heart failure: the predominant clinical picture is indicated

| | Left heart failure | Right heart failure | Biventricular heart failure |
|---|---|---|---|
| **Myocardial dysfunction** | | | |
| Ischaemic heart disease | X | | |
| Systemic hypertension | X | | |
| Dilated cardiomyopathy | | | X |
| **Volume overload** | | | |
| Ventricular septal defect | X | | |
| Mitral regurgitation | X | | |
| Aortic regurgitation | X | | |
| Pulmonary regurgitation | | X | |
| Tricuspid regurgitation | | X | |
| **Outflow obstruction** | | | |
| Aortic stenosis | X | | |
| Pulmonary hypertension | | X | |
| Pulmonary embolism | | X | |
| Pulmonary stenosis | | X | |
| **Compromised ventricular filling** | | | |
| Constrictive pericarditis | | X | |
| Pericardial tamponade | | X | |
| Restrictive cardiomyopathy | | | X |
| **Arrhythmia** | | | |
| Severe bradycardia | | | X |
| Severe tachycardia | | | X |

- *Low-output failure* develops when the heart is unable to generate adequate output.
- *High-output failure* is uncommon and occurs when the heart is unable to meet the perfusion requirements of tissue metabolism, in spite of an increased cardiac output. Causes include anaemia, systemic to pulmonary shunts, thyrotoxicosis, Paget's disease and beri-beri (p. 714).

## Pathophysiology

When the heart fails, compensatory mechanisms attempt to maintain cardiac output and peripheral perfusion. However, as heart failure progresses the mechanisms are overwhelmed and become pathophysiological. These mechanisms involve:

**Sympathetic nervous system** Activation of the sympathetic nervous system improves ventricular function by increasing heart rate and myocardial contractility. Constriction of venous capacitance vessels redistributes flow centrally and the increased venous return to the heart (preload) further augments ventricular function via the Starling mechanism (Fig. 9.10). Sympathetic stimulation, however, also leads to arteriolar constriction, this increasing

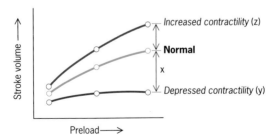

**Fig. 9.10 The Starling curve.** Starling's law states that the stroke volume is directly proportional to the diastolic filling (i.e. the preload or ventricular end-diastolic pressure). As the preload is increased, the stroke volume rises (normal). Increasing contractility (e.g. increased with sympathetic stimulation) shifts the curve upwards and to the left (z). If the ventricle is overstretched the stroke volume will fall (x). In heart failure (y) the ventricular function curve is relatively flat so that increasing the preload has only a small effect on cardiac output.

the afterload which would eventually reduce cardiac output.

***Renin–angiotensin system*** The fall in cardiac output and increased sympathetic tone lead to diminished renal perfusion, activation of the renin–angiotensin system, and hence increased fluid retention. Salt and water retention further increases venous pressure and maintains stroke volume by the Starling mechanism (Fig. 9.10). As salt and water retention increases, however, peripheral and pulmonary congestion cause oedema and contribute to dyspnoea. Angiotensin II also causes arteriolar constriction, thus increasing the afterload and the work of the heart.

***Atrial natriuretic peptides (ANPs)*** Distension of the atria leads to release of these peptides, which have vasodilator and natriuretic properties. The effect of their action may represent a beneficial, albeit inadequate, compensatory response leading to reduced cardiac load (preload and afterload).

***Ventricular dilatation*** Myocardial failure leads to a reduction of the volume of blood ejected with each heartbeat, and thus an increase in the volume of blood remaining after systole. The increased diastolic volume stretches the myocardial fibres and, as Starling's law would suggest, myocardial contraction is restored. Once cardiac failure is established, however, the compensatory effects of cardiac dilatation become limited by the flattened contour of Starling's curve. Eventually the increased venous pressure contributes to the development of pulmonary and peripheral oedema. In addition, as ventricular diameter increases, greater tension is required in the myocardium to expel a given volume of blood, and oxygen requirements increase.

## Clinical features

It is clinically useful to divide heart failure into the syndromes of right, left and biventricular (congestive) cardiac failure (see Table 9.4), but it is rare for any one part of the heart to fail in isolation.

***Left heart failure*** The most common cause of left heart failure is coronary artery disease. Other causes are listed in Table 9.4. The clinical features are largely the result of pulmonary congestion, with symptoms of fatigue, exertional dyspnoea, orthopnoea and paroxysmal nocturnal dyspnoea (p. 365). Physical signs include tachypnoea, tachycardia, a displaced apex beat and basal lung crackles. A third heart sound occurs and is the result of rapid filling of the ventricles. In severe failure, dilatation of the mitral annulus results in functional mitral regurgitation.

***Right heart failure*** The most frequent cause of chronic right heart failure is secondary to left heart failure. Other causes are indicated in Table 9.4. There is jugular venous distension, hepatomegaly and dependent pitting oedema (over the ankles and calves in ambulant patients, over the sacrum in bed-bound patients). Less frequently ascites or pleural transudates occur. Dilatation of the right ventricle may give rise to functional tricuspid incompetence, with giant 'V' waves in the JVP and a tender pulsatile liver. Non-specific features include fatigue, anorexia and nausea.

***Biventricular failure (congestive)*** This term is used variously but is best restricted to cases where right heart failure is a result of pre-existing left heart failure. The physical signs are thus a combination of the above syndromes.

389

***Acute heart failure*** This is a medical emergency, with left or right heart failure developing over minutes or hours. It most commonly occurs in the setting of myocardial infarction and can also occur following an acute pulmonary embolus or cardiac tamponade.

## Investigations
A clinical diagnosis of heart failure should always be confirmed by objective measures of structure and function. The underlying cause should be established in all patients.

- Radiology. The chest X-ray is usually unhelpful in determining the cause of heart failure, but shows cardiac enlargement (cardiothoracic ratio > 50% on a postero-anterior chest film) and characteristic appearances in left heart failure (Fig. 9.11).

- ECG may show evidence of underlying causes, e.g. arrhythmias, ischaemia, left ventricular hypertrophy in hypertension.
- Echocardiography is the most useful diagnostic investigation. It allows an assessment of left ventricular function, and identifies valvular abnormalities and pericardial effusion. An ejection fraction of < 0.45 is usually accepted as evidence for systolic dysfunction.
- Blood tests. These include full blood count, urea and electrolytes, and sometimes thyroid function tests.

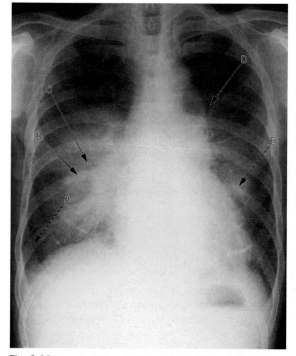

**Fig. 9.11 The chest X-ray in left ventricular failure.** A, Kerley B lines; B, hilar haziness; C, fluid in the right horizontal interlobar fissure; D, upper lobe venous engorgement; E, cardiomegaly.

- Other investigations. Resting and stress radionuclide angiography (MUGA) will estimate ejection fraction (p. 802), and identify regional wall motion abnormality. Cardiac catheterization is usually reserved for the small proportion of patients with a surgically correctable lesion, e.g. aortic or mitral valve abnormalities. In such cases the surgeon requires precise definition of the lesion and demonstration of the coronary anatomy.

### Treatment of chronic heart failure

Treatment is aimed at relieving symptoms, retarding disease progression and improving survival (Table 9.5).

### General treatment

During exacerbations of heart failure, bed rest is encouraged as it reduces the demands of the heart and promotes a diuresis. Low level endurance exercise is encouraged in compensated heart failure to reverse deconditioning of

---

**Table 9.5**
The management of chronic heart failure

**General measures**
Reduction of physical activity during exacerbations, thus reducing the work of the heart
Low-level exercise (20–30 min walks 3–5 times weekly) encouraged in patients with compensated heart failure
Reduction of salt intake: no added salt at meals
Avoid alcohol which has negative inotropic effects
Correct aggravating factors, e.g. arrhythmias, anaemia, hypertension, pulmonary infections
Vaccinate against pneumococcal disease and influenza
If possible discontinue aggravating drugs, e.g. NSAIDs

**Specific therapy**

| | |
|---|---|
| Drugs | Diuretics |
| | Vasodilators |
| | β-Adrenoceptor blockers |
| | Inotropic agents |
| | Antiarrhythmic drugs |
| Surgery | Coronary artery bypass graft |
| | Replacement of diseased valves |
| | Cardiac transplantation |
| | Repair of congenital heart disease |

NSAIDs, non-steroidal anti-inflammatory drugs

peripheral muscle metabolism. Large meals and alcohol should be avoided and salt restriction encouraged.

## Drug treatment

**Diuretics** These are the first line of treatment in patients with heart failure. They act by promoting renal sodium excretion, with enhanced water excretion as a secondary effect. The resulting loss of fluid reduces ventricular filling pressures (preload) and thus decreases pulmonary and systemic congestion.

- *Loop diuretics*, e.g. furosemide (frusemide) and bumetanide, inhibit sodium reabsorption in the ascending limb of the loop of Henle. They are potent diuretics used in moderate/severe heart failure. These drugs produce marked renal potassium loss and promote hyperuricaemia. When given intravenously, they also induce arteriolar vasodilatation, a beneficial action independent of their diuretic effect.
- *Thiazide diuretics*, e.g. bendroflumethiazide (bendrofluazide), are mild diuretics that inhibit sodium reabsorption in the distal renal tubule. The exception is metolazone, which causes a profound diuresis and is used in severe heart failure unresponsive to large doses of loop diuretics. The major side-effects of the thiazides are hypokalaemia, hyperglycaemia and hyperuricaemia.
- *Potassium-sparing diuretics*. Spironolactone is a relatively weak diuretic with a potassium-sparing action. Low-dose spirinolactone (25–50 mg daily) in combination with conventional treatment reduces mortality in patients with moderate to severe heart failure and should be given to all patients. Amiloride and triamterene have a direct action on ion transport in the distal renal tubule and are useful in combination with loop diuretics. They increase renal sodium loss and reduce potassium loss but have not been shown to have a prognostic effect as yet.

**Vasodilator therapy** Vasodilators have a beneficial effect in heart failure by reducing venous constriction (reduction of preload) and/or arteriolar constriction (reduction of afterload).

- *Angiotensin-converting enzyme inhibitors (ACEI)*, e.g. captopril, enalapril, lisinopril and quinapril, inhibit the production of angiotensin II, a potent vasoconstrictor, and increase concentrations of the vasodilator bradykinin. They enhance renal salt and water excretion and increase cardiac output by reducing afterload. They improve symptoms, limit the development of progressive heart failure and prolong survival, and should be given to all patients with heart failure, in addition to diuretic therapy. The major side-effect is first-dose hypotension, which is a particular risk in those with severe heart failure receiving large doses of diuretics. Patients should stop potassium supplements and omit or reduce the dose of diuretics for 24 hours before the first dose of ACE inhibitor at bedtime. They should start with a low dose followed by gradual increments every 1–2 weeks with a check on serum potassium and renal function. Other side-effects are prerenal renal failure (p. 341), hyperkalaemia, rash, angioedema and persistent cough due to inhibition of bradykinin metabolism.

- *Angiotensin II type 1 receptor antagonists (AII)*, such as losartan, specifically block the binding of angiotensin II to the type 1 receptor (AT1). In contrast the ACE inhibitors inhibit production of angiotensin II and consequently diminish the activity of both AT1 and AT2 receptors. One important consequence of this difference is that angiotensin II receptor antagonists do not affect kinin metabolism and do not cause cough. Both ACE inhibitors and AII receptor antagonists are contraindicated in patients with bilateral renal artery stenosis.

- *Other vasodilators.* The combination of isosorbide mononitrate (a vasodilator) and hydralazine (arteriolar vasodilator) improves symptoms and survival, and is used when ACE inhibitors are not tolerated or their use is contraindicated. Calcium-channel blockers, e.g. nifedipine, diltiazem, also reduce afterload but may have a detrimental effect on left ventricular function.

The second-generation calcium antagonist amlodipine is safe in heart failure but not of prognostic benefit. Other vasodilators, used less commonly, include prazosin and nitroprusside.

- *β-Blockers.* Metoprolol, bisoprolol and carvedilol, improve symptoms and exercise tolerance in patients with chronic stable heart failure, in addition to improving mortality. This effect is thought to arise through blockade of the chronically activated sympathetic system. These drugs are restricted to those with chronic stable heart failure and introduced cautiously because of the potential to cause heart failure decompensation.

### Inotropic agents

- *Digoxin* is of benefit in patients with congestive heart failure and atrial fibrillation. In combination with ACE inhibitors and diuretics, digoxin reduces death and hospitalization rates from progressive heart failure in patients in sinus rhythm.
- *Sympathomimetic agents.* Dopamine and dobutamine are intravenous adrenergic agonists. They are used in cardiogenic shock (p. 396). Xamoterol is an orally acting β-adrenoceptor agonist. It is effective in improving cardiac performance but its use is very limited because it may precipitate an acute deterioration in patients with severe heart failure.

**Antiarrhythmic drugs** Arrhythmias are frequent in heart failure and are implicated in sudden death, though the evidence that medical treatment of complex arrhythmias reduces mortality is conflicting. The insertion of an implantable cardioverter–defibrillator (ICD) may be the optimal treatment for patients who have experienced episodes of life-threatening arrhythmias.

**Summary of treatment** All patients with clinical heart failure should receive treatment with diuretics, ACE inhibitors, spirinolactone and, in some cases, β-blockers.

### Prognosis

There is usually a gradual deterioration necessitating increased doses of diuretics, and sometimes admission to hospital. The prognosis is poor in those with severe heart failure (i.e. breathless at rest or on minimal exertion), with a 1-year survival rate of 50%.

### Cardiac transplantation (K&C p. 764)

This has become the treatment of choice for younger patients with severe intractable heart failure. The expected 1-year survival following transplantation is over 90%, with 75% alive at 5 years. Death is usually the result of operative mortality, organ rejection and overwhelming infection secondary to immunosuppressive treatment. After this time the greatest threat to health is accelerated coronary atherosclerosis, the cause of which is unknown.

## Pulmonary oedema (K&C p. 764)

This is a very frightening life-threatening emergency characterized by the rapid onset of extreme breathlessness. Causes include acute, severe left ventricular failure (e.g. myocardial infarction, acute mitral and aortic regurgitation), mitral stenosis and arrhythmias. An acute elevation of left atrial pressure produces corresponding elevation of the pulmonary capillary pressure and increased transudation of fluid into the pulmonary interstitium and alveoli (cardiogenic pulmonary oedema). *Non-cardiogenic pulmonary oedema* (acute lung injury) is seen in very ill patients and is discussed on page 520.

### Clinical features

The patient is acutely breathless, wheezing and anxious. There is often a cough productive of frothy blood-tinged (pink) sputum. Increased sympathoadrenal activity leads to profuse sweating, tachycardia and peripheral circulatory shutdown. On auscultation there is a gallop rhythm, and wheezes and crackles are heard throughout the chest.

### Investigations

- Radiology. The chest X-ray shows distension of the upper lobe veins (indicating a raised pulmonary venous pressure) and bilateral perihilar shadowing in a 'butterfly' or 'bat's wing' distribution caused by alveolar fluid. Interstitial pulmonary oedema produces Kerley B lines (see Fig. 9.11).

- ECG and cardiac enzymes may show evidence of a myocardial infarction as the precipitating event.
- Arterial blood gases show hypoxaemia. Initially the $P_aCO_2$ falls because of overbreathing, but later increases because of impaired gas exchange.

### Management

In many cases the patient is so unwell that treatment (Emergency Box 9.2) must begin before investigations are completed. Intravenous opiates, e.g. morphine, and diuretics are the first-line agents. Morphine relieves dyspnoea by a combination of vasodilatation and relief of anxiety. Respiratory depression can occur with large doses (> 10 mg). Diuretics produce immediate vasodilatation in addition to the more delayed diuretic response. If the patient does not improve and is not hypotensive, intravenous nitrates such as glyceryl trinitrate may be used to reduce the preload. Occasionally, in severe cases which do not respond to treatment, ventilation is necessary.

## Cardiogenic shock (K&C p. 765)

Cardiogenic shock (pump failure) is an extreme type of cardiac failure characterized by hypotension, a low cardiac

 **Emergency Box 9.2**

### Management of pulmonary oedema

Sit the patient up
60% oxygen by face mask
Furosemide (frusemide) 40–80 mg i.v.
Morphine 2.5–10 mg i.v. + an antiemetic, e.g. metoclopramide 10 mg i.v.
Consider
   Intravenous GTN infusion (2–10 mg/h)
   Intravenous aminophylline (250 mg over 10 min) to relieve bronchospasm
Treat exacerbating and precipitating factors
   Hypertension
   Pulmonary infection
   Arrhythmias
Mechanical ventilation if no response to treatment

output and signs of poor tissue perfusion, such as oliguria, cold extremities and poor cerebral function. The most common cause is massive myocardial infarction, and management is discussed on page 510.

# Ischaemic heart disease (K&C p. 766)

Myocardial ischaemia results from an imbalance between the supply of oxygen to cardiac muscle and myocardial demand. The most common cause is coronary artery atheroma (coronary artery disease), which results in a fixed obstruction to coronary blood flow. Other causes of ischaemia include coronary artery thrombosis, spasm or, rarely, arteritis (e.g. polyarteritis). Increased demand for oxygen due to an increase in cardiac output may occur in thyrotoxicosis or myocardial hypertrophy (e.g. from aortic stenosis or hypertension).

Coronary artery disease (CAD) is the single largest cause of death in the UK, resulting in approximately 60 deaths per 100 000 population.

Atheroma consists of atherosclerotic plaques (seen postmortem as raised yellow-white areas covering the intimal surface of the artery) rich in cholesterol and other lipids, surrounded by smooth muscle cells and fibrous tissue. CAD gives rise to a wide variety of clinical presentations, ranging from stable angina to the acute coronary syndromes of unstable angina and myocardial infarction. A number of risk factors have been identified for CAD, some of which are irreversible and some of which can be modified.

397

## Irreversible risk factors

*Age* CAD rate increases with age. It rarely presents in the young, except in familial hyperlipidaemia (p. 625).

*Gender* Men are more often affected than premenopausal women, although the incidence in women after the menopause is similar to that in men. The cause for this difference is poorly understood, but probably relates to the loss of the protective effect of oestrogen.

**Family history** CAD is often present in several members of the same family. It is unclear, however, whether family history is an independent risk factor as so many other factors are familial. A number of genetic risk factors have been associated with CAD. For example, a specific genotype of the *ACE* gene associated with higher circulating ACE levels may be significantly associated with a predisposition to CAD and myocardial infarction.

## Potentially reversible risk factors

**Hyperlipidaemia** Elevated cholesterol levels increase the risk of premature atherosclerosis, particularly when associated with low levels of high-density lipoproteins (HDLs). There is increasing evidence that high triglyceride levels are independently linked with coronary atheroma. Lowering serum cholesterol not only slows the progression of coronary atherosclerosis, but may also cause regression of the disease.

**Smoking** In men the risk of developing CAD is directly related to the number of cigarettes smoked. In women this relationship, although still important, is less clear. Stopping smoking reduces the risk but does not eliminate it.

**Hypertension** Both elevated systolic and elevated diastolic hypertension are linked to an increased incidence of CAD.

**Homocysteine** This has emerged as a potential major risk factor in the pathogenesis of CAD, probably because of its adverse effects on vascular endothelium. Folic acid in low doses may ameliorate this process.

**Other factors** Diabetes mellitus, lack of exercise and obesity have all been linked to an increased incidence of atheroma. A number of other factors, including high levels of fibrinogen, C-reactive protein, and lipoprotein (a) in the blood, have been linked to atherosclerosis, although it is unclear whether they are directly linked to the pathogenesis of the disease.

## Angina (K&C p. 769)
Angina pectoris is a descriptive term for chest pain arising from the heart as a result of myocardial ischaemia.

## Clinical features

Angina is usually described as central, crushing, retro-sternal chest pain, coming on with exertion and relieved by rest within a few minutes. It is often exacerbated by cold weather, anger and excitement, and it frequently radiates to the arms and neck. Variants of classic angina include:

- *Decubitus angina* (occurs on lying down).
- *Variant (Prinzmetal's) angina* is caused by coronary artery spasm and results in angina that occurs without provocation, usually at rest.
- *Unstable angina.* Angina which increases rapidly in severity, occurs at rest, or is of recent onset. It is due to transient subtotal obstruction due to a platelet-rich clot over a fissured atherosclerotic plaque.
- *Cardiac syndrome X* refers to those patients with symptoms of angina, a positive exercise test and normal coronary arteries on angiogram. It is thought to result from functional abnormalities of the coronary microcirculation.

Physical examination in patients with angina is often normal but must include a search for risk factors (e.g. hypertension and xanthelasma occurring in hyperlipidaemia).

## Diagnosis

The primary diagnosis is clinical because investigations may be normal. Occasionally chest wall pain or oeso-phageal reflux causes diagnostic confusion (p. 366).

399

## Investigations

- Resting ECG typically shows ST segment depression and T-wave flattening or inversion during an attack. The ECG is usually normal between attacks.
- Exercise ECG testing is positive (p. 372) in about 75% of people with severe CAD; a normal test does not exclude the diagnosis. ST segment depression (> 1 mm) at a low workload or a paradoxical fall in blood pressure with exercise usually indicates severe coronary artery disease, and these patients should be considered for coronary angiography.
- Radioisotope studies (thallium-201 perfusion scan, (p. 802) are particularly useful in those with equivocal

exercise tests. Ischaemic areas show as 'cold spots' during exercise (*K&C* p. 727).

- Coronary angiography is occasionally used when the cause of pain is unclear. More commonly the test is performed to delineate the exact coronary anatomy before coronary artery surgery is considered (*K&C* p. 728)

## Management

**General** Underlying problems such as obesity, thyrotoxicosis, hypercholesterolaemia, anaemia or aortic valve disease should be identified and treated. Smoking should be discouraged, other risk factors evaluated and steps taken to correct them.

### Prognostic therapies
- Aspirin (75 mg daily) inhibits platelet cyclo-oxygenase, an enzyme involved in the formation of the aggregating agent thromboxane $A_2$. Aspirin reduces the risk of coronary events in patients with CAD.
- Lipid-lowering agents have been shown to reduce death rates and incidence of myocardial infarction in patients with CAD and should be used in patients with a cholesterol level of greater than 4.8 mmol/L. Guidelines on introduction of lipid-lowering therapy are illustrated on page 628.

**Symptomatic treatment** Acute attacks are treated with sublingual glyceryl trinitrate. Patients should be encouraged to use this before exertion, rather than waiting for the pain to develop. The main side-effect is a severe bursting headache, which is relieved by inactivating the tablet either by swallowing or spitting it out.

When angina occurs frequently or with only modest exertion, regular prophylactic therapy should be employed. Nitrates, β-blockers or calcium antagonists are most commonly used, with treatment being tailored to the individual patient.

- *β-Adrenergic blocking drugs,* e.g. atenolol 50–100 mg daily and metoprolol 25–50 mg twice daily, reduce heart rate and the force of ventricular contraction, both of which reduce myocardial oxygen demand. They are contraindicated in asthma, and relatively contraindicated in peripheral vascular disease.

- *Calcium antagonists*, e.g. diltiazem, amlodipine, block calcium influx into the cell and the utilization of calcium within the cell. They relax the coronary arteries and reduce the force of left ventricular contraction, thereby reducing oxygen demand. The side-effects (postural dizziness, headache, ankle oedema) are the result of systemic vasodilatation. High-dose nifedipine increases mortality and should not be used in this situation.
- *Nitrates* reduce venous and intracardiac diastolic pressure, reduce impedance to the emptying of the left ventricle, and dilate coronary arteries. They are available in a variety of slow-release preparations, including infiltrated skin plasters, buccal pellets and long-acting oral nitrate preparations, e.g. isosorbide mononitrate, isosorbide dinitrate. The major side-effect is headache, which tends to diminish with continued use.
- *Nicorandil* combines nitrate-like activity with potassium channel blockade. It can be useful when there are contraindications to the above agents or in refractory unstable angina.

When angina persists or worsens in spite of general measures and optimal medical treatment, patients should be considered for coronary artery bypass grafting (CABG) or angioplasty.

***Coronary angioplasty*** Localized atheromatous lesions are dilated at cardiac catheterization using small inflatable balloons. This technique is widely applied for angina resulting from isolated, proximal, non-calcified atheromatous plaques. Complications include acute occlusion in 2–4% of cases (necessitating full surgical back-up) and restenosis (30% in the first 6 months).

Intracoronary stents reduce the risk of restenosis but increase the cost of the procedure. Aspirin and other antiplatelet drugs, e.g. clopidigrel, are routinely given, and the use of monoclonal antibodies to the glycoprotein IIb/IIIa platelet receptor (the final common pathway of aggregation) in selected high-risk cases may reduce periprocedural complications.

***Surgery*** The left or right internal mammary artery is used to bypass stenoses in the left anterior descending or right coronary artery respectively. Less commonly, the saphenous vein from the leg is anastomosed to the proximal aorta, and coronary artery distal to the obstruction. Surgery successfully relieves angina in about 90% of cases and, when performed for left main stem obstruction or three-vessel disease, an improved lifespan and quality of life can be expected. Operative mortality rate is less than 1%. In most patients the angina eventually recurs because of accelerated atherosclerosis in the graft (particularly vein grafts), which can be treated by stenting.

## Prognosis

The average annual mortality rate for patients with stable angina is 4% a year, with the worst prognosis in those with extensive coronary artery disease.

## Acute coronary syndromes (ACS) (*K&C* p. 773)

ACS (also called *unstable angina*) and *myocardial infarction without ST segment elevation* are clinical features of coronary artery disease which lie between stable angina and myocardial infarction with ST segment elevation or sudden death. They are medical emergencies with a risk of myocardial infarction with ST segment elevation if treatment is inadequate. Immediate investigations are the same as for myocardial infarction (p. 401). Management involves admission to hospital, bed rest, low-molecular-weight heparin, aspirin and a combination of all three classes of antianginal drugs. Platelet glycoprotein IIb/IIIa receptor inhibitors, e.g. abciximab, are sometimes added for high-risk patients (e.g. ST segment depression on the ECG, refractory angina, raised serum troponin I/T levels, diabetes mellitus). Early coronary angiography with a view to surgery or angioplasty is recommended in patients who do not improve in spite of optimum medical treatment.

# Myocardial infarction (*K&C* p. 774)

Myocardial infarction (MI) is now the most common cause of death in developed countries. It is almost always the result of rupture of an atherosclerotic plaque, with the development of thrombosis and total occlusion of the artery.

## Clinical features

Central chest pain similar to that occurring in angina is the most common presenting symptom. Unlike angina it usually occurs at rest, is more severe and lasts for some hours. The pain is often associated with sweating, breathlessness, nausea, vomiting and restlessness. There may be no physical signs unless complications develop (see later), although the patient often appears pale, sweaty and grey. About 20% of patients have no pain, and such 'silent' infarctions either go unnoticed or present with hypotension, arrhythmias or pulmonary oedema. This occurs most commonly in elderly patients or those with diabetes or hypertension.

## Investigations

In most cases the diagnosis is made on the basis of the clinical history and early ECG appearances. Serial changes (over 3 days) in the ECG and serum levels of cardiac markers confirm the diagnosis and allow an assessment of infarct size (on the magnitude of the enzyme and protein rise and extent of ECG changes). A normal ECG in the early stages does not exclude the diagnosis.

**The ECG** usually shows a characteristic pattern. Within hours there is ST segment elevation (> 1 mm in two or more contiguous leads) followed by T-wave flattening or inversion (Fig. 9.12). Pathological Q waves are broad (> 1 mm) and deep (> 2 mm, or > 25% of the amplitude of the following R wave) negative deflections that start the QRS complex. They are seen once full-thickness infarction (as opposed to non-Q-wave or subendocardial infarction) has occurred. They develop because the infarcted muscle is electrically silent so that the recording leads 'look through' the infarcted area. This means that the electrical activity

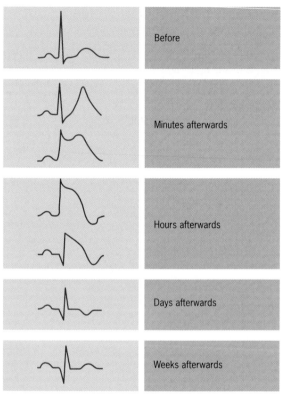

**Fig. 9.12 Electrocardiographic evolution of myocardial infarction.**
After the first few minutes the T waves become tall, pointed and upright
and there is ST segment elevation. After the first few hours the T waves
invert, the R wave voltage is decreased and Q waves develop. After a few
days the ST segment returns to normal. After weeks or months the T wave
may return to upright but the Q wave remains.

being recorded (on the opposite ventricular wall) is moving
away from the electrode and is therefore negative.

Typically ECG changes are confined to the leads that
'face' the infarct. Leads II, III and AVF are involved in inferior infarcts; I, II and AVL in lateral infarcts; and V$_2$–V$_6$ in
anterior infarcts. As there are no posterior leads a posterior
wall infarct is diagnosed by the appearance of reciprocal

changes in $V_1$ and $V_2$ (i.e. the development of tall initial R waves, ST segment depression and tall upright T waves).

***Cardiac markers*** Necrotic cardiac muscle releases several enzymes and proteins into the systemic circulation.

- Troponin T and troponin I are regulatory proteins, highly specific for cardiac muscle damage. They are released early and persist for several days and are more sensitive and cardiac specific than CK-MB. Measurement of these proteins can be performed at the bedside.
- Creatine kinase (CK), which is also produced by damaged skeletal muscle and brain. The myocardial-bound (MB) isoenzyme fraction of CK is specific for heart muscle damage and the size of the enzyme rise is broadly proportional to the infarct size.
- Aspartate aminotransferase (AST) and lactic dehydrogenase (LDH) are now rarely used for the diagnosis of infarction, but because serum levels remain elevated for up to 10 days after infarction, measurement may be useful in a patient presenting several days after an episode of chest pain.

There is a characteristic time course for the release of the enzymes into the blood, and thus they are usually measured for 3 days following suspected myocardial infarction (Fig. 9.13).

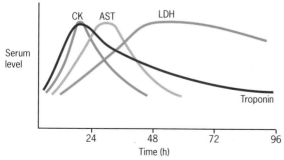

**Fig. 9.13 The cardiac enzyme and protein profile in acute myocardial infarction.** CK, creatine kinase; AST, aspartate aminotransferase; LDH, lactic dehydrogenase.

***Other investigations*** These include a chest X-ray, full blood count, serum urea and electrolytes, blood glucose and lipids (lipids taken within the first 12 hours reflect pre-infarction levels, but after this time they are altered for up to 6 weeks).

## Management
The aims of treatment are relief of pain, limitation of infarct size and treatment of complications (Emergency Box 9.3).

***Acute management*** Thrombolytic therapy is indicated in patients with chest pain consistent with myocardial infarction and ST segment elevation on the ECG. These agents can achieve early reperfusion in 50–70% of patients (compared to a spontaneous reperfusion of less than 30%) and reduce mortality and the extent of myocardial damage. They should be given as soon as possible, although benefit may occur for up to 12 hours after the onset of symptoms. Commonly used thrombolytic agents are streptokinase and recombinant tissue-type plasminogen activator (t-PA). Streptokinase is the cheapest and most commonly used, but may induce the development of antistreptokinase antibodies. This puts the patient at risk of allergic reactions and reduces the effectiveness of subsequent thrombolysis with streptokinase. t-PA is preferred in patients under 50 years of age with anterior MIs, in patients previously treated with streptokinase or when the systolic blood pressure is less than 100 mmHg. t-PA must be followed by intravenous heparin. The side-effects and contraindications to thrombolysis are discussed on page 215.

Aspirin (150 mg chewed) enhances the benefits of thrombolysis and should be given immediately and continued indefinitely as secondary prophylaxis.

Following initiation of thrombolysis, the patient should be transferred to the coronary care unit where close ECG monitoring and immediate resuscitation are possible. Mortality is increased in diabetic patients with MI, largely owing to the high incidence of cardiac failure. This is due in part to metabolic changes which occur in the early stages of MI, and is reduced by rigorous control of blood glucose with insulin infusion, and monitoring with 2-hourly BM

### Emergency Box 9.3

## Summary of the management of myocardial infarction

### Immediate management

- Aspirin: 300 mg to be chewed
- Insert intravenous cannula. Take blood for cardiac proteins, blood count, urea and electrolytes, glucose and lipids
- Attach patient to a cardiac monitor
- Pain relief: diamorphine (2.5–5 mg i.v.). Repeat after 15 minutes if necessary; half the dose in the elderly. Antiemetic, e.g. metoclopramide 10 mg i.v prevents nausea and vomiting
- 60% oxygen by face mask or nasal cannula. Discontinue if arterial oxygen saturation is normal
- Streptokinase: 1.5 million units in 100 mL 0.9% sodium chloride over 1 h by intravenous infusion pump
- Metoprolol 5 mg slow i.v. injection if systolic HR > 100 b.p.m. Repeat every 15 min, titrated against heart rate and BP. Do not give if hypotension, heart failure, bradycardia, asthma
- Insulin infusion if admission blood glucose > 11 mmol/L, aim for blood glucose of 7–10 mmol/L
- Treat complications (pp. 408–411)
- Treat persistent pain with glyceryl trinitrate infusion 2–10 mg/h titrated against the response; consider angiography and possible angioplasty

### Subsequent management of uncomplicated infarction

- Repeat ECG, serum cardiac markers and electrolytes at 24 and 48 hours after admission
- Initiate secondary prevention therapy
- ACE inhibitors, e.g. captopril 6.25 mg with dose titrated up to 25 mg three times daily; aspirin 150 mg daily; β-blockers, e.g. metoprolol 25–50 mg three times daily; warfarin in selected patients (p. 410). Stop smoking. Start lipid-lowering therapy if blood cholesterol > 4.8 mmol/L
- Transfer from CCU to medical ward after 48 h
- Mobilize gradually after 24–48 h if pain-free
- Discharge from hospital after 6 days
- Submaximal exercise test prior to discharge. Consider angiography if ischaemic ECG changes or chest pain in early stages
- Refer to rehabilitation nurse. No driving for 1 month; special assessment is required for heavy goods or public service licence holder before driving. Usually return to work in 2 months

Stix. This regimen is also indicated in patients not known to be diabetic who have an admission blood glucose of > 11 mmol/L.

β-Blockers reduce infarct size and the incidence of sudden death. Metoprolol (5–10 mg i.v) should be given, particularly if the heart rate is greater than 100 b.p.m. and there is persistent pain. β-Blocker therapy should be continued for at least 1 year unless contraindicated.

Recanalization of the infarct-related artery may also be achieved by primary (direct) angioplasty without prior or concomitant thrombolytic therapy; in experienced hands the results are equal or superior to thrombolysis. It is only a therapeutic option when rapid access to a catheterization laboratory is possible, the cardiologist is experienced in interventional cardiology and a full support team is immediately available. Therefore, it is not usually used in preference to thrombolysis but should be considered in patients when thrombolytic therapy is contraindicated (p. 216), or in patients who have received thrombolysis and who seem on clinical grounds not to have reperfused (ongoing chest pain and persistent ST elevation).

**Subsequent management** In selected patients, ACE inhibitors reduce mortality and prevent the development of heart failure. They should be started on the first day after MI in patients with extensive anterior infarction, impaired left ventricular ejection fraction (< 35%) on echocardiography, or who experience heart failure in the acute event. Treatment with ACE inhibitors and aspirin is continued indefinitely. Gradual mobilization takes place on the second day and if the patient is fully ambulant and pain free, a sub-maximal exercise tolerance test is performed (70% of age-predicted maximal heart rate) before hospital discharge on day 5 or 6 in uncomplicated cases. Patients with test results suggesting ischaemia are referred for coronary angiography.

## Complications
The common complications are listed in Table 9.6.

**Disturbances of rate, rhythm and conduction** See page 372, and web site http://www.resus.org.uk/pages/periarst.htm.

**Table 9.6**
Complications associated with myocardial infarction

| Early (within 2–3 days) | Late |
|---|---|
| Arrhythmias | Mitral valve regurgitation |
| Cardiac failure | Rupture of ventricular septum or wall |
| Heart block | Dressler's syndrome |
| Pericarditis | Ventricular aneurysm |
| Myocardial rupture (usually fatal) | Recurrent arrhythmias |
| Thromboembolism | Thromboembolism |

- *Atrial arrhythmias.* Sinus tachycardia is common; treatment is that of the underlying cause, particularly pain, anxiety and heart failure. Sinus bradycardia is especially associated with acute inferior wall myocardial infarction. Treatment is initially with intravenous atropine (500 μg repeated to a maximum of 3 mg) or temporary pacing if there are adverse signs (heart failure, hypotension, ventricular arrhythmias). Atrial fibrillation occurs in about 10% of cases and is usually a transient rhythm disturbance. Treatment with intravenous digoxin or amiodarone is indicated if the fast rate is exacerbating ischaemia or causing heart failure.

- *Ventricular arrhythmias.* Ventricular ectopic beats are very common and may precede the development of ventricular tachycardia or fibrillation. Antiarrhythmic drug treatment has not been shown to affect progression to these more serious arrhythmias. Ventricular tachycardia (VT) may degenerate into ventricular fibrillation (p. 383) or may itself produce shock or cardiac failure. Treatment of VT is with intravenous lidocaine (lignocaine) (p. 382) or direct current cardioversion if there is severe hypotension. Ventricular fibrillation (VF) may be primary (occurring in the first 24–48 hours) or secondary (occurring late after infarction and associated with large infarcts and heart failure). Treatment is with immediate DC cardioversion. Recurrences may be prevented with intravenous lidocaine or amiodarone. Late VF is associated with a poor prognosis and a high incidence of sudden death, and prophylactic antiarrhythmic treatment must be continued long term.

- *Heart block occurring with inferior infarction* is common and usually resolves spontaneously. Some patients respond to intravenous atropine, but a temporary pacemaker may be necessary if the rhythm is very slow or producing symptoms.

- *Complete heart block occurring with anterior wall infarction* indicates the involvement of both bundle branches by extensive myocardial necrosis, and hence a very poor prognosis. The ventricular rhythm in this case is unreliable and a temporary pacing wire is necessary. Heart block is often permanent and a permanent pacing wire may be necessary.

**Cardiac failure** in a mild form occurs in up to 40% of patients following myocardial infarction. Extensive infarction may cause pulmonary oedema (see Emergency Box 9.2), which may also occur following rupture of the ventricular septum or mitral valve papillary muscle. Both conditions present with worsening heart failure, a systolic thrill and a loud pansystolic murmur. Mortality is high and urgent surgical correction is often needed. Hypotension with a raised JVP is usually a complication of right ventricular infarction, which may occur with inferior wall infarcts. Initial treatment is with volume expansion, and pericardial effusion (which produces similar signs) ruled out on an echocardiogram.

**Thromboembolism** occurs most commonly following prolonged bed rest and with cardiac failure. Patients at risk of embolism from left ventricular or left atrial clot (those with severe left ventricular dysfunction, persistent AF or mural thrombus on echocardiography) should be anticoagulated with warfarin to achieve a target INR of 2–3.

**Pericarditis** is characterized by sharp chest pain and a pericardial rub. Treatment is with non-steroidal anti-inflammatory drugs until spontaneous resolution occurs within 1–2 days. Late pericarditis (2–12 weeks after) with fever and a pericardial effusion (Dressler's syndrome) is rare and corticosteroids may be necessary in some patients.

## Prognosis

Prognosis is variable depending on factors such as age and size of infarct. Fifty per cent of patients die during the acute event, many before reaching hospital. A further 10% die in hospital, and of the survivors a further 10% die in the next 2 years.

# Rheumatic fever

Rheumatic fever is an inflammatory disease that occurs in children and young adults (the first attack usually occurs between 5 and 15 years of age) as a result of infection with group A streptococci. It is a complication of less than 1% of streptococcal pharyngitis, developing 2–3 weeks after the onset of sore throat. It is thought to develop because of an autoimmune reaction triggered by the streptococci, and is not the result of direct infection of the heart.

## Epidemiology

The incidence in developed countries has decreased dramatically since the 1920s. This is thought to be the result of improved sanitation, a change in the virulence of the organism and the use of antibiotics.

## Clinical features

The disease presents suddenly with fever, joint pains and loss of appetite. The major clinical features are as follows:

411

- Changing heart murmurs, mitral and aortic regurgitation, cardiac failure and chest pain, caused by carditis affecting all three layers of the heart
- Polyarthritis which is classically fleeting and affects the large joints, e.g. knees, ankles and elbows
- Skin manifestations include erythema marginatum (transient pink coalescent rings develop on the trunk) and small non-tender subcutaneous nodules which occur over tendons, joints and bony prominences
- Sydenham's chorea ('St Vitus' dance') refers to involvement of the central nervous system. It develops late after a streptococcal infection. Sufferers are noticeably 'fidgety' and display spasmodic, unintentional movements.

### Investigations

**Blood count** shows a leucocytosis and a raised ESR.

The diagnosis is based on the revised Duckett Jones criteria, which depend on the combination of certain clinical features and evidence of recent streptococcal infection.

### Treatment

Treatment is with complete bed rest and high-dose aspirin. Penicillin is given to eradicate residual streptococcal infection, and then long term to all patients with persistent cardiac damage.

## Chronic rheumatic heart disease

More than 50% of those who suffer acute rheumatic fever with carditis will later (after 10–20 years) develop chronic rheumatic valvular disease, predominantly affecting the mitral and aortic valves (see below).

## Valvular heart disease

Cardiac valves may be incompetent (regurgitant), stenotic or both. The most common problems are acquired left-sided valvular lesions: aortic stenosis, mitral stenosis, mitral regurgitation and aortic regurgitation. Abnormal valves produce turbulent blood flow, which is heard as a murmur on auscultation; a few murmurs are also felt as a thrill on palpation. Murmurs may sometimes be heard with normal hearts ('innocent murmurs'), often reflecting a hyperdynamic circulation, e.g. in pregnancy, anaemia and thyrotoxicosis. Benign murmurs are soft, short, systolic, may vary with posture, and are not associated with signs of organic heart disease (*K&C* p. 715).

Diagnosis of valve dysfunction is made clinically and by echocardiography (*K&C* p. 722). The severity is assessed by Doppler echocardiography, which measures the direction and velocity of blood flow and allows a calculation to be made of the pressure across a stenotic valve. Transoesophageal echocardiography and invasive cardiac catheterization are usually only necessary to assess complex situations such as coexisting valvular and ischaemic heart disease, or suspected dysfunction of a prosthetic valve. Treatment of valve dysfunction is both medical and surgical; this may be valve replacement, valve repair (some incompetent valves) or valvotomy (the fused cusps of a stenotic valve are separated along the commissures). The timing of surgery is critical and must not be delayed until there is irreversible ventricular dysfunction or pulmonary hypertension.

### Prosthetic heart valves

Prosthetic heart valves may be either tissue or mechanical. Tissue valves are usually fashioned from pig aortic valves (a porcine xenograft), but occasionally a human aortic valve is used (homograft). Tissue valves tend to degenerate within about 10 years but patients do not need long-term anticoagulation. These valves are often used in elderly patients. Mechanical valves last much longer but patients need lifelong anticoagulation. There are several types: a ball-and-cage design (Starr–Edwards valve), a tilting disc (Björk–Shiley valve) or a double tilting disc (St Jude valve). Valves are susceptible to infection and thrombosis and may cause haemolysis or systemic emboli.

The individual valve lesions are considered separately below, but disease may affect more than one valve (particularly in rheumatic heart disease and infective endocarditis), when a combination of clinical features is produced. Damaged and prosthetic valves are at risk of infection during an episode of bacteraemia (e.g. after tooth extraction, endoscopy or surgery) and patients should always receive prophylactic antibiotics to cover these procedures (see p. 425).

## Mitral stenosis (K&C p. 783)

### Aetiology

Most cases of mitral stenosis are a result of rheumatic heart disease that primarily affects women. However, a reliable history of rheumatic fever is not always obtained.

### Pathophysiology

Valve thickening and cusp fusion leads to progressive immobility of the valve cusps and a narrowed (stenotic) valve orifice. Symptoms are the result of increased left atrial pressure and reduced cardiac output, caused by the mechanical obstruction of filling of the left ventricle. An increase in left atrial pressure leads to left atrial hypertrophy and dilatation. Thrombus may form in the dilated atrium, which is also prone to fibrillate and give rise to systemic emboli (e.g. to the brain, resulting in a stroke). Chronically elevated left atrial pressure leads to an increase in pulmonary capillary pressure and pulmonary oedema. Pulmonary arterial vasoconstriction leads to pulmonary hypertension and eventually right ventricular hypertrophy, dilatation and failure.

## Symptoms

Exertional dyspnoea which becomes progressively more severe is usually the first symptom. A cough productive of blood-tinged sputum is common, and frank haemoptysis may occasionally occur. The onset of atrial fibrillation may produce an abrupt deterioration and precipitate pulmonary oedema.

## Signs

- Cyanotic or dusky-pink discoloration on the upper cheeks produces the so-called mitral facies or malar flush that occurs with severe stenosis.
- The pulse is often irregular as a result of atrial fibrillation.
- The apex beat is 'tapping' in quality as a result of a combination of a palpable first heart sound and left ventricular backward displacement produced by an enlarging right ventricle.
- Auscultation at the apex reveals a loud first heart sound, an opening snap (when the mitral valve opens) in early diastole, followed by a rumbling mid-diastolic murmur. If the patient is in sinus rhythm the murmur becomes louder when atrial systole occurs (presystolic accentuation), as a result of increased flow across the narrowed valve.

The presence of a loud second heart sound, parasternal heave, elevated JVP, ascites and peripheral oedema indicates that pulmonary hypertension producing right ventricular overload has developed.

414

## Investigations

Investigations are performed to confirm the diagnosis, to estimate the severity of valve stenosis and to look for pulmonary hypertension.

***Chest X-ray*** appearances of mitral stenosis are indicated diagrammatically in Figure 9.14.

***ECG*** usually shows atrial fibrillation. In patients in sinus rhythm left atrial hypertrophy results in a bifid P wave ('P mitrale').

***Echocardiography*** is the most useful investigation to confirm the diagnosis and to assess the severity.

## Management

***General*** Treatment is often not required for mild mitral stenosis. Complications are treated medically, e.g. digoxin for atrial fibrillation, diuretics for heart failure and anticoagulation in patients with atrial fibrillation to prevent clot formation and embolization.

***Specific*** If symptoms are more than mild, or if there is evidence that pulmonary hypertension is beginning to develop, mechanical relief of the mitral stenosis is indicated. In many cases closed balloon valvotomy (access to the mitral valve is obtained via a catheter passed through

415

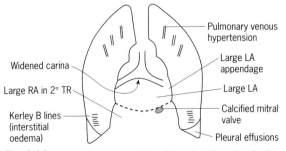

**Fig. 9.14 Schematic representation of the chest X-ray in mitral stenosis.** LA, left atrium; RA, right atrium; TR, tricuspid regurgitation.

the femoral vein, right atrium and interatrial septum, and a balloon inflated across the valve to split the commissures) provides relief of symptoms. In other cases open commissurotomy, valve reconstruction or mitral valve replacement is necessary.

# Mitral regurgitation (K&C p. 786)

## Aetiology

Rheumatic heart disease and a prolapsing mitral valve are the most common causes of mitral regurgitation (Table 9.7).

## Pathophysiology

The circulatory changes depend on the speed of onset and severity of regurgitation. Long-standing regurgitation produces little increase in the left atrial pressure because flow is accommodated by an enlarged left atrium. With acute mitral regurgitation there is a rise in left atrial pressure, resulting in an increase in pulmonary venous pressure and pulmonary oedema. The left ventricle dilates, but more so with chronic regurgitation.

## Symptoms

Acute regurgitation presents as pulmonary oedema. Chronic regurgitation causes progressive exertional dyspnoea, fatigue and lethargy (resulting from reduced cardiac output). Thromboembolism is less common than with

**Table 9.7**
Causes of mitral regurgitation

Rheumatic heart disease
Mitral valve prolapse
Infective endocarditis*
Ruptured chordae tendineae*
Rupture of the papillary muscle* complicating myocardial infarction
Papillary muscle dysfunction
Dilating left ventricle disease causing 'functional' mitral regurgitation
Hypertrophic cardiomyopathy
Rarely: systemic lupus erythematosus, Marfan's syndrome
Ehlers–Danlos syndrome

*These disorders may produce acute regurgitation

mitral stenosis, although infective endocarditis is much more common.

## Signs

- The apex beat is displaced laterally, with a diffuse thrusting character.
- The first heart sound is soft.
- There is a pansystolic murmur (palpated as a thrill), loudest at the apex and radiating widely over the precordium and into the axilla.
- A third heart sound is often present, caused by rapid filling of the dilated left ventricle in early diastole.

## Investigations

- Chest X-ray and ECG changes are not sensitive or specific for the diagnosis of mitral regurgitation. On both, evidence of enlargement of the left atrium, the left ventricle or both, is seen late in the course of the disease.
- Echocardiography confirms the diagnosis and may indicate the cause. The severity of the lesion can usually be assessed from Doppler studies without the need to resort to cardiac catheterization.

## Management

Mild mitral regurgitation in the absence of symptoms can be managed conservatively by following the patient with serial echocardiograms every 1–5 years depending on the severity. Patients should be referred for surgery (mitral valve replacement or repair) if more than mild symptoms develop or there is evidence of left ventricular dysfunction (ventricular dilatation or reduced ejection fraction).

## Prolapsing mitral valve (K&C p. 788)

This is a common condition occurring mainly in young women. One or more of the mitral valve leaflets prolapses back into the left atrium during ventricular systole, producing mitral regurgitation in a few cases.

## Aetiology

The cause is unknown but it may be associated with Marfan's syndrome, thyrotoxicosis, and rheumatic or ischaemic heart disease.

## Clinical features
Most patients are asymptomatic. Atypical chest pain is the most common symptom. Some patients complain of palpitations caused by atrial and ventricular arrhythmias. The typical finding on examination is a mid-systolic click, which may be followed by a murmur. Occasionally there are features of mitral regurgitation.

## Investigation
Echocardiography is diagnostic and shows the prolapsing valve cusps.

## Management
Chest pain and palpitations are treated with β-blockers. Anticoagulation to prevent thromboembolism is indicated if there is significant mitral regurgitation and atrial fibrillation. Prophylaxis against endocarditis is advised if there is significant mitral valve regurgitation.

# Aortic stenosis (K&C p. 788)
## Aetiology
There are three causes of aortic valve stenosis:
- Degeneration and calcification of a normal tricuspid valve – presenting in the elderly
- Calcification of a congenital bicuspid valve – presenting in middle age
- Rheumatic heart disease.

## Pathophysiology
Obstruction to left ventricular emptying results in left ventricular hypertrophy. In turn this results in increased myocardial oxygen demand, relative ischaemia of the myocardium and consequent angina, arrhythmias and eventually left ventricular failure.

## Symptoms
There are usually no symptoms until the stenosis is moderately severe (aortic orifice reduced to a third of its normal size). The classic symptoms are angina, exertional syncope and the symptoms of congestive heart failure. Ventricular arrhythmias may cause sudden death.

## Signs

The carotid pulse is slow rising (plateau pulse) and the apex beat thrusting. There is a harsh systolic ejection murmur (palpated as a thrill) at the right upper sternal border and radiating to the neck. The murmur may be preceded by an ejection click, which is the result of sudden opening of a deformed but mobile valve.

## Investigations

- Chest X-ray shows a normal heart size, prominence of the ascending aorta (post-stenotic dilatation) and there may be valvular calcification.
- ECG may show evidence of left ventricular hypertrophy.
- Echocardiography is diagnostic in most cases. Doppler examination of the valve allows an assessment of the pressure gradient across the valve during systole.
- Cardiac catheterization and coronary angiography are used particularly in patients with angina to exclude coronary artery disease, which may coexist in this predominantly elderly population.

## Management

The onset of symptoms in a patient with aortic stenosis is an ominous sign: 75% of patients will be dead within 3 years unless the valve is replaced. Thus aortic valve replacement is usually indicated in symptomatic patients or for severe stenosis (valve gradient of more than 50 mmHg), irrespective of symptoms. Balloon aortic valvotomy is sometimes used as a 'bridge' to valve replacement in very sick patients.

# Aortic regurgitation (K&C p. 791)

## Aetiology

Aortic regurgitation results from either disease of the valve cusps or dilatation of the aortic root and valve ring. The most common causes are rheumatic fever, and infective endocarditis complicating an already damaged valve (Table 9.8).

## Pathophysiology

Chronic regurgitation volume loads the left ventricle and results in hypertrophy and dilatation. The stroke volume is

Valvular heart disease

> **Table 9.8**
> Causes and associations of aortic regurgitation
>
> Damage to the aortic valve cusps
> Infective endocarditis*
> Acute rheumatic fever*
> Chronic rheumatic heart disease
> Bicuspid aortic valve
> Dilatation of aorta and valve ring
>
> Dissection of the aorta*
> Syphilis
> Arthritides
> Reiter's syndrome
> Ankylosing spondylitis
> Rheumatoid arthritis
> Severe hypertension
> Aortic endocarditis
> Marfan's syndrome
> Osteogenesis imperfecta

\* These conditions may produce acute aortic regurgitation

increased, which results in an increased pulse pressure and the myriad clinical signs described below. Eventually contraction of the ventricle deteriorates, resulting in left ventricular failure. The adaptations to the volume load entering the left ventricle do not occur with acute regurgitation and patients may present with pulmonary oedema and a reduced stroke volume (hence many of the signs of chronic regurgitation are absent).

### Symptoms
In chronic regurgitation patients remain asymptomatic for many years before developing dyspnoea, orthopnoea and fatigue as a result of left ventricular failure.

### Signs
- A 'collapsing' (water-hammer) pulse with wide pulse pressure is pathognomonic.
- The apex beat is displaced laterally and is thrusting in quality.
- A blowing early diastolic murmur is heard at the left sternal edge in the fourth intercostal space. It is accentuated when the patient sits forward with the breath held in expiration. Increased stroke volume

produces turbulent flow across the aortic valve, heard as a mid-systolic murmur.

- A mid-diastolic murmur (Austin Flint murmur) may be heard over the cardiac apex and is thought to be produced as a result of the aortic jet impinging on the mitral valve, producing premature closure of the valve and physiological stenosis.

## Investigations

- Chest X-ray shows a large heart and dilatation of the ascending aorta.
- ECG shows evidence of left ventricular hypertrophy.
- Echocardiography with Doppler examination of the aortic valve helps estimate the severity of regurgitation.
- Aortography during cardiac catheterization helps confirm the severity of the disease.

## Management

Mild symptoms may respond to the reduction of afterload with vasodilators and diuretics. The timing of surgery and valve replacement is critical and must not be delayed until there is irreversible left ventricular dysfunction.

# Tricuspid and pulmonary valve disease

(K&C p. 792)

Tricuspid and pulmonary valve disease are both uncommon. Tricuspid stenosis is almost always the result of rheumatic fever and is frequently associated with mitral and aortic valve disease, which tends to dominate the clinical picture.

Tricuspid regurgitation is usually functional and secondary to dilatation of the right ventricle (and hence tricuspid valve ring) in severe right ventricular failure. Much less commonly it is caused by rheumatic heart disease, infective endocarditis or carcinoid syndrome (p. 82). On examination there is a pansystolic murmur heard at the lower left sternal edge, the jugular venous pressure is elevated, with giant 'v' waves (produced by the regurgitant jet through the tricuspid valve in systole), and the liver is enlarged and pulsates in systole. There may be severe peripheral oedema and ascites. In functional tricuspid regurgitation these signs improve with diuretic therapy.

Pulmonary regurgitation results from pulmonary hypertension and dilatation of the valve ring. Occasionally it is the result of endocarditis (usually in intravenous drug abusers). Auscultation reveals an early diastolic murmur heard at the upper left sternal edge (Graham–Steell murmur), similar to that of aortic regurgitation. Usually there are no symptoms and treatment is rarely required. Pulmonary stenosis is usually a congenital lesion but may present in adult life with fatigue, syncope and right ventricular failure.

# Infective endocarditis

Infective endocarditis is an infection of the endocardium or vascular endothelium of the heart. It may occur as a fulminating or acute infection, but more commonly runs an insidious course and is known as subacute (bacterial) endocarditis (SBE).

Infection occurs in the following:

- On valves which have a congenital or acquired defect (usually on the left side of the heart). Right-sided endocarditis is more common in intravenous drug addicts.
- On normal valves (acute infection only).
- On prosthetic valves, when infection may be 'early' (acquired at surgery) or 'late' (following bacteraemia). Infected prosthetic valves often need to be replaced.
- In association with a ventricular septal defect or persistent ductus arteriosus.

## Aetiology

The most common organisms causing endocarditis are:

- *Streptococcus mutans* and *sanguis* (up to 50% of cases). These organisms are normal commensals of the upper respiratory tract; bacteraemia occurs following dental extractions, tonsillectomy and bronchoscopy. However, most patients have no history of recent surgery.
- *Enterococcus faecalis* is implicated in endocarditis particularly following genitourinary or gastrointestinal instrumentation.

- *Staphylococcus aureus.* This often produces an acute fulminating illness, seen particularly in intravenous drug addicts (using dirty needles) and in patients with central venous lines. It is also common in prosthetic valve infections (50%).
- *Uncommon organisms.* Bacteria (*Strep. bovis*) fungi (*Candida albicans*), *Coxiella burnetii* (causative organism of Q fever, p. 472) and *Chlamydia psittaci.*

## Pathology

A mass of fibrin, platelets and infectious organisms forms vegetations along the edges of the valve. Virulent organisms destroy the valve, producing regurgitation and worsening heart failure.

## Clinical features

Symptoms and signs result from:

- Systemic features of infection, such as malaise, fever, night sweats, weight loss and anaemia. Slight splenomegaly is common. Clubbing is rare and occurs late.
- Valve destruction, leading to heart failure and new or changing heart murmurs (in 90% of cases).
- Embolization of vegetations and metastatic abscess formation in the brain, spleen and kidney. Embolization from right-sided endocarditis causes pulmonary infarction and pneumonia.
- Immune complex deposition in blood vessels producing a vasculitis and petechial haemorrhages in the skin, under the nails (splinter haemorrhages) and in the retinae (Roth's spots). Osler's nodes (tender subcutaneous nodules in the fingers) and Janeway lesions (painless erythematous macules on the palms) are uncommon. Immune complex deposition in the joints causes arthralgia and, in the kidney, acute glomerulonephritis. Microscopic haematuria occurs in 70% of cases but renal failure is uncommon.

Endocarditis should always be considered in any patient with a heart murmur and fever.

## Investigation

- Blood cultures must be taken before antibiotics are started. Three sets (i.e. six bottles) taken over 24 hours will identify the organism in 75% of cases. Special culture techniques and serological tests are occasionally necessary if blood cultures are negative and unusual organisms suspected.
- Echocardiography identifies vegetations and underlying valvular dysfunction. Small vegetations may be missed and a normal echocardiogram does not exclude endocarditis. Transoesophageal echocardiography is more sensitive (but not 100%) particularly in cases of suspected prosthetic valve endocarditis.
- Serological tests may be helpful if unusual organisms are suspected e.g. *Coxiella*, *Bartonella*, *Legionella*.
- Chest X-ray may show heart failure or emboli in right-sided endocarditis.
- ECG may show myocardial infarction (emboli) or conduction defects.
- Blood count shows a normochromic, normocytic anaemia with a raised ESR and often a leucocytosis.
- Urine Stix testing shows haematuria in most cases.
- Serum immunoglobulins are increased and complement levels decreased as a result of immune complex formation.

## Management

**Drug therapy** Treatment is with bactericidal antibiotics, given intravenously for the first 2 weeks and by mouth for a further 2–4 weeks. While awaiting the results of blood cultures a combination of intravenous benzylpenicillin and gentamicin is given unless staphylococcal endocarditis is suspected, when vancomycin should be substituted for penicillin. Subsequent treatment depends on the results of blood cultures and the antibiotic sensitivity of the organism. Antibiotic doses are adjusted to ensure adequate bactericidal activity (microbiological assays of minimum bactericidal concentrations). Surgery to replace the valve should be considered when there is severe heart failure, early infection of prosthetic material, worsening renal failure and extensive damage to the valve.

### *Prophylaxis*

Patients at risk of endocarditis should receive antibiotic therapy before undergoing a procedure likely to result in bacteraemia. The choice of antibiotic depends on the procedure and the likelihood of endocarditis.

## Pulmonary heart disease

## Pulmonary hypertension *(K&C p. 808)*

Elevation of the pulmonary artery pressure (pulmonary hypertension) occurs with chronic lung disease, increased pulmonary blood flow (which occurs with atrial septal defect, ventricular septal defect and patent ductus arteriosus), left ventricular failure, mitral stenosis, recurrent pulmonary emboli and primary pulmonary hypertension. The latter is a rare condition of unknown aetiology predominantly affecting young women. In primary disease, medial hypertrophy and intimal fibrosis of the small pulmonary vessels leads to vascular obstruction, increased pulmonary vascular resistance and pulmonary hypertension.

### *Clinical features*

Chest pain, fatigue, dyspnoea and syncope are common symptoms. The physical signs include a right parasternal heave (caused by right ventricular hypertrophy) and a loud pulmonary second sound. In advanced disease there is right heart failure. There are also features of the underlying disease.

### *Investigations*

- Chest X-ray shows enlarged proximal pulmonary arteries which taper distally. It may also reveal the underlying cause (e.g. emphysema, calcified mitral valve).
- ECG shows right ventricular hypertrophy and P pulmonale. Echocardiography shows right ventricular hypertrophy and dilatation, and may reveal the underlying cause of pulmonary hypertension. Pulmonary artery pressure can be measured indirectly with Doppler echocardiography.

## Management

The treatment is that of the cause. In primary pulmonary hypertension there is a progressive downhill course which in some patients can be slowed by a combination of warfarin and oral calcium-channel blockers as pulmonary vasodilators. Continuous (a year or more) intravenous infusions of prostacyclin reduce pulmonary resistance and improve symptoms. However, many patients ultimately require heart and lung transplantation.

# Pulmonary embolism (K&C p. 804)

Pulmonary embolism is a common condition and usually a consequence of thrombosis in the iliofemoral veins (deep venous thrombosis, p. 441). The risk factors for thromboembolism are listed on page 216. Rarely pulmonary embolism results from clot formation in the right atrium in patients with right-sided cardiac failure, particularly if there is atrial fibrillation.

## Pathology

After pulmonary embolism lung tissue is ventilated but not perfused, resulting in impaired gas exchange. A *massive* embolism obstructs the right ventricular outflow tract and therefore suddenly increases pulmonary vascular resistance, causing acute right heart failure. A *small* embolus impacts in a terminal, peripheral pulmonary vessel and may be clinically silent unless it causes pulmonary infarction.

## Clinical features

- Small/medium pulmonary emboli present with dyspnoea, pleuritic chest pain, and haemoptysis if there is pulmonary infarction. On examination the patient may be tachypnoeic and have a pleural rub.
- Massive pulmonary embolism presents as a medical emergency: the patient has severe central chest pain and suddenly becomes shocked, pale and sweaty, with marked tachypnoea and tachycardia. Syncope and death may follow rapidly. On examination the patient is shocked, with central cyanosis. There is elevation of the jugular venous pressure, a right ventricular heave, accentuation of the second heart sound and a gallop rhythm (acute right heart failure).

- Multiple recurrent pulmonary emboli present with symptoms and signs of pulmonary hypertension (see above), developing over weeks to months.

## Investigations

- Chest X-ray, ECG and blood gases may all be normal with small/medium pulmonary emboli and any abnormalities with massive emboli are non-specific. The chest X-ray and ECG are useful to exclude other conditions that may present similarly. The chest X-ray may show decreased vascular markings and a raised hemidiaphragm (caused by loss of lung volume). With pulmonary infarction a late feature is the development of a wedge-shaped opacity adjacent to the pleural edge, sometimes with a pleural effusion. The commonest ECG finding is sinus tachycardia. The features of acute right heart strain may be seen: tall peaked P waves in lead II, right axis deviation and right bundle branch block. Blood gases show hypoxaemia and hypocapnia.
- Plasma D-dimers are a subset of fibrinogen degradation products released into the circulation when a clot begins to dissolve. Undetectable levels exclude a diagnosis of pulmonary embolism.
- Radionuclide lung scan ($\dot{V}/\dot{Q}$ scan) demonstrates areas of ventilated lung with perfusion defects (ventilation–perfusion defects). It is usually the initial diagnostic investigation. Up to 50% of $\dot{V}/\dot{Q}$ scans are non-diagnostic and may be normal, or show matched defects which can also be seen with some chronic lung diseases, e.g. emphysema.
- Ultrasound will detect clots in the pelvic or iliofemoral veins.
- Spiral CT images the pulmonary vessels directly and has approximately 90% sensitivity and specificity for medium/large pulmonary emboli. It is particularly useful if the $\dot{V}/\dot{Q}$ scan is equivocal or if urgent investigation is necessary. This technique is currently unable to exclude small emboli.
- MRI gives similar results and is used if CT is contraindicated.
- Pulmonary angiography is sometimes undertaken if surgery is considered in acute massive embolism. It

shows obstructed vessels or obvious filling defects in the artery.

## Management

Treatment (Emergency Box 9.4) should be started on the basis of clinical suspicion pending investigation.

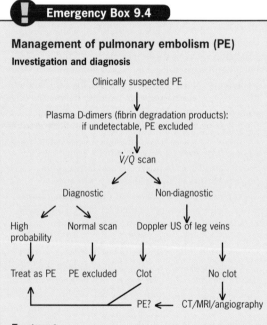

**Emergency Box 9.4**

### Management of pulmonary embolism (PE)

**Investigation and diagnosis**

Clinically suspected PE

↓

Plasma D-dimers (fibrin degradation products):
if undetectable, PE excluded

↓

V̇/Q̇ scan

Diagnostic ← → Non-diagnostic

High probability ← Normal scan — Doppler US of leg veins ← Non-diagnostic

Treat as PE — PE excluded — Clot — No clot

PE? ← CT/MRI/angiography

**Treatment**
60% oxygen if hypoxaemic
Dissolution of the thrombus
  Consider for massive embolism with hypotension and signs of acute right heart strain
  Streptokinase: 250 000 U by i.v. infusion over 30 minutes, followed by 100 000 U/h for 24 h
Analgesia
  Morphine (5–10 mg i.v.) to relieve pain and anxiety
Prevention of further thrombi
  Intravenous heparin and oral warfarin (p. 217)
Intravenous fluids (to raise the filling pressure) ± inotropes for patients presenting with moderate/severe embolism

Anticoagulation is continued for 6 weeks to 6 months depending on the likelihood of recurrence of thromboembolism, and lifelong treatment is indicated for recurrent emboli. Insertion of a vena caval filter is used to prevent further emboli when emboli recur despite adequate anticoagulation, or in high-risk individuals where anticoagulation is contraindicated. Surgery is rarely necessary but may be employed in severe cases of acute massive embolism.

## Chronic cor pulmonale (K&C p. 804)

Cor pulmonale is right heart failure resulting from chronic pulmonary hypertension.

### Aetiology

Chronic obstructive pulmonary disease caused by bronchitis and emphysema is responsible for most cases (Table 9.9). Pulmonary vascular resistance is increased because of destruction of the pulmonary vascular bed and pulmonary vasoconstriction caused by acidosis and hypoxia. Eventually, increased resistance leads to right heart strain and right ventricular failure.

### Treatment

Treatment is directed towards the underlying pulmonary disease as well as right ventricular failure. Acute chest infections must be treated promptly. Oxygen therapy over a long period may reduce established pulmonary hypertension, with an improvement in overall prognosis (p. 455).

429

**Table 9.9**
Causes of cor pulmonale

Intrinsic lung disease, e.g. COPD, pulmonary fibrosis
Recurrent pulmonary emboli
Skeletal abnormalities, e.g. kyphoscoliosis
Hypoventilation, e.g. morbid obesity
Neuromuscular disease, e.g. poliomyelitis, myasthenia gravis
Obstruction, e.g. sleep apnoea syndrome

# Myocardial disease

## Myocarditis (K&C p. 810)

Myocarditis is an inflammation of the myocardium. The most common cause in the UK is viral, particularly Coxsackie virus infection, but it may also occur with diphtheria, rheumatic fever, radiation injury and some drugs.

### Clinical features

Patients present with an acute illness characterized by fever and varying degrees of biventricular failure. Cardiac arrhythmias and pericarditis may also occur.

### Investigations

- Chest X-ray may show cardiac enlargement.
- ECG shows non-specific T-wave and ST changes.
- The diagnosis is supported by demonstration of an increase in serum viral titres and inflammation on cardiac biopsy. The findings rarely influence management and biopsy is not usually performed.

### Management

Treatment is with bed rest and treatment of cardiac failure. The prognosis is generally good.

# Cardiomyopathy (K&C p. 810)

Cardiomyopathies are myocardial disorders that are not secondary to coronary artery disease, hypertension, or congenital, valvular or pericardial abnormalities.

There are four main types:

- Dilated
- Hypertrophic
- Restrictive
- Arrhythmogenic right ventricular.

## Dilated cardiomyopathy (K&C p. 811)

Dilated cardiomyopathy (DCM) is characterized by a dilated left ventricle which contracts poorly. In about 25% of patients it is a familial disease.

## Clinical features

Shortness of breath is usually the first complaint; less often patients present with embolism (from mural thrombus) or arrhythmia. Subsequently there is progressive heart failure with the symptoms and signs of biventricular failure.

## Investigations

- Chest X-ray may show cardiac enlargement.
- ECG is often abnormal. The changes are non-specific and include arrhythmias and T-wave flattening.
- Echocardiography shows dilated ventricles with global hypokinesis (compare with ischaemia with regional contractile impairment).

Other tests such as coronary arteriography, viral and autoimmune screen, and endomyocardial biopsy may be needed to exclude other diseases (Table 9.10) which present with the clinical features of DCM.

## Management

Heart failure and atrial fibrillation are treated in the conventional way (pp. 391, 379). Ventricular tachycardia is not prevented with antiarrhythmic drugs and is best treated with an internal cardioverter–defibrillator. A history of embolization or AF is an indication for anticoagulation. Severe cardiomyopathy is treated with cardiac transplantation.

431

# Hypertrophic cardiomyopathy (*K&C* p. 812)

Hyertrophic cardiomyopathy is characterized by marked ventricular hypertrophy of unknown cause, usually with disproportionate involvement of the interventricular

---

**Table 9.10**
Heart muscle disease presenting with features of DCM

Ischaemia
Hypertension
Congenital heart disease
Peripartum cardiomyopathy
Infections, e.g. cytomegalovirus, HIV
Alcohol
Muscular dystrophy
Amyloidosis
Haemochromatosis

septum. The hypertrophic non-compliant ventricles impair diastolic filling, so that stroke volume is reduced. Most cases are familial, autosomal dominant, and caused by mutations in genes coding for proteins that regulate contraction, e.g. troponin T and β-myosin.

### Clinical features

Patients may be symptom-free or have dyspnoea, angina or syncope. Atrial and ventricular arrhythmias are common; ventricular tachyarrhythmias are the major cause of sudden death, which is most common in adolescence and young adulthood. The carotid pulse is jerky because of rapid ejection and sudden obstruction to the ventricular outflow during systole. An ejection systolic murmur occurs because of left ventricular outflow obstruction, and the pansystolic murmur of functional mitral regurgitation may also be heard.

### Investigations

- ECG is almost always abnormal. A pattern of left ventricular hypertrophy with no discernible cause is diagnostic.
- Echocardiography shows ventricular hypertrophy with disproportionate involvement of the septum.

### Management

The risk of arrhythmias and sudden death is reduced by amiodarone, but survivors of cardiac arrest need to be fitted with an internal defibrillator. Chest pain and dyspnoea are treated with β-blockers and verapamil. In selected cases outflow tract gradients are reduced by surgical resection or alcohol ablation of the septum, or by dual-chamber pacing.

Family members should be screened for evidence of disease by ECG and echocardiography.

## Restrictive cardiomyopathy (K&C p. 814)

The rigid myocardium restricts diastolic ventricular filling and the clinical features resemble those of constrictive pericarditis (see later). In the UK the most common cause is amyloidosis. The ECG, chest X-ray and echocardiogram are often abnormal, but the findings are non-specific. Diagnosis is by cardiac catheterization, which shows characteristic pressure changes. An endomyocardial biopsy may be taken during the catheter procedure, thus providing histological diagnosis. There is no specific treatment and the prognosis is poor, with most patients dying less than a year after diagnosis. Cardiac transplantation is performed in selected cases.

## Arrhythmogenic right ventricular cardiomyopathy (K&C p. 814)

There is progressive fibro-adipose replacement of the wall of the right ventricle. The typical presentation is ventricular tachycardia or sudden death in a young man.

## Pericardial disease

### Acute pericarditis (K&C p. 815)

#### Aetiology

Acute inflammation of the pericardium is usually caused by Coxsackie viral infection or follows acute myocardial infarction. Other causes include uraemia, connective tissue diseases, trauma, tuberculosis and malignancy (breast, lung, leukaemia and lymphoma).

#### Clinical features

There is sharp retrosternal chest pain which is characteristically relieved by leaning forward. Pain may be worse on inspiration and radiate to the neck and shoulders. The cardinal clinical sign is a pericardial friction rub, which may be transient.

#### Diagnosis

The ECG is diagnostic showing ST segment elevation in all the leads except AVR and $V_1$. The elevated ST segments are characteristically concave upwards (convex upwards in infarction) and return towards baseline as inflammation subsides.

#### Management

Treatment is of the underlying disorder plus NSAIDs. Systemic corticosteroids are used in resistant cases.

433

# Pericardial effusion and tamponade (K&C p. 817)

Pericardial effusion is an accumulation of fluid in the pericardial sac which may result from any of the causes of pericarditis. Pericardial tamponade is a medical emergency and occurs when a large amount of pericardial fluid (which has often accumulated rapidly) restricts diastolic ventricular filling and causes a marked reduction in cardiac output.

## Clinical features

The effusion obscures the apex beat and the heart sounds are soft. The signs of pericardial tamponade are hypotension, tachycardia and an elevated jugular venous pressure, which paradoxically rises with inspiration (Kussmaul's sign). There is invariably pulsus paradoxus (a fall in blood pressure of more than 10 mmHg on inspiration). This is the result of increased venous return to the right side of the heart during inspiration. The increased right ventricular volume thus occupies more space within the rigid pericardium and impairs left ventricular filling.

## Investigations

- Chest X-ray shows a large globular heart.
- ECG shows low-voltage complexes.
- Echocardiography is diagnostic, showing an echo-free space around the heart.

## Management

The treatment of tamponade is emergency pericardiocentesis. Pericardial fluid is drained percutaneously by introducing a needle into the pericardial sac. If the effusion recurs, in spite of treatment of the underlying cause, excision of a pericardial segment may be necessary. Fluid is then absorbed through the pleural and mediastinal lymphatics.

# Constrictive pericarditis (K&C p. 818)

In the UK most cases of constrictive pericarditis are idiopathic in origin or result from intrapericardial haemorrhage during heart surgery. Tuberculous infection is no longer the most common cause.

## Clinical features

The heart becomes encased within a rigid fibrotic pericardial sac which prevents adequate diastolic filling of the ventricles. The clinical features resemble those of right-sided cardiac failure, with jugular venous distension, dependent oedema, hepatomegaly and ascites. Kussmaul's sign (JVP rises paradoxically with inspiration) is usually present and there may be pulsus paradoxus, atrial fibrillation and, on auscultation, a pericardial knock caused by rapid ventricular filling.

## Investigations

A chest X-ray shows a normal heart size and pericardial calcification (best seen on the lateral film). Diagnosis is made by CT, which shows pericardial thickening and calcification.

## Management

Treatment is by surgical excision of the pericardium.

# Systemic hypertension

The level of blood pressure can be said to be abnormal when it is associated with a clear increase in morbidity and mortality from heart disease, stroke and renal failure. This level varies with age, sex, race and country. The definition varies, but recent guidelines from the USA recommend a definition of hypertension as over 140/90 mmHg, based on at least two readings on separate occasions. The validity of a single blood pressure measurement is unclear (blood pressure rises acutely in certain situations, e.g. visiting the doctor) and usually several readings are required to confirm a diagnosis of hypertension. Occasionally, ambulatory blood pressure monitoring (blood pressure measured over a 24-hour period using a non-invasive technique) is used if there is doubt as to the level of blood pressure.

## Aetiology

**Essential hypertension** More than 90% of cases of hypertension have no known underlying cause, and the terms 'primary' or 'essential' hypertension are used. Several factors may play an aetiological role:

- Genetic factors
- Low birthweight
- Obesity
- High alcohol intake
- High salt intake – controversial
- Insulin resistance (hyperinsulinaemia, glucose intolerance, low HDL cholesterol and central obesity – sometimes known as syndrome X).

**Secondary hypertension** This should always be considered, particularly in those presenting under the age of 35. Causes of secondary hypertension are the following:

- Renal disease, which accounts for over 80% of cases of secondary hypertension: chronic glomerulonephritis, reflux nephropathy, congenital polycystic kidneys and renal artery stenosis are the diseases usually involved
- Endocrine disease (p. 590): Conn's syndrome, Cushing's syndrome, phaeochromocytoma and acromegaly
- Coarctation of the aorta (narrowing of the aorta)
- Pre-eclampsia occurring in the third trimester of pregnancy
- Drugs, including oestrogen-containing oral contraceptives, other steroids and vasopressin.

436

## Clinical features

Hypertension is generally asymptomatic, although malignant or accelerated hypertension (usually BP > 200/140 mmHg) may present with characteristic symptoms. These include visual impairment, nausea, vomiting, fits, headaches or symptoms of acute cardiac failure. Secondary causes of hypertension may be suggested by specific features, such as attacks of sweating and tachycardia in phaeochromocytoma.

**Examination** In most patients the only finding is high blood pressure, but in others signs relating to the cause (e.g. abdominal bruit in renal artery stenosis, delayed femoral pulses in coarctation of the aorta) or the end-organ effects of hypertension may be present, e.g. loud second heart sound, left ventricular heave, fourth heart sound in hypertensive heart disease, and retinal abnormalities. The latter are graded according to severity:

- Grade 1 – increased tortuosity and reflectiveness of the retinal arteries (silver wiring)
- Grade 2 – grade 1 plus arteriovenous nipping
- Grade 3 – grade 2 plus flame-shaped haemorrhages and soft 'cotton wool' exudates
- Grade 4 – grade 3 plus papilloedema.

## Investigations

Investigations are carried out to identify end-organ damage and those patients with secondary causes of hypertension.

- Chest X-ray may show heart failure. Rib notching indicates coarctation of the aorta.
- ECG may show evidence of left ventricular hypertrophy or myocardial ischaemia.
- Serum urea and electrolytes may show evidence of renal impairment, in which case more specific renal investigations are indicated. Hypokalaemia occurs in Conn's syndrome.
- Urine Stix testing is performed to look for haematuria and proteinuria, which may indicate renal disease (either the cause or the effect of hypertension).

Young patients with hypertension (< 35 years) or those where a secondary cause is suspected (e.g. from clinical examination or abnormal baseline investigations) should undergo further investigation, e.g. urinary/plasma catecholamines for phaeochromocytoma, investigation for renovascular hypertension (p. 331).

## Management

Treatment of moderate-to-severe hypertension reduces the incidence of stroke, cardiac events and renal damage but has less effect on coronary artery disease. General measures include weight reduction, reduction of heavy alcohol consumption, no added salt diet and regular exercise.

437

Systemic hypertension

***Drug therapy*** Indications for drug treatment are:
- Sustained systolic blood pressure (BP) > 160 mmHg, or sustained diastolic BP = 100 mmHg.
- Sustained systolic BP > 140 mmHg or sustained diastolic BP > 90 mmHg if there is evidence of end-organ damage or other risk factors, e.g. diabetes, or age > 60 years.

A large number of drugs may be used in treatment and the most appropriate 'first-line' treatment depends on the basis of efficacy, tolerance and co-morbidity, e.g. β-blockers or calcium-channel blockers for patients with coexistent angina, ACE inhibitors for patients with diabetic nephropathy. Single agents are used initially, but combination treatment may be needed in patients not controlled with one drug. Particularly effective combinations include an ACE inhibitor or β-blocker with a diuretic, and the combination of a calcium antagonist with a β-blocker.

*Diuretics* increase renal sodium and water excretion and directly dilate arterioles. Loop diuretics, e.g. furosemide (frusemide), and thiazide diuretics, e.g. bendroflumethiazide (bendrofluazide), are equally effective in lowering blood pressure, although thiazides are usually preferred, as the duration of action is longer, the diuresis is not so severe and they are cheaper. The major concern with thiazide diuretics is their adverse metabolic effects: increased serum cholesterol, hypokalaemia, hyperuricaemia (may precipitate gout) and impairment of glucose tolerance.

*β-Adrenergic blocking agents* The mechanism of action of these agents is unclear. Although they reduce the force of cardiac contraction and renin production, they probably act predominantly via the central nervous system. There are a wide range of β-blocking agents with different properties, such as cardioselectivity, intrinsic sympathomimetic activity and lipid solubility. Complications include bradycardia, bronchospasm, cold extremities, fatigue and weakness.

*ACE inhibitors*, e.g. captopril, enalapril lisinopril, and ramipril, block the conversion of angiotensin I to angiotensin II, which is a potent vasoconstrictor, and block degradation of bradykinin, which is a vasodilator. Side-effects include first-dose hypotension and cough, proteinuria, rashes and leucopenia in high doses. ACE inhibitors are contraindicated in renal artery stenosis because inhibition of the renin–angiotensin system in this instance may lead to loss of renal blood flow and infarction of the kidney.

*Angiotensin II receptor antagonists*, e.g. losartan, valsartan, irbesartan and candesartan, selectively block receptors for angiotensin II. They share some of the actions of ACE inhibitors and are useful in patients who cannot tolerate ACE inhibitors because of cough.

*Calcium antagonists*, e.g. amlodipine and nifedipine, are increasingly used and act predominantly by dilatation of peripheral arterioles. Side-effects are few and include bradycardia and cardiac conduction defects (verapamil and diltiazem), headaches, flushing and fluid retention.

*Other agents* α-Blocking agents (e.g. doxazosin), hydralazine, and centrally acting agents (e.g. clonidine, moxonidine) may be indicated in specific circumstances.

## Management of severe hypertension

Patients with severe hypertension (diastolic BP > 140 mmHg) or those with severe hypertensive complications such as encephalopathy or cardiac failure should be admitted to hospital for treatment. The aim should be to reduce the diastolic blood pressure slowly (over 24–48 hours) to about 100–110 mmHg and this is usually achieved with oral antihypertensives, e.g. atenolol or amlodipine. Sublingual and intravenous antihypertensives are not recommended because they may produce a precipitous fall in blood pressure leading to cerebral infarction.

When rapid control of blood pressure is required (e.g. aortic dissection), the agent of choice is intravenous sodium nitroprusside (starting dose 0.3 μg/kg/min, i.e. 100 mg nitroprusside in 250 mL saline at 2–5 mL/h). Alternatively, intravenous labetolol can be used.

# Arterial and venous disease

## Aortic aneurysms (K&C P. 829)

An aneurysm refers to an increase in 50% or greater of the normal diameter of the vessel. Aortic aneurysms are usually abdominal and result from atheroma.

***Abdominal*** Abdominal aortic aneurysms may be asymptomatic and found as a pulsating mass on abdominal examination or as calcification on a plain X-ray. An expanding aneurysm may cause epigastric or back pain. A ruptured aortic aneurysm is a surgical emergency presenting with epigastric pain radiating to the back, and hypovolaemic shock. Diagnosis is by ultrasonography or CT scan. Surgical replacement of the aneurysmal segment with a prosthetic graft is indicated for a symptomatic aneurysm or large asymptomatic aneurysms (> 5 cm).

***Thoracic*** Cystic medial necrosis and atherosclerosis are the usual causes of thoracic aneurysms. Cardiovascular syphilis is no longer a common cause. Thoracic aneurysms may be asymptomatic, cause pressure on local structures (causing back pain, dysphagia and cough) or result in aortic regurgitation if the aortic root is involved.

***Dissecting aortic aneurysm*** Aortic dissection results from a tear in the intima: blood under high pressure creates a false lumen in the diseased media. Typically there is an abrupt onset of severe, tearing central chest pain, radiating through to the back. Involvement of branch arteries may produce neurological signs, absent pulses and unequal blood pressure in the arms. The chest X-ray shows a widened mediastinum and the diagnosis is confirmed by CT scanning and transoesophageal echocardiography or MRI. Management involves urgent control of blood pressure (p. 439) and surgical repair for proximal aortic dissection.

## Raynaud's disease and phenomenon (K&C p. 831)

Raynaud's phenomenon consists of intermittent spasm in the arteries supplying the fingers and toes. It is usually precipitated by cold and relieved by heat. There is initial pallor (resulting from vasoconstriction) followed by cyanosis and, finally, redness from hyperaemia. Raynaud's disease (no underlying disorder) occurs most commonly in young women and must be differentiated from secondary causes of Raynaud's phenomenon, e.g. connective tissue diseases and β-blockers. Treatment is by keeping the hands and feet warm, stopping smoking and stopping β-blockers. Medical treatment includes oral nifedipine and occasionally prostacyclin infusions. Lumbar sympathectomy may help lower limb symptoms.

## Venous disease (K&C p. 831)

**Superficial thrombophlebitis** This usually occurs in the leg. The vein is painful, tender and hard, with overlying redness. Treatment is with simple analgesia, e.g. NSAIDs. Anticoagulation is not necessary as embolism does not occur.

**Deep venous thrombosis** Thrombosis can occur in any vein, but those of the pelvis and leg are the most common sites. The risk factors for deep vein thrombosis (DVT) are listed on page 216.

### Clinical features
DVT is often asymptomatic but the leg may be warm and swollen, with calf tenderness and superficial venous distension. The differential diagnosis includes ruptured Baker's cyst, oedema from other causes and cellulitis.

441

### Investigations
Diagnosis of iliofemoral thrombosis is made by Doppler ultrasonography. This method is not reliable for calf vein thrombosis, which is diagnosed by venography.

### Management
This is discussed on page 217.

The main aim of therapy is to prevent pulmonary embolism, and all patients with thrombi above the knee must be anticoagulated. Anticoagulation for below-knee thrombi is controversial but is usually recommended for

6 weeks to reduce proximal extension. Anticoagulation is initially with heparin and subsequently with warfarin, continued for 3 months unless there had been a definite risk factor prior to presentation, e.g. bed rest, when treatment is usually for 4 weeks. Thrombolytic therapy is occasionally used for patients with a large iliofemoral thrombosis.

The main complications of DVT are pulmonary embolus, post-thrombotic syndrome (permanent pain, swelling, oedema and sometimes venous eczema may result from destruction of the deep-vein valves) and recurrence of thrombosis. Elastic support stockings are used for the post-thrombotic syndrome.

# 10

# Respiratory disease

## Symptoms of respiratory disease

The common symptoms of respiratory disease are cough, sputum production, chest pain (p. 366), breathlessness, haemoptysis and wheeze.

**Cough** is a non-specific symptom and the most common manifestation of lower respiratory tract disease. It is initiated by stimulation of cough receptors on the epithelium of the upper and lower respiratory tract and in the pericardium, oesophagus and diaphragm. Cough receptors are stimulated by mechanical (e.g. touch and displacement) and chemical (e.g. noxious fumes) stimuli and impulses carried by afferent nerves to a 'cough centre' in the medulla. This generates efferent signals to expiratory musculature to generate a cough. Estimating the duration of cough is useful in making a diagnosis (Table 10.1).

**Table 10.1**
Causes of cough

| Acute<br><3 weeks' duration | Chronic<br>>3 weeks' duration |
|---|---|
| Upper respiratory tract infection<br>Exacerbation of COPD<br>Sinusitis<br>Allergic rhinitis | Postnasal drip*<br>Asthma*<br>Gastro-oesophageal reflux disease*<br>Lung airway disease: COPD, bronchiectasis, tumour, foreign body<br>Lung parenchymal disease: interstitial lung disease, lung abscess<br>Drugs: ACE inhibitors |

* These causes are responsible for 90% of cases of chronic cough; and responsible for 99% of cases who are non-smokers, not taking ACE inhibitors and with a normal chest X-ray
COPD, chronic obstructive pulmonary disease; ACE, angiotensin-converting enzyme

Postnasal drip is the most common cause of persistent cough. Underlying reasons for postnasal drip include rhinitis, acute nasopharyngitis and sinusitis. Symptoms of postnasal drip, other than cough, include nasal discharge, a sensation of liquid dripping back into the throat, and frequent throat clearing. Cough due to asthma is frequently accompanied by intermittent wheezing and breathlessness but it may be the only symptom, when it is typically worse at night, on waking and after exercise. Similarly, gastro-oesophageal reflux disease may present with a cough as the only symptom. A chronic cough, sometimes accompanied by sputum production, is common in smokers; however, a worsening cough may be the presenting symptom of bronchial carcinoma and needs investigation.

**Dyspnoea** This is the subjective sensation of shortness of breath. *Orthopnoea* is breathlessness that occurs when lying flat and is the result both of abdominal contents pushing the diaphragm into the thorax and of redistribution of blood from the lower extremities to the lungs. *Paroxysmal nocturnal dyspnoea* is a manifestation of left heart failure: the patient wakes up gasping for breath and finds some relief by sitting upright. The mechanism is similar to orthopnoea, but because sensory awareness is depressed during sleep, severe interstitial pulmonary oedema can accumulate.

The speed of onset of breathlessness is useful when formulating a differential diagnosis (Table 10.2). The clinical history and examination will often suggest a probable cause, particularly with sudden and acute breathlessness. In acute breathlessness appropriate initial investigations include a chest X-ray, pulse oximetry and sometimes arterial blood gases, electrocardiogram, full blood count, serum urea and electrolytes, and blood glucose. Pulmonary embolism can be a difficult diagnosis to make and chest X-ray, blood gases and ECG may be normal. Simple lung function tests and a chest X-ray are the initial investigations for most patients with chronic breathlessness.

**Wheeze** Wheezing is the result of airflow limitation of any cause. It may be due to localized obstruction of the

**Table 10.2**
Differential diagnosis of dyspnoea

| Sudden | Acute: over hours | Over days/months | Intermittent |
|---|---|---|---|
| Upper airway obstruction: inhaled foreign body anaphylaxis Pneumothorax Pulmonary embolism Asthma | Asthma Pneumonia Pulmonary oedema Extrinsic allergic alveolitis Cardiac tamponade | Asthma COPD Diffuse parenchymal lung disease Heart failure Pleural effusion Cancer of the bronchus/trachea Anaemia | Asthma Pulmonary oedema |

COPD, chronic obstructive pulmonary disease

airways, e.g. cancer, foreign body, or to generalized obstruction, of which the commonest causes are asthma and chronic obstructive pulmonary disease. Asthma is a common cause of wheezing and considered likely when patients present with episodic wheezing, cough and dyspnoea which responds favourably to inhaled bronchodilators. Wheeze should be distinguished from stridor which is a harsh inspiratory wheezing sound caused by obstruction of the trachea or major bronchi, e.g. by tumour.

**Haemoptysis** (coughing blood) requires thorough investigation. The common causes are bronchiectasis, bronchial carcinoma, pulmonary infarction, bronchitis and lung infections including pneumonia, abscess and tuberculosis. Pulmonary oedema is associated with the production of pink frothy sputum. Rust-coloured sputum may occur with pneumococcal pneumonia but haemoptysis should not be attributed to infection without investigation. Less common causes include benign tumour, bleeding disorder and, rarely, Wegener's granulomatosis (p. 486) and Goodpasture's syndrome (p. 317). A chest X-ray should be performed in all patients, and subsequent investigations (e.g. bronchoscopy, CT of the thorax, isotope lung scan) decided from the history and examination.

Massive haemoptysis (more than 200 mL in 24 h) is often due to bronchiectasis, TB or cancer. It may be life-threatening due to asphyxiation and is an indication for hospital admission. The initial management includes administration of oxygen, placement of a large-bore intravenous catheter, blood samples (for full blood count, clotting screen, urea and electrolytes), arterial blood gases and chest X-ray. There should be early referral to a respiratory physician and thoracic surgeon.

**Chest pain** (p. 366) The most common chest pain encountered in respiratory disease is a localized sharp pain, typically made worse by deep breathing or coughing. It is commonly referred to as pleuritic pain and is most commonly caused by infection or by pleural irritation from a pulmonary embolism.

# Simple investigations of respiratory disease

## Sputum (K&C p. 843 & p. 846)

Sputum samples are obtained during the investigation of pneumonia, tuberculosis and bronchial carcinoma. A 5% saline nebulizer will encourage productive coughing if sputum is difficult to obtain. Inspection of the sputum may indicate infection (yellow/green) or haemoptysis (blood-stained). Sputum is commonly sent for microbiology (Gram stain and culture, Ziehl–Nielsen stain) and cytology (malignant cells).

## Chest X-ray (K&C p.847)

Routine films are taken postero-anteriorly (PA), i.e. the film is placed in front of the patient with the X-ray source behind. AP films are taken only in patients who are unable to stand; the cardiac outline appears bigger and the scapulae cannot be moved out of the way. The following should be noted:

- Patient's name and date of the film
- Contour of diaphragm and outline of rib cage (? pleural effusion, pneumothorax, raised hemidiaphragm, air under the diaphragm)
- Bony structure (ribs, clavicles, spine)
- Size, shape and position of the heart (enlarged heart is > 50% of maximum distance between ribs)
- Position of trachea (? deviated from midline; a rotated patient will also make the trachea look deviated)
- Mediastinum (? widened, ? lymphadenopathy)
- Hilar shadows (? enlarged pulmonary arteries and veins)
- Lungs (? opacities, consolidation, fluid, nodules).

## Respiratory function tests (K&C p. 849)

Respiratory function tests can be simple outpatient investigations carried out to assess airflow limitation and lung volumes. The normal values vary for age, sex and height, and between individuals.

**Peak expiratory flow rate (PEFR)** is measured with a peak flow meter. This records the maximum expiratory flow rate during a forced expiration after full inspiration. It is useful in detecting airflow limitation and in monitoring the response to treatment of acute asthma. It is simple to perform and many patients will monitor their own PEFR at home.

**Forced expiratory volume (FEV) and forced vital capacity (FVC)** are measured with a spirometer. The patient exhales as fast and as long as possible from a full inspiration; the volume expired in the first second is the $FEV_1$ and the total volume expired is the FVC. The ratio $FEV_1 : FVC$ is a measure of airflow limitation and is normally about 75%.

- Airflow limitation: $FEV_1 : FVC < 75\%$
- Restrictive lung disease: $FEV_1 : FVC > 75\%$.

More sophisticated techniques allow the measurement of total lung capacity (TLC) and residual volume (RV). These are increased in obstructive lung disease, e.g. asthma or COPD, because of air trapping, and reduced in lung fibrosis. Transfer factor ($T_{CO}$) measures the transfer of a low concentration of added carbon monoxide in the inspired air to haemoglobin. The transfer coefficient ($K_{CO}$) is the value corrected for differences in lung volume. Gas transfer is reduced early on in emphysema and lung fibrosis.

Assessment of lung function is also made by measuring arterial blood gases (p. 737) and with exercise tests to assess walking distance in a 6-minute period.

## Arterial blood gases and pulse oximetry
(*K&C* p. 852)
See page 516.

# Diseases of the upper respiratory tract

## The common cold (acute coryza) (*K&C* p. 856)
The common cold is caused by infection with one of the many strains of rhinovirus. Spread is by droplets and close

personal contact. After an incubation period of 12 hours to 5 days the major symptoms are malaise, slight pyrexia, a sore throat and a watery nasal discharge, which becomes mucopurulent after a few days. Treatment is symptomatic. The differential diagnosis is mainly from rhinitis.

## Sinusitis (K&C p. 857)

Sinusitis is an infection of one of the paranasal sinuses (maxillary, frontal or ethmoid) and may complicate allergic rhinitis or an upper respiratory tract infection (caused by mucosal oedema and blockage of the ostium). Acute infections are usually caused by *Streptococcus pneumoniae* or *Haemophilus influenzae*. Symptoms are frontal headache, facial pain and tenderness, and nasal discharge. The diagnosis is usually clinical and treatment is with antibiotics, e.g. cefaclor, and nasal treatment with decongestants, e.g. xylometazoline. Rare complications include local and cerebral abscesses. Chronic sinusitis can be a cause of headaches.

## Rhinitis (K&C p. 857)

The symptoms of rhinitis are sneezing, a watery nasal discharge and nasal blockage. *Perennial rhinitis* occurs throughout the year and may be allergic (the allergens are similar to those for asthma) or non-allergic. Some of these patients develop nasal polyps which may cause nasal obstruction, loss of smell and taste, and mouth breathing. *Seasonal allergic rhinitis* (hay fever) occurs during the summer months and is caused by allergy to grass and tree pollen and a variety of mould spores (e.g. *Aspergillus fumigatus*) which grow on cultivated plants. The diagnosis of rhinitis is clinical. Skin-prick testing or measurement of specific serum IgE antibody against the particular antigen (RAST test) in conjunction with a detailed clinical history will identify causal antigens. The management involves avoidance of allergens if practical, antihistamines, e.g. cetirizine tablets, decongestants and topical steroids, e.g. beclometasone spray twice daily. A 2-week course of low-dose oral prednisolone (5–10 mg daily) may be necessary when other treatments fail.

# Acute pharyngitis (K&C p. 860)

Viruses, particularly from the adenovirus group, are the most common cause of acute pharyngitis. Symptoms are a sore throat and fever which are self-limiting and only require symptomatic treatment. More persistent and severe pharyngitis may imply bacterial infection, often secondary invaders, of which the most common organisms are haemolytic *Streptococcus*, *Haemophilus influenzae* and *Staphylococcus aureus*. This requires antibiotic treatment such as oral cefaclor.

# Acute laryngotracheobronchitis (K&C p. 860)

This is usually the result of infection with one of the parainfluenza viruses or measles virus. Symptoms are most severe in children under 3 years of age. Inflammatory oedema involving the larynx causes a hoarse voice, barking cough (croup) and stridor. Tracheitis produces a burning retrosternal pain. Treatment is with oxygen and inhaled steam; tracheostomy is needed in severe cases.

# Influenza (K&C p. 860)

The influenza virus belongs to the orthomyxovirus group and exists in two main forms, A and B. The surface of the virion is coated with haemagglutinin (H) and an enzyme, neuraminidase (N), which are necessary for attachment to the host respiratory epithelium. Human immunity develops against the H and N antigens. Influenza A has the capacity to undergo antigenic 'shift', and major changes in the H and N antigens are associated with pandemic infections which may cause millions of deaths world-wide. Minor antigenic 'drifts' are associated with less severe epidemics.

## Clinical features

After an incubation period of 1–3 days there is an abrupt onset of fever, myalgia, headache, sore throat and dry cough, which may last several weeks.

## Diagnosis

Laboratory diagnosis is not always necessary, but serology shows a fourfold rise in antibody titre over a 2-week period or the virus can be demonstrated in throat or nasal secretion.

## Management
Treatment is usually symptomatic (aspirin, bed rest, maintenance of fluid intake), together with antibiotics for individuals with chronic bronchitis, or heart or renal disease. Neuraminidase inhibitors, e.g. zanamivir and oseltamivir, shorten the duration of symptoms in patients with influenza. They are recommended in the UK for patients over the age of 65 years with suspected influenza and 'at-risk' adults (i.e. with co-morbid disease).

## Complications
Pneumonia is the most common complication. This is either viral or the result of secondary infection with bacteria, of which *Staphylococcus aureus* is the most serious, with a mortality rate of up to 20%.

## Prophylaxis
Influenza vaccine is prepared from current strains. It is effective in 70% of people and lasts for about a year. It is recommended for all individuals over 65 years of age, and also for younger people with chronic heart or lung disease, diabetes mellitus, chronic renal failure, immunosuppressed individuals and medical staff during a pandemic.

# Inhalation of foreign bodies (K&P p. 861)
Children inhale foreign bodies – frequently peanuts – more often than adults. In adults inhalation is usually associated with a depressed conscious level, such as after an alcoholic binge. A large object may totally occlude the airways and rapidly result in death. Smaller objects impact more peripherally (usually in the right main bronchus, because it is more vertical than the left) and cause choking or persistent wheeze, or patients may present at a later stage with persistent suppurative pneumonia or lung abscess. In an emergency the foreign body is dislodged from the airway using the Heimlich manoeuvre: the subject is gripped from behind with the arms around the upper abdomen, a sharp forceful squeeze pushes the diaphragm into the thorax and

the rapid airflow generated may be sufficient to force the foreign body out of the trachea or bronchus. In the non-emergency situation bronchoscopy is used to remove the foreign body.

# Diseases of the lower respiratory tract

## Acute bronchitis (K&C p. 861)

Acute bronchitis is usually viral but may be complicated by bacterial infection, particularly in smokers and in patients with chronic airflow limitation. Symptoms are cough, retrosternal discomfort, chest tightness and wheezing, which usually resolve spontaneously over 4–8 days.

## Chronic obstructive pulmonary disease – COPD (K&C p. 862)

COPD is a group of disorders characterized by a poorly reversible limitation of airflow that is usually progressive and associated with a persistent inflammatory response of the lungs. The term encompasses chronic bronchitis accompanied by the hypersecretion of mucus, and emphysema with destruction of alveolar walls. Chronic bronchitis is defined *symptomatically* as cough productive of sputum on most days for at least 3 months of the year for more than 1 year. Emphysema is a *pathological diagnosis* and is defined as dilatation and destruction of the lung tissue distal to the terminal bronchioles. Although it has been suggested that these definitions separate patients into two different clinical groups (the 'pink puffers' with predominant emphysema and the 'blue bloaters' with predominant chronic bronchitis), most have both emphysema and chronic bronchitis, irrespective of the clinical signs.

### Epidemiology

COPD develops over many years and patients are rarely symptomatic before middle age. It is common (18% of male and 14% of female smokers) in the UK, where it is one of the leading causes of lost working days.

## Pathology

In chronic bronchitis there is airway narrowing, and hence airflow limitation, as a result of hypertrophy and hyperplasia of mucus-secreting glands of the bronchial tree, bronchial wall inflammation and mucosal oedema. The epithelial cell layer may ulcerate and, when the ulcers heal, squamous epithelium may replace columnar epithelium (squamous metaplasia).

Emphysematous changes lead to loss of elastic recoil, which normally keeps airways open during expiration; this is associated with expiratory airflow limitation and air trapping.

## Aetiology and pathogenesis

- *Smoking* is the dominant causal agent. Cigarette smoke activates macrophages and airway epithelial cells in the respiratory tract, which release neutrophil chemotactic factors, including interleukin-8 and leukotriene $B_4$. Neutrophils and macrophages then release proteases that break down connective tissue in the lung parenchyma resulting in emphysema, and also stimulate mucus hypersecretion. Proteases are normally counteracted by protease inhibitors, including $\alpha_1$-antitrypsin, but in COPD the balance is tipped in favour of proteolysis. In contrast to asthma (see p. 464) the bronchiole wall infiltrate is predominantly CD8+ (cytotoxic) T cells. The role of cytotoxic T cells is not yet clear.
- *Atmospheric pollution* plays a minor role compared to smoking.
- $\alpha_1$-Antitrypsin deficiency (p. 147) is a rare cause of early-onset emphysema.

## Clinical features

The characteristic symptoms of COPD are cough with the production of sputum, wheeze and breathlessness following many years of a smoker's cough. Frequent infective exacerbations occur, giving purulent sputum. On examination the patient with severe disease is breathless at rest, with prolonged expiration and using the accessory muscles of respiration; chest expansion is poor and the lungs are hyperinflated. There may be a wheeze or quiet breath sounds. In 'pink puffers' breathlessness is the predominant problem; they are not cyanosed. 'Blue bloaters' hypoventilate; they are cyanosed, may be oedematous and have features of $CO_2$ retention (warm peripheries with a bounding pulse, flapping tremor of the outstretched hands and confusion in severe cases).

## Investigations

The diagnosis is usually clinical. There is a history of breathlessness and sputum production in a lifetime smoker.

- Lung function tests. The ratio of $FEV_1$ to FVC is reduced (< 70%) and the PEFR is low. Some patients have partially reversible airflow limitation with an increase in $FEV_1$ (usually < 15%) following inhalation of a $\beta_2$ agonist. Lung volumes are normal or increased, and the loss of alveoli with emphysema results in a decreased gas transfer coefficient of carbon monoxide.
- Chest X-ray. Typical features are hyperinflation indicated by a low flat diaphragm and a long narrow heart shadow. There are reduced peripheral lung markings and bullae, although the chest X-ray may be normal.
- Haemoglobin and PCV may be high as a result of persistent hypoxaemia and secondary polycythaemia (p. 194).
- Arterial blood gases may be normal or show hypoxia and hypercapnia in advanced cases.

## Complications
- Respiratory failure (p. 515)
- Cor pulmonale, i.e. right heart failure secondary to lung disease (p. 429).

## Management

**Cessation of smoking**  The most important aspect of management is to persuade the patient to stop smoking, which is the only measure that will slow the rate of deterioration. Smoking withdrawal clinics, nicotine replacement (gum, transdermal patch, or inhaler) or bupropion tablets may help.

***Bronchodilators*** Drug therapy is similar to that for asthma (p. 467). Inhaled $\beta_2$ agonists and the anticholinergic agent ipratropium bromide may produce symptomatic improvement even with little change in lung function tests.

***Corticosteroids*** Assessment of reversibility is made with a 2-week course of oral prednisolone (30 mg daily), with measurement of lung function before and after the treatment period. If there is objective evidence of benefit (> 15% improvement in $FEV_1$) oral steroids are gradually reduced and replaced with inhaled steroids.

***Prevention of infection*** Acute exacerbations of COPD are commonly due to bacterial or viral infection. Patients should receive influenza and pneumococcal vaccine.

***Oxygen*** Long-term domiciliary oxygen therapy will reduce mortality if given for 19 hours per day (every day) at a flow rate of 1–3 L/min via nasal prongs to increase arterial oxygen saturation to > 90%. It is prescribed to patients who no longer smoke and who have an $FEV_1$ < 1.5 L/min and a $P_aO_2$ < 7.3 kPa.

***Additional treatments*** include venesection for polycythaemia, diuretics for oedema, and exercise training to improve sense of well-being and breathlessness.

## Acute exacerbation of COPD

Patients with COPD are prone to acute exacerbations which are diagnosed on the basis of increased breathlessness, wheeze and production of increased volume of purulent sputum. The major complication is respiratory failure. Exacerbations are usually the result of a superimposed viral or bacterial (often *Haemophilus influenzae*) respiratory tract infection and are treated in a similar manner to asthma (p. 470). However, these patients often depend on a degree of hypoxaemia to maintain respiratory drive and therefore, if oxygen is necessary, low concentrations (24%) are given, via a Venturi mask (fixed-performance mask), so as not to reduce respiratory drive. The oxygen concentration may be increased in increments (28% and then 35%) if clinical examination and repeated arterial blood gases do not show hypoventilation and carbon dioxide retention. Salbutamol and ipratropium bromide are given via an air-driven nebulizer. Antibiotics, e.g. cefaclor or co-amoxiclav, should be given promptly for all exacerbations and patients should be encouraged to cough up sputum, initially with the help of a physiotherapist. Antibiotic treatment may be modified depending on sputum culture results. Exacerbations of COPD are occasionally the result of pneumothorax, heart failure or pulmonary embolism, and these must be considered and excluded. Some patients with an acute exacerbation and respiratory failure will require respiratory support; non-invasive positive-pressure ventilation (NIPPV) is often used (p. 517).

## Prognosis

Fifty per cent of patients with severe breathlessness due to COPD die within 5 years.

# Obstructive sleep apnoea (K&C p. 869)

Obstructive sleep apnoea (OSA) is characterized by repetitive apnoea (cessation of breathing for 10 seconds or more) as a result of obstruction of the upper airway during sleep.

## Epidemiology

OSA affects about 2% of the population and is most common in overweight middle-aged men. It can also occur in children, particularly those with enlarged tonsils.

## Aetiology

Apnoea occurs if the upper airway at the back of the throat is sucked closed when the patient breathes in. This occurs during sleep because the muscles that hold the airway open are hypotonic. Airway closure continues until the patient is woken up by the struggle to breathe against a blocked throat. Contributing factors include alcohol ingestion before sleep, obesity and COPD. It is more common in hypothyroidism and acromegaly.

## Clinical features

The major symptoms are loud snoring, apnoeas witnessed by bed partners, and excessive daytime sleepiness, which may lead to impairment of work performance and driving.

Other symptoms are irritability, personality change, morning headaches, impotence and nocturnal choking. Patients with sleep apnoea have an increased risk of hypertension, heart failure, myocardial infarction and stroke.

## Diagnosis

*Overnight oximetry* (transcutaneous measurement of oxygen saturation) shows frequent falls in arteriolar oxygen saturation in some, but not all, patients.

*Polysomnography* is a detailed sleep study performed in a sleep laboratory and provides a definitive diagnosis. It includes measurement of sleep quality, nasal and oral airflow, thoracoabdominal movements and arterial oxygen saturation. The diagnosis of sleep apnoea/hypopnoea is confirmed if there are more than 15 apnoeas or hypopnoeas in any 1 hour of sleep.

## Management
- Predisposing factors, e.g. obesity, tonsillar hypertrophy and facial deformities, should be corrected. Alcohol and sedatives should be avoided.
- CPAP (continuous positive airway pressure) to the airway via a tight-fitting nasal mask – nasal CPAP – during sleep keeps the pharyngeal walls open and is a very effective treatment.

457

## Bronchiectasis (K&C p. 869)
Bronchiectasis is defined as permanent dilatation of the bronchi. It may be localized to a lobe or generalized throughout the bronchial tree. There is impaired clearance of bronchial secretions with secondary bacterial infection.

## Aetiology
Cystic fibrosis (p. 459) is the most common cause in developed countries. Other causes are:

- *Idiopathic* in which there is progressive bronchiectasis with no underlying cause.
- *Inflammatory*. Infective processes, e.g. measles, whooping cough, *Klebsiella* pneumonia, may damage

and weaken the bronchial wall, leading to dilatation and ciliary damage.

- *Obstruction.* Proximal obstruction of an airway, e.g. inhaled foreign body, enlarged tuberculous lymph nodes, leads to distal accumulation of secretions which then become infected, resulting in localized bronchiectasis.

- *Congenital factors.* Other than cystic fibrosis, causes include Kartagener's syndrome (bronchiectasis associated with immotile cilia, transposition of viscera and sinusitis) and immunoglobulin deficiencies which lead to recurrent infections.

## Epidemiology

Most cases arise in childhood, but the incidence has decreased in all age groups with effective antibiotic treatment of pneumonia.

## Clinical features

Cough and sputum production are the most common symptoms. In severe bronchiectasis there is production of copious amounts of thick, foul-smelling green sputum. Other symptoms are haemoptysis (which may be massive and life-threatening), breathlessness and wheeze. On examination there is clubbing and coarse crackles over the affected area, usually the lung bases.

## Investigations

- Radiology. The chest X-ray may be normal or show dilated bronchi with thickened bronchial walls, and sometimes multiple cysts containing fluid. High-resolution CT (slices are between 1 and 2 mm thick, compared to conventional CT slice of 10 mm) is the investigation of choice and may show bronchial wall thickening that is not shown on a standard chest X-ray. Inspiratory and expiratory scans show air trapping in small airways. Bronchography is only used to assess the extent of disease before surgery (see Management).

- Sputum culture is essential during an infective exacerbation. The common organisms are

*Staphylococcus aureus*, *Pseudomonas aeruginosa* and *Haemophilus influenzae*.
- Further investigations, e.g. serum immunoglobulins, sweat test, in patients where an underlying cause is suspected.

## Management
- Physiotherapy and daily postural drainage are of vital importance. The patient is taught to carry them out at home.
- Antibiotics. In mild cases intermittent chemotherapy with cefaclor 500 mg three times daily may be the only therapy needed. Flucloxacillin is the best treatment if *Staph. aureus* is isolated on sputum culture. If the sputum remains yellow or green despite regular physiotherapy and antibiotics it is probable that there is infection with *Pseudomonas aeruginosa*, which requires specific antibiotics, e.g. ceftazidime, administered by aerosol or parenterally. Oral ciprofloxacin is an alternative.
- Bronchodilators are used for those with demonstrable airflow limitation.
- Inhaled or oral steroids can decrease the rate of progression.
- Surgery is reserved for the very small minority with localized disease. Severe disease sometimes requires lung or heart–lung transplantation.

## Complications
The main complications are pneumonia, haemoptysis which may be life-threatening, and cerebral abscess. Most patients with severe bronchiectasis will eventually develop respiratory failure.

# Cystic fibrosis *(K&C p. 871)*
Cystic fibrosis (CF) is an autosomal recessive condition occurring in 1:2000 live births. It is caused by mutations in a single gene on the long arm of chromosome 7 that encodes the cystic fibrosis transmembrane conductance regulator (CFTR). Mutations in the *CFTR* gene result in the production of a defective transmembrane protein

which is involved in chloride transport across epithelial cell membranes in the pancreas and respiratory, gastro-intestinal and reproductive tracts. The decreased chloride transport is accompanied by decreased transport of sodium and water, resulting in dehydrated viscous secretions that are associated with luminal obstruction and destruction and scarring of exocrine glands. The most common mutation is $\Delta F_{508}$ (deletion, phenylalanine at position 508).

### Clinical features

Although the lungs of babies born with CF are normal at birth, respiratory symptoms are usually the presenting features. Bronchiectasis and obstructive pulmonary disease are the primary causes of morbidity and mortality in patients with CF. Infants with CF have persistent endo-bronchial infections due initially to *Staphylococcus aureus*, *Haemophilus influenzae* and Gram-negative bacilli. By the end of the first decade of life *Pseudomonas aeruginosa* is the predominant pathogen (p. 476). The resultant inflammatory response damages the airway, leading to progressive bronchiectasis and eventually respiratory failure. Finger clubbing is seen in patients with moderate or advanced disease. Other abnormalities in the respiratory system include pansinusitis and nasal polyps. Meconium ileus is the presenting problem in about one-fifth of newborns with CF and is virtually pathognomonic of the diagnosis. Episodes of small bowel obstruction may also occur in later life and have been called the meconium ileus equivalent (MIE) syndrome. There may be steatorrhoea and diabetes mellitus as a result of pancreatic insufficiency. Males are infertile because of failure of development of the vas deferens. Chronic ill health in children leads to impaired growth and delayed puberty.

### Investigations

- Sweat testing alone (a high sweat sodium > 60 mmol/L) may be sufficient to diagnose or rule out cystic fibrosis in patients with typical gastrointestinal or pulmonary disease (classic cystic fibrosis). In patients with suspicious clinical findings and a normal sweat test

genotyping is indicated; the commercially available probes will identify more than 90% of all CF genes.
- Genetic screening for the carrier state should be offered to persons or couples with a family history of CF, together with counselling.

## Management

Management of bronchiectasis and exocrine pancreatic insufficiency has been described on pages 459 and 162. An understanding of the basic defect and pathogenesis of cystic fibrosis has led to newer treatments, which are described in Table 10.3. Some patients with severe respiratory disease have received lung or heart–lung transplantations (*K&C* p. 873)

The emergence of *Burkholderia cepacia* infection is a problem for patients and doctors alike. It is associated with accelerated lung disease and resistance to antibiotics in some strains. Close contact promotes cross-infection, so siblings and fellow sufferers with cystic fibrosis may pass the organism from one to another.

## Prognosis

Ninety per cent of children now survive into their teens and the median survival for those born after 1990 is estimated at 40 years. Most mortality is the result of pulmonary disease.

## Asthma (*K&C* p. 874)

Asthma is a common chronic inflammatory condition of the lung airways, whose cause is incompletely understood. It has three characteristics: airflow limitation which is usually reversible, airway hyperresponsiveness to a range of stimuli, and inflammation of the bronchi.

## Epidemiology

The prevalence of asthma is increasing, particularly in the second decade of life, when 10–15% of the population are affected. There is a geographical variation: asthma is more common in New Zealand and much rarer in Far Eastern countries.

**Table 10.3**
Pathogenesis and approaches to treatment of respiratory disease in cystic fibrosis. Amiloride, adenosine or uridine triphosphates (ATP and UTP), DNAase and $\alpha_1$-antitrypsin are given by aerosol

| Pathogenesis | Treatment |
|---|---|
| Defective gene | Introduction of the normal *CFTR* gene into respiratory epithelium. *But studies are in the early stages, owing to difficulties in establishing an effective vector to deliver the gene* |
| Defective protein – CFTR | |
| Abnormal epithelial cell transport | Amiloride blocks sodium reabsorption, ATP and UTP stimulate chloride secretion through channels other than CFTR |
| Viscous intraluminal secretions | |
| Chronic bacterial colonization and infections | Prompt treatment with antibiotics for exacerbations |
| Accumulation of chronic inflammatory cells and release of proteolytic enzymes | Oral steroids for anti-inflammatory effects. Antiproteases |
| Release of DNA from degraded cells | DNAase to digest extracellular DNA |

## Aetiology

There are two major factors involved in the development of asthma:

- *Atopy.* This is the term used in individuals who readily develop antibodies of immunoglobulin E (IgE) class against common environmental antigens such as the house-dust mite, grass pollen and fungal spores from *Aspergillus fumigatus*. Genetic and environmental factors affect serum IgE levels. Included in the genetic influence is the cytokine gene complex on chromosome 5, the interleukin-4 (IL-4) gene cluster, which controls the production of IL-3, IL-4, IL-5 and IL-13. Environmental factors include childhood exposure to respiratory irritants such as tobacco smoke, and intestinal bacterial and childhood infections. There is evidence that growing up in a relatively clean environment may predispose towards an IgE response to allergens.
- *Increased responsiveness of the airways of the lung* (as measured by a fall in $FEV_1$) to stimuli such as inhaled histamine and methacholine (bronchial provocation tests, see below).

Asthma has traditionally been divided into extrinsic (atopic) and intrinsic (non-atopic) on the basis that in extrinsic asthma allergens can be identified by positive skin-prick reactions to common inhaled allergens. It is now recognized that almost all asthmatic patients show some degree of atopy, and this classification is used less often.

## Pathogenesis

The primary abnormality in asthma is narrowing of the airway, which is due to smooth muscle contraction, thickening of the airway wall by cellular infiltration and inflammation, and the presence of secretions within the airway lumen. The pathogenesis of asthma is complex and not fully understood. It involves a number of cells, mediators, nerves and vascular leakage which can be activated by several mechanisms, of which exposure to allergens is the most relevant.

*Inflammation* The cellular component of the inflammatory response includes eosinophils, T lymphocytes, macrophages and mast cells, which release a number of inflammatory mediators. Macrophages may have a role in the initial uptake and presentation of allergens to lymphocytes. Lymphocytes infiltrating the asthmatic airway primarily bear the Th2 phenotype. These lymphocytes, when stimulated by the appropriate antigen, release a restricted panel of cytokines: IL-3, IL-4, IL-5 and GM-CSF which play a part in the migration and activation of mast cells and eosinophils. In addition, production of IL-4 leads to the maintenance of the allergic (Th2) T cell phenotype, favouring switching of antibody production by B lymphocytes to IgE. These IgE molecules attach to mast cells via high-affinity receptors which in turn release a number of powerful mediators acting on smooth muscle and small blood vessels, such as histamine, tryptase, prostaglandin $D_2$ and leukotriene $C_4$, which cause the immediate asthmatic reaction. Activation of eosinophils, by IgE binding, leads to release of a variety of mediators, such as eosinophilic cationic protein, which are predominantly toxic to airway cells.

*Remodelling* Airway smooth muscle undergoes hypertrophy and hyperplasia leading to a larger fraction of the wall being occupied by smooth muscle tissue. The airway wall is further thickened by deposition of repair collagens and matrix proteins below the basement membrane. The airway epithelium is damaged, with loss of the ciliated columnar cells into the lumen. The epithelium undergoes metaplasia with an increase in the number of mucus-secreting goblet cells.

## Precipitating factors

The major allergen (Der p1) is contained in the faecal particles of the house-dust mite, *Dermatophagoides pteronnysinus*, which is found in dust throughout the house. Non-specific factors which may cause wheezing are viral infections, cold air, exercise, irritant dusts, vapours and fumes (cigarette smoke, perfume, exhaust fumes), emotion and drugs (NSAID, aspirin and β-blockers).

Over 200 materials encountered at the workplace may give rise to wheezing, which typically improves on days away from work and during holidays (occupational asthma). Common occupations associated with asthma are veterinary medicine and animal handling (allergens are mouse, rat and rabbit urine and fur), bakery (wheat, rye) and laundry work (biological enzymes).

A rare cause of asthma is the airborne spores of *Aspergillus fumigatus*, a soil mould. There are fleeting shadows on the chest X-ray and peripheral blood eosinophilia (allergic bronchopulmonary aspergillosis, not to be confused with the severe aspergillus pneumonia occurring in the immunocompromised).

## Clinical features

Symptoms are episodic wheezing, cough and shortness of breath which are typically worse at night and in the early morning. A cough may be the only presenting symptom. Some patients have just one or two attacks a year, whereas others have chronic symptoms. Asthma may be precipitated by all the factors discussed previously. On examination, during an attack, there is reduced chest expansion, prolonged expiratory time and expiratory polyphonic wheezes.

## Investigations

The diagnosis of asthma is often made on the history and response to bronchodilators. There is no single satisfactory diagnostic test for all asthmatic patients.

- Peak expiratory flow charts. Measurement of PEFR by the patient on waking, during the day and before bed shows the characteristic variability in airflow limitation. Most asthmatic individuals will show obvious diurnal variation, with lowest values occurring in the early morning (the 'morning dip', Fig. 10.1).
- Lung function tests. Demonstration of a greater than 15% improvement in $FEV_1$ or PEFR following inhalation of a bronchodilator ('reversibility').
- Histamine or methacholine bronchial provocation tests are used to indicate the presence of airway hyperresponsiveness, a feature found in most asthmatics. Bronchial hyperreactivity is demonstrated

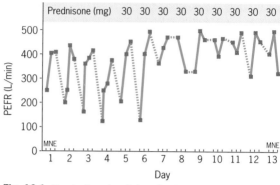

**Fig. 10.1 Classic diurnal variation of asthma, showing the effect of steroids.** The arrows indicate the morning 'dips'. M, morning; N, noon; E, evening.

by asking the patient to inhale gradually increasing doses of histamine or methacholine and demonstrating a fall in $FEV_1$. The test should not be performed on individuals who have poor lung function ($FEV_1$ < 1.5 L) or a history of 'brittle' asthma.

- Skin-prick tests are used to identify allergens to which the patient is sensitive. A weal develops 15 minutes after allergen injection in the epidermis of the forearm.
- Chest X-ray is performed at diagnosis and usually only repeated in an acute severe asthma attack.
- Serum. *Aspergillus* antibody titres should be measured in those with a marked blood eosinophilia or transient shadowing on the chest X-ray.
- A trial of steroids (prednisolone 30 mg daily for 2 weeks) should be given to everyone with severe airflow limitation. An improvement in $FEV_1$ of > 15% confirms some reversibility and indicates that inhaled steroids may prove beneficial.

## Management

The effective management of asthma centres on patient and family education, antismoking advice, the avoidance of precipitating factors and specific drug treatment. Self-management programmes have been incorporated into patient care. These programmes involve individualized self-treatment plans based on monitoring of PEFR and symptoms and a written action plan showing patients how to act early in exacerbations.

**Avoidance of precipitating factors**  Patients should be discouraged from smoking and avoid allergens, e.g. household pets, which have been shown to provoke attacks. Avoidance of the house-dust mite may be possible with frequent house cleaning and the use of effective covers for bedding. It is necessary to identify occupational asthma because early diagnosis and removal of the patient from exposure may cure the asthma. Continued exposure may lead to severe asthma, which continues even when exposure ceases. β-blockers in any form are absolutely contraindicated in patients with asthma.

**Specific drug treatment**  Most drugs are delivered directly into the lungs as aerosols or powders, which means that lower doses can be used and systemic side-effects are reduced compared to oral treatment. Asthma is managed with a stepwise approach which depends partly on repeated measurements of PEFR by the patient (Table 10.4). The aim is that the patient starts treatment at the step most appropriate to the initial severity, and when control of symptoms is achieved, treatment is gradually reduced to the previous step over a period of 3–6 months. The aim is to have minimal symptoms with few exacerbations and minimal need for relieving bronchodilators. Ideally a PEFR > 80% of predicted or the patient's best should be achieved with less than 20% circadian variation.

- $\beta_2$-Adrenoceptor agonists, e.g. salbutamol, terbutaline and the longer-acting salmeterol and formoterol, relax bronchial smooth muscle and cause bronchial dilatation.
- Anticholinergic bronchodilators, e.g. ipratropium bromide or oxitropium bromide, cause bronchodilatation and may be additive to adrenoceptor stimulants.
- Corticosteroids are powerful anti-inflammatory agents. Inhaled steroids, e.g. beclometasone dipropionate, budesonide and fluticasone propionate, are used as maintenance treatment in all but very mild

**Table 10.4**
The stepwise management of chronic asthma in adults

| Step | PEFR (% predicted) | Treatment |
|------|------|------|
| 1. Occasional symptoms, less frequent than daily | 100 | Inhaled short-acting β₂ agonist as required<br>If needed > once daily move to step 2 |
| 2. Daily symptoms | ≤ 80 | Low-dose inhaled corticosteroid:<br>Beclometasone or budesonide up to 400 µg twice daily<br>Fluticasone up to 200 µg twice daily |
| 3. Severe symptoms | 50–80 | High-dose inhaled corticosteroid via a large volume spacer:<br>Beclometasone or budesonide up to 1000 µg twice daily<br>Fluticasone up to 500 µg twice daily or low-dose inhaled<br>corticosteroid plus salmeterol 50 µg twice daily |
| 4. Severe symptoms uncontrolled at step 3 | 50–80 | Add in long-acting β₂ agonist (e.g. salmeterol or formoterol) |
| 5. Severe symptoms deteriorating | ≤ 50 | Add oral prednisolone 40 mg daily |

- Patient measures PEFR at home to guide treatment
- Short-acting inhaled β agonist taken at any step as needed for symptom relief
- A rescue of oral steroids may be needed at any time and at any step
- Check inhaler technique and compliance before any increase in treatment
- Decrease treatment after 1–3 months of stability

asthmatic individuals. Side-effects of inhaled steroids are oral candidiasis, hoarseness and rarely cataract formation. Oral steroids are occasionally necessary in those patients not controlled on inhaled steroids. Side-effects are listed on page 577.

- Anti-inflammatory agents, e.g. sodium cromoglicate, prevent activation of inflammatory cells and may be useful in mild asthma.`
- Leukotriene receptor antagonists (LTRA), e.g. montelukast and zafirlukast, are given orally. Leukotrienes are inflammatory mediators released by mast cells which cause bronchoconstriction and increased production of mucus. LTRA are particularly useful in patients who still have symptoms despite taking high-dose inhaled or oral corticosteroids, and in patients with asthma induced by aspirin.
- The immunosuppressive drug methotrexate in low doses has been used in severely asthmatic individuals as a steroid-sparing agent.
- Intravenous aminophylline is sometimes used in acute severe asthma.

## Acute severe asthma

Acute severe asthma is diagnosed when a patient has severe progressive asthmatic symptoms over a number of hours or days. It is a medical emergency that must be recognized and treated immediately at home, with subsequent transfer to hospital (Emergency Box 10.1). In the UK, 1500 patients still die annually from this condition.

### Clinical features

Features of acute severe asthma are:

- Inability to complete a sentence in one breath
- Respiratory rate ≥ 25 breaths/min
- Tachycardia > 110 beats/min
- PEFR < 50% of predicted value or < 50% of patient's best.

Life-threatening features are:

- Silent chest, cyanosis or feeble respiratory effort
- Exhaustion, confusion or coma

Acute severe asthma

> ## ! Emergency Box 10.1
>
> ## Management of acute severe asthma in hospital
>
> - 60% oxygen
> - Salbutamol 5 mg or terbutaline 10 mg via oxygen-driven nebulizer
> - Hydrocortisone 200 mg intravenously
> - No sedatives of any kind
> - Antibiotics if definite evidence of infection: focal shadowing on the chest X-ray, purulent sputum
> - Chest X-ray to exclude pneumothorax or pneumonia
>
> **Monitor in all patients**
>
> - Arterial oxygen saturation by pulse oximetry
> - Arterial blood gases only if $P_aO_2 < 92\%$ or life-threatening features
> - PEFR 30 min after starting treatment, and then before and after $\beta_2$ agonist treatment
> - Consider repeat blood gases 2 hours after starting treatment
> - Fluid intake, aim for 2.5–3 L/day, intravenously if necessary
> - Urea and electrolytes daily, steroids and salbutamol may result in hypokalaemia

**If improved – continue**
60% oxygen
Hydrocortisone 200 mg
6-hourly i.v., change to oral
prednisolone 40 mg after
24 hours
Nebulized $\beta_2$ agonist 4-hourly

**After 24 hours – consider**
Adding in high-dose inhaled
corticosteroid
Change nebulized to inhaled $\beta_2$
agonist

**Discharge from hospital**
When PEFR > 75% predicted or
patient's best and diurnal
variability < 25%
When stable on discharge
treatment for 24 hours
Check inhaler technique
Determine reason for
exacerbation

**Life-threatening features
present or poor response to
treatment**
60% oxygen
Hydrocortisone 200 mg 6-hourly
intravenously
Repeat nebulized $\beta_2$ agonist every
15–30 min
Add ipratropium 0.5 mg to the
nebulizer
Consider intravenous:

Salbutamol. Add 5 mg to 500 ml
normal saline or 5% dextrose
(i.e. 10 mg/ml). Give a loading
dose of 250 µg (25 ml) over
10 min and continue at
10–30 µg (1–3 ml/min)
Aminophylline. Loading dose of
250 mg over 10 min and
continue at 0.5 µg/kg/h. Omit
loading dose if patient has been
taking oral aminophylline.
Monitor blood concentrations if
continued for 24 h, therapeutic
range 10–20 mg/L

If poor response within 1 hour
transfer to ITU for possible
intubation and mechanical
ventilation

- Bradycardia or hypotension
- PEFR < 30% of predicted or best (approximately 150 L/min in adults)
- Blood gas markers of a very severe attack are $P_aCO_2 > 6$ kPa, $P_aO_2 < 8$ kPa, and pH < 7.35.

The management of acute severe asthma is summarized in Emergency Box 10.1. Patients with moderate asthma (defined as a PEFR 50–75% of predicted and with none of the above features) who present to hospital are treated with a nebulized β-agonist. Provided they improve and are then stable for at least 1 hour, they may be discharged with a tapering dose of prednisolone (e.g. starting at 40 mg daily). Oral prednisolone should be given until the acute attack has completely resolved.

## Pneumonia (K&C p. 885)

Pneumonia is defined as an inflammation of the substance of the lungs and is usually caused by bacteria. Pneumonia can be classified both anatomically, e.g. lobar (affecting the whole of one lobe) and bronchopneumonia (affecting the lobules and bronchi), or on the basis of aetiology. However, the most useful classification to guide management is based on the clinical circumstances under which the pneumonia is acquired (Table 10.5). *Mycobacterium tuberculosis* is one cause of pneumonia; it is considered separately, as both mode of presentation and treatment are different from the other pneumonias.

### Clinical features
Symptoms and signs vary according to the infecting agent and to the immune state of the patient. Most commonly there is pyrexia, combined with respiratory symptoms such as cough, sputum production, pleurisy and dyspnoea. Signs of consolidation and a pleural rub may be present. There may be a pleural effusion. Elderly patients often have fewer symptoms than younger patients or may present with a confusional state. The criteria for the diagnosis of severe community-acquired pneumonia are listed

**Table 10.5**
Aetiology of pneumonia in the UK based on clinical circumstances

| Microbial agent or cause | Prevalence (%) |
| --- | --- |
| **Community acquired** | |
| Bacteria | |
| Streptococcus pneumonia | 60–75 |
| Haemophilus influenzae | 4–5 |
| Legionella | 2–5 |
| Staphylococcus aureus | 1–5 |
| Gram-negative bacilli | 0–8 |
| Miscellaneous | 1–2 |
| Other agents | |
| Mycoplasma pneumonia | 5–18 |
| Chlamydia sp. | 5–10 |
| Coxiella burnetii | Rare |
| Viruses | Uncommon* |
| **Hospital acquired (nosocomial)** | |
| Gram-negative bacteria | 50 |
| Staphylococcus aureus | < 25 |
| Anaerobes | |
| **Aspiration** | |
| Gastric acid | |
| Oropharyngeal bacteria – multiple bacteria including anaerobes | |
| **In the immunosuppressed** | |
| Pneumocystis carinii | |
| Mycobacterium tuberculosis | |
| Mycobacterium avium-intracellulare | |
| Aspergillus fumigatus | |
| Cytomegalovirus | |
| Bacteria (as in other groups) | |

* Pneumonia due to viral infection per se is uncommon, most is due to secondary bacterial infection

in Table 10.6. Precipitating factors for pneumonia are underlying lung disease, smoking, alcohol abuse, immunosuppression and other chronic illnesses. The clinical history should enquire about contact with birds (possible psittacosis), contact with farm animals (*Coxiella burnetii*, causative organism of Q fever), recent stays in large hotels or institutions (*Legionella pneumophila*), chronic alcohol abuse (*Mycobacterium tuberculosis*), intravenous drug abuse (*Staphylococcus aureus*, *Mycobacterium tuberculosis*) and contact with other patients with pneumonia.

> **Table 10.6**
> Criteria for the diagnosis of severe community-acquired
> pneumonia
>
> **Clinical features**
> Respiratory rate $\geq$ 30/min
> Diastolic blood pressure $\leq$ 60 mmHg
> Confusion
> 65 years or over
> Underlying lung disease or other co-morbidity
>
> **Investigations**
> Chest X-ray – more than one lobe involved
> $P_aO_2$ < 8 kPa
> Serum albumin < 35 g/L
> White cell count < 4 or > $20 \times 10^9$/L
> Raised serum urea > 7 mmol/L
> Blood culture – positive

## Investigations

Many otherwise fit patients with community-acquired pneumonia are treated as outpatients and the only investigation needed is a chest X-ray, which should be repeated 6–8 weeks after clinical recovery to confirm resolution. Patients admitted to hospital require investigations to identify the cause and severity of the pneumonia (Table 10.6).

- Sputum should be sent for Gram stain and culture, although negative results are reported for 30–60% of cultures of expectorated sputum.
- Blood count. A white cell count above $15 \times 10^9$/L suggests bacterial infection. The white cell count is > $15 \times 10^9$/L in only 10% of patients with *Legionella* pneumonia, and sometimes there is lymphopenia. Marked red cell agglutination on the blood film suggests the presence of cold agglutinins (immunoglobulins that agglutinate reds cells at 4°C), which are raised in 50% of patients with *Mycoplasma* pneumonia.
- Liver biochemistry and serum electrolytes. Liver biochemistry may be non-specifically abnormal. Raised serum urea and hypoalbuminaemia indicate severe pneumonia.
- Blood culture is positive in 15–25% of cases even if the sputum is negative, and indicates a poorer prognosis.

- Serology. Some organisms, e.g. mycoplasma, causing pneumonia can be diagnosed by detection of a raised IgM antibody by immunofluorescent tests or by a fourfold rise in antibody titre from blood taken early in the clinical course and 10–14 days later.
- Chest X-ray confirms consolidation, but these changes may lag behind the clinical course. A chest X-ray which remains persistently abnormal (> 6 weeks) suggests an underlying abnormality, usually a carcinoma.
- Arterial blood gases. $P_aO_2 < 8$ kPa or rising $P_aCO_2$ indicates severe pneumonia.
- Pneumococcal antigen in sputum, urine or serum (more sensitive than sputum or blood culture).

## Differential diagnosis

This includes pulmonary embolism, pulmonary oedema, pulmonary haemorrhage, bronchial carcinoma, acute extrinsic allergic alveolitis and cryptogenic organizing pneumonia (pneumonia of unknown aetiology, no infective agent has been described).

## Management

In mild cases of community-acquired pneumonia treatment can be started immediately with oral amoxicillin, 500 mg 8-hourly for 7 days. Oral erythromycin or azithromycin is an alternative for patients allergic to penicillin. More severe cases are admitted to hospital and treated with a combination of oral amoxicillin and erythromycin, or intravenous treatment in severe cases. If *Staph. aureus* infection is suspected or proven on culture, intravenous flucloxacillin ± sodium fusidate is added. Pleuritic pain requires analgesia, and humidified oxygen is given if there is hypoxaemia. Fluids are encouraged, to avoid dehydration. Physiotherapy is needed to help and encourage the patient to cough. Treatment should be modified in the light of culture and serology results. Patients with severe pneumonia are best managed on an intensive care unit. Treatment of other types of pneumonia depend of the clinical circumstances and likely organisms.

## Prognosis

Complications of pneumonia include lung abscess and empyema. In elderly patients the mortality rate may be as high as 25%.

## Specific forms of pneumonia

**Mycoplasma pneumoniae** (*K&C* p. 887) *Mycoplasma* pneumonia commonly presents in young adults with generalized features such as headaches and malaise, which may precede chest symptoms by 1–5 days. Physical signs in the chest may be scanty, and chest X-ray appearances frequently do not correlate with the clinical state of the patient. Treatment is with erythromycin or clarithromycin. Extrapulmonary complications (myocarditis, erythema multiforme, haemolytic anaemia and meningoencephalitis) will occasionally dominate the clinical picture.

**Haemophilus influenzae** (*K&C* p. 887) This is commonly the cause of pneumonia in patients with COPD. There are no other features to differentiate it from other causes of bacterial pneumonia. Treatment is with oral cefaclor.

**Chlamydia** (*K&C* p. 887) *Chlamydia pneumoniae* accounts for 5–10% of cases of community-acquired pneumonia. Patients with *C. psittaci* pneumonia may give a history of contact with infected birds, particularly parrots. Symptoms include malaise, fever, cough and muscular pains, which may be low grade and protracted over many months. Occasionally the presentation mimics meningitis, with a high fever, prostration, photophobia and neck stiffness. Diagnosis of *Chlamydia* infection is made by demonstrating a rising serum titre of complement-fixing antibody. *C. pneumoniae* is distinguished from *C. psittaci* infection by type-specific immunofluoresence tests. Treatment of *Chlamydia* infection is with erythromycin or tetracycline.

**Staphylococcus aureus** (*K&C* p. 887) usually causes pneumonia only after a preceding influenza viral illness, in intravenous drug users or in patients with central venous catheters. It results in patchy areas of consolidation which can break down to form abscesses that appear as cysts on the chest X-ray. Pneumothorax, effusions and empyemas are frequent, and septicaemia may develop with metastatic abscesses in other organs. All patients with this form of pneumonia are extremely ill and the mortality rate is in excess of 25%. Treatment is with intravenous flucloxacillin.

***Legionellosis*** (*K&C* p. 888) Legionnaire's disease can be acquired by the inhalation of aerosols or microaspiration of infected water containing legionella. Infection is linked to contamination of water distribution systems in hotels, hospitals and workplaces. Most cases of legionellosis are due to infection with *L. pneumophila* which causes more severe disease than most other pathogens associated with community-acquired pneumonia. The clinical and radio-logical presentation of legionnaire's disease cannot be reliably distinguished from other forms of pneumonia, although a prodromal virus-like illness, temperature of up to 40°C and the presence of diarrhoea, confusion, lym-phopenia and hyponatraemia can be clues. Diagnosis is by direct fluorescent antibody staining of the organism in the pleural fluid, sputum or bronchial washings, or by detec-tion of *L. pneumophila* antigen in the urine. Treatment is with clarithromycin, ciprofloxacin or rifampicin for 14–21 days.

***Pseudomonas aeruginosa*** (*K&C* p. 888) is seen in the immunocompromised and in patients with cystic fibrosis, in whom its presence is associated with a worsening of the clinical condition and increasing mortality. Treatment includes intravenous ceftazidime, ciprofloxacin, tobramycin or ticarcillin. Tobramycin and ticarcillin can be inhaled directly into the lung in patients with CF.

***Pneumocystis carinii*** is the most common opportunistic infection in patients with AIDS. The clinical features and treatment of this and other opportunistic infection are described on page 48.

***Aspiration pneumonia*** (*K&C* p. 890) Aspiration of gastric contents into the lungs can produce a severe destructive pneumonia as a result of the corrosive effect of gastric acid – Mendelson's syndrome. Aspiration usually occurs into the posterior segment of the right lower lobe because of the bronchial anatomy. It is associated with periods of impaired consciousness, structural abnormalities, such as tracheo-oesophageal fistulae or oesophageal strictures, and bulbar palsy. Infection is often due to anaerobes, and treatment must include metronidazole.

## Complications of pneumonia: lung abscess and empyema (K&C p. 891)

A lung abscess results from localized suppuration of the lung associated with cavity formation, often with a fluid level on the chest X-ray. Empyema means the presence of pus in the pleural cavity, usually from rupture of a lung abscess into the pleural cavity, or from bacterial spread from a severe pneumonia.

A lung abscess develops in the following circumstances:

- Complicating aspiration pneumonia or bacterial pneumonia caused by *Staphylococcus aureus* or *Klebsiella pneumoniae*
- Secondary to bronchial obstruction by tumour or foreign body
- From septic emboli from a focus elsewhere (usually *Staphylococcus aureus*)
- Secondary to infarction.

### Clinical features

Lung abscess presents with persisting or worsening pneumonia, often with the production of copious amounts of foul-smelling sputum. With empyema the patient is usually very ill, with a high fever and neutrophil leucocytosis. There may be malaise, weight loss and clubbing of the digits.

### Investigations

Bacteriological investigation is best conducted on specimens obtained by transtracheal aspiration, bronchoscopy or percutaneous transthoracic aspiration. Bronchoscopy is helpful to exclude carcinomas and foreign bodies.

## Management

Antibiotics are given to cover both aerobic and anaerobic organisms. Intravenous cefuroxime, erythromycin and metronidazole are given for 5 days, followed by oral cefaclor and metronidazole for several weeks. Empyemas should be treated by prompt tube drainage or rib resection and drainage of the empyema cavity. Abscesses occasionally require surgery.

## Tuberculosis ND (K&C p. 892)

### Epidemiology

Tuberculosis (TB) is the most common cause of death world-wide from a single infectious disease, and is on the increase in most parts of the world. This results primarily from inadequate programmes for disease control, multiple drug resistance, co-infection with HIV and a rapid rise in the world population of young adults, the group with the highest mortality from tuberculosis. In the UK the incidence of tuberculosis is much higher in Asian and West Indian immigrants than in the native white population.

### Pathology

The initial infection with *Mycobacterium tuberculosis* is known as primary tuberculosis. It usually occurs in the lung but may occur in the gastrointestinal tract, particularly the ileocaecal region. The primary focus in the lung is subpleural in the mid to upper zones (Fig. 10.2), and is characterized by exudation and infiltration with neutrophil granulocytes. These are replaced by macrophages which engulf the bacilli and result in the typical granulomatous lesions, which consist of central areas of caseation surrounded by epithelioid cells and Langhans' giant cells (both derived from the macrophage). The primary focus is almost always accompanied by caseous lesions in the regional lymph nodes (mediastinal and cervical). In most people the primary infection and the lymph nodes heal completely and become calcified. Some of these calcified primary lesions harbour tubercle bacilli, which may become reactivated if there is depression of the host defence system.

Occasionally there is dissemination of the primary infection, producing miliary tuberculosis.

Reactivation results in typical post-primary tuberculosis. Post-primary tuberculosis refers to all forms of tuberculosis that develop after the first few weeks of the primary infection when immunity to the mycobacteria has developed.

## Clinical features

Primary TB is usually symptomless; occasionally there may be erythema nodosum (p. 728), a small pleural effusion or pulmonary collapse caused by compression of a lobar bronchus by enlarged nodes (Fig. 10.2). Most commonly clinical tuberculosis represents delayed reactivation. Symptoms begin insidiously, with malaise, anorexia, weight loss, fever and cough. Sputum is mucoid purulent or blood-stained, but night sweats are uncommon. There are often no physical signs, although occasionally signs of a pneumonia or pleural effusion may be present. The liver and spleen may be enlarged in miliary tuberculosis. Choroidal tubercles (yellowy/white raised lesions about one-quarter the diameter of the optic disc) are occasionally seen in the eye.

## Investigations

- Chest X-ray typically shows patchy or nodular shadows in the upper zones, with loss of volume, and fibrosis with or without cavitation. With miliary tuberculosis the chest X-ray may be normal or show miliary shadows 1–2 mm in diameter throughout the lung.

479

- Sputum is stained with Ziehl–Nielsen (ZN) stain for acid- and alcohol-fast bacilli and cultured on Ogana or Lowenstein–Jensen medium. This takes 4–8 weeks.
- Bronchoscopy with washings of the affected lobes is useful if no sputum is available.
- Mantoux test is positive except in some patients with very severe disease or in the first 4–7 weeks after primary infection. The diameter of the area of induration is measured 48–72 hours after the intradermal injection of tuberculin (purified protein derivative) into the dorsal surface of the forearm. An area of induration of 5–15 mm (depending on clinical

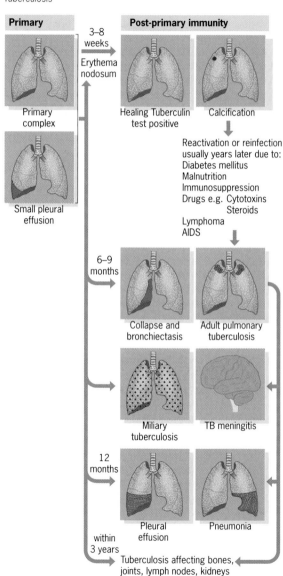

**Fig. 10.2 The manifestations of primary and post-primary tuberculosis.**

circumstances) indicates infection with *M. tuberculosis*. A positive test also occurs with previously treated infection or after BCG vaccination.

- Biopsy with histological examination and culture of pleura, lymph nodes and solid lesions within the lung (tuberculomas) may be required for diagnosis.

Direct testing of sputum and other fluids for *M. tuberculosis* DNA using the polymerase chain reaction may allow rapid diagnosis (within 48 hours) of infection, though the technique is still not entirely reliable and should not be considered diagnostic in the 'difficult' case.

## Management

Pulmonary and lymph node tuberculosis assumed to be caused by sensitive organisms is treated with rifampicin and isoniazid for 6 months, along with pyrazinamide for the first 2 months until drug sensitivities are available. Treatment duration should be extended to 9 months for bone tuberculosis and to 12 months for tuberculous meningitis. Pyridoxine is given to reduce the risk of isoniazid-induced neuropathy. Ethambutol is included in a treatment regimen if resistance is suspected. Streptomycin is now rarely used in the UK, but it may be added if the organism is resistant to isoniazid. Significant side-effects are uncommon and are listed in Table 10.7. A transient asymptomatic rise in the serum transferase level may occur with rifampicin, but treatment is only stopped if hepatitis develops. Multidrug resistance is a major problem and occurs mainly in HIV-infected patients. Three drugs to which the organism is sensitive are used for up to 2 years. A variety of second-line drugs, including capreomycin, clarithromycin, azithromycin and ciprofloxacin, are used for these patients.

The major causes of treatment failure are incorrect prescribing by the doctor and inadequate compliance by the patient. Treatment should be supervised by a specialist physician. All cases of TB must be notified to the local Public Health Authority so that contact tracing and screening can be arranged. Close contacts of a case are screened for evidence of disease with a chest X-ray and a Mantoux test. Antituberculous treatment is given if the chest X-ray

**Table 10.7**
Side-effects of antituberculous drug treatment

| | |
|---|---|
| Rifampicin | Stains body secretions and urine pink |
| | Induces liver enzymes and accelerates metabolism of some drugs resulting in reduced efficacy, e.g. phenytoin, warfarin, and oestrogen-containing contraceptive pill |
| | Elevation of liver enzymes and hepatitis |
| | Rarely thrombocytopenia |
| Isoniazid | Polyneuropathy – rare and prevented by co-administration of pyridoxine |
| | Allergic reactions – skin rash and fever |
| | Hepatitis |
| Pyrazinamide | Hepatitis – rarely |
| | Hyperuricaemia and gout |
| | Rash and arthralgia |
| Ethambutol | Optic retrobulbar neuritis presenting with colour blindness, reduced visual acuity and central scotoma. Patients are asked to report visual problems and to undergo regular specialist ophthalmic examination |

shows evidence of disease, or if the Mantoux test is negative initially but becomes positive on repeat testing 6 weeks later. In adults, an initial positive tuberculin test with a normal chest X-ray is not usually taken as indication of infection.

## Prevention

Immunization with BCG (bacille Calmette–Guérin) reduces the risk of developing tuberculosis by about 50%. It is a bovine strain of *M. tuberculosis* which has lost its virulence after growth in the laboratory for many years. Routine immunization is becoming less common in the UK as the incidence of tuberculosis is decreasing in the indigenous population. Immunization produces cellular immunity and a positive tuberculin test, and is the main reason why the Mantoux test is now of little value for diagnosis of active disease in the UK. BCG immunization of the newborn is still given in developing countries, where TB is more prevalent.

## Chemoprophylaxis

Patients with chest X-ray changes compatible with previous tuberculosis and who are about to undergo treatment with an immunosuppressive agent should receive chemo-prophylaxis with isoniazid.

# Diffuse diseases of the lung parenchyma

A wide variety of diseases can affect the parenchyma of the lung. They are often classified together because of similar clinical, radiographic, physiological or pathogenic manifestations. Sarcoidosis and cryptogenic fibrosing alveolitis are the commonest forms of diffuse parenchymal lung diseases (DPLD) and are of unknown cause. The commonest identifiable causes of DPLD are related to occupational and environmental exposure often to a variety of dusts. Patients with DPLD commonly present with shortness of breath on exertion, a persistent non-productive cough, with an abnormal chest X-ray or with pulmonary symptoms associated with another disease such as a connective tissue disease.

## Granulomatous lung disease

A granuloma is a mass or nodule of chronic inflammatory tissue formed by the response of macrophages and histiocytes to a slowly soluble antigen or irritant. It is characterized by the presence of epithelioid multinucleate giant cells. Sarcoidosis is the most common cause of lung granulomas.

### Sarcoidosis (*K&C* p. 897 & p. 1300)

Sarcoidosis is a multisystem granulomatous disorder of unknown aetiology that commonly affects young adults and usually presents with bilateral hilar lymphadenopathy (BHL), pulmonary infiltrations and skin or eye lesions. In about half of cases, the disease is detected incidentally on a routine chest X-ray in an asymptomatic individual.

### *Epidemiology*

The disease has been identified in all ethnic groups but is uncommon in Japan. The course of the disease is more severe in African blacks than in whites. The peak incidence is in the third and forth decades with a female preponderance.

## Immunopathology

- The typical non-caseating (compare with TB) sarcoid granuloma consists of a focal accumulation of epithelioid cells, macrophages and lymphocytes, mainly T cells.
- There is a depressed cell-mediated immunity to antigens, such as tuberculin and *Candida albicans*, and an overall lymphopenia with low circulating T cells, as a result of sequestration of lymphocytes within the lung and slightly increased B cells.
- There is an increased number of cells in the bronchoalveolar lavage, particularly CD4 helper cells.
- Transbronchial biopsies show infiltration of alveolar walls and interstitial spaces with mononuclear cells before granuloma formation.

## Clinical features

The most common presentation is with bilateral hilar lymphadenopathy, which may be found incidentally on a routine chest X-ray or be associated with mild fever, malaise, arthralgia and erythema nodosum (p. 728). Pulmonary infiltration may predominate, and, in a minority of patients there is progressive fibrosis resulting in increasing effort dyspnoea, cor pulmonale and death. The chest X-ray is negative at presentation in up to 20% of non-respiratory cases. Skin and ocular sarcoidosis are the most common extrapulmonary problems (Table 10.8). Asymptomatic hypercalcaemia is found on routine blood tests in 10% of established cases, but is less commonly a clinical problem. Hepatitis and hepatosplenomegaly are uncommon, but granulomas may often be found if a liver biopsy is performed. Cardiac involvement is rare.

## Investigations

Diagnosis depends on a compatible clinical picture, exclusion of other causes of granulomatous diseases, such as tuberculosis and beryllium poisoning, and histological evidence of non-caseating granulomas.

- Chest X-ray may show typical features (see above). CT scanning is essential for assessment of diffuse lung involvement.

**Table 10.8**
Extrapulmonary features of sarcoidosis

| | |
|---|---|
| Skin | Erythema nodosum, skin papules, lupus pernio (red/blue infiltration of the nose) |
| Eye | Anterior uveitis, conjunctivitis, keratoconjunctivitis sicca, uveoparotid fever (bilateral uveitis, parotid gland enlargement and facial nerve palsy) |
| Bone | Arthralgias, bone cysts |
| Metabolic | Hypercalcaemia as a result of high circulating levels of $1,25\text{-}(OH_2)D_3$ from activated sarcoid macrophages |
| Liver | Granulomatous hepatitis, hepatosplenomegaly |
| CNS | VIIth cranial nerve palsy, hypothalamic involvement, hypopituitarism |
| Heart | Ventricular arrhythmias, conduction defects, cardiomyopathy with cardiac failure |

- Transbronchial biopsy is the most useful investigation and gives positive histological evidence in 90% of cases of pulmonary sarcoidosis.
- Lung function tests in pulmonary infiltration show a restrictive lung defect with a decreased total lung capacity, $FEV_1$, FVC and gas transfer.
- Serum angiotensin-converting enzyme (ACE) is raised in 75% of patients. It is useful in assessing the activity of disease and response to treatment, but is not of diagnostic value because it is also elevated in patients with lymphoma, tuberculosis, asbestosis, silicosis and Gaucher's disease.
- Tuberculin test is negative in 80% of patients. It is of interest but of no diagnostic value.
- Biopsy and histological examination of involved lymph nodes, liver or skin lesions is sometimes necessary for diagnosis.

## Differential diagnosis

The differential diagnosis of bilateral hilar lymphadenopathy includes lymphoma, pulmonary tuberculosis and bronchial carcinoma with secondary spread. The combination of symmetrical bilateral hilar lymphadenopathy and erythema nodosum only occurs in sarcoidosis.

## Management

The requirement for treatment and the role of steroids are presently contested in many aspects of this disease. Hilar lymphadenopathy with no other evidence of lung involvement on chest X-ray or lung function testing does not require treatment. Infiltration or abnormal lung function tests that persist for 6 months after diagnosis should be treated with 30 mg prednisolone for 6 weeks, reducing to 15 mg on alternate days for 6–12 months. Most patients with hypercalcaemia or other evidence of extrapulmonary sarcoidosis probably require treatment with prednisolone. Topical steroids are used for eye involvement.

## Prognosis

In patients of African origin the mortality rate may be up to 10%, but is less than 5% in Caucasians. Death is mainly as a result of respiratory failure or renal damage from hypercalciuria. The prognosis is best in those with BHL and no infiltration on the chest X-ray: the disease remits within 2 years in over two-thirds of patients.

# Pulmonary vasculitis and granulomatosis

(*K&C* p. 900)

There are two main groups:

- Pulmonary vasculitis associated with systemic connective tissue diseases including rheumatoid arthritis, systemic lupus erythematosus and systemic sclerosis (Ch. 6).
- The vasculitides associated with the presence of antineutrophil cytoplasmic antibodies (ANCAs) including Churg–Strauss syndrome, microscopic polyangiitis (p. 264) and Wegener's granulomatosis.

Wegener's granulomatosis is a vasculitis of unknown aetiology characterized by lesions involving the upper respiratory tract, the lungs and the kidneys. The disease often starts with rhinorrhoea, with subsequent nasal mucosal ulceration, cough, haemoptysis and pleuritic pain. Chest X-ray shows nodular masses or pneumonic infiltrates with cavitation which often show a migratory pattern.

Antineutrophil cytoplasmic antibodies are found in the serum in over 90% of cases with active disease, and measurement is useful both diagnostically and as a guide to disease activity in the treated patient. Typical histological changes are best shown in the kidney, where there is a necrotizing glomerulonephritis. Treatment is with cyclophosphamide.

# Pulmonary fibrosis and honeycomb lung

(*K&C* p. 904)

Pulmonary fibrosis is the end result of many diseases of the respiratory tract. It may be one of the following types:

- Localized, e.g. following unresolved pneumonia
- Bilateral, e.g. in TB
- Widespread, e.g. in cryptogenic fibrosing alveolitis.

Honeycomb lung is the radiological appearance seen with widespread fibrosis. Dilated and thickened terminal and respiratory bronchioles produce cystic airspaces, giving a honeycomb appearance on chest X-ray.

## Cryptogenic fibrosing alveolitis (*K&C* p. 904)

Cryptogenic fibrosing alveolitis (CFA) is a rare disorder of unknown aetiology characterized by sequential acute lung injury with subsequent scarring and end-stage lung disease. It presents in late middle age.

### Clinical features

Patients with CFA typically present with exertional dyspnoea and a non-productive cough. Eventually there is respiratory failure, pulmonary hypertension and cor pulmonale. Finger clubbing occurs in two-thirds of cases, and fine inspiratory basal crackles are heard on auscultation. Rarely, an acute form known as the Hamman–Rich syndrome occurs.

### Investigations

- Chest X-ray appearances are initially of a ground-glass appearance, progressing to fibrosis and honeycomb lung. These changes are most prominent in the lower lung zones.

- High-resolution CT scan (sampling lung parenchyma with scans of 1–2 mm thickness at intervals of 10–20 mm) is the most sensitive imaging technique, and shows irregular linear opacities and honeycombing.
- Respiratory function tests show a restrictive defect (p. 447) with low lung volumes and impaired gas transfer.
- Blood gases show hypoxaemia with a normal $P_a\text{CO}_2$.
- Histological confirmation with transbronchial or open lung biopsies may be required in younger people.
- Autoantibodies, such as antinuclear factor and rheumatoid factor, are present in one-third of patients.

## Differential diagnosis

This is from other causes of lung fibrosis: rheumatoid arthritis, systemic lupus erythematosus, systemic sclerosis, sarcoidosis, radiation, pneumoconiosis, chronic extrinsic allergic alveolitis and drugs (amiodarone, busulfan, bleomycin, methysergide, cyclophosphamide). A detailed occupational exposure history and drug history are required to exclude other causes of pulmonary fibrosis.

The diagnosis of CFA is usually made in a patient presenting with the above signs and characteristic CT changes. The differential diagnosis of the chest X-ray appearance includes extrinsic allergic alveolitis, bronchiectasis, chronic left heart failure, industrial lung disease and lymphangitis carcinomatosa.

## Treatment

Large doses of prednisolone are used (30 mg daily); azathioprine and cyclophosphamide may also be tried. Single lung transplantation is now an established treatment for some individuals, and current survival rate figures are 60% at 1 year after transplantation.

## Prognosis

The median survival without lung transplantation is approximately 5 years.

## Extrinsic allergic alveolitis (*K&C p. 905*)

Extrinsic allergic alveolitis is characterized by a widespread diffuse inflammatory reaction in the alveoli and small airways of the lung as a response to inhalation of a range of different antigens (Table 10.9). By far the most common is farmer's lung, which affects up to 1 in 10 of the farming community in poor wet areas around the world.

### Clinical features

There is fever, malaise, cough and shortness of breath several hours after exposure to the causative antigen. Physical examination reveals tachypnoea, and coarse end-inspiratory crackles and wheezes. Continuing exposure leads to a chronic illness with weight loss, effort dyspnoea, cough and the features of fibrosing alveolitis.

### Investigations

- Chest X-ray shows fluffy nodular shadowing with the subsequent development of streaky shadows, particularly in the upper zones.
- Full blood count shows a raised white cell count in acute cases.
- Lung function tests show a restrictive defect with a decrease in gas transfer.
- Precipitating antibodies to causative antigens are present in the serum (these are evidence of exposure and not disease).
- Bronchoalveolar lavage shows increased lymphocytes and granulocytes.

### Management

Prevention is the aim, with avoidance of exposure to the antigen if possible. Prednisolone in large doses (30–60 mg daily) may be required to cause regression of the disease in the early stages.

## Occupational lung disease (*K&C p. 907*)

Exposure to dusts, gases, vapours and fumes at work can lead to the following types of lung disease:

**Table 10.9**
Extrinsic allergic bronchiolar alveolitis

| Disease | Situation | Antigens |
|---|---|---|
| Farmer's lung | Forking mouldy hay or other vegetable material | *Faenia rectivirgula* (*Micropolyspora faeni*) |
| Bird fancier's lung | Handling pigeons, cleaning lofts or budgerigar cages | Proteins present in feathers and excreta |
| Malt worker's lung | Turning germinating barley | *Aspergillus clavatus* |
| Humidifier fever | Contaminated humidifying systems in air conditioners or humidifiers | A variety of bacteria or amoebae |

- Acute bronchitis and pulmonary oedema from irritants such as sulphur dioxide, chlorine, ammonia or oxides of nitrogen
- Pulmonary fibrosis due to mineral dust such as coal, silica, asbestos, iron and tin
- Occupational asthma – this is the commonest industrial lung disease in the developed world
- Extrinsic allergic alveolitis (p. 489)
- Bronchial carcinoma due to asbestos, polycyclic hydrocarbons and radon in mines.

## Coal worker's pneumoconiosis (K&C p. 908)

Most inhaled particles cause no damage to the lung because they are trapped in the nose, removed by the mucociliary clearance system or destroyed by alveolar macrophages. Small inorganic dust particles that reach the acinus and damage macrophages initiate an inflammatory reaction and subsequent fibrosis. Coal worker's pneumoconiosis is the term used for the accumulation of coal dust in the lungs and the reaction of the lung tissue to its presence. Improved working conditions and reduction in the coal industry has led to a considerable reduction in the number of cases of pneumoconiosis. The disease is subdivided into simple pneumoconiosis and progressive massive fibrosis (PMF). Simple pneumoconiosis produces small (< 1.5 mm) pulmonary nodules on the chest X-ray. The importance of simple pneumoconiosis is that it may lead to the development of PMF with continued exposure. PMF is characterized by large (1–10 cm) fibrotic masses, predominantly in the upper lobes. Unlike simple pneumoconiosis the disease may progress after exposure to coal dust has ceased. Symptoms are dyspnoea and cough productive of black sputum. Eventually respiratory failure may supervene. There is no specific treatment and further exposure must be prevented. Patients with PMF and some with simple pneumoconiosis (depending on the severity of radiological changes) are eligible for disability benefit in the UK.

## Asbestosis (K&C p. 908)

Asbestos is a mixture of fibrous silicates which have the common properties of resistance to heat, acid and alkali, hence their widespread use at one time. Chrysotile or white asbestos comprises 90% of the world production and is less fibrogenic than the other forms – crocidolite (blue asbestos) and amosite (brown asbestos). The diseases caused by asbestos (Table 10.10) are all characterized by a long latency period (20–40 years) between exposure and disease.

# Carcinoma of the lung (K&C p. 911)

## Epidemiology
Bronchial carcinoma is the most common malignant tumour in the western world and in the UK is the third most common cause of death after heart disease and pneumonia. There is a 3 : 1 male : female ratio, but although the rising mortality of this disease has levelled off in men, it continues to rise in women.

## Aetiology
Smoking is by far the most common aetiological factor, although there is a higher incidence in urban areas than in rural areas even when allowances are made for smoking. Other aetiological factors are passive smoking, exposure to asbestos, and possibly also contact with arsenic, chromium, iron oxides and the products of coal combustion.

## Pathology
These are broadly divided into small cell and non-small cell cancer. Non-small cell tumours are further subdivided as shown in Table 10.11.

## Clinical features

**Local effects of tumour within a bronchus** Cough, chest pain, haemoptysis and breathlessness are typical symptoms.

**Spread within the chest** Tumour may directly involve the pleura and ribs, causing pain and bone fractures. Spread to involve the brachial plexus causes pain in the shoulder and inner arm (Pancoast's tumour), spread to the sympathetic ganglion causes Horner's syndrome (p. 651), and spread to

**Table 10.10**
The effects of asbestos on the lung

| Disease | Pathology and clinical features |
|---------|--------------------------------|
| Asbestos bodies in the lung | They produce no symptoms or change in lung function and serve only as a marker of exposure |
| Pleural plaques | Fibrotic plaques on the parietal pleura which usually produce no symptoms |
| Pleural effusion | Recurrent effusions produce pleuritic pain and dyspnoea |
| Bilateral diffuse pleural thickening* | Thickening of the parietal and visceral pleura which produces effort dyspnoea and a restrictive ventilatory defect |
| Mesothelioma* | Tumour arising from mesothelial cells of the pleura, peritoneum and pericardium. Often presents with a pleural effusion. There is no treatment and median survival is 2 years |
| Asbestosis* | Characterized by progressive dyspnoea associated with finger clubbing and bilateral basal end-inspiratory crackles. There is a restrictive ventilatory defect on lung function testing |
| Lung cancer, often adenocarcinoma* | Presentation and treatment is that of lung cancer (see pp. 491–492) |

* The diseases indicated are all eligible for compensation under the Social Security Act of 1975

494

**Table 10.11**
Types of bronchial carcinoma

| Cell type | % Lung tumours | Characteristics |
|---|---|---|
| **Non-small cell** | | |
| Squamous | 40 | Most present as obstructive lesion leading to infection<br>Occasionally cavitates<br>Local spread common, widespread metastases occur late |
| Large cell | 25 | Less well-differentiated tumour that metastasizes early |
| Adenocarcinoma | 10 | Proportionately more common in non-smokers. Most common bronchial carcinoma associated with asbestos exposure. Usually occurs peripherally. Local and distant metastases |
| Alveolar cell | 1–2 | Presents as a peripheral solitary nodule or as diffuse nodular lesions of multicentric origin |
| **Small cell** | 20–30 | Arises from endocrine cells (Kulchitsky cells) which often secrete polypeptide hormones. These enhance tumour cell growth and result in paraneoplastic syndromes, e.g. production of ACTH and Cushing's syndrome. Early development of widespread metastases. Responds to chemotherapy |

the left recurrent laryngeal nerve causes hoarseness and a bovine cough. In addition the tumour may directly involve the oesophagus, heart or superior vena cava (causing upper limb oedema, facial congestion and distended neck veins).

**Metastatic disease** Metastases present as bone pain, epilepsy or with focal neurological signs.

**Non-metastatic manifestations** These are rare apart from finger clubbing (Table 10.12). There may, in addition, be non-specific features such as malaise, lethargy and weight loss. On examination of the chest there are often no physical signs, although lymphadenopathy, signs of a pleural effusion, lobar collapse or unresolved pneumonia may be present.

## Investigations

The aim of investigation is to confirm the diagnosis, determine the histology and assess tumour spread as a guide to treatment.

**Confirm the diagnosis** Chest X-ray is the most valuable initial test, although tumours need to be between 1 and 2 cm to be recognized reliably. They usually appear as a round shadow, the edge of which often has a fluffy or spiked appearance. There may be evidence of cavitation, lobar collapse, a pleural effusion or secondary pneumonia. Spread through the lymphatic channels gives rise to lymphangitis carcinomatosis, appearing as streaky shadowing throughout the lung.

**Determine the histology** Sputum is examined by a cytologist for malignant cells. Bronchoscopy is used to obtain biopsies for histological investigation and washings for cytology. Transthoracic fine needle aspiration biopsy under radiographic or CT screening is useful for obtaining tissue diagnosis from peripheral lesions.

**Assess spread of the tumour** At bronchoscopy involvement of the first 2 cm of either main bronchus or of the recurrent laryngeal nerve (vocal cord paresis) indicates inoperability. CT is useful for assessing the mediastinum and the extent of tumour spread. Magnetic resonance imaging is also used for

**Table 10.12**
Non-metastatic extrapulmonary manifestations of bronchial carcinoma

| | |
|---|---|
| Endocrine | Ectopic secretion of:<br>ACTH causing Cushing's syndrome<br>ADH causing dilutional hyponatraemia<br>PTH-like substance causing hypercalcaemia |
| Neurological | Cerebellar degeneration<br>Myopathy, polyneuropathies<br>Myasthenic syndrome (Eaton–Lambert syndrome) |
| Vascular/haematological | Thrombophlebitis migrans<br>Non-bacterial thrombotic endocarditis<br>Anaemia<br>Disseminated intravascular coagulation |
| Skeletal | Clubbing<br>Hypertrophic pulmonary osteoarthropathy (clubbing, painful wrists and ankles) |
| Cutaneous | Dermatomyositis<br>Acanthosis nigricans (pigmented overgrowth of skin in axillae or groin)<br>Herpes zoster |

staging and provides better images of the mediastinum than CT. Mediastinoscopy and lymph node biopsy may be necessary before surgery if the scan shows lymphadenopathy, which can be reactive or involved by tumour. The presence of bony and liver metastases is determined by serum alkaline phosphatase and other liver biochemistry. Liver ultrasonography and isotope bone scanning are only necessary if these screening tests are abnormal.

*Determine patient suitability for major operation* Physical examination and respiratory function tests.

## Treatment

- Surgery is the only treatment of any curative value for non-small cell cancer. In the 20% of cases that are suitable for resection the 5-year survival rate is 25–30%.
- Radiotherapy in high doses can produce results that are equal to surgery in patients with localized tumours but who are otherwise unfit for surgery, e.g. poor lung function testing. Palliative radiotherapy is useful for bone pain, haemoptysis and superior vena cava obstruction.
- Chemotherapy (*K&C* p. 503). In small cell cancer this has resulted in a fivefold increase in median survival, from 2 to 10 months. A small number of patients achieve several years of remission.

  In non-small cell lung cancer the response is less satisfactory, though newer agents, e.g. gemcitabine, achieve response rates of greater than 20% and significantly extend median survival.
- Local treatment. Endoscopic laser therapy, endobronchial irradiation and transbronchial stenting are being increasingly employed to deal with distressing symptoms in inoperable cases. Malignant pleural effusions should be aspirated to dryness and a sclerosing agent (e.g. tetracycline, bleomycin) instilled into the pleural space. In the terminal stages the quality of life must be maintained as far as possible. In addition to general nursing, counselling and medical care, patients may need oral or intravenous opiates for pain (given with laxatives to prevent constipation), and prednisolone may improve the appetite.

### Differential diagnosis

In most cases the diagnosis is straightforward. A solitary round shadow on the chest X-ray may also be the result of a benign growth (*K&C* p. 910), a primary bronchial carcinoid, a secondary deposit, tuberculoma or hydatid cyst.

## Metastatic tumours in the lung (*K&C* p. 914)

Metastases in the lung are common, usually presenting as round shadows 1.5–3 cm in diameter. The most common primary sites are the kidney, prostate, breast, bone, gastro-intestinal tract, cervix or ovary.

## Diseases of the pleura

### Dry pleurisy (*K&C* p. 915)

Dry pleurisy is the term used to describe inflammation of the pleura when there is no effusion. This results in local-ized sharp pain made worse on deep inspiration, coughing and bending or twisting movements. Common causes are pneumonia, pulmonary infarct and carcinoma.

Epidemic myalgia (Bornholm disease) is the result of infection with Coxsackie B virus. It is characterized by an upper respiratory tract infection followed by pleuritic pain and abdominal pain with tender muscles. The chest X-ray remains normal and the illness clears in 1 week.

### Pleural effusion (*K&C* p. 916)

A pleural effusion is an excessive accumulation of fluid in the pleural space. It can be detected clinically when there are more than 500 mL present, and by X-ray when there are more than 300 mL. A pleural effusion may be asymptomatic (if small) or cause breathlessness. The physical signs and chest X-ray appearances are shown in Figure 10.3.

### Aetiology

Serous effusions may be transudates (protein content < 30 g/L) or exudates (> 30 g/L). The causes of a serous effusion are shown in Table 10.13. More rarely, effusions consist of blood (haemothorax), pus (empyema) or lymph

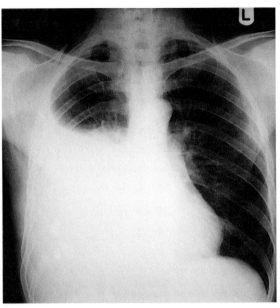

**Fig. 10.3 The chest radiographic appearances of a pleural effusion.** Physical signs on the affected side:
- Reduced chest wall movement
- Dull ('stony dull') to percussion
- Absent breath sounds
- Reduced vocal resonance
- Mediastinum shifted away.

(chylothorax). Chylous effusions are caused by leakage of lymph from the thoracic duct as a result of trauma or infiltration by carcinoma.

## Investigations

Diagnosis is by pleural aspiration and pleural biopsy (p. 743). Fluid is sent for the following:

- Protein estimation
- Lactic dehydrogenase
- Bacteriological examination: Gram stain and culture, Ziehl–Nielsen stain and culture
- Cytology for malignant cells
- Occasionally: amylase, rheumatoid factor, glucose.

Table 10.13
Causes of a pleural effusion

| Transudate | Exudate |
|---|---|
| Protein < 30 g/L<br>Lactic dehydrogenase < 200 IU/L | Protein > 30 g/L<br>Lactic dehydrogenase > 200 IU/L |
| Heart failure<br>Hypoproteinaemia<br>Constrictive pericarditis<br>Hypothyroidism<br>Meigs' syndrome (ovarian fibroma with right-sided pleural effusion and ascites) | Bacterial pneumonia<br>Carcinoma of the bronchus<br>Pulmonary infarction<br>Tuberculosis<br>Connective tissue disease<br>Rare causes:<br>Post-myocardial infarction syndrome<br>Acute pancreatitis<br>Mesothelioma<br>Sarcoidosis |

## Management

This depends on the underlying cause. Exudates are usually drained and transudates are managed by treatment of the underlying cause. Malignant effusions usually reaccumulate after drainage. They can be treated by aspiration to dryness followed by instillation into the pleural space of a sclerosing agent such as tetracycline or bleomycin.

# Pneumothorax (K&C p. 917)

Pneumothorax means the presence of air in the pleural space, and this may occur spontaneously or secondary to chest trauma. A 'tension pneumothorax' is rare unless the patient is on positive-pressure ventilation. In this situation the pleural tear acts as a one-way valve through which air passes only during inspiration. Positive pressure builds up, causing increasing cardiorespiratory embarrassment and eventually cardiac arrest. Treatment is immediate decompression by needle thoracocentesis (2nd intercostal space, mid-clavicular line) and then intercostal tube drainage.

## Aetiology

Spontaneous pneumothorax typically occurs in tall, thin boys and men between the ages of 10 and 30 years and is the result of rupture of a subpleural bleb. A bleb is thought to be a congenital defect in the connective tissue of the alveolar wall, which may occur in both lungs with equal frequency. In patients over 40 years of age the usual cause is underlying COPD.

## Clinical features

There is a sudden onset of pleuritic pain with increasing breathlessness. The physical signs and chest X-ray appearances are shown in Figure 10.4.

## Management

Treatment depends on four factors: the size of the pneumothorax, severity of symptoms, coexistent lung disease and whether there is a persistent air leak. With a small pneumothorax (< 20% of the hemithorax), patients without coexistent lung disease may have minimal symptoms and

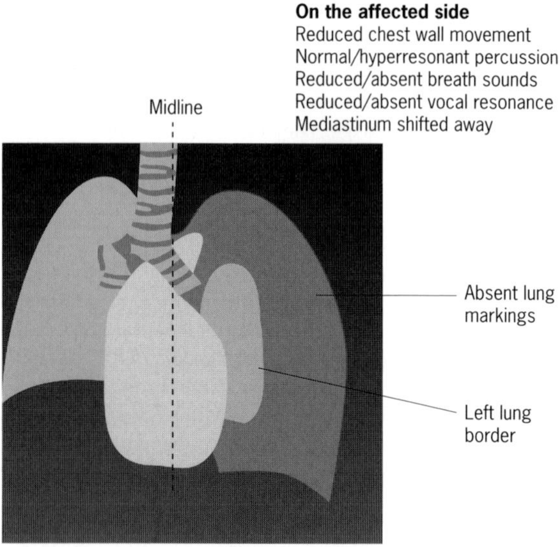

Disorders of the diaphragm

**On the affected side**
Reduced chest wall movement
Normal/hyperresonant percussion
Reduced/absent breath sounds
Reduced/absent vocal resonance
Mediastinum shifted away

Midline

Absent lung
markings

Left lung
border

**Fig. 10.4 Schematic representation of the chest radiographic
appearances and physical signs of a pneumothorax.** The chest
radiograph shows a large pneumothorax (> 50% radiographic volume).
Sometimes with a large pneumothorax there is a shift of the trachea and
mediastinum.

can be managed at home, returning for a repeat chest
X-ray in 2 weeks. All patients with coexistent lung disease
should remain in hospital. Larger pneumothoraxes
should be drained by simple aspiration with a plastic
intravenous catheter (p. 43). Insertion of a chest tube may
be necessary if this fails. The application of suction (pressure of 20 cm of water) to the chest drain can help where
there is failure of re-expansion or with ongoing air leaks.
Persistent air leaks are, however, usually an indication for
surgery.

# Disorders of the diaphragm (K&C p. 917)

The most common cause of unilateral diaphragmatic paralysis is the result of involvement of the phrenic nerve

(C2–C4) in the thorax by a bronchial carcinoma. Other common causes of phrenic paralysis are trauma, surgery and motor neurone disease. Unilateral paralysis produces no symptoms.

The characteristic features of bilateral diaphragmatic weakness are orthopnoea, paradoxical (inward) movement of the abdominal wall on inspiration and a large fall in FVC on lying down. It may be the result of trauma or occur as part of a generalized muscular or neurological condition, such as motor neurone disease, muscular dystrophy or Guillain–Barré syndrome. Treatment is either diaphragmatic pacing or night-time assisted ventilation.

## USEFUL WEB SITES

http://www.brit-thoracic.org.uk
British Thoracic Society: guidelines for the management of many respiratory diseases including asthma

http://www.ginaasthma.com
Global Initiative for Asthma: advice on the management and prevention of asthma

http://www.nhlbi.nih.gov/guidelines/asthma/asthgdln.htm
National Asthma Education and Prevention Program: guidelines for the diagnosis and management of asthma

http://www.goldcopd.com
WHO global initiative for COPD: diagnosis, treatment and prevention of COPD

# 11

# Intensive care medicine

Intensive care medicine (or 'critical care medicine') is concerned mainly with the management of patients with acute life-threatening conditions ('the critically ill') in a specialized unit. It also encompasses the resuscitation and transport of those who become acutely ill, or are injured, either elsewhere in the hospital or in the community. An intensive care unit (ICU) has the facilities and expertise to provide cardiorespiratory support to these sick patients, some of whom also have kidney or liver failure, and management of this is described in the relevant chapters.

All patients admitted to the ICU require skilled nursing care (patient to nurse ratio of 1:1) and physiotherapy. Many require nutritional support. General medical management includes the prevention of venous thrombosis (p. 217), pressure sores and constipation. A number of scoring systems, such as the APACHE score, are in use to evaluate the severity of the patient's illness.

## Acute disturbances of haemodynamic function (shock) (K&C p. 926)

505

The term 'shock' is used to describe acute circulatory failure with inadequate or inappropriately distributed tissue perfusion resulting in generalized cellular hypoxia. The causes of shock are listed in Table 11.1. Shock is often the result of a combination of these factors.

### Pathophysiology

**Sympathoadrenal** In response to hypotension there is a reflex increase in sympathetic nervous activity and catecholamine release from the adrenal medulla. The resulting vasoconstriction, increased myocardial contractility and heart rate help restore blood pressure and cardiac output. Activation of the renin–angiotensin system leads to

**Table 11.1**
Causes of shock

Hypovolaemic
    Exogenous losses (e.g. haemorrhage, burns)
    Endogenous losses (e.g. sepsis, anaphylaxis)
Cardiogenic
    Myocardial infarction
    Myocarditis
    Rupture of a valve cusp
Obstructive
    Obstruction to outflow (e.g. pulmonary embolus)
    Restricted cardiac filling (e.g. cardiac tamponade)
Distributive
    Vascular dilatation (e.g. drugs, sepsis)
    Arteriovenous shunting
    Maldistribution of flow (e.g. sepsis, anaphylaxis)

vasoconstriction and salt and water retention, which help to restore circulating volume.

**Neuroendocrine response** There is release of anterior pituitary hormones and glucagon, which are insulin antagonists. They raise blood sugar and may be responsible for some of the cardiovascular changes.

**Release of mediators** In septic shock components of microorganisms (e.g. endotoxin of Gram-negative bacteria) release cytokines (tumour necrosis factor, interleukin-1 and interferon-$\gamma$) from macrophages and white cells, activate the complement system and cause the release of vasoactive mediators (e.g. prostacyclin, endothelin-1 and nitric oxide) from vascular endothelium. The end result of these processes is vasodilatation, increased vascular permeability, endothelial cell damage and platelet aggregation. Vasodilatation and increased vascular permeability are also seen in shock secondary to anaphylaxis.

A similar widespread inflammatory response may occur with non-infectious processes, e.g. trauma and acute pancreatitis, and is referred to as the *systemic inflammatory response syndrome* (SIRS). The clinical features are pyrexia, tachycardia, tachypnoea and a raised white cell count.

***Microcirculatory changes*** In the early stages of septic shock there is vasodilatation, increased capillary permeability with interstitial oedema, and arteriovenous shunting. Vasodilatation and increased capillary permeability also occur in anaphylactic shock. In the initial stages of other forms of shock, and in the later stages of sepsis and anaphylaxis, there is capillary sequestration of blood. Fluid is forced into the extravascular space, causing interstitial oedema, haemoconcentration and an increase in plasma viscosity.

In all forms of shock there may be activation of the coagulation pathway, with the development of disseminated intravascular coagulation (DIC, see p. 213). The disseminated inflammatory response and microcirculatory changes may lead to progressive organ failure (*multiple organ dysfunction syndrome* (MODS), also known as multiple organ failure (MOF)); the lungs are usually affected first, with the development of the *acute respiratory distress syndrome* (ARDS). The mortality in MODS is high and treatment is supportive.

## Clinical features

The history will often indicate the cause of shock, e.g. a patient with major injuries (often internal and thus concealed) will often develop hypovolaemic shock. A patient with a history of peptic ulceration may now be bleeding into the gastrointestinal tract, and rectal examination will show melaena. Anaphylactic shock may develop in susceptible individuals after insect stings and eating certain foods, e.g. peanuts.

***Hypovolaemic shock*** Inadequate tissue perfusion causes blue cold skin with slow capillary refill. The blood pressure (particularly when supine) may be maintained initially, but later hypotension supervenes (systolic BP < 100 mmHg) with oliguria (< 30 mL of urine/h), confusion and restlessness. Increased sympathetic tone causes tachycardia (pulse > 100/min) and sweating.

***Cardiogenic shock*** Additional clinical features are those of myocardial failure, e.g. raised jugular venous pressure

(JVP), pulsus alternans (alternating strong and weak pulses) and/or a 'gallop' rhythm (p. 389).

**Mechanical shock** Muffled heart sounds, pulsus paradoxus (pulse fades on inspiration), elevated JVP and Kussmaul's sign (JVP increases on inspiration) occur in cardiac tamponade. In pulmonary embolism there are signs of right heart strain, with a raised JVP with prominent 'a' waves, right ventricular heave and a loud pulmonary second sound.

**Anaphylactic shock** Profound vasodilatation leads to warm peripheries and low blood pressure. Erythema, urticaria, angio-oedema, bronchospasm, and oedema of the face and larynx may all be present.

**Septic shock** In the early stages there is vasodilatation, pyrexia and rigors. At a later stage there are features of hypovolaemic shock. Sepsis in elderly people or in the immunosuppressed is common without the classic clinical features.

## Management (K&C p. 937)
This is summarized in Emergency Box 11.1. The underlying cause must be identified and treated appropriately. Whatever the aetiology of shock, tissue blood flow and blood pressure must be restored as quickly as possible to avoid the development of MOF.

**Expansion of the circulating volume** Volume replacement is obviously important in hypovolaemic shock, but also in anaphylactic and septic shock, where there is vasodilatation, sequestration of blood and loss of circulating volume secondary to capillary leakage. High filling pressures may also be needed in mechanical shock. Care must be taken to prevent volume overload, which leads to a reduction in stroke volume and a rise in left atrial pressure with a risk of pulmonary oedema. The choice of fluid depends on the clinical situation:

- Whole blood is the fluid of choice for haemorrhage. Crossmatched blood must be used if possible, but in

## Emergency Box 11.1

### Management of shock

**Ensure adequate oxygenation and ventilation**
- Maintain patent airway: use oropharyngeal airway or endotracheal tube if necessary.
- Administer 100% oxygen via tight-fitting face mask.
- Monitor respiratory rate, blood gases and chest X-ray.

**Restore cardiac output and BP**
- Lay patient flat or head-down.
- Expand circulating volume with appropriate fluids given quickly via large-bore cannulae.
- Monitor skin colour, pulse and blood pressure, peripheral temperature, urine output, ECG.

CVP monitoring is required in most cases, Swan–Ganz catheter in selected cases.

**Investigations**
- FBC, U+E, glucose, liver biochemistry, and blood gases in all cases.
- Infection screen, lactate levels, fibrinogen degradation products and crossmatch blood in selected cases. Echocardiogram in post-MI patients to identify patients with intra- or extramyocardial rupture.

**Treat underlying cause**
- Haemorrhage
- Sepsis
- Anaphylaxis.

**Treat complications**
- e.g. Coagulopathy, renal failure.

509

extreme emergencies the 'universal donor' group O rhesus-negative blood is used. Complications of massive blood transfusion are hypothermia, thrombocytopenia, hypocalcaemia and depletion of clotting factors.

- Colloidal solutions increase colloid osmotic pressure and produce a greater and more sustained increase in plasma volume than crystalloid solutions. They are used to replace fluid in hypovolaemic patients and are useful for the maintenance of blood volume, but have no oxygen-carrying capacity. Polygelatin solutions (e.g. Gelofusin and Haemaccel) are the most widely used. Human albumin solution and dextrans are less commonly used because of the expense (albumin) and higher complication rate (dextrans). Colloid solutions are often used for acute blood loss before whole blood becomes available, and for volume replacement in anaphylactic and septic shock.

- Crystalloids, e.g. 5% dextrose, 0.9% saline, are readily available and cheap. Once in the circulation they quickly redistribute into the interstitial fluid; therefore large volumes are needed to restore circulating volume and the excess fluid in the interstitial space may contribute to pulmonary oedema. Large volumes of crystalloid (> 2 litres) as a treatment for shock are best avoided. However, crystalloids are frequently used for volume replacement with diarrhoea and vomiting, and sometimes with burns.

***Myocardial contractility and inotropic agents*** Myocardial contractility is impaired in cardiogenic shock and at a later stage in other forms of shock as a result of hypoxaemia, acidosis and the release of mediators. It is recommended that the treatment of acidosis should concentrate on correcting the cause; intravenous bicarbonate should only be administered to correct extreme (pH < 7.0) persistent metabolic acidosis. Drugs that impair cardiac performance, e.g. β-blockers, should be stopped. When a patient remains hypotensive despite adequate volume replacement inotropic agents are administered. This must be via a large central vein and the effects carefully monitored. The inotropic agents used and their clinical effects are shown in Table 11.2. Many consider dopamine to be the inotrope of choice in critically ill patients, but dobutamine is a better choice when vasconstriction caused by dopamine could be dangerous. Norepinephrine (noradrenaline) in combination with dobutamine (depending on the cardiac output) is used for shocked patients with a low peripheral resistance, e.g. septic patients.

***Additional treatment*** Vasodilators, e.g. sodium nitroprusside and isosorbide dinitrate, may be useful in selected

**Table 11.2**
Inotropic agents used in the management of shock: the effect of each inotrope on the adrenergic and dopaminergic receptors is shown

| (Dose, μg/kg/min) | $\beta_1$ | $\beta_2$ | $\alpha_1$ | $\alpha_2$ | $DA_1$ | $DA_2$ | Comments |
|---|---|---|---|---|---|---|---|
| Epinephrine (adrenaline) <br> Low dose (0.06–0.1) <br> Moderate dose (0.1–0.18) <br> High dose (>0.18) | ++ <br> ++ <br> ++(+) | + <br> + <br> + | + <br> ++ <br> +++ | + <br> + <br> +++ | 0 <br> 0 <br> 0 | 0 <br> 0 <br> 0 | A potent inotrope used in patients not responding to dobutamine or dopamine. At high doses vasoconstriction may increase renal perfusion pressure and urine output, but as dose is further increased marked vasoconstriction leads to decreased cardiac output, oliguria and peripheral gangrene. Agent of choice in septic shock when haemodynamic monitoring not available |
| Norepinephrine (noradrenaline) | ++ | 0 | +++ | +++ | 0 | 0 | Particularly useful in septic shock as administration leads to increased inotropy and an increase in peripheral vascular resistance. Requires full haemodynamic monitoring |
| Isoprenaline | +++ | +++ | 0 | 0 | 0 | 0 | Rarely used |

**Table 11.2**
(continued)

| (Dose, µg/kg/min) | β₁ | β₂ | α₁ | α₂ | DA₁ | DA₂ | Comments |
|---|---|---|---|---|---|---|---|
| **Dopamine** | | | | | | | At low dose general vasodilatory action which may increase urine output and preserve function of vital organs. Increases cardiac output at all doses, but at high doses this beneficial effect may be offset by vasoconstriction, thus increasing afterload and ventricular filling pressure |
| Low dose (1–3) | + | 0 | 0 | + | ++ | + | |
| Moderate (3–10) | ++ | + | ++ | + | ++(+) | + | |
| High dose (> 10) | +++ | ++ | +++ | + | ++(+) | + | |
| Dopexamine | + | +++ | 0 | 0 | ++ | | Dopamine analogue. Most useful in patients with a low cardiac output and peripheral vasoconstriction |
| Dobutamine | ++ | + | + | 0 | 0 | | Similar actions to dopexamine, useful in patients with cardiogenic shock |
| Enoximone | Phosphodiesterase inhibitor with inotropic and vasodilator actions | | Occasionally useful in acute heart failure | | | | |

0, no agonism; + mild agonism; ++, moderate agonism; +++, profound agonism; α, α-adrenergic receptors; β, β-adrenergic receptors; DA, dopamine receptors

patients who remain vasoconstricted and oliguric despite adequate volume replacement and a satisfactory blood pressure. Finally, in patients with a potentially reversible depression of left ventricular function (e.g. cardiogenic shock secondary to a ruptured interventricular septum), intra-aortic balloon counterpulsation (IABCP) may be used as a temporary measure to maintain life until definitive surgical treatment can be carried out.

**Specific treatment of the cause** In all cases the cause of shock must be identified if possible and specific treatment given when indicated.

- *Septic shock.* Antibiotic therapy should be directed towards the probable cause. In the absence of helpful clinical guidelines, 'blind' intravenous antibiotic therapy (e.g. cefuroxime and gentamicin) should be started after performing an infection screen: chest X-ray and culture of blood, urine and sputum. Lumbar puncture, ultrasonography and CT of the chest and abdomen are useful in selected cases. Abscesses require drainage. Steroids have no role in the treatment of septic shock.
- *Anaphylactic shock* must be identified and treated immediately (Emergency Box 11.2).

## Monitoring (K&C p. 932)
This is by both clinical and invasive means.

**Clinical** An assessment of skin perfusion, measurement of pulse, BP, JVP and urinary flow rate will guide treatment in a straightforward case. Additional invasive monitoring will be required in seriously ill patients who do not respond to initial treatment.

### Invasive
- *Blood pressure.* A continuous recording may be made with an intra-arterial cannula, usually in the radial artery.
- *Central venous pressure* (CVP) is related to right ventricular end-diastolic pressure, which depends on circulating blood volume, venous tone, intrathoracic

## Emergency Box 11.2

### Management of anaphylactic shock

Remove the precipitating cause, e.g. stop administration of the offending drug.

Administer:

    0.5 mg epinephrine (adrenaline) intramuscularly,* i.e. 5 mL of a 1 in 10 000 solution

    Colloid, e.g. Haemaccel, 1 L rapid i.v. infusion and continue depending on response

    High concentration inhaled oxygen

    Antihistamine, e.g. chlorphenamine (chlorpheniramine) 10 mg i.v over 1–2 min

    Hydrocortisone 200 mg i.v.

    Repeat epinephrine every 10 minutes until improvement occurs.

\* Give intravenous epinephrine (0.5 mg over 5 minutes) with full ECG monitoring if patient is extremely unwell with hypotension and severe dyspnoea. There is a risk of relapse even after full recovery. Admit patient to hospital for 24 hours for monitoring and treatment with hydrocortisone and chlorphenamine.

Patients who have had an attack of anaphylaxis and who are at risk of developing another should carry a preloaded syringe of epinephrine for subcutaneous self-administration (e.g. Epipen device) and wear an appropriate information bracelet (e.g. MedicAlert).

---

pressure and right ventricular function. CVP is measured by inserting a catheter percutaneously into the superior vena cava and connecting it to a manometer system (p. 740). The normal range is 0–4 cmH$_2$O above the manubriosternal angle in a supine patient. In shock CVP may be normal, because in spite of hypovolaemia there is increased venous tone. A better guide to circulating volume is the response to a fluid challenge (Fig. 11.1).

- *Left atrial pressure.* In uncomplicated cases the CVP is an adequate guide to the filling pressures of both sides of the heart. However, if there is disparity in function between the two ventricles (e.g. infarction of the left ventricle), left atrial pressure must be measured. A Swan–Ganz catheter is introduced percutaneously into a central vein and then guided through the chambers

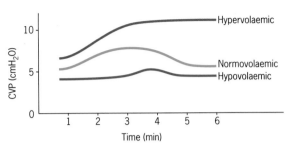

**Fig. 11.1 The effect of rapid administration (200 mL of 0.9% saline over 1–3 minutes) of a fluid challenge to patients with a CVP within the normal range.** (From Sykes MK (1963) Venous pressure as a clinical indication of adequacy of transfusion. Annals of the Royal College of Surgeons of England 33: 185–197.)

of the heart into the pulmonary artery. By inflating a balloon at the tip of the catheter, pulmonary artery wedge pressure (PAWP) is measured, which is a reflection of left atrial pressure.

- *Cardiac output* is measured, using a modified Swan–Ganz catheter, by recording temperature changes in the pulmonary artery after injecting a bolus of cold dextrose into the right atrium.

## Respiratory failure (K&C p. 944)

Respiratory failure occurs when pulmonary gas exchange is sufficiently impaired to cause hypoxaemia with or without hypercapnia.

It can be divided into two types (Table 11.3):

- Type 1 respiratory failure is caused by a diffusion defect in the gas exchange area of the lung, ventilation/perfusion mismatch or right-to-left shunts (e.g. with cyanotic congenital heart disease). The $P_aO_2$ is low (< 8 kPa) and the $P_aCO_2$ is normal or low.
- Type 2 respiratory failure is caused by hypoventilation. The $P_aO_2$ is low and the $P_aCO_2$ is high (> 7 kPa).

### Monitoring

**Clinical** Assessment should be made on the following criteria: tachypnoea, tachycardia, sweating, pulsus paradoxus,

**Table 11.3**
Causes of respiratory failure

| Type 1 | Type 2 |
| --- | --- |
| Pulmonary oedema | COPD |
| Pneumonia | Severe asthma |
| Asthma | Muscle weakness, e.g. |
| COPD | Guillain–Barré syndrome |
| Pulmonary embolism | Respiratory centre depression, e.g. |
| Acute respiratory distress | with sedatives |
| syndrome | Chest wall deformities |
| Fibrosing alveolitis | |
| Right-to-left cardiac shunts | |

use of accessory muscles of respiration, and inability to speak. Signs of carbon dioxide retention may be present, such as asterixis (coarse tremor), bounding pulse, warm peripheries and papilloedema.

**Pulse oximetry** Lightweight oximeters placed on an earlobe or finger can give a continuous reading of oxygen saturation by measuring the changing amount of light transmitted through arterial blood. In general, if the saturation is greater than 90% oxygenation can be considered to be adequate. Although simple and reliable, these instruments are not very sensitive to changes in oxygenation. They also give no indication of carbon dioxide retention.

**Arterial blood gas analysis** Analysis of arterial blood gives definitive measurements of $P_aO_2$, $P_aCO_2$, oxygen saturation, pH and bicarbonate (p. 738). In type 2 respiratory failure, retention of carbon dioxide causes $P_aCO_2$ and $[H^+]$ to rise, resulting in respiratory acidosis. The kidney compensates by retaining bicarbonate, reducing the $[H^+]$ towards normal. In type 1 respiratory failure or in hyperventilation there may be a fall in $P_aCO_2$ and $[H^+]$, resulting in respiratory alkalosis. Other abnormalities of acid–base balance are discussed on page 302.

**Capnography** This allows the continuous breath-by-breath analysis of expired carbon dioxide concentrations, and is mandatory in patients having tracheal intubation outside the ITU.

## Management

This includes the administration of supplemental oxygen, control of secretions, treatment of pulmonary infection, control of airway obstruction and limiting pulmonary oedema. In most patients oxygen is given by a face mask or nasal cannulae. With these devices, inspired oxygen concentration varies from 35% to 55%, with flow rates between 6 and 10 litres. However, in patients with chronically elevated carbon dioxide (e.g. COPD), hypoxia rather than hypercapnia maintains the respiratory drive and thus fixed-performance masks (e.g. Venturi masks) should be used, in which the concentration of oxygen can be accurately controlled. Respiratory stimulants such as doxapram have a very limited role in treatment.

**Respiratory support** Respiratory support should be considered when the above measures are not sufficient. The type depends on the underlying disorder and its clinical severity. Careful consideration should be given to ventilating patients with severe chronic lung disease, as those who are severely incapacitated may be difficult to wean from the ventilator.

- *Continuous positive airway pressure (CPAP)*. Oxygen is delivered to the spontaneously breathing patient under pressure via a tightly fitting face mask (non-invasive positive-pressure ventilation, NIPPV) or endotracheal tube. Oxygenation and vital capacity improve and the lungs become less stiff.

- *NIPPV* has been shown to be of use in patients with hypercapnic respiratory failure secondary to acute exacerbations of COPD who do not require immediate intubation and ventilation. NIPPV should be instituted at an early stage in the hospital admission when the pH falls below 7.35 and the respiratory rate exceeds 30 breaths per minute. NIPPV is usually given for at least 6 hours a day, and oxygen is administered to maintain arterial oxygen saturation above 90%. NIPPV reduces the need for intubation, complications, mortality and hospital stay.

- *Intermittent positive-pressure ventilation (IPPV)*. IPPV requires tracheal intubation and therefore anaesthesia if the patient is conscious. The beneficial effects of IPPV (Table 11.4) include improved carbon dioxide elimination, improved oxygenation, and relief from exhaustion as the work of ventilation is removed. High concentrations of oxygen (up to 100%) may be administered accurately. If adequate oxygenation cannot be achieved, a positive airway pressure can be maintained at a chosen level throughout expiration by attaching a threshold resistor valve to the expiratory limb of the circuit. This is known as positive end-expiratory pressure (PEEP), and its primary effect is to re-expand underventilated lung areas, thereby reducing shunts and increasing $P_aO_2$.

- *Intermittent mandatory ventilation (IMV)*. This technique allows the ventilated patient to breathe spontaneously between mandatory tidal volumes delivered by the ventilator. These coincide with the patient's own respiratory effort. It is used as a method of weaning patients from artificial ventilation, or as an alternative to IPPV.

The major complications of intubation and assisted ventilation are:

- Trauma to the upper respiratory tract from the endotracheal tube
- Secondary pulmonary infection
- Barotrauma – overdistension of the lungs and alveolar rupture may present with pneumothorax (p. 501) and surgical emphysema
- Reduction in cardiac output – the increase in intrathoracic pressures during controlled ventilation impedes cardiac filling and lowers cardiac output.

**Table 11.4**
Indications for IPPV

| Indication | Comment |
|---|---|
| Acute respiratory failure | Particularly when exhaustion, confusion, agitation or decreased consciousness are present |
| Acute ventilatory failure, e.g. myasthenia gravis, Guillain–Barré syndrome | Institute when vital capacity fallen to 10–15 mL/kg |
| Prophylactic postoperative ventilation | In poor-risk patients |
| Head injury | With acute brain oedema. Intracranial pressure is decreased by elective hyperventilation as this reduces cerebral blood flow |
| Trauma | e.g. Chest injury and lung contusion |
| Severe left ventricular failure | |
| Coma with breathing difficulties | e.g. Following drug overdose |

## Acute lung injury/acute respiratory distress syndrome (*K&C* p. 951)

Acute lung injury (ALI) and acute respiratory distress syndrome (ARDS) are defined as respiratory distress occurring with stiff lungs, diffuse bilateral pulmonary infiltrates, refractory hypoxaemia, in the presence of a recognized precipitating cause and in the absence of cardiogenic pulmonary oedema (i.e. the pulmonary capillary wedge pressure is less than 16 mmHg).

### Aetiology

The commonest precipitating factor is sepsis. Other causes include trauma, burns, pancreatitis, fat or amniotic fluid embolism, aspiration pneumonia or cardiopulmonary bypass.

### Pathophysiology

The cardinal feature is pulmonary oedema as a result of increased vascular permeability caused by the release of inflammatory mediators. Oedema may induce vascular compression resulting in pulmonary hypertension, which is later exacerbated by vasoconstriction in response to increased autonomic nervous activity. A haemorrhagic intra-alveolar exudate forms which is rich in platelets, fibrin and clotting factors. This inactivates surfactant, stimulates inflammation and promotes hyaline membrane formation. These changes may result in progressive pulmonary fibrosis.

### Clinical features

Tachypnoea, increasing hypoxia and laboured breathing are the initial features. The chest X-ray shows diffuse bilateral shadowing, which may progress to a complete 'white-out'.

## Management
This is based on the treatment of the underlying condition. Pulmonary oedema should be limited with fluid restriction, diuretics, and haemofiltration if these measures fail.

Steroids currently have no role in the prophylaxis of this condition, but may be beneficial when administered during the late fibroproliferative phase. Aerosolized surfactant, inhaled nitric oxide and aerosolized prostacyclin are experimental treatments whose exact role in the management of ARDS is unclear.

## Prognosis
Although the mortality has fallen over the last decade, it remains at 30–40%, most patients dying from sepsis. The prognosis is very dependent on the underlying cause, and rises steeply with age and with the development of multi-organ failure.

# Poisoning, drug and alcohol abuse

In many hospitals in the developed world, acute poisoning is one of the most common reasons for acute admission to a medical ward. Such poisoning may be:

- Deliberate self-administration of an excess quantity of prescribed and over-the-counter medicines, or illicit drugs
- Occupational exposure to chemicals
- Iatrogenic, e.g. digoxin toxicity
- In children due to accidental ingestion or Münchausen's syndrome by proxy.

Self-poisoning is the most common way by which people commit or attempt suicide (these categories are encompassed by the term 'deliberate self-harm'); other means are usually by violent methods, e.g. hanging, shooting or drowning (*K&C* p. 1249). Attempted suicide by a violent method is associated with future suicide and these patients must be assessed by a psychiatrist. In adults with self-poisoning admitted to hospital in the UK the most common drugs taken are paracetamol and benzodiazepines, followed by antidepressants, non-steroidal anti-inflammatory drugs (NSAIDs) and aspirin. In many cases more than one substance is taken; alcohol is frequently a secondary poison. Outside hospital, where most deaths occur, the commonest causes are deliberate carbon monoxide poisoning from inhalation of vehicle exhaust fumes. This is also seen in cases of accidental poisoning with faulty appliances using natural gas. In the developing world ingestion of pesticides, heating fuels, antimalarials and traditional medicines is more common.

The majority of cases (80%) of self-poisoning do not require intensive medical management but all require a sympathetic and caring approach to their problems. Both the patient and the family may require psychiatric help (see p. 527) and the social services should be contacted to help with social and domestic problems.

## *Clinical features* (K&C p. 974)

Eighty per cent of adults are conscious on arrival at hospital and the diagnosis of self-poisoning can usually be made easily from the history. In the unconscious patient a history from friends or relatives is helpful, and the diagnosis can often be inferred from tablet bottles or a suicide note brought by the ambulance attendants. In any patient with an altered conscious level drug overdose must always be considered in the differential diagnosis. On arrival at hospital the patient must be assessed urgently in the accident and emergency department. A full physical examination must include an assessment of cardiorespiratory status and conscious level (p. 659).

The physical signs that may aid identification of the agents responsible for poisoning are shown in Figure 12.1.

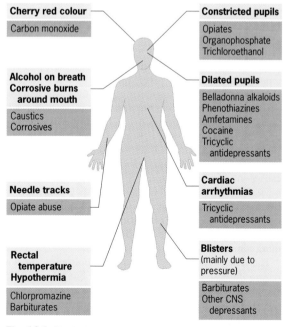

**Cherry red colour**
Carbon monoxide

**Constricted pupils**
Opiates
Organophosphate
Trichloroethanol

**Alcohol on breath
Corrosive burns
around mouth**
Caustics
Corrosives

**Dilated pupils**
Belladonna alkaloids
Phenothiazines
Amfetamines
Cocaine
Tricyclic
    antidepressants

**Needle tracks**
Opiate abuse

**Cardiac
arrhythmias**
Tricyclic
    antidepressants

**Rectal
    temperature
Hypothermia**
Chlorpromazine
Barbiturates

**Blisters**
(mainly due to
pressure)
Barbiturates
Other CNS
    depressants

**Fig. 12.1 Physical signs of poisoning.**

## Investigations

Blood and urine samples should always be taken on admission for the determination of drug levels, as these are invaluable for the management of certain poisons, e.g. paracetamol and salicylates, and are helpful in legal disputes. Drug screens of blood and urine are also occasionally helpful in the seriously ill unconscious patient in whom the cause of coma is unknown. Further investigations depend on the drugs ingested and clinical assessment of the patient, e.g. arterial blood gases in the comatose patient.

## Management (K&C p. 975)

Most patients with self-poisoning require only general care and support of the vital systems. However, for a few drugs additional therapy is required. In the UK the Regional Poisons Centre provides a round-the-clock service for advice about the management of overdose; the telephone number is found in the *British National Formulary*. The management of a patient with overdose is summarized in Table 12.1.

---

**Table 12.1**
Principles of management of patients with self-poisoning

1. Emergency resuscitation
2. Prevent further drug absorption
3. Increase drug elimination
4. Administration of specific drug antidotes
5. Psychiatric assessment

---

### Emergency resuscitation

- Nurse the patient in the lateral position with the lower leg straight and the upper leg flexed; this reduces the risk of aspiration.
- Clear the airway and intubate if the gag reflex is absent.
- Administer 60% oxygen by face mask in patients not intubated.
- Artificial ventilation is sometimes necessary if ventilation is inadequate (p. 518).
- Treat hypotension (p. 508), arrhythmias (p. 372) and convulsions (p. 678).

Management

- Respiratory function (arterial blood gas analysis or pulse oximetry) and ECG monitoring in selected patients.
- Measure temperature with a low-reading rectal thermometer and treat hypothermia (< 35°C) with 'space blankets', warm (37°C) intravenous fluids and inspired gases.

**Prevention of further drug absorption** Most patients coming to hospital after an overdose are not at serious risk. These measures are usually reserved for those who have taken a potentially serious overdose.

- *Gastric lavage* is used to remove the drug from the stomach. It should only be considered if a patient has ingested a potentially life-threatening amount of a poison and the procedure can be undertaken within 1 hour of ingestion. The main danger of gastric lavage is aspiration, and the unconscious patient must be intubated with a cuffed endotracheal tube if the gag reflex is absent. Lavage is contraindicated for some poisons, e.g. corrosives, petrol or paraffin, because of the risk of pneumonitis.
- *Whole bowel irrigation* is considered for potentially toxic ingestions of sustained-release or enteric-coated drugs. Polyethylene glycol electrolyte solution (2000 mL/h) is infused via a nasogastric tube until the rectal effluent is clear.
- *Activated charcoal* administered by mouth adsorbs unabsorbed poison still present in the gut. *Single-dose administration* (50 g) is considered if a patient has ingested a potentially toxic amount of a drug absorbed by charcoal (e.g. aspirin, digoxin, paracetamol, barbiturates) up to 1 hour previously. *Multiple-dose administration* (50 g initially followed by 50 g 4-hourly until charcoal appears in the faeces or recovery occurs) is considered if a patient has ingested a life-threatening amount of carbamazepine, phenobarbital, quinine, or theophylline. It increases drug elimination by interrupting the enterohepatic circulation and adsorbing the drug that has diffused into intestinal juices.

- *Induction of vomiting* with ipecacuanha syrup is no longer used in the management of poisoning.

### Increasing drug elimination

- *Urinary alkalinization* depends on the principle that ionization of acid drugs is increased in alkaline urine and thus renal tubular reabsorption is reduced (as only lipophilic non-ionized drugs cross the lipid membrane readily). In practice urine alkalinization is only employed commonly in salicylate intoxication (p. 528).
- *Dialysis* (peritoneal or haemodialysis) is used with some drugs in cases of severe poisoning, e.g. lithium, methyl or ethyl alcohols, and patients with severe salicylate poisoning (blood salicylate level > 700 mg/L, or 5.07 mmol/L) refractory to urine alkalization.

**Antagonizing the effects of poisons**  Specific antidotes are available for a small number of drugs; these will be considered under the individual drugs.

**Psychiatric assessment**  All suicide attempts must be taken seriously and an assessment made of suicidal intent (Table 12.2). In some patients, often young females, the act was not premeditated, they have no wish to die and the tablets were taken in response to an acute situation, e.g. an argument with the boyfriend. The risk of suicide is low and formal psychiatric assessment is not always necessary. In

---

**Table 12.2**
Factors associated with increased risk of suicide and need for psychiatric referral (SAD PERSONS scale)

- **S**  Sex (male)
- **A**  Age (> 45 years)
- **D**  Depression/hopelessness
- **P**  Previous deliberate self-harm
- **E**  Excessive alcohol or drug abuse
- **R**  Rational thinking, loss of
- **S**  Separated, widowed, divorced
- **O**  Organized or serious attempt (e.g. well thought out, suicide note, changed will)
- **N**  No social supports (no close/reliable family friends or siblings)
- **S**  Stated future intention to self-harm

the absence of potential medical problems these patients may not necessarily need to be admitted to hospital, provided there is the necessary social and emotional back-up at home. In other patients there is clear suicidal intent: the act was planned, a suicide note was written and efforts were made not to be discovered. These patients must be assessed by a psychiatrist before they leave hospital.

## Specific drug problems

In this section only specific treatment regimens will be discussed. The general principles of management of self-poisoning should always be applied.

### Aspirin (*K&C* p. 979)

Overdosage of aspirin (salicylate) stimulates the respiratory centre, directly increasing the depth and rate of respiration and thereby producing a respiratory alkalosis. Compensatory mechanisms include renal excretion of bicarbonate and potassium, which results in a metabolic acidosis, and a fall in arterial pH indicates serious poisoning. Salicylates also interfere with carbohydrate, fat and protein metabolism, as well as with oxidative phosphorylation. This gives rise to increased lactate, pyruvate and ketone bodies, all of which contribute to the acidosis.

#### Clinical features

Symptoms and signs of aspirin poisoning include tinnitus, nausea and vomiting, overbreathing, hyperpyrexia and sweating with a tachycardia. Alternatively, the patient may appear completely well, even with high plasma concentrations of salicylate. Ingestion of 10–20 g of aspirin by an adult (or one-tenth of this amount for a child) is likely to cause moderate or severe toxicity.

In severe poisoning (plasma salicylate concentration > 700 mg/L; 5.07 mmol/L) there may be cerebral and pulmonary oedema resulting from increased capillary permeability. Coma and respiratory depression may be seen with severe poisoning, but more frequently are due to the ingestion of a second drug or alcohol.

## Investigations

- Plasma salicylate concentration to determine the severity of poisoning. Initial and repeat levels after 2–4 hours should be performed.
- Serum urea and electrolytes.
- Blood glucose (hypoglycaemia may occur).
- Prothrombin time (may be prolonged).
- Arterial blood gases.
- Chest X-ray.

## Management

- Correct dehydration and hypokalaemia with intravenous fluids.
- Intravenous vitamin K (10 mg) to correct hypoprothrombinaemia.
- Consider gastric lavage or activated charcoal (50 g) in a patient who has taken a large amount of aspirin less than 1 hour previously.
- Urine alkalinization for moderately severe poisoning (plasma salicylate poisoning 500–700 mg/L, 3.62–5.07 mmol/L). Approximately 225 ml of an 8.4% (1 mmol bicarbonate/mL) solution of sodium bicarbonate is infused intravenously over 1 hour to ensure a urinary pH (measured by narrow range indicator paper or pH meter) of more than 7.5 and preferably close to 8.5.
- Haemodialysis is indicated for severe poisoning (plasma salicylate > 700 mg/L (5.07 mmol/L)).

# Paracetamol (acetaminophen) (K&C p. 985)

529

Paracetamol in overdose may cause fatal hepatic necrosis and is the commonest form of poisoning encountered in the UK today. Paracetamol is converted to a toxic metabolite, $N$-acetyl-$p$-benzoquinoneimine, which is normally inactivated by conjugation with reduced glutathione. After a large overdose glutathione is depleted and the toxic metabolite binds covalently with sulphydryl groups on liver cell membranes, causing necrosis. Marked liver cell necrosis can occur with as little as 7.5 g (15 tablets) and death with 15 g. The prothrombin time or international normalized ratio (INR) is the best guide to the severity of the liver damage.

## Clinical features

The main danger is liver failure, which usually becomes apparent in 72–96 hours after drug ingestion. Initial symptoms include malaise, nausea and vomiting, with preserved consciousness unless another drug has also been taken. Acute renal failure may occur in the absence of severe liver failure.

## Management

Treatment depends on the interval between overdose and presentation and on the plasma concentrations of paracetamol. The investigation and management of paracetamol poisoning are summarized in Emergency Box 12.1 and Figure 12.2. The two antidotes in use for paracetamol poisoning increase the availability of glutathione.

 **Emergency Box 12.1**

### Management of paracetamol poisoning

- Take blood for paracetamol levels (at or after 4 h since ingestion), full blood count, INR and ALT/AST, U+E and glucose
- Gastric lavage or activated charcoal if patient presents early (within 1 hour of ingestion)
- Give intravenous NAC if potentially serious overdose taken (> 10 g or > 150 mg/kg)
    150 mg/kg in 200 ml 5% dextrose over 15 min, then
    50 mg/kg in 500 ml 5% dextrose over 4 h, then
    100 mg/kg in 1 litre 5% dextrose over 16 h.
- Make decision to continue treatment based on nomogram (Fig. 12.2). Discontinue treatment if the plasma paracetamol concentration is below the relevant treatment line and there is no abnormality of INR, plasma creatinine or ALT
- If patient presents > 15 h following ingestion Figure 12.2 is unreliable. Give NAC if a potentially serious overdose was taken. Repeat investigations (PT, AST/ALT) and consider continuing NAC treatment (100 mg/kg in 1 litre 5% dextrose over 16 h repeated until recovery)
- Repeat blood investigations (except paracetamol) at the end of NAC treatment. If the patient is asymptomatic and the investigations are normal, there is little risk of serious complications and the patient can be discharged.

NAC, *N*-acetylcysteine

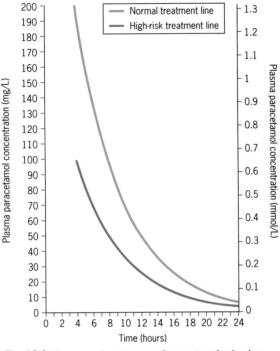

**Fig. 12.2 Nomogram for treatment of paracetamol poisoning.**
(From British National Formulary (1998) with permission.) Use the high-risk
(lower) treatment line in patients with:
- High alcohol intake
- Poor nutrition
- Anorexia nervosa
- HIV infection
- Pre-existing liver disease
  Hepatic enzyme induction from treatment with carbamazepine,
  phenobarbital, phenytoin and rifampicin.

Intravenous *N*-acetylcysteine (NAC) is the treatment of
choice; there are few side-effects other than occasional
hypersensitivity reactions. Oral methionine (four doses of
2.5 g at 4-hour intervals) is an alternative, but absorption
and efficacy are erratic if the patient is vomiting. Patients
who develop liver damage with a raised INR should
remain in hospital until the values are returning to normal.
Fresh frozen plasma should not normally be given to

patients with a raised INR, as the trend in the INR is important in assessing prognosis and in determining the need for possible transplantation. A poor prognosis is indicated by an INR value above 3, raised serum creatinine concentration or a blood pH below 7.3 recorded more than 24 hours after the overdose and after correction of hypovolaemia. If any of these abnormalities is present, advice should be sought from a specialist liver unit. Patients with severe hepatic damage may require liver transplantation.

## Co-proxamol

Combinations of paracetamol and the opioid analgesic dextropropoxyphene (co-proxamol) are frequently taken in overdose. The initial features are those of opioid overdose (see later); patients may die from respiratory depression and acute heart failure unless they are given naloxone as an antidote to the dextropropoxyphene. Paracetamol hepatotoxicity may develop later and should be anticipated and treated as indicated above.

## Other drugs (K&C p. 979)

Table 12.3 outlines the clinical features and management of the other drugs that are commonly taken in cases of overdose. For all of those that are taken by mouth the initial management should include gastric lavage and activated charcoal if the patient presents in time.

## Carbon monoxide (K&C p. 981)

Carbon monoxide (CO) poisoning is usually the result of inhalation of smoke, car exhaust or fumes from improperly maintained and ventilated heating systems. Methylene chloride, a component of paint remover, is readily absorbed and metabolized to CO by the liver and may lead to poisoning. CO combines readily with haemoglobin to form carboxyhaemoglobin, thus preventing the formation of oxyhaemoglobin. The clinical features include headache, mental impairment and, in severe cases, convulsions, coma and cardiac arrest. In spite of hypoxaemia the skin is pink. Carboxyhaemoglobin (COHb) levels should be measured in a venous blood sample although they do not correlate precisely with clinical outcome. Treatment consists of

**Table 12.3**
Clinical features and specific management for certain drugs taken in overdose

| Drug | Clinical features | Management |
|---|---|---|
| Tricyclic antidepressants | Tachycardia, hypotension, fixed dilated pupils, convulsions, urinary retention, arrhythmias, decreased conscious level | Treat convulsions with diazepam. Supraventricular and ventricular tachycardia is treated with intravenous sodium bicarbonate (8.4%) 50 mmol (50 ml) over 20 min, even in the absence of acidosis |
| Benzodiazepines | Drowsiness, ataxia, dysarthria respiratory depression and coma. Potentiate the effects of other CNS depressants taken concomitantly | Flumazenil (0.5 mg i.v. and repeated if necessary) a benzodiazepine antagonist is used if respiratory depression is present |
| Phenothiazines | Hypotension, hypothermia, arrhythmias. Depression of consciousness and respiration. Convulsion and dystonic reactions | Symptomatic treatment of complications, e.g. diazepam for convulsions. Dystonic reactions treated with i.v. benzatropine |
| NSAIDs | Coma, convulsions, metabolic acidosis and renal failure | Treatment is symptomatic and supportive |
| β-Blockers | Bradycardia and hypotension. Coma, convulsions and hypoglycaemia with severe overdose | Atropine (0.6–1.2 mg i.v.) for bradycardia. In resistant cases i.v. glucagon (5–10 mg followed by an infusion of 1–5 mg/h) has a positive inotropic action on the heart |

removing the patient from the CO source and giving 100% oxygen via a tightly fitting face mask. Referral for hyperbaric oxygen treatment should be considered if the victim is, or has been, unconscious or has a blood carboxyhaemoglobin concentration of more than 40%.

## Alcohol

Acute intoxication with alcohol produces severe depression of consciousness and hypoglycaemia, particularly in children. Treatment usually only consists of gastric lavage with an endotracheal tube in position. Blood glucose is measured and glucose given if indicated.

## Drug abuse (K&C p. 1259)

Under the Misuse of Drugs Regulations of 1985, drugs with a high abuse potential, drugs of addiction and other drugs with non-therapeutic psychotropic activity are categorized as controlled drugs. These include opiates, cocaine, barbiturates, lysergide, amfetamines and related drugs. Any patient who is believed to be dependent on or addicted to controlled drugs must, by law, be notified to the Home Office.

## Opioids

Opioid drugs, e.g. diamorphine (heroin), codeine and buprenorphine, produce physical dependency, such that an acute withdrawal syndrome develops ('cold turkey') if the drugs are stopped. These severe symptoms – profuse sweating, tachycardia, dilated pupils, leg cramps, diarrhoea and vomiting – may be reduced by giving methadone, a pharmaceutical preparation of an opioid.

Drug addicts frequently overdose themselves, causing varying degrees of coma, respiratory depression and pinpoint pupils. Treatment is with intravenous naloxone, an opiate antagonist, 1.2 mg i.v. every 2 minutes until breathing is adequate. The drug is short acting and repeated doses or an infusion may be necessary, with the rate titrated according to the clinical response.

## Cannabis

Cannabis is usually smoked and is often taken casually. It is a mild hallucinogen, seldom accompanied by a desire to increase the dose; withdrawal symptoms are uncommon.

## Lysergide

Lysergic acid diethylamine (LSD) is a much more potent hallucinogen; its use can lead to severe psychotic states in which life may be at risk. Even in overdose severe physiological reactions do not seem to occur. Adverse reactions are treated with repeated reassurance; a sedative, e.g. diazepam, is sometimes necessary. Phenothiazines may be necessary in severe cases.

## Cocaine

Cocaine can be taken by injection, inhalation ('crack') or ingestion. It stimulates the central nervous system, producing euphoria, agitation and tachycardia. Convulsions, pyrexia and cardiorespiratory depression may occur in severe cases of overdose and management is supportive.

## Amfetamines

Amfetamines are taken for their stimulatory effect. In overdose there is confusion, delirium, hallucinations and violent behaviour. Cardiac arrhythmias can be a major problem. Treatment is with sedatives, such as diazepam. Forced acid diuresis may be used but is rarely required.

Ecstasy (MDMA, 3,4-methylenedioxy-methamfetamine) is a synthetic amfetamine derivative taken orally as tablets or capsules. In Britain it is used almost exclusively as a 'dance drug' and the adverse effects are the result of the drug's pharmacological properties compounded by physical exertion. Serious acute complications are convulsions, hyperpyrexia, coagulopathy, rhabdomyolysis, renal and liver failure and death. Treatment is rehydration, diazepam for severe agitation and dantrolene for hyperthermia.

## Solvents

The inhalation of organic solvents has become a common problem, particularly in teenagers. The patient presents

535

either in the acute intoxicated state (with euphoria and excitement) or as a chronic abuser with excoriation and rashes over the face and a peripheral neuropathy. Sudden death can occur and is probably the result of cardiac arrhythmias.

# Alcohol abuse (K&C p. 1256)

Drinking-related problems have increased in recent years. Approximately one in five male admissions to acute medical wards is directly or indirectly the result of alcohol. Over the past 20 years admissions to psychiatric hospitals for the treatment of alcohol-related problems has increased 25-fold.

A number of medical, social and psychiatric problems are related to alcohol abuse (see below) and may be seen in the absence of actual physiological dependence. Alcohol dependence has seven essential elements:

- A compulsive need to drink
- A regular (daily) drinking routine to avoid or relieve withdrawal symptoms
- Drinking takes priority over other activities
- Increased tolerance to alcohol
- Repeated withdrawal symptoms often worse on waking in the morning
- Early-morning drinking to avoid withdrawal symptoms (nausea, sweating, agitation)
- Reinstatement after abstinence.

Guidelines for safe limits of drinking are 21 units per week in men and 14 units in women (one unit = a measure of spirits, a glass of wine or half a pint of standard-strength beer). A slightly higher intake is probably unlikely to lead to harm, but more than 36 units per week in men and 24 units in women increases the risk to health. An elevated serum γ-GT (γ-glutamyl transpeptidase) (p. 115) and raised red cell mean corpuscular volume (MCV, p. 176) are useful screening tests for alcohol abuse and are helpful in monitoring progress. Blood and urine alcohol levels are sometimes measured to demonstrate high intake.

# Consequences of alcohol abuse and dependence

## Physical complications

These usually occur after a long period of heavy drinking, e.g. 10 years. Problems are generally seen earlier in women than in men. Damage is the result of direct tissue toxicity and the effects of malnutrition and vitamin deficiency which often accompany alcohol abuse.

- *Cardiovascular.* A direct toxic effect in the heart leads to a cardiomyopathy and arrhythmias.
- *Neurological.* Acute intoxication leads to ataxia, falls and head injury with intracranial bleeds. Long-term complications include polyneuropathy (p. 711), myopathy, cerebellar degeneration (p. 645), dementia (p. 719) and epilepsy.

  Wernicke's encephalopathy (WE) is the result of vitamin $B_1$ deficiency (thiamin) and thus may also be seen in severe starvation and prolonged vomiting. The clinical features include an acute onset of confusion, ataxia, nystagmus and ophthalmoplegia, usually with VIth nerve palsies or defects of conjugate gaze (p.652). Untreated, the patient becomes increasingly drowsy, lapses into a coma and dies. The diagnosis is clinical. As in a patient presenting with these features the alcohol history may be unknown, a high index of suspicion and a low threshold for making a presumptive diagnosis are appropriate. Treatment is with an intravenous complex of B vitamins (e.g. two pairs of ampoules of Pabrinex three times daily for 3 days followed by one pair of ampoules daily for 5 days), which may reverse some of the early changes. Inappropriately managed, WE is fatal in 20% of patients. Of survivors many will develop long-term brain damage (Korsakoff's syndrome) with a gross defect of short-term memory, associated with confabulation.
- *Gastrointestinal effects.* These include liver damage (p. 148), pancreatitis (p. 158), oesophagitis and an increased incidence of oesophageal carcinoma.

- *Haematology.* These include thrombocytopenia (alcohol inhibits platelet maturation and release from bone marrow), a raised MCV and anaemia caused by dietary folate deficiency.
- *Psychiatric complications.* There is an increased incidence of depression and deliberate self-harm among alcoholics. In these patients attempted suicide must always be taken seriously and psychiatric referral considered (p. 527).
- *Social complications.* These include marital and sexual difficulties, employment problems, financial difficulties and homelessness.

### Alcohol withdrawal

Most heavy drinkers will experience some form of withdrawal symptoms if they attempt to reduce or stop drinking.

- Early mild features occur within 6–12 hours and include tremor, nausea and sweating. Treatment is with a reducing dose of diazepam or alternative drug

### Emergency Box 12.2

#### Management of delirium tremens

- Admit the patient to a medical bed
- Prevent or treat established Wernicke's encephalopathy by administration of intravenous B vitamin complex (see text). Give before administration of glucose-containing i.v. fluids
- Treat infection
- Correct dehydration and electrolyte imbalance
- Give prophylactic phenytoin or carbamazepine, if previous history of withdrawal fits
- Give diazepam 10–20 mg or chlordiazepoxide 30–60 mg *or* lorazepam 2–4 mg and repeat after 1 hour depending on response
- Continue maintenance treatment:
  - Diazepam, 10 mg every 6 hours for 4 doses then 5 mg every 6 hours for 8 doses *or*
  - Chlordiazepoxide, 30 mg every 6 hours for 4 doses then 15 mg every 6 hours for 8 doses *or*
  - Lorazepam, 2 mg every 6 hours for 4 doses then 1 mg every 6 hours for 8 doses

(see Emergency Box 12.2). In mild cases this can be on an outpatient basis as long as the patient attends daily for medication and monitoring and has good social support.

- Late major features usually occur within 2–3 days but may take up to 2 weeks:
  - Generalized tonic–clonic seizures (p. 678)
  - Delirium tremens with fever, tremor, tachycardia, agitation and visual hallucinations ('pink elephants'). Treatment must be given urgently (see Emergency Box 12.2).

After alcohol withdrawal it is essential that relapse is prevented. This involves local alcohol services, specialist psychiatry and the alcohol nurse specialist. Oral acamprosate, a GABA analogue, reduces relapses by 50%.

**USEFUL WEBSITE**

http://www.doh.gov.uk/cmo/cmo0202.htm
Department of Health: detailed information on CO poisoning

# 13 Endocrinology

Hormones were traditionally thought of as chemical messengers, released from endocrine cells into the circulation and acting at a site distant from their site of secretion. However, the situation is more complex and hormones may also act as:

- Neurotransmitters
- A local hormone with action on adjacent cells (paracrine action)
- Directly on the cell of origin (autocrine).

Hormones act by binding to specific receptors either on the target cell surface or within the cell (e.g. thyroid hormones, cortisol) (*K&C* p. 999). The result is a cascade of intracellular reactions within the target cell which frequently amplifies the original stimulus and leads ultimately to a response by the target cell. Some hormones, e.g. growth hormone and thyroxine, act on most tissues of the body. Others act on only one tissue, e.g. thyroid-stimulating hormone (TSH) and adrenocorticotrophin (ACTH) are secreted by the anterior pituitary and have specific target tissues, namely the thyroid gland and the adrenal cortex.

## The hypothalamus and pituitary (*K&C* p. 1006)

The hypothalamus contains many vital centres for functions such as appetite, thirst, thermal regulation and sleep/waking. It also plays a role in circadian rhythm, the menstrual cycle, stress and mood. Releasing factors produced in the hypothalamus reach the pituitary via the portal system, which runs down the pituitary stalk. These releasing factors stimulate or inhibit the production of hormones from distinct cell types (e.g. production of growth hormone by acidophils), each of which secretes a specific hormone in response to unique hypothalamic stimulatory or inhibitory hormones. The anterior pituitary hormones, in turn, stimulate the peripheral glands and tissues. This pattern is illustrated in Figure 13.1. The posterior pituitary acts as a

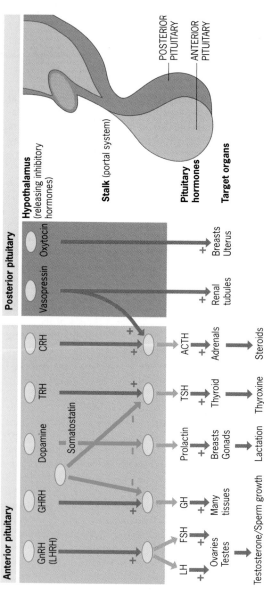

**Fig. 13.1 Hypothalamic releasing hormones and the pituitary trophic hormones.** See the text for abbreviations and explanation.

542

storage organ for antidiuretic hormone (ADH, vasopressin) and oxytocin, which are synthesized in the supraoptic and paraventricular nuclei in the anterior hypothalamus and pass to the posterior pituitary along a single axon in the pituitary stalk. ADH is discussed on page 581; oxytocin produces milk ejection and uterine myometrial contractions.

## Control and feedback (K&C p. 1000)

Most hormone systems are controlled by some form of feedback; an example is the hypothalamic–pituitary–thyroid axis (Fig. 13.2). Thyrotrophin-releasing hormone (TRH), secreted in the hypothalamus, stimulates TSH secretion from the anterior pituitary which, in turn, stimulates the synthesis and release of thyroid hormones from the thyroid gland. Circulating thyroid hormone feeds back on the pituitary, and possibly the hypothalamus, to suppress

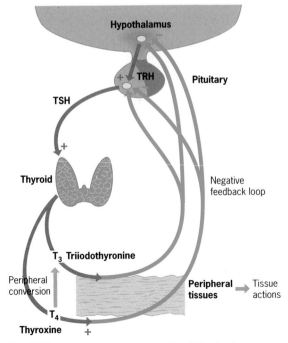

Fig. 13.2 The hypothalamic–pituitary–thyroid feedback system.

the production of TSH and TRH, and hence a fall in thyroid hormone secretion. This is known as a 'negative feedback' system and represents the most common mechanism for regulation of circulating hormone levels. Conversely, a fall in thyroid hormone secretion (e.g. after thyroidectomy) leads to increased secretion of TSH and TRH.

A patient with a hormone-producing tumour fails to show negative feedback and this is useful in diagnosis, e.g. the dexamethasone suppression test in the diagnosis of Cushing's syndrome.

## Common presenting symptoms in endocrine disease (K&C p. 1000)

Hormonal abnormalities have a wide range of clinical effects and there are many presenting symptoms and signs of endocrine disease, the commonest of which are shown in

---

**Table 13.1**
Common presenting complaints in endocrine disease

**Body size and shape**
Short stature
Tall stature
Excessive weight or weight gain
Loss of weight

**Metabolic effects**
Tiredness
Weakness
Increased appetite
Decreased appetite
Polydipsia/thirst
Polyuria/nocturia
Tremor
Palpitation
Anxiety

**Local effects**
Swelling in the neck
Carpal tunnel syndrome
Bone or muscle pain
Protrusion of eyes
Visual loss (acuity and/or fields)
Headache

**Skin**
Hirsutism
Hair thinning
Pigmentation
Dry skin
Excess sweating

**Reproduction/sex**
Loss or absence of libido
Impotence
Oligomenorrhoea/amenorrhoea
Subfertility
Galactorrhoea
Gynaecomastia
Delayed puberty
Precocious puberty

Table 13.1. Many of these are vague and non-specific, e.g. tiredness in hypothyroidism, weight loss or weight gain, anorexia and malaise in Addison's disease, and the differential diagnosis is often wide. Precocious puberty (< 9 years) or delayed puberty (> 15 years) is often the result of a familial tendency, although hypothalamic–pituitary disease may present in this way, and endocrine investigations are usually undertaken.

## Pituitary tumours (K&C p. 1009)

Benign pituitary tumours (adenomas) are the most common form of pituitary disease. Symptoms may arise as a result of inadequate hormone production, excess hormone secretion, or from pressure and local infiltration.

### Underproduction

This is the result of disease at either a hypothalamic or a pituitary level, and it results in the clinical features of hypopituitarism (p. 546).

### Overproduction

Overproduction of pituitary hormones may cause the following:

- Growth hormone (GH) excess, resulting in acromegaly or gigantism (usually acidophil adenomas)
- Prolactin excess (chromophobe adenomas)
- Cushing's disease, resulting from excess ACTH production (basophil adenomas or hyperplasia)
- Tumours producing luteinizing hormone (LH), follicle-stimulating hormone (FSH) or TSH are very rare.

### Local effects

Local infiltration of or pressure on surrounding structures (Fig. 13.3), may result in:

- Visual loss with field defects. This is typically a bitemporal hemianopia caused by pressure on the optic chiasm (p. 649).
- Headache produced by tumour involvement of the meninges and bony structures.
- Obesity and altered appetite and thirst. This is due to involvement of the hypothalamus. In children,

Common presenting symptoms in endocrine disease

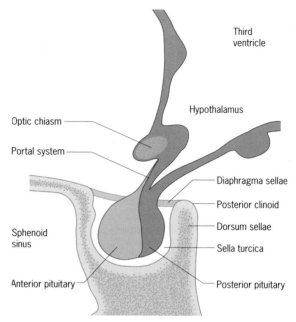

**Fig. 13.3 A sagittal section of the pituitary fossa, showing the important anatomical relationships.** The cavernous sinus lies lateral to the pituitary and is seen on a coronal view.

  hypothalamic involvement may lead to early puberty
  (precocious puberty).
- Hydrocephalus caused by interruption of
  cerebrospinal fluid flow.
- Cranial nerve lesions (III, IV and VI) by infiltration of
  the cavernous sinus.

## Hypopituitarism (K&C p. 1011)

Deficiency of hypothalamic-releasing hormones or pituitary hormones may be either selective or multiple. Multiple deficiencies usually result from tumour growth or other destructive lesions, and there is usually a progressive loss of function, with LH and FSH being affected first and TSH and ACTH last. Rather than prolactin deficiency, hyperprolactinaemia occurs relatively early because of loss of tonic inhibitory control by dopamine (see Fig. 13.1).

**Table 13.2**
Causes of hypopituitarism

| | |
|---|---|
| **Neoplastic**<br>Primary tumours<br>Secondary deposits<br>Craniopharyngioma | **Traumatic**<br>Skull fracture<br>Surgery |
| **Infective**<br>Meningitis<br>Encephalitis<br>Syphilis | **Infiltrations**<br>Sarcoidosis<br>Haemochromatosis |
| **Vascular**<br>Pituitary apoplexy<br>Sheehan's syndrome<br>'Empty sella' syndrome | **Others**<br>Radiation damage<br>Chemotherapy |
| **Immunological**<br>Pituitary antibodies | **Functional**<br>Anorexia<br>Starvation<br>Emotional deprivation |
| **Congenital**<br>Kallmann's syndrome | |

Panhypopituitarism is a deficiency of all anterior pituitary hormones. Vasopressin and oxytocin secretion will only be affected if the hypothalamus is involved by either hypothalamic tumour or by extension of a pituitary lesion.

## Aetiology

The causes of hypopituitarism are listed in Table 13.2. The commonest cause (> 70% of cases) is a pituitary tumour or treatment of the tumour either by surgical removal or radiotherapy.

## Clinical features

547

These depend on the extent of hypothalamic–pituitary deficiencies. Gonadotrophin deficiency results in loss of libido, amenorrhoea (absent menstruation) and impotence, whereas hyperprolactinaemia results in galactorrhoea (breast milk secretion unrelated to pregnancy) and hypogonadism. Growth hormone deficiency is usually clinically silent except in children, although it may impair well-being in adults. Secondary hypothyroidism and adrenal failure lead to tiredness, slowness of thought and action, and mild hypotension. Long-standing hypopituitarism may give the classic picture of pallor with hairlessness (alabaster skin). Particular syndromes related to hypopituitarism are:

- *Kallmann's syndrome.* Isolated gonadotrophin deficiency with anosmia (absent sense of smell), colour blindness, midline facial deformities and renal abnormalities.
- *Sheehan's syndrome.* This situation, now rare, is pituitary infarction following severe postpartum haemorrhage.
- *Pituitary apoplexy.* Infarction or haemorrhage into a pituitary tumour which may result in life-threatening hypopituitarism. Additional features include severe headaches, visual loss and cranial nerve palsy.
- *'Empty sella' syndrome.* The sella turcica appears radiologically devoid of pituitary tissue; the pituitary is actually placed eccentrically and function is usually normal.

### Investigation

Each axis of the hypothalamic–pituitary system requires separate investigation. The presence of normal gonadal function (ovulatory menstruation or normal libido/erections) suggests that multiple defects of the anterior pituitary are unlikely. Tests range from measurement of basal hormone levels to stimulatory tests of the pituitary and tests of feedback for the hypothalamus.

### Management

Steroid and thyroid hormones are essential for life and are given as oral replacement drugs (e.g. 15–40 mg hydrocortisone daily in divided doses, 100–150 μg thyroxine daily) with the aim of restoring clinical and biochemical normality. Androgens and oestrogens are replaced for symptomatic control. If fertility is desired, LH and FSH analogues are used. GH therapy should be given to the growing child under appropriate specialist supervision and it may also produce substantial benefits to the GH-deficient adult in terms of work capacity and psychological well-being.

Two warnings are necessary:

- Thyroid replacement should not commence until normal glucocorticoid function has been demonstrated or replacement steroid therapy initiated, as an adrenal 'crisis' may otherwise be precipitated.

- Glucocorticoid deficiency masks impaired urine concentrating ability. Diabetes insipidus is apparent after steroid replacement, the steroids being necessary for excretion of a water load.

# Male reproduction and sex (K&C p. 1014)

Luteinizing hormone-releasing hormone (LHRH, also called gonadotrophin-releasing hormone, GnRH) is synthesized in the hypothalamus. It is released episodically into the pituitary portal circulation (during and after puberty) and stimulates LH and FSH secretion from the anterior pituitary gland. LH and FSH stimulate the production of testosterone and sperm respectively from the testes.

## Male hypogonadism (K&C p. 1019)

Male hypogonadism is a descriptive term for the clinical features associated with androgen deficiency. The presentation depends on the age of onset of hypogonadism (Table 13.3). In prepubertal onset the patient presents with delayed puberty and eunuchoid body proportions resulting from the continued growth of long bones, which occurs because of delayed fusion of the epiphyses.

A large number of diseases can lead to destruction or malfunction of the hypothalamic–pituitary–testicular axis (Table 13.4).

---

**Table 13.3**
Consequences of androgen deficiency in the male

**Prepubertal onset with eunuchoidism**
Increased height and arm span
Lack of adult hair distribution
High-pitched voice
Small penis, testes and scrotum
Decreased muscle mass

**Hypogonadism beginning after puberty**
Decreased prostate size
Diminished rate of growth of beard and body hair
Fine feminine skin
Decreased potency and libido

---

Table 13.4
Causes of male hypogonadism

**Hypothalamic – pituitary disorder**
Hypopituitarism
Selective gonadotrophin deficiency (Kallmann's syndrome)
Severe systemic illness
Severe malnourishment
Hyperprolactinaemia (interferes with pulsatile secretion of LH and FSH)

**Primary gonadal disease**
Congenital: Klinefelter's syndrome, anorchia, Leydig cell agenesis, failure of testicular descent
Acquired: trauma, torsion, chemotherapy, radiation

**Target tissues**
Androgen-receptor deficiency

**Klinefelter's syndrome** is the most common cause of male hypogonadism, with an incidence of 1 in 1000 live births. It is the result of the presence of an extra X chromosome (47, XXY). Accelerated atrophy of the testicular germ cells gives rise to sterility and small firm testes. The clinical picture varies: in the most severely affected there is complete failure of sexual maturation, eunuchoid body proportions, gynaecomastia and learning difficulties.

## Investigations

Measurement of basal serum testosterone, LH and FSH will confirm the diagnosis and allow the distinction between primary gonadal (testicular) failure and hypothalamic–pituitary disease. In testicular failure testosterone levels will be low but LH/FSH levels high, as a result of loss of the negative feedback of testosterone on the hypothalamus–pituitary axis. Further investigations, e.g. serum prolactin, chromosomal analysis, pituitary MRI scan and pituitary function tests, will depend on the likely site of the defect.

## Management

The cause can rarely be reversed and the mainstay of treatment is androgen replacement. Although hypogonadotrophic patients have the potential for fertility, LH and FSH or pulsatile GnRH are only used (instead of testosterone) when fertility is desired, as these regimens are expensive and complex.

## Loss of libido and impotence (K&C p. 1021)

Erectile impotence is defined as failure to initiate an erection or to maintain an erection until ejaculation. Erection is the result of increased vascularity of the penis controlled via the sacral parasympathetic outflow; it may be impaired by vascular disease, autonomic neuropathy and nerve damage after pelvic surgery. The nervous pathways for ejaculation are centred on the lumbar sympathetics, and abnormalities may occur with autonomic neuropathy (most commonly with diabetes mellitus) and traumatic nerve damage. Psychological factors, endocrine factors (causes of hypogonadism described above), alcohol and drugs, e.g. cannabis, and diuretics, may cause abnormalities of both parasympathetic and sympathetic nerves. A careful history and examination will identify the cause in many patients. The presence of nocturnal emissions and morning erections is suggestive of psychogenic impotence.

Apart from cessation of the offending drug, methods of treatment include oral sildenafil citrate, a phosphodiesterase inhibitor which increases penile blood flow, the use of intracavernosal injections of alprostadil, papaverine or phentolamine, penile implants and vacuum expanders.

Many cases are the result of psychological factors and the patient may respond to psychosexual counselling.

## Gynaecomastia (K&C p. 1021)

551

The development of benign breast tissue in the male is the result of an increase in the oestrogen:androgen ratio (Table 13.5) and is most commonly a result of liver disease or drug side-effects. Gynaecomastia is common in early puberty as a result of relative oestrogen excess, and usually resolves spontaneously. Unexplained gynaecomastia occurs, especially in elderly people, and is a diagnosis of exclusion after thorough examination and investigation. The treatment is either of the underlying cause or by removal of the drug if possible. Occasionally surgery is needed.

**Table 13.5**
Causes of gynaecomastia

**Physiological**
Neonatal, resulting from the influence of maternal hormones
Pubertal
Old age

**Deficient testosterone secretion**
Any cause of hypogonadism (see Table 13.4)

**Oestrogen-producing tumours**
Of the testis or adrenal gland

**HCG-producing tumours**
Of the testis or the lung

**Drugs**
Digitalis
Spironolactone
Cyproterone
Cimetidine
Oestrogens
Cannabis
Heroin

**Other**
Hyperthyroidism
Liver disease

HCG, human chorionic gonadotrophin

# Female reproduction and sex

(*K&C* p. 1015)

In the adult female higher brain centres impose a menstrual cycle of 28 days upon the activity of hypothalamic GnRH. Pulses of GnRH stimulate the release of pituitary LH and FSH. LH stimulates ovarian androgen production and FSH stimulates follicular development and aromatase activity (an enzyme required to convert ovarian androgens to oestrogens). Oestrogens are necessary for normal pubertal development and, together with progesterone, for maintenance of the menstrual cycle; they also have effects on a variety of tissues.

## The menopause (*K&C* p. 1017)

The menopause, or cessation of periods, naturally occurs about the age of 45–55 years. During the late 40s, first FSH and then LH concentrations begin to rise, probably as a result of diminishing follicle supply. Oestrogen levels fall and the cycle becomes disrupted. Menopause may also occur surgically, with radiotherapy to the ovaries and with ovarian disease (e.g. premature menopause in the 20s and 30s). Symptoms of the menopause are hot flushes, vaginal dryness and breast atrophy. There may also be vague symptoms of depression, loss of libido and weight gain. There is loss of bone density (osteoporosis, p. 278) and the premenopausal protection against ischaemic heart disease disappears. Most of these effects may be reduced by hormone replacement therapy (HRT), which is now given long term to most women with menopausal symptoms. Other effects of hormone replacement therapy include:

- protection from osteoporosis
- possible reduction in the risk of Alzheimer's disease and colon cancer
- detrimental effect of an increase in mortality from ischaemic heart disease and cerebrovascular disease.

HRT is always given to women with premature ovarian failure. Oestrogens, when given alone, increase the risk of endometrial cancer and so combination treatment with pro-gestogens is given to women with an intact uterus.

Selective oestrogen receptor modulators, SERMs (e.g. raloxifene) have the potential advantage of positive oestrogen effects on the cardiovascular system and bone while having no effect on oestrogen receptors of breast and uterus.

## Female hypogonadism and amenorrhoea
(K&C p. 1021)

Amenorrhoea is the absence of menstruation. It is often physiological, e.g. during pregnancy and lactation, and after the menopause. Primary amenorrhoea is failure to start spontaneous menstruation by the age of 16 years. Secondary amenorrhoea is the absence of menstruation for 3 months in a woman who has previously had menstrual cycles. In the female, hypogonadism almost always presents as amenorrhoea or oligomenorrhoea (irregular periods with long cycles). The other features of oestrogen deficiency include atrophy of the breasts and vagina, loss of pubic hair and osteoporosis.

## Aetiology

The causes of amenorrhoea are listed in Table 13.6. Polycystic ovary syndrome is the most common cause of oligomenorrhoea and amenorrhoea in clinical practice, though one should always consider pregnancy as a possible cause. Severe weight loss (e.g. anorexia nervosa) has long been associated with amenorrhoea, but it is now recognized that less severe forms of weight loss, produced by dieting and exercise, are a common cause of amenorrhoea caused by abnormal secretion of GnRH.

## Investigations

The cause of amenorrhoea may be apparent after a full history and examination. Basal levels of serum FSH, LH, oestrogen and prolactin will allow a distinction between

**Table 13.6**
Pathological causes of amenorrhoea

**Hypothalamic**
GnRH deficiency (isolated or as part of Kallmann's syndrome)*
Weight loss, physical exercise, stress
Post oral contraceptive therapy

**Pituitary**
Hyperprolactinaemia
Hypopituitarism

**Gonadal**
Polycystic ovary syndrome
Premature ovarian failure – autoimmune basis
Defective ovarian development (dysgenesis)*
Androgen-secreting ovarian tumours
Radiotherapy

**Other diseases**
Thyroid dysfunction
Cushing's syndrome
Adrenal tumours
Severe illness

**Uterine/vaginal abnormality**
Imperforate hymen or absent uterus*

*Presents as primary amenorrhoea

554

primary gonadal and hypothalamic–pituitary causes. Further investigations, e.g. ultrasonography of the ovaries, laparoscopy and ovarian biopsy, pituitary MRI and measurement of serum testosterone, will depend on the probable site of the defect and the findings on clinical examination.

### Management

Treatment is of the cause where possible, e.g. increase weight, treat hypothyroidism and hyperprolactinaemia. In patients where the underlying defect cannot be corrected, cyclical oestrogens are given to reverse the symptoms of oestrogen deficiency and prevent early osteoporosis. Patients with isolated GnRH deficiency or hypopituitarism are treated with human FSH/LH. The management of polycystic ovaries is discussed on page 557.

## Hirsutism and polycystic ovary syndrome (PCOS) (K&C p. 1022)

Hirsutism is an excess growth of hair in a male pattern (androgen dependent): beard area, abdominal wall, thigh and around the nipples. There is, however, considerable variation in normal hair growth between individuals, families and races, being more extensive in the Mediterranean and some Asian Indian subcontinent populations.

In clinical practice the majority of patients with signs of androgen-dependent hirsutism will have PCOS, and investigation is mainly required to exclude rarer and more serious causes (Table 13.7) of virilization (male secondary sexual characteristics).

PCOS is characterized by multiple small cysts within the ovary and by excess androgen production from the ovaries and, to a lesser extent, from the adrenals, although whether the basic defect is in the ovary, adrenal or pituitary remains unknown. The ovarian 'cysts' represent arrested follicular development. PCOS is associated with anovulation and insulin resistance, which may also be associated with hypertension and hyperlipidaemia. The precise mechanisms that link this syndrome remain to be elucidated, but may play a role in the causation of macrovascular disease in women.

> **Table 13.7**
> Causes of hirsutism
>
> **Familial and racial**
> Ovarian
> Polycystic ovary syndrome
> Androgen-secreting tumours
>
> **Adrenal**
> Androgen-secreting tumours
> Congenital adrenal hyperplasia
>
> **Androgenic drugs**
> Androgens
> Phenytoin
> Minoxidil
> Ciclosporin
>
> **Idiopathic**
> Target organ hypersensitivity

## Clinical features

Typically, PCOS presents with amenorrhoea/oligomenorrhoea, hirsutism and acne, usually beginning shortly after menarche. It is sometimes associated with marked obesity, but weight may be normal. Mild virilization occurs in severe cases. A short history, accompanying virilization, and severe menstrual disturbance are suggestive of significant androgen secretion with a more serious underlying cause, e.g. adrenal tumour.

## Investigations

The diagnosis of PCOS is made on a clinical basis supported by:

- Serum testosterone concentrations are increased
- Serum LH concentrations are increased or normal
- Serum FSH concentrations are normal
- Ovarian ultrasound shows a thickened capsule with multiple cysts.

Other investigations in a patient presenting with hirsutism include measurement of serum androgens and CT/MRI of the adrenal glands to exclude other causes of hirsutism.

## Management

The management is to identify and treat the underlying cause. Excess hair can be removed or disguised by shaving, bleaching and waxing. Other potentially useful treatments for hirsutism include:

- Cyproterone acetate (an *antiandrogen*)
- Oestrogens which reduce free androgens by increasing levels of the sex hormone-binding globulin
- Spironolactone which has an antiandrogen activity
- Finasteride, a 5α-reductase inhibitor, inhibits dihydrotestosterone formation in skin.

Patients with PCOS who require induction of ovulation are treated with the anti-oestrogen, clomifene. For those not concerned with fertility, menstrual irregularity can be managed with oral contraceptives. Symptoms of hyperandrogenism can be managed by antiandrogens such as cyproterone acetate.

## Hyperprolactinaemia (*K&C* p. 1027)

Unlike other pituitary hormones, prolactin release is tonically inhibited by dopamine from the hypothalamus via the pituitary stalk (Fig. 13.1). There is a physiological increase in prolactin during pregnancy and postpartum breastfeeding.

### Aetiology

The commonest cause of pathological hyperprolactinaemia is a prolactin-secreting pituitary adenoma (prolactinoma). Other pituitary or hypothalamic tumours may also cause hyperprolactinaemia by interfering with dopamine inhibition of prolactin release. Other causes include primary hypothyroidism (high TRH levels stimulate prolactin) and drugs, metoclopramide and phenothiazines (caused by inhibition of dopamine), oestrogens and cimetidine.

### Clinical features

Prolactinomas are rarely diagnosed in men. The cardinal feature is galactorrhoea. Other features such as oligo- or amenorrhoea, subfertility and impotence occur as a result of inhibition of GnRH by high levels of prolactin. If there is a pituitary tumour there may be headache and visual field defects.

## Investigations

- Serum prolactin level. At least three measurements should be taken. Further tests are appropriate after physiological and drug causes have been excluded.
- Thyroid function tests, as hypothyroidism is a cause of hyperprolactinaemia.
- Magnetic resonance imaging of the pituitary.
- Pituitary function should be checked if a pituitary tumour is suspected.
- Visual fields should be checked by clinical assessment and plotted formally by perimetry (p. 647) if a pituitary tumour is the cause.

## Management

Causative drugs should be withdrawn if possible and hypothyroidism treated. In the case of a prolactinoma, the dopamine agonist bromocriptine will reduce plasma prolactin concentrations and produce some shrinkage in tumour size. Definitive therapy is controversial and depends on the size of the tumour, the patient's wish for fertility and the facilities available. Surgical removal of the tumour via a trans-sphenoidal approach, combined with postoperative radiotherapy for large tumours, often restores normoprolactinaemia but there is a high late recurrence rate (50% at 5 years). Small tumours (microadenomas) in asymptomatic patients may only need observation.

# The growth axis (K&C p. 1031)

Growth hormone (GH) is secreted from the anterior pituitary and its tissue effects are mediated by insulin-like growth factor (IGF-1) synthesized in the liver and other tissues. Deficiency of GH produces short stature in children but in adults it is often clinically silent, although it may result in significant impairment in well-being and work capacity. Excessive GH production leads to gigantism in children (if acquired before fusion of the epiphyses of the long bones) and acromegaly in adults.

# Acromegaly

Acromegaly is rare and caused by a benign pituitary adenoma in almost all cases. Males and females are affected equally and the incidence is highest in middle age.

## Clinical features

Symptoms and signs are shown in Figure 13.4. One-third of patients present with changes in appearance and 10% with visual field defects or headaches. Old photographs of the patient may be useful to demonstrate a change in appearance and physical features. Inadequately treated acromegaly is associated with an increased mortality rate particularly from cardiovascular disease and cancer.

## Investigations

- Glucose tolerance test is diagnostic. In a positive test there is failure of the normal suppression of serum GH below 1 mU/L in response to a glucose load. Some show a paradoxical rise. Twenty-five per cent of individuals with acromegaly have a diabetic glucose tolerance test.

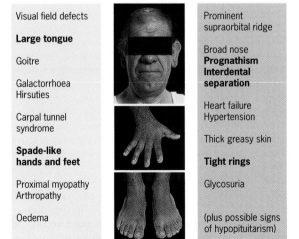

Visual field defects

**Large tongue**

Goitre

Galactorrhoea
Hirsuties

Carpal tunnel syndrome

**Spade-like hands and feet**

Proximal myopathy
Arthropathy

Oedema

Prominent supraorbital ridge

Broad nose
**Prognathism
Interdental separation**

Heart failure
Hypertension

Thick greasy skin

**Tight rings**

Glycosuria

(plus possible signs of hypopituitarism)

**Fig. 13.4 The symptoms and signs of acromegaly.** Bold type indicates signs of greater discriminant value.

- Serum GH levels are usually elevated, but levels fluctuate and a single normal level does not exclude the diagnosis.
- Serum IGF-1 levels are almost always raised in acromegaly, and fluctuate less than those of GH.
- MRI scan of the pituitary will almost always reveal the adenoma.
- Visual field defects are common and should be plotted by perimetry.
- Pituitary function testing usually shows evidence of hypopituitarism.
- Hyperprolactinaemia occurs in 30%.

## Management

Treatment is indicated in all except elderly people or those with minimal abnormalities, because untreated acromegaly is associated with markedly reduced survival. Most deaths result from heart failure, coronary artery disease and hypertension-related causes. The aim of therapy should be to reduce mean GH level to below 5 mU/L after a glucose load, which has been shown to reduce mortality to normal levels. The preferred treatment is controversial and complete cure, if possible, is often slow. The choice lies among the following:

*Surgery* This is the treatment of choice in suitable cases and may be trans-sphenoidal, or transfrontal if the tumour is large. Surgery is often combined with radiotherapy because excision is rarely complete with large tumours (macroadenomas, i.e. > 1 cm in diameter).

*External beam radiotherapy* is normally used after pituitary surgery fails to normalize GH levels, rather than as primary therapy. It may take 1–10 years to be effective when used alone.

*Drugs* Octreotide and the long-acting preparation, lanreotide, are analogues of somatostatin (GH-inhibitory hormone) and are given by subcutaneous injection in resistant cases. They are given to shrink tumours before definitive treatment or to control symptoms. Bromocriptine is usually reserved for elderly and frail people.

Pegvisomant, a GH-receptor antagonist, is a new agent which is likely to be of value in patients where GH levels cannot be safely lowered with somatostatin analogues alone.

## The thyroid axis (K&C p. 1035)

The thyroid gland secretes predominantly thyroxine ($T_4$) and only a small amount of the biologically active hormone triiodothyronine ($T_3$). These hormones control the metabolic rate of many tissues. Most circulating $T_3$ is produced by peripheral conversion of $T_4$. Over 99% of $T_4$ and $T_3$ circulate bound to plasma proteins, mainly thyroxine-binding globulin (TBG). The feedback pathway that controls the secretion of TSH is discussed on page 543. Thyroid function is assessed by measurement of:

- Serum TSH concentration
- Serum free $T_4$ (or $T_3$) concentration.

Free hormone concentrations are measured in preference to total hormone concentrations (i.e. bound and free) because free hormone is that which is available for uptake by cells and interaction with nuclear receptors. Drugs and illness can alter the concentrations of binding proteins or interaction of the binding hormones with $T_4$ and $T_3$. Thus free and total hormone concentrations may not be concordant. For instance, oestrogens (e.g. in pregnancy and in women taking the oral contraceptive pill) increase concentrations of TBG and hence total $T_4$ but the physiologically important free $T_4$ concentrations are normal.

561

## Hypothyroidism (K&C p. 1037)

Underactivity of the thyroid gland may be primary, from disease of the thyroid gland, or, much less commonly, secondary to hypothalamic–pituitary disease.

### Aetiology

**Atrophic (autoimmune) hypothyroidism** This is the most common cause of hypothyroidism and is associated with thyroid microsomal antibodies and lymphoid infiltration of the gland, with eventual fibrosis and atrophy. It is six times more common in females and the incidence increases with age. It is associated with other autoimmune conditions, such as pernicious anaemia and Addison's disease.

**Hashimoto's thyroiditis** This autoimmune thyroiditis, also associated with thyroid microsomal antibodies, produces atrophic changes with regeneration leading to goitre formation. It is more common in females and in late middle age. Patients may be hypothyroid, euthyroid, or go through an initial toxic phase.

**Iatrogenic** Forty per cent are hypothyroid by 25 years following radioactive iodine or surgery for hyperthyroidism.

**Iodine deficiency** This still exists in some areas, particularly mountainous areas (Alps, Himalayas, South America). Goitre, occasionally massive, is common. The patient may be euthyroid or hypothyroid, depending on the severity of the iodine deficiency.

**Dyshormonogenesis** This rare condition is caused by genetic defects in the synthesis of thyroid hormones.

### Clinical features
Symptoms and signs of hypothyroidism are illustrated in Figure 13.5. The term myxoedema refers to the accumulation of mucopolysaccharide in subcutaneous tissues. Features are often difficult to distinguish in elderly people and young women. Hypothyroidism should be excluded in all patients with oligomenorrhoea/amenorrhoea, menorrhagia, infertility and hyperprolactinaemia. Many cases are detected on routine biochemical screening.

### Investigations
Measurement of serum TSH is the investigation of choice. A high TSH with a compatible clinical picture confirms primary hypothyroidism.

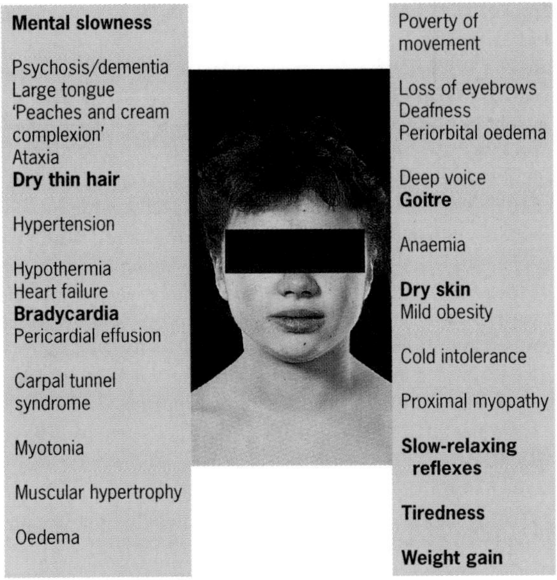

Mental slowness

Psychosis/dementia
Large tongue
'Peaches and cream complexion'
Ataxia
**Dry thin hair**

Hypertension

Hypothermia
Heart failure
**Bradycardia**
Pericardial effusion

Carpal tunnel syndrome

Myotonia

Muscular hypertrophy

Oedema

Poverty of movement

Loss of eyebrows
Deafness
Periorbital oedema

Deep voice
**Goitre**

Anaemia

**Dry skin**
Mild obesity

Cold intolerance

Proximal myopathy

**Slow-relaxing reflexes**

**Tiredness**

**Weight gain**

Fig. 13.5 **The symptoms and signs of hypothyroidism.** Bold type indicates signs of greater discriminant value.

- Serum free $T_4$ levels are low.
- Thyroid antibodies and other organ-specific antibodies may be present in the serum.
- Other features include anaemia (normocytic or macrocytic), hypercholesterolaemia and hyponatraemia (due to increased antidiuretic hormone and impaired clearance of free water).
- Creatine kinase levels may be increased with associated myopathy.

## Management

Replacement therapy with thyroxine (100–200 µg/day) is required for life. The starting dose is 100 µg/day (50 µg/day in elderly people) and the adequacy of replacement is assessed clinically and by thyroid function tests after at least 6 weeks on a steady dose. In patients with ischaemic heart disease, starting doses should be even lower

(25 µg/day) and increased at intervals of 2–6 weeks if ischaemic symptoms do not deteriorate.

## Myxoedema coma

Severe hypothyroidism may rarely present with confusion and coma, particularly in elderly people. Typical features include hypothermia (p. 595), cardiac failure, hypoventilation, hypoglycaemia and hyponatraemia. The optimal treatment is controversial and data are lacking, but a summary is given in Emergency Box 13.1. Treatment should be begun on the basis of clinical suspicion without waiting for the results of laboratory tests. Clues to the possible presence of myxoedema coma include a previous history of thyroid disease and a history from family members suggesting antecedent symptoms of thyroid dysfunction.

## Myxoedema madness

Depression is common but occasionally, with severe hypothyroidism in elderly people, the patient may become frankly demented or psychotic, sometimes with striking delusions. This may occur shortly after starting thyroxine replacement.

### Emergency Box 13.1

**Management of myxoedema coma**

**Investigations**
- TSH, $T_4$ and cortisol before thyroid hormone is given
- Full blood count, serum urea and electrolytes, blood glucose and blood cultures

**Treatment**
- Oxygen (by mechanical ventilation if necessary)
- Gradual rewarming (Emergency Box 13.5)
- Intravenous $T_3$ 2.5–10 µg 8-hourly, depending on patient's age and coexistent cardiovascular disease
- Intravenous hydrocortisone 100 mg 8-hourly (in case hypothyroidism is a manifestation of hypopituitarism)
- Intravenous dextrose to prevent hypoglycaemia
- Supportive management of the comatose patient (p. 661)
- Swap to oral maintenance treatment after clinical improvement and patient stable

# Hyperthyroidism (K&C p. 1039)

Hyperthyroidism (thyroid overactivity, thyrotoxicosis) is common, affecting 2–5% of all women at some time, mainly between the ages of 20 and 40 years. Three intrinsic thyroid disorders account for the vast majority of cases of hyperthyroidism: Graves' disease, toxic adenoma and toxic multinodular goitre. Rarer causes include de Quervain's thyroiditis, thyroiditis factitia (surreptitious $T_4$ consumption), drugs (amiodarone), metastatic differentiated thyroid carcinoma and TSH-secreting tumours (e.g. of the pituitary).

***Graves' disease*** Graves' disease is the most common cause of hyperthyroidism and is the result of IgG antibodies binding to the TSH receptor and stimulating thyroid hormone production. It is associated with typical eye changes (see below), vitiligo, pretibial myxoedema and, rarely, lymphadenopathy and splenomegaly. It is also associated with other autoimmune diseases, such as pernicious anaemia and myasthenia gravis.

***Toxic multinodular goitre*** Many patients with toxic multinodular goitre have been euthyroid for several years before the development of nodular autonomy. Toxic multinodular goitre commonly occurs in older women, and drug therapy is rarely successful in inducing a prolonged remission.

***Solitary toxic nodule (Plummer's disease)*** This is responsible for about 5% of cases. Prolonged remission is again rarely induced by drug therapy.

***de Quervain's thyroiditis*** Transient hyperthyroidism sometimes results from acute inflammation of the gland, probably as a result of viral infection. It is usually accompanied by fever, malaise and pain in the neck. Treatment is with aspirin, reserving prednisolone for severely symptomatic cases.

## Clinical features

Typical symptoms and signs of hyperthyroidism are shown in Figure 13.6.

Clinical features vary with age and the underlying aetiology. Ophthalmopathy (see below), pretibial myxoedema

565

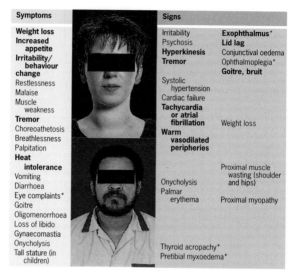

| Symptoms | | Signs | |
|---|---|---|---|
| **Weight loss** | | Irritability | **Exophthalmus*** |
| **Increased** | | Psychosis | Lid lag |
| **appetite** | | **Hyperkinesis** | Conjunctival oedema |
| **Irritability/** | | **Tremor** | Ophthalmoplegia* |
| **behaviour** | | | **Goitre, bruit** |
| **change** | | | |
| Restlessness | | Systolic | |
| Malaise | | hypertension | |
| Muscle | | Cardiac failure | |
| weakness | | **Tachycardia** | |
| **Tremor** | | **or atrial** | |
| Choreoathetosis | | **fibrillation** | Weight loss |
| Breathlessness | | **Warm** | |
| Palpitation | | **vasodilated** | |
| **Heat** | | **peripheries** | |
| **intolerance** | | | Proximal muscle |
| Vomiting | | | wasting (shoulder |
| Diarrhoea | | Onycholysis | and hips) |
| Eye complaints* | | Palmar | |
| Goitre | | erythema | Proximal myopathy |
| Oligomenorrhoea | | | |
| Loss of libido | | | |
| Gynaecomastia | | Thyroid acropachy* | |
| Onycholysis | | Pretibial myxoedema* | |
| Tall stature (in | | | |
| children) | | | |

**Fig. 13.6 The symptoms and signs of hyperthyroidism.** Bold type indicates signs of greater discriminatory value. *, only in Graves' disease.

(raised, purple-red symmetrical skin lesions over antero-lateral aspects of the shins) and thyroid acropachy (clubbing, swollen fingers and periosteal new bone formation) occur only in Graves' disease. Elderly patients may present with atrial fibrillation and/or heart failure, or with a clinical picture resembling hypothyroidism ('apathetic thyrotoxicosis').

## Investigations

- Serum TSH is suppressed (< 0.05 mU/L).
- Serum free $T_4$ and $T_3$ are elevated. Occasionally $T_3$ alone is elevated ($T_3$ toxicosis).
- Serum microsomal and thyroglobulin antibodies are present in most cases of Graves' disease. TSH receptor antibodies are not measured routinely.
- Thyroid ultrasound will help differentiate Graves' disease from a toxic adenoma.

## Management

**Antithyroid drugs** Carbimazole (10–20 mg 8-hourly) blocks thyroid hormone biosynthesis and also has immuno-suppressive effects which will affect the Graves' disease process. As clinical benefit may not be apparent for 10–20 days, β-blockers may be used to provide rapid symp-tomatic control because many manifestations are mediated via the sympathetic system. Carbimazole is then reduced to maintain normal free $T_4$ levels over the next 12–18 months. Some physicians prefer the 'block and replace regimen', whereby full doses of carbimazole 30–45 mg/day are given for 18 months to suppress the thyroid completely, while replacing thyroid activity with thyroxine. Claimed advan-tages are avoidance of under- or overtreatment and better use of the immunosuppressive action. Fifty per cent of patients with Graves' disease will relapse on discontinu-ation of drug treatment, mostly within the following 2 years. The most severe side-effect of carbimazole is agranulocytosis. All patients starting treatment must be warned to stop carbimazole and seek an urgent blood count if they develop a sore throat or unexplained fever.

**Radioactive iodine** This treatment is now much more com-monly used than previously though it is contraindicated in pregnancy and while breast-feeding. $^{131}$I accumulates in the gland and destroys it by local irradiation and, though it takes several months to be fully effective, 75% of patients are rendered euthyroid in 4–12 weeks. If hyperthyroidism persists a further dose of $^{131}$I can be given, although this increases the rate of subsequent hypothyroidism.

**Surgery** Subtotal thyroidectomy should only be per-formed in patients who have been rendered euthyroid. Antithyroid drugs are stopped 10–14 days before the operation and replaced with oral potassium iodide, which inhibits thyroid hormone release and reduces the vascu-larity of the gland. Complications of surgery include hypocalcaemia, hypothyroidism, hypoparathyroidism, recurrent laryngeal nerve palsy and recurrent hyper-thyroidism.

The choice of therapy for hyperthyroidism depends on patient preference and local expertise. Radioiodine or surgical treatment is particularly indicated when there are persistent drug side-effects, poor compliance with drug therapy, or recurrent hyperthyroidism following drug treatment. Surgical treatment is particularly suited to patients with large goitres which are unlikely to remit after medical treatment.

# Thyroid crisis

Thyroid crisis or storm is a rare life-threatening condition in which there is a rapid deterioration of thyrotoxicosis with hyperpyrexia, tachycardia, extreme restlessness and eventually delirium, coma and death. It is most commonly precipitated by infection, stress, and surgery or radioactive iodine therapy in an unprepared patient. Management (Emergency Box 13.2) includes the administration of large doses of carbimazole and propranolol, iodine to block

## Emergency Box 13.2

### Management of thyroid crisis

**Investigations**
- Full blood count, blood glucose, serum urea and electrolytes, thyroid function tests, blood cultures
- Chest X-ray and ECG

**Give antithyroid drugs**
- Propranolol 5 mg i.v. 6-hourly or 80 mg orally 12-hourly (contraindicated in asthma or heart failure)
- Carbimazole 20 mg 8-hourly by mouth or nasogastric tube
- Potassium iodide by mouth or nasogastric tube 15 mg 6-hourly. Give after carbimazole. Stop after 1 week if clinical improvement
- Dexamethasone 2 mg i.v. 6-hourly

**Additional management**
- Heart failure is usually associated with rapid atrial fibrillation. Treat with intravenous digoxin, diuretics and heparin
- Supportive treatment, including oxygen, i.v. fluids and management of hyperpyrexia
- Search for and treat precipitating cause

acutely the release of thyroid hormone from the gland, and dexamethasone which inhibits peripheral conversion of $T_4$ to $T_3$.

## Thyroid eye disease (K&C p. 1044)

Lid retraction (white of sclera visible above the cornea as the patient looks forwards) and lid lag are a result of increased catecholamine sensitivity of the levator palpebrae superioris and may occur in any form of hyperthyroidism. Exophthalmos (proptosis, protruding eyeballs) and ophthalmoplegia (limitation of eye movements) only occur in patients with Graves' disease (ophthalmic Graves' disease).

### Aetiology

It is thought that the exophthalmos of Graves' disease, which may be unilateral or bilateral, is the result of specific antibodies causing retro-orbital inflammation, with swelling and oedema of the extraocular muscles leading to limitation of movement. TSH antibodies are found in the serum although their role in pathogenesis is not clear.

### Clinical features

The clinical appearances are characteristic. Exophthalmos and ophthalmoplegia are direct effects of retro-orbital inflammation, whereas conjunctival oedema (chemosis), lid lag and corneal scarring are secondary to the proptosis and lack of eye cover (Fig. 13.7). Eye manifestations do not parallel the clinical course of Graves' disease and may appear before the onset of hyperthyroidism. MRI of the orbits will exclude other causes of proptosis, e.g. retro-orbital tumour, and show enlarged muscles and oedema.

569

### Management

Thyroid status should be normalized and hypothyroidism avoided because this may exacerbate the eye problem. Smoking increases the severity of ophthalmopathy and patients should be advised to stop. Specific treatment includes methylcellulose eyedrops or, if more severe, high-dose systemic steroids to reduce inflammation. Lateral tarsorraphy will protect the cornea if the lids cannot be closed. Occasionally irradiation of the orbits or surgical decompression of the orbit(s) is required.

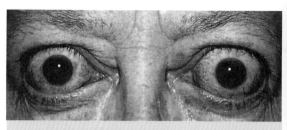

| Grade 0 | No signs or symptoms |
| Grade 1 | Only signs, no symptoms |
| Grade 2 | Soft tissue involvement |
| Grade 3 | Proptosis (measured with exophthalmometer) |
| Grade 4 | Extraocular muscle involvement |
| Grade 5 | Corneal involvement |
| Grade 6 | Sight loss with optic nerve involvement |

Fig. 13.7 **The eye signs of Graves' disease.**

## Goitre (thyroid enlargement) (K&C p. 1044)

Goitre is more common in women than in men and may be physiological or pathological in origin (Table 13.8). The presence of a goitre gives no indication about the thyroid status of the patient.

### Clinical features

It is usually noticed as a cosmetic defect, although discomfort and pain in the neck can occur, and occasionally oesophageal or tracheal compression produces dysphagia

Table 13.8
Causes of goitre

Physiological: puberty, pregnancy
Multinodular goitre
Autoimmune: Graves' disease, Hashimoto's disease
Thyroiditis: acute (de Quervain's thyroiditis), chronic fibrotic (Riedel's thyroiditis)
Iodine deficiency (endemic goitre)
Dyshormonogenesis
Diffuse goitre
Benign cysts, lymphoma, carcinoma

or difficulty in breathing. The gland may be diffusely enlarged, multinodular or possess a solitary nodule. A bruit may be present and occasionally there is lymphadenopathy.

### Investigations

- Thyroid function tests: TSH plus $T_4$ or $T_3$.
- Thyroid ultrasonography can delineate nodules and demonstrate whether they are solid or cystic.
- Fine needle aspiration for cytology should be performed for solitary nodules or a dominant nodule in a multinodular goitre because there is a 5% chance of malignancy.
- Radiography of the chest and thoracic inlet where appropriate to detect tracheal compression.
- Other tests are not usually required. Thyroid scan ($^{125}$I or $^{131}$I) distinguishes between a functioning ('hot') or non-functioning ('cold') nodule. Hot nodules are rarely malignant, whereas cold nodules are malignant in up to 10% of cases.

### Management

Treatment is usually not required, apart from inducing euthyroidism if necessary. Surgical intervention may be required for cosmetic reasons, pressure effects, or if there is a persisting concern of malignancy.

## Thyroid carcinoma (K&C p. 1046)

Thyroid cancer is relatively uncommon, being responsible for 400 deaths annually in the UK. Characteristics are listed in Table 13.9. Most differentiated thyroid cancers present as asymptomatic thyroid nodules, but the first sign of disease is occasionally lymph-node metastases or, in rare cases, lung or bone metastases. Features that suggest carcinoma in a patient presenting with a thyroid nodule are a history of progressive increase in size, a hard and irregular nodule, and the presence of enlarged lymph nodes on examination. Fine needle aspiration cytology is the best test for distinguishing between benign and malignant thyroid nodules. Treatment of follicular and papillary cancers is surgical, with total thyroidectomy. Ablative radioactive iodine is subsequently given which will be taken up by remaining

**Table 13.9**
Characteristics of thyroid cancer

| Cell type | Frequency (%) | Behaviour | Spread | Prognosis |
|---|---|---|---|---|
| Papillary | 70 | Young people, slow growing | Local | Good |
| Follicular | 20 | More common in females | Lung/bone | Good if resected |
| Anaplastic | < 5 | Aggressive | Local | Very poor |
| Lymphoma | 2 | Variable | Variable* | Variable |
| Medullary cell | 5 | Often familial and part of MEN syndrome | Local/metastases | Poor |

* Sometimes responsive to radiotherapy
MEN, multiple endocrine neoplasia

thyroid tissue or metastatic lesions. Treatment of anaplastic carcinoma is largely palliative.

# The glucocorticoid axis (K&C p. 1047)

The adrenal gland consists of an outer cortex producing steroids (cortisol, aldosterone and androgens) and an inner medulla secreting catecholamines. Aldosterone secretion is under the control of the renin–angiotensin system (see later). Corticotropin-releasing hormone (CRH) from the hypothalamus stimulates ACTH (from the anterior pituitary), which stimulates cortisol production by the adrenal cortex. The cortisol secreted feeds back on the hypothalamus and pituitary to inhibit further CRH/ACTH release. CRH release, and hence cortisol release, is in response to a circadian rhythm (light–dark), stress and other factors. Random 'one-off' serum cortisol measurements may therefore be misleading in the diagnosis of hypoadrenalism or Cushing's syndrome. Cortisol has many effects, particularly on carbohydrate metabolism. It leads to increased protein catabolism, increased deposition of fat and glycogen, sodium retention, increased renal potassium loss and a diminished host response to infection.

## Addison's disease – primary hypoadrenalism (K&C p. 1050)

This is an uncommon condition in which there is destruction of the entire adrenal cortex.

### Aetiology

More than 90% of cases result from destruction of the adrenal cortex by organ-specific autoantibodies. This is associated with other autoimmune conditions, e.g. Hashimoto's thyroiditis, Graves' disease, pernicious anaemia and type 1 diabetes mellitus. Rarer causes are adrenal gland tuberculosis, surgical removal, haemorrhage (in meningococcal septicaemia), malignant infiltration and secondary adrenocortical failure as a result of pituitary disease (p. 546).

## Clinical features

Adrenal insufficiency has an insidious presentation with lethargy, depression, anorexia and weight loss. It may also present as an emergency (Addisonian crisis), with vomiting, abdominal pain, profound weakness and hypovolaemic shock. The important signs are hypotension (which may only be postural) caused by salt and water loss, and hyperpigmentation (buccal mucosa, pressure points, skin creases and recent scars) resulting from stimulation of melanocytes by excess ACTH. There may be vitiligo and loss of body hair in women because of the dependence on adrenal androgens.

## Investigations

- Serum urea and electrolytes may be normal but classically there is hyponatraemia, hyperkalaemia, a raised urea and hypoglycaemia.
- Blood count shows a neutrophil leucocytosis and eosinophilia.
- Adrenal antibodies are detected in most cases of autoimmune adrenalitis.
- Radiographs of the chest and abdomen may show evidence of tuberculosis, with calcified adrenals.

The diagnosis is usually made using the short tetracosactide (synacthen or synthetic ACTH) test (Table 13.10). Addisonian crisis is a life-threatening emergency that requires immediate treatment before full investigation (Emergency Box 13.3). Treatment should be begun on the basis of clinical suspicion without waiting for the results of laboratory results.

574

## Management

This is with lifelong steroid replacement taken as tablets.

- *Hydrocortisone.* The usual dose is 20 mg on waking and 10 mg in the evening, which mimics the normal diurnal rhythm. The dose is best monitored by measuring a series of cortisol levels throughout the day.
- *Fludrocortisone*, a synthetic mineralocorticoid, 0.05–0.4 mg daily. The dose is adequate when there is no postural drop in blood pressure and plasma renin levels are suppressed to within the normal range.

**Table 13.10**
Tetracosactide (synacthen tests)

| | |
|---|---|
| Short test | 1. Take blood for measurement of plasma cortisol |
| | 2. Administer tetracosactide 250 μg i.m./i.v. |
| | 3. Take blood for measurement of cortisol at 30 and 60 minutes |
| | 4. Interpretation: adrenal failure is excluded if the basal plasma cortisol exceeds 170 nmol/L and rises by at least 330 nmol/L to 690 nmol/L. An inadequate rise in plasma cortisol is due either to primary adrenal failure or to secondary adrenocortical failure. A long test is then performed to differentiate between these |
| Long test | 1. Take blood for measurement of plasma cortisol |
| | 2. Administer tetracosactide 1 mg i.m. |
| | 3. Take blood for cortisol at 1, 4, 8 and 24 hours |
| | 4. Interpretation: patients with normal adrenal glands reach a plasma cortisol concentration of over 1000 nmol/L by 4 hours. In patients with Addison's disease the cortisol response is impaired throughout, and in secondary adrenal insufficiency a delayed but normal response is seen |

In a normal individual stress of any type, e.g. infection, trauma and surgery, causes an immediate and marked increase in ACTH and hence in cortisol. This is a necessary response and therefore it is very important in patients on steroid replacement that the dose is increased when they are placed in any of these situations. The usual dose is 100 mg hydrocortisone intramuscularly for minor surgery and, for major surgery, 100 mg hydrocortisone 6-hourly until oral medication is resumed.

## Uses and problems of therapeutic steroid therapy (K&C p. 1055)

In addition to their use as therapeutic replacement for deficiency states, steroids are widely used for a variety of non-endocrine conditions such as inflammatory bowel disease, asthma and rheumatological conditions. Long-term steroid use may be associated with significant side-effects (Table 13.11) and may also result in suppression of the adrenal axis if used continually for more than 3–4 weeks. All patients

### Emergency Box 13.3

## Management of Addisonian crisis

### Investigations

- Take blood for plasma cortisol (will be inappropriately low) and ACTH (will be high because of loss of negative feedback) before administration of hydrocortisone
- Full blood count, urea and electrolytes, blood glucose and blood cultures

### Immediate

- Hydrocortisone 100 mg intravenously
- 0.9% saline, 1 litre over 30–60 minutes
- 50 mL of 50% dextrose if hypoglycaemic
- Search for precipitating cause, e.g. infection, gastroenteritis

### Subsequent

- Hydrocortisone 100 mg intramuscular 6-hourly until BP stable and vomiting ceased
- 0.9% saline 2–4 litres intravenously in 12–24 hours; monitor by JVP or CVP
- Expect recovery, with normal BP, blood glucose and serum sodium, within 12–24 hours
- When stable, convert to oral maintenance treatment (see pp. 514–575) continued lifelong

receiving steroids should carry a 'Steroid Card' and should be made aware of the following points:

- Long-term steroid therapy must never be stopped suddenly.
- Doses should be reduced very gradually.
- Doses should be doubled in times of serious intercurrent illness.
- Other physicians, anaesthetists and dentists must be told about steroid therapy.

Patients should also be informed of potential side-effects and all this information should be documented in the patient records.

## Secondary hypoadrenalism (K&C p. 1051)

This may arise from hypothalamic–pituitary disease or from long-term steroid therapy leading to hypothalamic–

**Table 13.11**
Adverse effects of corticosteroids

**Physiological**
Adrenal and/or pituitary
suppression

**Pathological**

*Cardiovascular*
Increased blood pressure

*Gastrointestinal*
Peptic ulceration
  exacerbation (possibly)
Acute pancreatitis

*Renal*
Polyuria
Nocturia

*Central nervous*
Depression
Euphoria
Psychosis
Insomnia

*Increased susceptibility
to infection*
(signs and fever are
frequently masked)
Septicaemia
Reactivation of tuberculosis
Skin (e.g. fungi)

*Endocrine*
Weight gain
Glycosuria, hyperglycaemia
  (diabetes mellitus)
Impaired growth in children

*Bone and muscle*
Osteoporosis
Proximal myopathy and wasting
Aseptic necrosis of the hip
Pathological fractures

*Skin*
Thinning
Easy bruising

*Eyes*
Cataracts (including with inhaled
drugs)

pituitary–adrenal suppression. The clinical features are the same as those of Addison's disease but there is no pigmentation because ACTH levels are low and, in pituitary disease, there are usually features of failure of other pituitary hormones. A long tetracosactide (synacthen) test (see Table 13.10) will differentiate between primary and secondary adrenal failure. Treatment is with hydrocortisone; fludrocortisone is unnecessary. If adrenal failure is secondary to long-term steroid therapy, the adrenals will recover if steroids are withdrawn very slowly.

## Cushing's syndrome (K&C p. 1052)

Cushing's syndrome is caused by persistently and inappropriately elevated glucocorticoid levels. Most cases result from administration of steroids for the treatment of medical

**Table 13.12**
Aetiology of spontaneous Cushing's syndrome

|  | % of cases |
| --- | --- |
| **ACTH-dependent causes** |  |
| Pituitary disease (Cushing's disease) | 60–70 |
| Ectopic ACTH-producing tumours |  |
|    (small-cell lung cancer, carcinoid tumours) | 15 |
| **Non-ACTH-dependent causes** |  |
| Adrenal adenomas | 9 |
| Adrenal carcinomas | 7 |
| **Rare causes, e.g. adrenal hyperplasia** |  |

conditions, e.g. asthma. Spontaneous Cushing's syndrome is rare (Table 13.12). Cushing's disease must be distinguished from Cushing's syndrome. The latter is a general term which refers to the abnormalities resulting from a chronic excess of glucocorticoids whatever the cause, whereas Cushing's disease specifically refers to excess glucocorticoids resulting from inappropriate ACTH secretion from the pituitary (usually a microadenoma, less often corticotroph hyperplasia). Alcohol excess mimics Cushing's syndrome clinically and biochemically (pseudo-Cushing's syndrome). The pathogenesis is incompletely understood but the features resolve when alcohol is stopped.

### Clinical features
Patients are obese: fat distribution is typically central, affecting the trunk, abdomen and neck (buffalo hump). They have a plethoric complexion with a moon face. Many of the features are the result of the protein-catabolic effects of cortisol: the skin is thin and bruises easily, and there are purple striae on the abdomen, breasts and thighs (Fig. 13.8). Pigmentation occurs with ACTH-dependent cases. Patients with ectopic production of ACTH tend to have rapidly progressive symptoms and signs, and may have evidence of the primary tumour.

### Investigations
In a patient with suspected spontaneous Cushing's syndrome the purpose of investigation is firstly to confirm

| Symptoms | Signs | |
|---|---|---|
| Weight gain (central) | Depression/ psychosis | Frontal balding (female) |
| Change of appearance | Acne, hirsuties | |
| Depression | **Thin skin** | Moon face |
| Psychosis | **Bruising** | **Plethora** |
| Insomnia | **Hypertension** | 'Buffalo-hump' |
| Amenorrhoea/ oligomenorrhoea | | Kyphosis |
| Poor libido | Rib fractures | |
| Thin skin/ easy bruising | Osteoporosis | Centripetal obesity |
| Hair growth/acne | | Pigmentation |
| Muscular weakness | **Pathological fractures** | **Striae (purple)** |
| Growth arrest in children | | |
| Back pain | Poor wound healing | Skin infections |
| Polyuria/polydipsia | | Glycosuria |
| Old photographs may be useful | Proximal muscle wasting | |
| Symptoms of hypopituitarism are rare | **Proximal myopathy** | |
| | Oedema | |

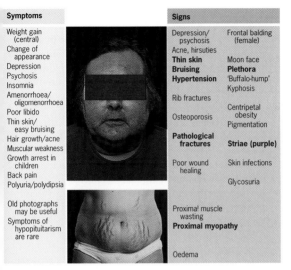

**Fig. 13.8 The symptoms and signs of Cushing's syndrome.** Bold type indicates signs of most value in discriminating Cushing's syndrome from simple obesity and hirsutes.

the presence of cortisol excess, and secondly to determine the cause.

### Confirm raised cortisol

- The *48-hour low-dose dexamethasone suppression test* is the most reliable screening test. Dexamethasone (a potent synthetic glucocorticoid) 0.5 mg 6-hourly is given orally for 48 hours. Normal individuals suppress plasma cortisol by 48 hours.
- *Urinary free cortisol* is raised (normal < 700 nmol/24 h).
- *Circadian rhythm studies* show loss of the normal circadian fall of plasma cortisol at 24 hours in patients with Cushing's syndrome.

### Establishing the cause of Cushing's syndrome

- Adrenal CT or MRI will detect adrenal adenomas and carcinomas, as those which produce Cushing's syndrome are usually large.

579

- Pituitary MRI and CT will detect some, but not all, pituitary adenomas.
- *Plasma ACTH levels* are low or undetectable in adrenal gland disease (non-ACTH dependent) and should lead to adrenal imaging. High or inappropriately normal values suggest pituitary disease or ectopic production of ACTH.
- *High-dose dexamethasone suppression test.* Dexamethasone 2.0 mg 6-hourly is given orally for 48 hours. Most patients with pituitary-dependent Cushing's disease suppress plasma cortisol by 48 hours. Failure of suppression suggests an ectopic source of ACTH or an adrenal tumour.
- *Corticotropin-releasing hormone test.* An exaggerated plasma ACTH response to exogenous CRH (bolus given intravenously) suggests pituitary-dependent Cushing's disease.
- *Other tests* will depend on the probable cause of Cushing's syndrome, which has been established from the above tests. Chest radiography, bronchoscopy and CT of the body may localize ectopic ACTH-producing tumours. Selective venous sampling for ACTH will localize pituitary tumours and an otherwise occult ectopic ACTH-producing tumour.
- *Radiolabelled octreotide* ($^{111}$In octreotide) shows promise in locating ectopic ACTH sites.

## Management

Surgical removal is indicated for most pituitary (usually a trans-sphenoidal approach) and adrenal tumours and may be appropriate for many cases of ectopic ACTH-producing tumours.

Drugs which inhibit cortisol synthesis (metyrapone, keto-conazole or aminoglutethimide) may be useful in cases not amenable to surgery.

External-beam irradiation of the pituitary produces a very slow response and is restricted to cases where surgery is unsuccessful, contraindicated or unacceptable to the patient.

Iatrogenic Cushing's syndrome responds to a reduction in steroid dosage when possible. Immunosuppressant drugs such as azathioprine may be used in conjunction with steroids to enable lower doses to be used to control the underlying disease.

## Incidental adrenal tumours

With the advent of improved abdominal imaging, unsuspected adrenal masses have been discovered in about 1% of scans. These include primary tumours, metastases and cysts. If found, functional tests to exclude secretory activity should be performed; if none is found then most authorities recommend surgical removal of large (> 4–5 cm) and functional tumours but observation of smaller hormonally inactive lesions.

## The thirst axis (K&C p. 1057)

The secretion of antidiuretic hormone (ADH, vasopressin) from the posterior pituitary gland is determined principally by the plasma osmolality. ADH secretion is suppressed at levels below 280 mmol/kg, thus allowing maximal water diuresis. Secretion increases to a maximum at a plasma osmolality of 295 mmol/kg. Large falls in blood pressure or volume also stimulate vasopressin secretion. The major hormonal action is on the collecting tubule of the kidney to cause water reabsorption. At high concentrations vasopressin also causes vasoconstriction.

## Syndrome of inappropriate ADH secretion (SIADH) (K&C p. 1059)

There is continued ADH secretion in spite of plasma hypotonicity and a normal or expanded plasma volume.

### Aetiology

SIADH is caused by ectopic production of ADH, e.g. small-cell lung cancer or disordered hypothalamic–pituitary secretion (Table 13.13).

### Clinical features

There is nausea, irritability and headache with mild dilutional hyponatraemia (115–125 mmol/L). Fits and coma may occur with severe hyponatraemia (< 115 mmol/L).

**Table 13.13**
Causes of syndrome of inappropriate ADH

| | |
|---|---|
| **Cancer** | Many tumours, of which the most common is small-cell cancer of the lung |
| **Brain** | Meningitis, cerebral abscess, head injury, tumour |
| **Lung** | Pneumonia, tuberculosis, lung abscess |
| **Metabolic** | Porphyria, alcohol withdrawal |
| **Drugs** | Opiates, chlorpropamide, carbamazepine, vincristine |

### Investigations

SIADH must be differentiated from other causes of dilutional hyponatraemia (p. 295). The criteria for diagnosis are:

- Low serum sodium (< 125 mmol/L)
- Low plasma osmolality
- Urine osmolality 'inappropriately' higher than plasma osmolality
- Continued urinary sodium excretion (> 30 mmol/L)
- Absence of hypotension and hypovolaemia
- Normal renal, adrenal and thyroid function.

### Management

Mild asymptomatic cases need no treatment other than that of the underlying cause. For symptomatic cases the options are:

- Water restriction: 500–1000 mL in 24 hours
- Dimethylchlorotetracycline (demeclocycline) inhibits the action of vasopressin on the kidney and may be useful if water restriction is poorly tolerated or ineffective
- Hypertonic saline, with furosemide (frusemide) to prevent circulatory overload, may be necessary in severe cases (Emergency Box 7.1, p. 296).

## Diabetes insipidus (K&C p. 1057)

Impaired vasopressin secretion (cranial diabetes insipidus, CDI) or renal resistance to its action (nephrogenic diabetes insipidus, NDI) leads to polyuria (dilute urine in excess of 3 L/24 h), nocturia and compensatory polydipsia. It must be distinguished from primary polydipsia, which is a psychiatric disturbance characterized by excessive intake of water, and other causes of polyuria and polydipsia, e.g. hyperglycaemia.

## Aetiology

The causes are listed in Table 13.14.

## Clinical features

There is polyuria (as much as 15 L in 24 h) and polydipsia. Patients depend on a normal thirst mechanism and access to water to maintain normonatraemia.

## Investigations

- Urine volume must be measured to confirm polyuria.
- Plasma biochemistry shows high or high–normal sodium concentration and osmolality. Blood glucose, serum potassium and calcium should be measured to exclude common causes of polyuria.
- Urine osmolality is inappropriately low for the high plasma osmolality.
- A water deprivation test with exogenous desmopressin (a synthetic vasopressin analogue) is the

**Table 13.14**
Causes of diabetes insipidus

| Cranial diabetes insipidus | Nephrogenic diabetes insipidus |
| --- | --- |
| Familial | Familial |
| Idiopathic* | Renal tubular acidosis |
| Head injury* | Metabolic |
| Surgery transfrontal, trans-sphenoidal* |    Hypercalcaemia |
| Hypothalamic – pituitary tumours |    Hypokalaemia* |
| | Prolonged polyuria of any cause |
| Granulomas: sarcoidosis, histiocytosis | Drugs* |
| |    Lithium chloride |
| Infections: meningitis, encephalitis |    Dimethylchlorotetracycline |
| |    Glibenclamide |
| Vascular: haemorrhage, thrombosis | |

* Indicate the most common causes. Diabetes insipidus after surgery may only be transient

**Table 13.15**
Response to fluid deprivation and desmopressin in polyuric patients

| Urine osmolality (mmol/kg) | | Diagnosis |
|---|---|---|
| **After 8 h fluid deprivation** | **After desmopressin** | |
| < 300 | > 800 | CDI |
| < 300 | < 300 | NDI |
| > 800 | > 800 | Primary polydipsia |

usual investigation for polyuric patients with normal blood glucose and serum electrolytes. It confirms the diagnosis of DI and will usually distinguish between CDI, NDI and primary polydipsia (Table 13.15). Water is restricted for 8 hours, during which time blood and urine osmolality are measured hourly. Patients are weighed hourly and the test stopped if bodyweight drops by 5%, as this indicates significant dehydration. In equivocal cases the measurement of plasma vasopressin during water deprivation provides a definitive diagnosis, but this test is not routinely available.

- MRI of the pituitary and hypothalamus is performed in cases of CDI.

### Management

Treatment of the underlying condition seldom improves established CDI. In mild cases (3–4 L urine per day) no specific treatment is necessary. Desmopressin, administered orally, nasally or intramuscularly, is useful for more severe cases. Treatment of the cause will usually improve NDI.

## Calcium and the parathyroids
(K&C p. 1059)

The control of calcium and bone metabolism is discussed on page 276. Total plasma calcium is normally 2.2–2.6 mmol/L.

584

Usually only 40% of total plasma calcium is ionized and physiologically relevant; the remainder is bound to albumin and thus unavailable to the tissues. Routine analytical methods measure total plasma calcium and this must be corrected for the serum albumin concentration: add or subtract 0.02 mmol/L for every g/L by which the simultaneous albumin lies below or above 40 g/L. For critical measurements samples should be taken in the fasting state without the use of an occluding cuff, which may increase the local plasma protein concentration.

## Hypercalcaemia (K&C p. 1060)

Mild asymptomatic hypercalcaemia occurs in about 1 in 1000 of the population, especially elderly women, and is usually the result of primary hyperparathyroidism.

### Aetiology

Primary hyperparathyroidism and malignancy account for 80–90% of cases (Table 13.16). Tumour-related hypercalcaemia is caused by the secretion of a peptide with PTH-like activity, or by direct invasion of bone and production of local factors that mobilize calcium. Ectopic PTH secretion by tumours is very rare.

Hyperparathyroidism may be primary, secondary or tertiary.

***Primary hyperparathyroidism*** affects about 0.1% of the population and is usually caused by a single adenoma, occasionally hyperplasia, and rarely carcinoma.

***Secondary hyperparathyroidism*** is a physiological response to hypocalcaemia (e.g. in renal failure or vitamin D deficiency). Calcium is low or low–normal.

***Tertiary hyperparathyroidism*** is the development of apparently autonomous parathyroid hyperplasia after long-standing secondary hyperparathyroidism, most often in renal disease. Plasma calcium and PTH are both raised. Treatment is parathyroidectomy.

Table 13.16
Causes of hypercalcaemia

**Excess PTH**
Primary hyperparathyroidism (commonest cause)*
Tertiary hyperparathyroidism
Ectopic PTH (very rare)

**Excess action of vitamin D**
Self-administered vitamin D[+]
Sarcoidosis

**Excess calcium intake**
'Milk–alkali' syndrome

**Malignant disease***[+]

| | |
|---|---|
| Multiple myeloma | Prostate |
| Breast cancer | Renal cell |
| Bronchus | Lymphoma |
| Thyroid | |

**Other endocrine disease**
Thyrotoxicosis
Addison's disease

**Drugs**
Thiazides

**Miscellaneous**
Long-term immobility

* Indicates commonest causes of hypercalcaemia
[+] Conditions causing severe hypercalcaemia (> 3.5 mmol/L)

## Clinical features

Mild hypercalcaemia (adjusted serum calcium < 3 mmol/L) is often asymptomatic and discovered on biochemical screening. More severe hypercalcaemia produces symptoms such as general malaise and depression, bone pain, abdominal pain, nausea and constipation. Calcium deposition in the renal tubules causes polyuria and nocturia. Renal calculi and renal failure may develop. With very high levels (> 3.8 mmol/L) there is dehydration, confusion, clouding of consciousness and a risk of cardiac arrest.

## Investigations

- Several fasting serum calcium and phosphate samples should be performed.

586

- Serum PTH levels. Detectable levels during hypercalcaemia are inappropriate and imply hyperparathyroidism.
- Radiology. Subperiosteal erosions in the phalanges are seen in hyperparathyroidism.
- If PTH is undetectable or equivocal the following tests should be considered:
  - Protein electrophoresis for myeloma
  - TSH to exclude hyperthyroidism
  - Synacthen test to exclude Addison's disease.

## *Management*

This involves lowering of the calcium levels to near normal and treatment of the underlying cause. Severe hypercalcaemia (> 3.5 mmol/L) is a medical emergency which must be treated aggressively whatever the underlying cause (Emergency Box 13.4). Treatment is based on the corrected calcium value.

### Emergency Box 13.4

**Management of acute hypercalcaemia**

- **Rehydrate with intravenous fluid (0.9% saline)**
  4–6 litres of intravenous saline over 24 h and then 3–4 litres for several days thereafter
  Amount and rate depend on clinical assessment and measurement of serum urea and electrolytes
- **After minimum of 2 litres of intravenous fluids give bisphosphonate infusion**
  Pamidronate disodium 15–60 mg as an intravenous infusion in 0.5 litre 0.9% saline over 2–8 h
- **Measure**
  Serum urea and electrolytes at least daily
  Do not measure serum calcium for a least 48 h after initiation of treatment, normalization may take 3–5 days
- **Prednisolone (30–60 mg daily)**
  May be useful in some cases (myeloma, sarcoidosis and vitamin D excess) but in most cases ineffective
- **Prevent recurrence**
  Treat underlying cause if possible
  With untreatable malignancy consider maintenance treatment with bisphosphonates

### Treatment of primary hyperparathyroidism

The treatment of a symptomatic parathyroid adenoma is surgical removal. Conservative therapy may be indicated in asymptomatic patients with mildly raised serum calcium levels (2.65–3 mmol/L). In those with parathyroid hyperplasia all four glands are removed.

## Hypocalcaemia and hypoparathyroidism

(*K&C* p. 1062)

### Aetiology

The causes of hypocalcaemia are listed in Table 13.17. Renal failure is the most common cause of hypocalcaemia, which results from the inadequate production of active vitamin D and renal phosphate retention, leading to microprecipitation of calcium phosphate in the tissues. Mild transient hypocalcaemia often occurs after parathyroid-

**Table 13.17**
Causes of hypocalcaemia

**Increased serum phosphate levels**
Chronic renal failure*
Phosphate therapy

**Hypoparathyroidism**
Post-thyroidectomy and parathyroidectomy (usually transient)*
Congenital deficiency (DiGeorge syndrome)
Idiopathic hypoparathyroidism (autoimmune)
Severe hypomagnesaemia (inhibits PTH release)

**Vitamin D deficiency**
Osteomalacia
Resistance

**End-organ resistance to PTH**
Pseudohypoparathyroidism

**Drugs**
Calcitonin
Bisphosphonates

**Miscellaneous**
Acute pancreatitis*
Citrated blood in massive transfusion

* Indicates common cause of hypocalcaemia

ectomy, and a few patients develop long-standing hypoparathyroidism.

## Clinical features

Hypocalcaemia causes increased excitability of nerves. There is numbness around the mouth and in the extremities, followed by cramps, tetany (carpopedal spasm: opposition of the thumb, extension of the interphalangeal and flexion of the metacarpophalangeal joints), convulsions and death if untreated. Two important physical signs are Chvostek's sign (tapping over the facial nerve in the region of the parotid gland causes twitching of the facial muscles) and Trousseau's sign (carpopedal spasm induced by inflation of the sphygmomanometer cuff to a level above systolic blood pressure). With prolonged hypocalcaemia there may be cataract formation and rarely papilloedema.

Tetany may also develop in the presence of alkalosis, and potassium and magnesium deficiency as well as in hypocalcaemia. Hyperventilation alters the protein binding of calcium such that the ionized fraction is decreased, and may therefore cause hypocalcaemic tetany even with a normal plasma total calcium.

## Investigations

The clinical picture is usually diagnostic and is confirmed by a low corrected serum calcium. Additional tests identify the cause:

- Serum urea and creatinine for renal disease
- Serum PTH levels, which are absent or low in hypoparathyroidism and elevated in other causes of hypocalcaemia
- Serum parathyroid antibodies – present in autoimmune disease
- Serum 25-hydroxyvitamin D level.

## Management

Acute (e.g. with tetany): 10 mL of 10% calcium gluconate intravenously and repeated as necessary as an infusion over 4 hours.

Maintenance therapy is with alfacalcidol ($1\alpha$-OH-$D_3$).

# Endocrinology of blood pressure control (*K&C* p. 1063)

Blood pressure is determined by cardiac output and peripheral resistance and thus an increase in blood pressure may be due to an increase in one or both of these. In approximately 90% of cases no cause can be found (p. 435) and patients are said to have essential hypertension. In the remaining minority an underlying cause can be identified, and these include endocrine causes (Table 13.18). Young patients (< 35 years), those with an abnormal baseline screening test (p. 437) or patients with hypertension resistant to treatment should be screened for secondary causes.

## The renin–angiotensin system

The renin–angiotensin–aldosterone system is illustrated in Figure 13.9. *Angiotensin*, an $\alpha_2$-globulin of hepatic origin, circulates in plasma. The enzyme *renin* is secreted by the kidney in response to decreased renal perfusion pressure or flow; it cleaves the decapeptide *angiotensin I* from angiotensinogen. Angiotensin I is inactive but is further cleaved by converting enzyme (present in lung and vascular endothelium) into the active peptide, *angiotensin II*, which has two major actions:

- It causes powerful vasoconstriction (within seconds)
- It stimulates the adrenal zona glomerulosa to increase aldosterone production.

**Table 13.18**
Endocrine causes of hypertension

**Excessive production of**

| | |
|---|---|
| Renin | Renal artery stenosis, renin-secreting tumours |
| Aldosterone | Adrenal adenoma, adrenal hyperplasia |
| Mineralocorticoids | Cushing's syndrome (cortisol is a weak mineralocorticoid) |
| Catecholamines | Phaeochromocytoma |
| Growth hormone | Acromegaly |
| Oral contraceptive pill (mechanism unclear) | |

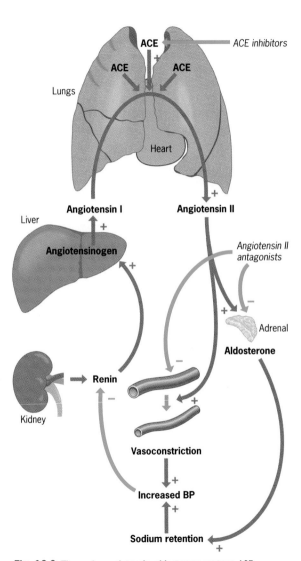

Fig. 13.9 **The renin–angiotensin–aldosterone system.** ACE, angiotensin-converting enzyme. Angiotensin II antagonists act on the adrenals and blood vessels.

*Aldosterone* causes sodium retention and urinary potassium loss (hours to days). This combination of changes leads to an increase in blood pressure, and the stimulus to renin production is reduced. Sodium deprivation or urinary loss also increases renin production, whereas dietary sodium excess will suppress production.

# Primary hyperaldosteronism (K&C p. 1065)

This is a rare condition (< 1% of all hypertension) where high aldosterone levels exist independently of the renin–angiotensin system. It is caused by an adrenal adenoma secreting aldosterone (Conn's syndrome, 60% of cases) or by bilateral adrenal hyperplasia.

## Clinical features

The major function of aldosterone is to cause an exchange transport of sodium and potassium in the distal renal tubule; that is, absorption of sodium (and hence water) and excretion of potassium. Therefore, hyperaldosteronism causes hypertension, resulting from expansion of intravascular volume, and hypokalaemia, which is rarely low enough to produce symptoms.

## Investigations

- Urea and electrolytes show a low serum potassium and normal or high sodium.
- The diagnosis is made by demonstrating increased plasma aldosterone levels that are not suppressed with saline infusion (300 mmol over 4 h) or fludrocortisone (a mineralocorticoid), associated with suppressed plasma renin levels.
- Antihypertensives, except bethanidine and prazosin, interfere with renin activity and should be stopped before these investigations.
- CT or MRI of the adrenals is used to differentiate adenomas from hyperplasia.

## Management

An adenoma is removed surgically. Hypertension resulting from hyperplasia is treated with the aldosterone antagonist spironolactone.

# Phaeochromocytoma (K&C p. 1066)

This is a rare (0.1% of hypertension) catecholamine-producing tumour of the sympathetic nervous system; 10% are malignant and 10% occur outside the adrenal gland. Some are associated with multiple endocrine neoplasia (see below).

## Clinical features

Symptoms may be episodic and include headache, palpitations, sweating, anxiety, nausea and weight loss. The signs, which may also be intermittent, include hypertension, tachycardia and pallor. There may be hyperglycaemia.

## Investigations

A 24-hour urine collection for urinary metanephrines (degradation products of epinephrine (adrenaline)) is a useful screening test; normal levels on three separate collections virtually exclude the diagnosis. Raised levels of plasma catecholamines confirm the diagnosis. The tumour is then localized by CT/MRI and scintigraphy using meta-[$^{131}$I]iodobenzylguanidine (mIBG), which is selectively taken up by adrenergic cells.

## Management

The treatment of choice is surgical excision of the tumour under α- and β-blockade using phenoxybenzamine and propranolol, which is started before the operation. These drugs can also be used long term where operation is not possible.

593

# Multiple endocrine neoplasia (K&C p. 1067)

The multiple endocrine neoplasia syndromes (MEN) are rare, but recognition is important both for treatment and for evaluation of family members. MEN is the name given to the synchronous or metachronous (i.e. occurring at different times) occurrence of tumours involving a number of endocrine glands (Table 13.19). MEN is subdivided into type 1, type 2a and type 2b. They are inherited in an autosomal dominant manner. MEN type 1 is due to a mutation in the menin gene on chromosome 11; the normal protein

**Table 13.19**
Multiple endocrine neoplasia (MEN) syndrome

| Organ | Frequency | Tumours/clinical manifestations |
|---|---|---|
| **Type 1** | | |
| Functioning adenomas in: | | |
| Parathyroid | 95% | Hypercalcaemia |
| Pituitary | 30% | Prolactinoma, acromegaly, Cushing's disease |
| Pancreatic islets | 60% | Gastrinoma, insulinoma, glucagonoma, VIPoma |
| Adrenal cortex | 40% | Non-functional adenomas |
| Thyroid | 20% | Adenomas – multiple or single |
| **Type 2A** | | |
| Medullary thyroid carcinoma | 95% | Thyroid mass, diarrhoea, raised plasma calcitonin |
| Adrenal | Most | Phaeochromocytoma, Cushing's syndrome |
| Parathyroid hyperplasia | 20% | Hypercalcaemia |
| **Type 2B** | | |
| Like type 2A (but parathyroid disease is rare) with a typical phenotypic appearance: slim body habitus and neuromas of lips, tongue, and gastrointestinal tract | | |

VIP, vasoactive intestinal polypeptide

product of this gene acts as a tumour suppressor. The genetic abnormality in MEN 2 lies within the *Ret* proto-oncogene on chromosome 10; the gene product plays an important role in central and peripheral nerve development and function. Management involves surgical excision of the tumours if possible and biochemical screening of first- and second-degree relatives. In a patient known to have MEN constant surveillance is required for additional features of the syndrome, which may develop many years after the initial presentation.

# Disorders of temperature regulation
(*K&C* p. 991)

Normal body temperature is 36.5–37.5°C and is controlled by temperature-sensitive cells within the hypothalamus which control heat generation and loss. Fever during an infection is due to cytokines, particularly interleukin-1, released from inflammatory cells acting in the hypothalamus affecting the thermoregulatory set-point.

## Hypothermia (*K&C* p. 992)
Hypothermia is defined as a drop in core (i.e. rectal) temperature to below 35°C. It is frequently fatal when the temperature falls below 32°C.

### Aetiology
Very young and elderly individuals are particularly prone to hypothermia, the latter having a reduced ability to feel the cold. Hypothyroidism, hypnotics, alcohol or intercurrent illness may contribute. In healthy individuals, prolonged exposure to extremes of temperature or prolonged immersion in cold water are the most common underlying causes.

### Clinical features
Mild hypothermia (32–35°C) causes shivering and a feeling of intense cold. More severe hypothermia leads progressively to altered consciousness and coma. This is usually associated with a fall in pulse rate and blood pressure,

muscle stiffness and depressed reflexes. As coma ensues the pupillary and other brainstem reflexes are lost. Ventricular arrhythmias or asystole are the usual causes of death.

### Diagnosis

Measurement of core temperature with a low-reading rectal thermometer makes the diagnosis. Alteration in consciousness usually indicates a core temperature of below 32°C; this is a medical emergency. With severe hypothermia there are ECG changes, including an increase in the PR interval, widening of the QRS complex and 'J' waves (deflections at the junction of the QRS complex and ST segment).

### Management

The principles of treatment are to rewarm the patient gradually while correcting metabolic abnormalities (if severe) and treating cardiac arrhythmias (Emergency Box 13.5). Hypothyroidism should always be looked for and, if suspected, should be treated with intravenous triiodothyronine. Clues to the presence of hypothyroidism include previous radioiodine treatment or surgery for thyrotoxicosis, and preceding symptoms of hypothyroidism (p. 562). Hypothermia may protect organs from ischaemia in patients with prolonged hypothermia-induced cardiopulmonary arrest. Therefore, it is usually recommended that resuscitation efforts are continued (maybe for some hours) until arrest persists after rewarming.

## Hyperthermia (hyperpyrexia) (K&C p. 991)

Hyperpyrexia is a body temperature above 41°C. Causes include:

- Injury to the hypothalamus (trauma, surgery, infection)
- Malignant hyperpyrexia – rare autosomal dominant condition in which skeletal muscle generates heat in the presence of certain anaesthetic drugs, e.g. suxamethonium

### Emergency Box 13.5

## Management of hypothermia

### Investigations
- Arterial blood gases
- Full blood count, urea and electrolytes, blood glucose, thyroid function tests, blood cultures
- Chest X-ray, ECG

### Treatment
- Give oxygen by face mask and attach an ECG monitor
- Search for and treat infection, pneumonia is common
- Intubate and ventilate patients who are comatose or in respiratory failure
- Warmed (37°C) intravenous fluids to achieve urine output 30–40 mL/h
- External warming if core temperature > 32°C:
  - Place patient in a warm room (27–29°C)
  - 'Space' blankets
  - Warm bath water
- Internal rewarming if core temperature < 32°C:
  - Humidified and warmed oxygen
  - Extracorporeal shunt (haemodialysis, arteriovenous or venovenous) rewarming
  - Cardiopulmonary bypass – treatment of choice for arrested hypothermic patients
- Monitor core temperature, oxygen saturation by pulse oximetry, urine output and central venous pressure

- Ingestion of 3,4-methylenedioxy-metamfetamine (Ecstasy)
- Neuroleptic malignant syndrome: idiosyncratic reaction to therapeutic dose of neuroleptic medication, e.g. phenothiazines.

Treatment includes stopping the offending drug, cooling, and the administration of dantrolene sodium.

# 14 Diabetes mellitus and other disorders of metabolism

## Diabetes mellitus

### Glucose metabolism (K&C p. 1069)

Blood glucose levels are closely regulated in health. The principal organ of glucose homeostasis is the liver, which absorbs and stores glucose (as glycogen) in the post-absorptive state and releases it into the circulation between meals to match the rate of glucose utilization by peripheral tissues. The liver also combines 3-carbon molecules derived from breakdown of fat (glycerol), muscle glycogen (lactate) and protein (e.g. alanine) into the 6-carbon glucose molecule by the process of gluconeogenesis. Insulin is the key hormone involved in the storage of nutrients in the form of glycogen in liver and muscle, and triglyceride in fat. During a meal insulin is released from the beta ($\beta$) cells of the pancreatic islets and facilitates glucose uptake by fat and muscle. In the fasting state the main action of insulin is to regulate glucose release by the liver. The counter-regulatory hormones, glucagon, epinephrine (adrenaline), cortisol and growth hormone oppose the actions of insulin and cause greater production of glucose from the liver and less utilization of glucose in fat and muscle for a given plasma level of insulin. The normal venous *whole blood glucose* concentration is between 3.5 and 8.0 mmol/L. It should be noted that whole blood values are about 10–15% lower than *plasma values*, and *capillary values* are about 7% higher than plasma values.

599

### Types of diabetes (K&C p. 1071)

Diabetes mellitus is a common group of metabolic disorders that are characterized by chronic hyperglycaemia resulting from relative insulin deficiency, insulin resistance or both. Diabetes is usually primary but may be secondary to other conditions, which include pancreatic (e.g. total pancreatectomy, chronic pancreatitis, haemochromatosis) and endocrine diseases (e.g. acromegaly and Cushing's syndrome). It may also be drug induced, most commonly by thiazide diuretics and corticosteroids.

Primary diabetes is divided into type 1 diabetes (insulin-dependent diabetes mellitus, IDDM) and the much more prevalent type 2 diabetes (non-insulin-dependent diabetes, NIDDM). Type 1 diabetes is most prevalent in Northern European countries, particularly Finland, and the incidence is increasing in most populations, particularly in young children. Type 2 diabetes is common in all populations enjoying an affluent lifestyle and, like type 1 diabetes, is increasing in frequency, particularly in adolescents.

In clinical terms these represent two ends of a spectrum (Table 14.1).

## Aetiology and pathogenesis

**Type 1 diabetes mellitus** is thought to be a polygenic disorder and the genes (as yet unknown) causing diabetes to be transmitted along with particular HLA types (Table 14.1). An autoimmune aetiology is suggested by:

- Antibodies directed against insulin and several islet cell antigens (e.g. glutamic acid decarboxylase) predating clinical onset by many years
- Infiltration of pancreatic islets by mononuclear cells (insulitis) resembling that in other autoimmune diseases, e.g. thyroiditis
- Association with other organ-specific autoimmune diseases, e.g. autoimmune thyroid disease, Addison's disease and pernicious anaemia.

**Type 2 diabetes mellitus** is a polygenic disorder and the genes responsible for the majority of cases have yet to be identified. However, the genetic causes of some of the rare forms of type 2 diabetes have been identified and include mutations of the insulin receptor and structural alterations of the insulin molecule. Environmental factors, notably central obesity, appear to trigger the disease in genetically susceptible individuals. The beta-cell mass is reduced to about 50% of normal at the time of diagnosis in type 2 diabetes. Hyperglycaemia is the result of reduced insulin secretion (inappropriately low for the glucose level) and peripheral insulin resistance.

**Table 14.1**
The spectrum of diabetes: a comparison of type 1 and type 2 diabetes

| | Type 1 | Type 2 |
|---|---|---|
| Epidemiology | Peak incidence around puberty, can present at any age<br>Usually lean<br>European extraction (usually) | Usually presents after age 40<br>Often overweight<br>All racial groups, commoner in African/Asian |
| Inheritance | HLA-DR3 and/or DR4 in >90%<br>30–50% concordance in identical twins | No HLA links<br>50% concordance in identical twins |
| Pathogenesis | Autoimmune beta-cell destruction<br>Insulin resistance | No evidence of immune disturbance |
| Clinical picture | Complete insulin deficiency<br>May develop ketoacidosis<br>Always need insulin treatment | Relative insulin deficiency, and insulin resistance<br>May develop non-ketotic hyperosmolar state<br>Sometimes need insulin |

## Clinical features (K&C p. 1076)

- *Acute presentation.* Young people present with a brief history (2–4 weeks) of thirst, polyuria, weight loss and lethargy. Polyuria is the result of an osmotic diuresis that results when blood glucose levels exceed the renal tubular reabsorptive capacity (the renal threshold). Fluid and electrolyte losses stimulate thirst. Weight loss is caused by fluid depletion and breakdown of fat and muscle as a result of insulin deficiency. Ketoacidosis (see later) is the presenting feature if these early symptoms are not recognized and treated.
- *Subacute presentation.* Older patients may present with the same symptoms, although less marked and extending over several months. They may also complain of lack of energy, visual problems and pruritus vulvae or balanitis due to *Candida* infection.
- *With complications* (see later).
- *In asymptomatic individuals* diagnosed at routine medical examinations, e.g. for insurance purposes.

## Investigations (K&C p. 1077)

The diagnosis of diabetes mellitus is made by demonstrating:

- Fasting (no calorie intake for last 8 hours) plasma glucose ≥ 7.0 mmol/L
- Random (without regard to time since last meal) plasma glucose ≥ 11.1 mmol/L
- One abnormal laboratory value is diagnostic in symptomatic individuals; two values are needed in asymptomatic people.

A glucose tolerance test (Table 14.2) is only used for borderline cases and for the diagnosis of gestational diabetes. Glycosuria does not necessarily indicate diabetes and may be the result of a low renal threshold for glucose excretion.

Other routine investigations at diagnosis include screening the urine for proteinuria (p. 312), full blood count, serum urea and electrolytes, liver biochemistry, and a fasting blood sample for cholesterol and triglyceride levels.

## Management (K&C p. 1078)

A multidisciplinary approach involving, among others, the hospital doctor, the general practitioner, nurse specialists,

**Table 14.2**
The oral glucose tolerance test

|  | Fasting venous plasma glucose (mmol/L) | 2-Hour plasma glucose (mmol/L) |
| --- | --- | --- |
| Normal | ≤ 6.1 | ≤ 7.8 |
| Diabetes mellitus | ≥ 7.0 | ≥ 11.1 |
| Impaired glucose tolerance (IGT) | 6.1–7.0 | 7.8–11.0 |

After an overnight fast 75 g of glucose is taken in 250–350 mL of water. Blood samples are taken before and 2 hours after the glucose has been given. Individuals with IGT have an increased risk of cardiovascular disease compared to the normal population and 2–4% yearly will go on to develop diabetes. Results are for venous plasma – whole blood values are lower

dieticians and chiropodists is important in the management of this condition. It is essential that the patient understands the risks of diabetes, the potential benefits of good glycaemic control and the importance of maintaining a lean weight, stopping smoking and taking care of the feet.

Management involves:

- Achieving good glycaemic control. In young patients with type 1 diabetes the aim is to maintain blood glucose concentrations as near normal as possible to minimize long-term complications.
- Advice regarding regular physical activity and reduction of bodyweight in the obese, both of which improve glycaemic control in type 2 diabetes.
- Aggressive treatment of hypertension and hyperlipidaemia, both of which are additional risk factors for long-term complications of diabetes.
- Regular checks of metabolic control and physical examination for evidence of diabetic complications (Table 14.3).

**Principles of treatment** All patients with diabetes require diet therapy. Regular exercise is encouraged to control weight and reduce cardiovascular risk. Insulin is always indicated in a patient who presents in ketoacidosis and is usually indicated in those under 40 years of age. Insulin is also indicated in other patients who do not achieve satisfactory control with

> **Table 14.3**
> Regular checks for patients with diabetes
>
> **Checked each visit**
> Review of monitoring results and current treatment
> Talk about targets and change where necessary
> Talk about any general or specific problems
> Continued education
>
> **Checked at least once a year**
> Biochemical assessment of metabolic control (e.g. glycosylated
> haemoglobin test)
> Measure bodyweight
> Measure blood pressure
> Measure plasma lipids (except in extreme old age)
> Measure visual acuity
> Examine state of retina (ophthalmoscope or retinal photo)
> Test urine for proteinuria
> Test blood for renal function (creatinine)
> Check condition of feet, pulses and neurology
> Review cardiovascular risk factors
> Review self-monitoring and injection techniques
> Review eating habits

oral hypoglycaemics. Treatment of type 2 diabetes is summarized in Figure 14.1.

*Diet* In older patients the first approach is by diet alone. The diet itself is no different from the normal healthy diet recommended for the rest of the population. Fat should be reduced to 30% of total energy intake and consist mainly of unsaturated fats. Protein should be 15% and carbohydrate 50–55% of total energy intake. Patients should eat complex carbohydrates (e.g. potato, pasta), which are absorbed relatively slowly from the gastrointestinal tract, thus preventing the rapid fluctuations in blood glucose that occur when simple sugars, such as sucrose or glucose, are eaten. The nutrient load should be spread throughout the day (three main meals with snacks in between times and at bedtime), which reduces swings in blood glucose.

*Tablet treatments for type 2 diabetes* These are used in association with dietary treatment when this alone has failed to control hyperglycaemia.

- *Sulphonylureas* promote insulin secretion.
  Glibenclamide is the most popular choice, but is best

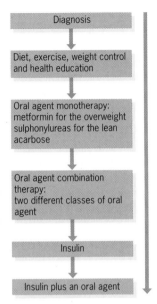

**Fig. 14.1 Treatment of type 2 diabetes.**

avoided in elderly people and in those with renal failure because of its relatively long duration of action (12–20 hours) and renal excretion. Tolbutamide, which is shorter acting and metabolized by the liver, is a better choice in these patient groups. The most common side-effect of this group of drugs is hypoglycaemia, which may be prolonged. All encourage weight gain and are not drugs of first choice in obese patients.

- *Biguanides*. Metformin reduces glucose production by the liver and sensitizes target tissues to insulin. It is used in combination with sulphonylureas when a single agent has failed to control diabetes. It is also used as the first-line agent in obese diabetic individuals because, unlike the sulphonylureas, appetite is not increased. Side-effects include anorexia and diarrhoea. Lactic acidosis has occurred in patients with severe hepatic or renal disease, in whom its use is contraindicated.

- *α-Glucosidase inhibitors.* Acarbose inhibits intestinal α-glucosidases, thus impairing carbohydrate digestion and slowing glucose absorption. Postprandial glucose peaks are reduced. Gastrointestinal side-effects, e.g. flatulence, bloating and diarrhoea, are common and limit the dose and acceptability of this treatment.
- *Thiazolidinediones,* e.g. rosiglitazone and pioglitazone, activate nuclear peroxisome proliferator activated receptor-gamma (PPAR-gamma), which is a nuclear receptor expressed predominantly in adipose tissue. Insulin action is improved through the increased transcription of genes involved in lipid metabolism and insulin action. In the UK these drugs are licensed for use in combination with metformin in obese patients with insufficient glycaemic control and in combination with sulphonylureas if metformin is either not tolerated or contraindicated. They are contraindicated in patients with hepatic impairment or cardiac failure (past or present).
- *Repaglinide* is a novel insulin-releasing agent developed from the non-sulphonylurea portion of glibenclamide. Rapid onset of action lowers postprandial hyperglycaemia.

*Insulin*  Almost all insulin now used in developed countries is synthetic (recombinant) human insulin.

There are three main types of insulin:

1. *Soluble insulins.* These insulins start working within 30–60 minutes and last for 4–6 hours. They are the only insulins to be used in emergencies such as ketoacidosis, or for surgical operations.

2. *Rapid-acting insulin analogues.* Modifications have been made to the insulin molecule to prevent it from forming dimers and other complexes (in contrast to regular insulin). As a result, the onset of action of these monomeric insulins (insulin lispro and insulin aspart) is quicker (within 15 minutes) and with a shorter duration of action (2–4 hours) than regular soluble insulin. They are the preferred insulin preparation for pre-meal bolus doses for patients who experience hypoglycaemia between meals on multiple injection regimens.

3. *Prolonged-acting insulins.* Insulins premixed with retarding agents (either protamine or zinc) that precipitate crystals of varying size according to the conditions employed. These insulins are intermediate (12–24 hours) or long acting (more than 24 hours). The protamine insulins are also known as isophane or NPH insulins, and the zinc insulins as lente insulins. Insulin glargine is a structurally modified insulin that precipitates in tissues and is then slowly released from the injection site.

In young patients a reasonable starting regimen is subcutaneous injection of an intermediate-acting insulin, 8–10 units administered half an hour before breakfast and before the evening meal. In many patients who present acutely with diabetes there is some recovery of endogenous insulin secretion soon after diagnosis ('the honeymoon period') and the insulin dose may need to be reduced. Requirements rise thereafter and a multiple injection regimen (often using a 'pen injector' device), which may improve control and allows greater meal flexibility, is then appropriate for most younger patients. An example of this is soluble insulin administered before each meal and an intermediate-acting insulin given at bedtime. Target blood values should normally be 4–7 mmol/L before meals and 4–10 mmol/L after meals. An alternative to multiple injections is to use a small pump strapped to the waist, which delivers a continuous subcutaneous insulin infusion (CSII). Meal-time doses are delivered when the patient presses a button on the side of the pump. This should only be used under the guidance of specialized centres.

In many patients with type 2 diabetes who eventually require insulin, a twice-daily regimen of premixed soluble and isophane insulin (e.g. Mixtard) is suitable.

The most common complications of insulin therapy are hypoglycaemia and weight gain.

## **Measuring control** (*K&C* p. 1085)

Patients may feel very well and be asymptomatic even if their blood glucose is consistently above the normal range. Self-monitoring at home is therefore necessary because of the immediate risks of hyper- and hypoglycaemia, and because it has been shown that persistently good control (i.e. near normoglycaemia) reduces the risk of progression to retinopathy, nephropathy and neuropathy in both type 1 and type 2 diabetes.

### Home testing

- Most patients, especially those on insulin, are taught to monitor control by testing finger-prick blood samples with enzyme-impregnated reagent strips, which change colour according to the capillary blood glucose level. Patients are asked to take regular profiles (e.g. four times daily samples on 2 days each week) and to note these in a diary or record book.
- Urine testing for glucose (using Stix) is a crude measure of glycaemic control because glycosuria only appears above the renal threshold for glucose (which varies between a blood glucose of 7 and 13 mmol/L) and because urine glucose lags behind blood glucose. It is usually reserved for the elderly patient in whom tight control is unnecessary.
- Urine ketones, also measured with Stix (Ketostix), are useful if the patient is unwell, because ketonuria indicates potentially serious metabolic derangement.

**Hospital testing** Single random blood glucose measurements, obtained at clinic visits, are of limited value.

- Glycosylated haemoglobin ($HbA_{1c}$) is produced by the attachment of glucose to Hb and measurement of this Hb fraction (normally 4–8%) is a useful measure of the average glucose concentration over the life of the Hb molecule (approximately 6 weeks).
- Glycosylated plasma proteins (fructosamine) are less reliable than $HbA_{1c}$ but may be useful in certain situations, e.g. thalassaemia where haemoglobin is abnormal.

608

# Diabetic metabolic emergencies

## Hypoglycaemia (blood glucose < 2.2 mmol/L)

This is the most common complication of insulin treatment and may also occur in patients taking sulphonylureas.

## Clinical features

Increased sympathetic activity causes hunger, sweating, pallor and tachycardia. Hours later there is personality change, fits, occasionally hemiparesis, and finally coma. In patients with long-standing diabetes and autonomic neuropathy the early 'adrenergic features' may be absent.

## Investigations

Immediate diagnosis and treatment are essential. A blood glucose confirms the diagnosis but treatment should begin immediately (while waiting for the result) if hypoglycaemia is suspected on clinical grounds.

## Management

A rapidly absorbed carbohydrate, e.g. sugary water, should be given orally if possible. In unconscious patients, treatment is with intravenous dextrose (50 mL of 50% dextrose into a large vein though a large-gauge needle) followed by a flush of normal saline, as concentrated dextrose is highly irritant. Intramuscular glucagon (1 mg) acts rapidly by mobilizing hepatic glycogen and is particularly useful where intravenous access is difficult. Oral glucose is given to replenish glycogen reserves once the patient revives. Hypoglycaemia may recur after treatment, particularly if it is a result of treatment with long-acting insulin preparations or oral hypoglycaemics. These patients should be monitored with hourly (4-hourly when stable) blood glucose readings and may require a 10% dextrose drip to prevent recurrent hypoglycaemia.

# Diabetic ketoacidosis (K&C p. 1088)

Diabetic ketoacidosis results from insulin deficiency and is the result of previously undiagnosed diabetes, the stress of intercurrent illness (e.g. infection or surgery) or the interruption of insulin therapy. A common error is for insulin to be reduced or stopped if the patient is ill and feels unable to eat. Insulin should never be stopped and most patients need a larger dose when ill.

## Pathogenesis

Ketoacidosis is a state of uncontrolled catabolism associated with insulin deficiency. In the absence of insulin there is an unrestrained increase in hepatic gluconeogenesis. High circulating glucose levels result in an osmotic diuresis by the kidneys and consequent dehydration. In addition, peripheral lipolysis leads to an increase in circulating free fatty acids, which are converted within the liver to acidic ketones, leading to a metabolic acidosis. These processes are accelerated by the 'stress hormones' – catecholamines, glucagon and cortisol – which are secreted in response to dehydration and intercurrent illness.

## Clinical features

There is profound dehydration secondary to water and electrolyte loss from the kidney. The eyes are sunken, tissue turgor is reduced, the tongue is dry and, in severe cases, the blood pressure is low. Kussmaul's respiration (deep rapid breathing) may be present, as a sign of respiratory compensation for metabolic acidosis, and the breath smells of ketones. Some disturbance of consciousness is common, but only 5% present in coma. Body temperature is often subnormal despite intercurrent infection. A few patients have abdominal pain and rarely this may cause confusion with a surgical acute abdomen.

## Investigations

The diagnosis is based on the demonstration of hyperglycaemia in combination with acidosis and ketosis.

- Blood glucose is elevated, usually > 20 mmol/L.
- Plasma ketones are easily detected by centrifuging a blood sample and testing the plasma obtained with a dipstick that measures ketones, which will usually show ++ or +++.
- Urine Stix testing shows heavy glycosuria and ketonuria.
- Arterial blood gases show a metabolic acidosis. Calculation shows a high-anion gap (p. 305).
- Serum urea and electrolytes. Urea and creatinine are often raised as a result of dehydration. The total body potassium is low as a result of osmotic diuresis, but the serum potassium concentration is often raised because of the absence of the action of insulin, which allows potassium to shift out of cells. Serum bicarbonate is low.

- Full blood count may show an elevated white cell count even in the absence of infection.
- Further investigations are directed towards identifying a precipitating cause: blood cultures, chest radiograph and urine microscopy and culture to look for evidence of infection, and an ECG to look for evidence of myocardial infarction.

## Management

Admission to the intensive care unit is recommended in the seriously ill. The aims of treatment are to replace fluid and electrolyte loss (Table 14.4), replace insulin, and restore acid–base balance over a period of about 24 hours. Therapy of diabetic ketoacidosis shifts potassium into cells, which may lead to profound hypokalaemia and death if not treated prospectively. A treatment regimen for a patient with severe ketoacidosis is set out in Emergency Box 14.1. Cerebral oedema (presenting with headache and reduced conscious level) may complicate therapy in some patients and results from rapid lowering of blood glucose and osmolality. When the patient has recovered it is necessary to determine the cause of the episode and provide advice and information to prevent recurrence.

## Non-ketotic hyperosmolar state (*K&C* p. 1091)

This condition, in which severe hyperglycaemia develops without significant ketosis, is the metabolic emergency characteristic of uncontrolled type 2 diabetes mellitus. It is often precipitated by consumption of glucose-rich fluids, concomitant medication such as thiazides or steroids or by intercurrent illness.

**Table 14.4**
Average loss of fluid and electrolytes in an adult with ketoacidosis

| | |
|---|---|
| Water | 6 L |
| Sodium | 500 mmol |
| Potassium | 400 mmol |

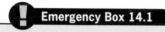

# Emergency Box 14.1

## Management of diabetic ketoacidosis

### Phase I management
- Insulin: soluble insulin i.v. 6 units/h by infusion, or 20 units i.m. stat. followed by 6 units i.m. hourly
- Fluid replacement: 0.9% sodium chloride with 20 mmol KCl per litre. An average regimen would be 1 litre in 30 minutes, then 1 litre in 1 hour, then 1 litre in 2 hours, then 1 litre in 4 hours, then 1 litre in 6 hours
- Adjust KCl concentration depending on results of 2 hours' blood K measurement. Temporarily delay if serum potassium > 5.0 mmol/L. Increase to 30–40 mmol/L if serum potassium is low, e.g. < 3.5 mmol/L

IF:

- Blood pressure below 90 mmHg, give plasma expander
- pH below 7.0 give 500 mL of sodium bicarbonate 1.26% plus 10 mmol KCl. Repeat if necessary to bring pH up to 7.0

### Phase 2 management
- When blood glucose falls to 10–12 mmol/L swap infusion fluid to 1 litre 5% dextrose plus 20 mmol KCl 6-hourly. Continue insulin with dose adjusted according to hourly blood glucose test results

### Phase 3 management
- Once stable and able to eat and drink normally, transfer patient to four-times-daily subcutaneous insulin regimen (based on previous 24 hours insulin consumption, and trend in consumption)

### Special measures
- Broad-spectrum antibiotic if infection likely
- Bladder catheter if no urine passed in 2 hours
- Nasogastric tube if drowsy
- Consider CVP pressure monitoring if shocked or if previous cardiac or renal impairment
- Consider s.c. prophylactic heparin in comatose, elderly or obese patients

### Subsequent management
- Monitor glucose hourly for 8 hours
- Monitor electrolytes 2-hourly for 8 hours
- Adjust K replacement according to results

*Note:* The regimen of fluid replacement set out above is a guide for patients with severe ketoacidosis. Excessive fluid can precipitate pulmonary and cerebral oedema; adequate replacement must therefore be tailored to the individual and monitored carefully throughout treatment.

## Clinical features

Endogenous insulin levels are reduced but are still sufficient to inhibit hepatic ketogenesis, whereas glucose production is unrestrained. Patients present with profound dehydration (secondary to an osmotic diuresis) and a decreased level of consciousness, which is directly related to the elevation of plasma osmolality. The main biochemical differences between ketoacidosis and hyperosmolar coma are illustrated in Table 14.5.

## Management

Investigations and treatment are the same as for ketoacidosis with the exception that a lower rate of insulin infusion (3 U/h) is often sufficient, as these patients are extremely sensitive to insulin. The rate may be doubled after 2–3 h if glucose is falling too slowly. The hyperosmolar state predisposes to stroke, myocardial infarction, or arterial thrombosis, and prophylactic subcutaneous heparin is given.

## Prognosis

Mortality rate is around 20–30%, mainly because of the advanced age of the patients and the frequency of intercurrent illness. Unlike ketoacidosis, non-ketotic hyperglycaemia is not an absolute indication for subsequent insulin therapy, and survivors may do well on diet and oral agents.

**Table 14.5**
The main biochemical differences between diabetic ketoacidosis and non-ketotic hyperosmolar coma

| Examples of blood values | Severe ketoacidosis | Non-ketotic hyperosmolar coma |
|---|---|---|
| $Na^+$ (mmol/L) | 140 | 155 |
| $K^+$ (mmol/L) | 5 | 5 |
| $Cl^-$ (mmol/L) | 100 | 110 |
| $HCO_3$ (mmol/L) | 5 | 30 |
| Urea (mmol/L) | 8 | 15 |
| Glucose (mmol/L) | 30 | 50 |
| Serum osmolality (mOsm/kg)* | 328 | 385 |
| Arterial pH | 7.0 | 7.35 |

* See page 283 for definition and discussion of plasma osmolality

# Lactic acidosis (K&C p. 1091)

Lactic acidosis is a rare complication in patients taking metformin. Patients present with severe metabolic acidosis without significant hyperglycaemia or ketosis. Treatment is rehydration with intravenous saline. Intravenous bicarbonate is used only in severe acidosis (pH < 7).

# Complications of diabetes

Patients with diabetes have a reduced life expectancy. In older studies, insulin-treated patients diagnosed before the age of 20 had only a 60–70% chance of living past the age of 50 years, the excess deaths being mainly the result of diabetic nephropathy. Heart disease, peripheral vascular disease and stroke are the major causes of death in patients over the age of 50.

## Vascular

### Macrovascular complications (K&C p. 1092)

Diabetes is a risk factor for atherosclerosis and this is additive with other risk factors for large vessel disease, e.g. smoking, hypertension and hyperlipidaemia. Atherosclerosis results in stroke, ischaemic heart disease and peripheral vascular disease.

### Microvascular complications (K&C p. 1092)

In contrast to macrovascular disease, microvascular disease is specific to diabetes. Small vessels throughout the body are affected, but the disease process is of particular danger in three sites: the retina, the renal glomerulus and the nerve sheath. Diabetic retinopathy, nephropathy and neuropathy tend to manifest 10–20 years after diagnosis in young patients. They present earlier in older patients, probably because they have had unrecognized diabetes for months or even years before diagnosis.

# Diabetic eye disease (K&C p. 1093)

About one-third of young diabetics develop visual problems and in the UK 5% have become blind after 30 years of diabetes. However, the prevalence is falling.

## Retinopathy

***Background retinopathy*** is the earliest feature of retinopathy. Capillary microaneurysms appear on ophthalmoscopy as tiny red dots, haemorrhages are seen as larger red spots (blot haemorrhages), and capillary leaks of fluid rich in lipid and protein give rise to hard exudates (yellow-white discrete patches). There is no specific treatment for background retinopathy, but patients should undergo regular eye examination by an ophthalmologist to look for any deterioration. Background retinopathy does not itself constitute a threat to vision, but may progress to two other distinct forms of retinopathy: maculopathy or proliferative retinopathy. Both are the consequence of damage to retinal blood vessels and resultant retinal ischaemia.

***Maculopathy*** Macular oedema is the first feature of maculopathy and will result in permanent damage if not treated early. It cannot be detected by standard ophthalmoscopy and the only sign may be deteriorating visual acuity detected by Snellen chart testing. At a later stage there are perimacular haemorrhages and hard exudates.

***Pre-proliferative retinopathy*** is characterized by 'cotton-wool spots', which are indistinct pale lesions and represent oedema from retinal infarcts. Venous beading and/or venous loops are other pre-proliferative changes.

***Proliferative retinopathy*** Hypoxia is thought to be the signal for new vessel formation. These are fragile and bleed easily, resulting in loss of vision because of vitreous haemorrhage. Fibrous tissue associated with new vessels may shrink and cause retinal detachment.

Maculopathy and proliferative retinopathy are indications for urgent referral to an ophthalmologist and are treated by laser photocoagulation of the retina. Effective early therapy of proliferative retinopathy reduces the risk of visual loss by about 50%.

## Other eye complications
- Blurred vision (caused by reversible osmotic changes in the lens in patients with acute hyperglycaemia)

- Cataracts
- Glaucoma
- External ocular palsies, especially of the VIth nerve can occur (a mononeuritis).

## The diabetic kidney (*K&C* p. 1095)

The kidney may be damaged by diabetes as a result of:

- Glomerular disease
- Ischaemic renal lesions
- Ascending urinary tract infection.

***Diabetic nephropathies*** Clinical nephropathy secondary to glomerular disease affects 25–30% of patients diagnosed under the age of 30 years. On histological investigation there is thickening of the glomerular basement membrane and later glomerulosclerosis, which may be a diffuse or nodular form (Kimmelstiel–Wilson lesion). The earliest evidence of glomerular damage is 'microalbuminuria' (defined as an increase above the normal range in urinary albumin excretion but undetectable by conventional dipsticks) which in turn may, after some years, progress to intermittent albuminuria followed by persistent proteinuria, sometimes with a frank nephrotic syndrome. At the stage of persistent proteinuria the plasma creatinine is normal but the average patient is only some 5–10 years from end-stage renal failure.

The urine of all patients should be checked regularly by dipsticks for the presence of protein. Most centres also screen for microalbuminuria, because meticulous glycaemic control and treatment with angiotensin-converting enzyme (ACE) inhibitors at this stage (even in the absence of hypertension) may delay the onset of frank proteinuria. Aggressive control of blood pressure (target below 135/85 mmHg) is the most important factor to reduce disease progression in those with established proteinuria, and ACE inhibitors are the treatment of choice. Many will develop end-stage renal failure and need dialysis and eventually renal transplantation.

***Ischaemic lesions*** Arteriolar lesions with hypertrophy and hyalinization of the vessels affect both afferent and efferent arterioles. The appearances are similar to those of hypertensive disease but are not necessarily related to the blood pressure in patients with diabetes.

***Infective lesions*** Urinary tract infections are common (p. 325). A rare complication is renal papillary necrosis, in which renal papillae are shed in the urine and may cause ureteral obstruction.

## Diabetic neuropathy (Table 14.6) (*K&C* p. 1097)

Diabetic neuropathy is thought to result from nerve ischaemia from occlusion of the vasa vasorum, or the accumulation of fructose and sorbitol (metabolized from glucose in peripheral nerves), which disrupts the structure and function of the nerve.

***Symmetrical mainly sensory neuropathy*** This is the most common form of neuropathy and first affects the most distal parts of the longest nerves, i.e. the toes and the soles of the feet. Symptoms consist of numbness, tingling and pain, which is typically worse at night. Involvement of the hands is less common and results in a 'stocking and glove' sensory loss. Complications include unrecognized trauma, beginning as blistering caused by an ill-fitting shoe or a hot-water bottle, and leading to ulceration. Abnormal mechanical stress and repeated minor trauma, usually prevented by pain, may lead to the development of a neuropathic arthropathy (Charcot's joints) in the ankle and knee, where the joint is grossly deformed and swollen. All patients with diabetic sensory neuropathy are at risk of insensitive foot ulceration. They should learn the principles of foot care (see below) and visit a chiropodist regularly.

**Table 14.6**
Diabetic neuropathies

| Progressive | Symmetrical sensory polyneuropathy |
| | Autonomic neuropathy |
| Reversible | Acute painful neuropathy |
| | Mononeuropathy and mononeuritis multiplex |
| | Cranial nerve lesions |
| | Isolated peripheral nerve lesions |
| | Diabetic amyotrophy |

**Autonomic neuropathy** may present with impotence (p. 551), postural hypotension, diarrhoea, and nausea and vomiting as a consequence of gastroparesis. In addition, bladder involvement may result in a neuropathic bladder with painless urinary retention.

**Acute painful neuropathy** The patient describes burning or crawling pains in the lower limbs. These symptoms are typically worse at night, and pressure from bedclothes may be intolerable. Treatment is with good diabetic control, tricyclic antidepressants, gabapentin and carbamazepine.

**Diabetic mononeuropathy** Individual nerves are affected. In some instances this relates to local pressure, e.g. carpal tunnel syndrome. In others it results from a localized nerve infarction: commonly the IIIrd and VIth cranial nerves are affected, resulting in diplopia (p. 652). More than one nerve may be affected: mononeuritis multiplex.

**Diabetic amyotrophy** This presents with painful wasting, usually asymmetrical, of the quadriceps muscles. The wasting may be very marked and knee reflexes are diminished or absent.

## The diabetic foot (K&C p. 1099)

Foot problems are a major cause of morbidity and mortality in patients with diabetes mellitus, with infection, ischaemia and neuropathy all contributing to produce tissue necrosis. On physical examination evidence of a neuropathy is demonstrated by reduced sensation to vibration, temperature and pin-prick. There may be evidence of Charcot arthropathy. Signs of vascular disease in the lower leg include thin skin and absence of hair, bluish discoloration of the skin, reduced skin temperature and absent foot pulses. Many diabetic foot ulcers are avoidable, so patients need to learn the principles of foot care: well-fitting lace-up shoes, regular chiropody, no 'bathroom' surgery, daily inspection of feet and early advice for any damage, and finally avoiding sources of heat, such as radiators and hot bath water. Management of foot lesions involves:

- Swabbing of ulcers for bacterial culture and early antibiotic treatment

- Good local wound care and, if necessary, surgical debridement of ulcers
- Evaluation for peripheral vascular disease by clinical examination, measurement of blood flow (by Doppler probe) and femoral angiography if clinically indicated
- Reconstructive vascular surgery for localized areas of arterial occlusion.

## Infections (K&C p. 1100)

Poorly controlled diabetes impairs the function of poly-morphonuclear leucocytes and confers an increased risk of infection, particularly of the urinary tract and skin, e.g. cellulitis, boils and abscesses. Tuberculosis and mucocuta-neous candidiasis are more common in diabetic individu-als. Infections may lead to loss of glycaemic control and are a common cause of ketoacidosis. Insulin-treated patients may need to increase their insulin therapy even if they feel nauseated and unable to eat. Non-insulin-treated patients may need insulin for the same reasons.

## The skin (K&C p. 1100 & p. 1301)

- Lipohypertrophy is where fat lumps develop at frequently used insulin injection sites, and may be avoided by varying the injection site from day to day.
- Necrobiosis lipoidica diabeticorum is an unusual complication of diabetes characterized by erythematous plaques, often over the shins, which gradually develop a brown waxy discoloration.
- Vitiligo is symmetrical white patches seen in diabetes mellitus and other organ-specific autoimmune diseases.
- Granuloma annulare, which presents as flesh-coloured rings and nodules, principally over the extensor surfaces of the fingers.

619

## Special situations

## Surgery (K&C p. 1100)

Smooth control of diabetes minimizes the risk of infection and balances the catabolic response to anaesthesia and surgery. If possible, diabetic patients should be admitted 1 or

2 days before surgery and glucose control optimized. They should be first on the operating list and a blood glucose of 6–11 mmol/L maintained during the perioperative period.

### Insulin-treated patients
- Stop long-acting insulins the day before surgery; substitute with soluble insulin.
- Start glucose/potassium/insulin infusion (GKI: 500 mL 10% glucose + 10 mmol KCl + 16 U soluble insulin over 5 hours) on the morning of surgery and continue until first meal.
- Check blood glucose levels 2-hourly and serum potassium every 4–6 hours.
- Increase or decrease insulin in GKI by 5 U if blood glucose > 11 or < 6 mmol/L respectively.
- Postoperatively, continue infusion until patient is able to eat.

### Non-insulin-treated patients
- Omit oral hypoglycaemics 2 days before operation.
- Check blood glucose 4-hourly.
- Patients with fasting blood glucose > 8 mmol/L: treat as for insulin-treated.
- Patients with fasting blood glucose < 8 mmol/L: treat as non-diabetic.
- Restart oral hypoglycaemics with first meal.

## Pregnancy and diabetes (*K&C* p. 1101)
Poorly controlled diabetes is associated with congenital malformations, macrosomia (large babies), hydramnios, pre-eclampsia and intrauterine death. In the neonatal period there is an increased risk of hyaline membrane disease and neonatal hypoglycaemia (unlike insulin, maternal glucose crosses the placenta and causes hypersecretion of insulin from the fetal islets, which continues when the umbilical cord is cut). Meticulous control of blood glucose levels achieves results comparable to those with non-diabetic pregnancies.

Gestational diabetes is diabetes that develops in the course of pregnancy and remits following delivery. Treatment is with diet in the first instance, but most patients require insulin cover during pregnancy. It is likely to recur in subsequent pregnancies, and diabetes may develop later in life.

## Brittle diabetes (K&C p. 1102)

There is no precise definition for this term, which is used to describe patients with recurrent ketoacidosis and/or recurrent hypoglycaemic coma. Of these, the largest group is made up of those who experience recurrent severe hypoglycaemia.

## Hypoglycaemia (K&C p. 1102)

The causes and mechanism of hypoglycaemia are listed in Table 14.7. Insulin or sulphonylurea therapy for diabetes accounts for the vast majority of cases of severe hypoglycaemia encountered in an accident and emergency department.

### Insulinomas

These are rare pancreatic islet cell tumours (usually benign) that secrete insulin. They may be part of the multiple endocrine neoplasia syndrome (p. 593).

#### Clinical features

The classic presentation is with fasting hypoglycaemia. Hypoglycaemia produces symptoms as a result of neuroglycopenia and stimulation of the sympathetic nervous system. These include sweating, palpitations, diplopia and weakness, progressing to confusion, abnormal behaviour, fits and coma.

#### Investigations

The diagnosis is made by demonstrating hypoglycaemia in association with inappropriate or excessive insulin secretion:

- Measurement of overnight fasting plasma glucose and insulin levels on three occasions
- Performing a prolonged 72-hour supervised fast if overnight testing is inconclusive and symptoms persist.

Further investigations are usually necessary to localize tumours before surgery as they are often very small. These include highly selective angiography, high-resolution CT

621

**Table 14.7**
Causes of hypoglycaemia

| Cause | Mechanism of hypoglycaemia |
|---|---|
| Drug induced: insulin, sulphonylureas, quinine, pentamidine and salicylates in overdose | Variety of mechanisms |
| Islet cell tumour of the pancreas (insulinoma) | Inappropriately high circulating insulin levels |
| Non-pancreatic tumours, e.g. sarcoma, hepatoma | Secretion of IGF-1 by some tumours |
| Endocrine causes: Addison's disease | Impaired counter-regulation to the action of insulin |
| Fulminant liver failure | Failure of hepatic gluconeogenesis |
| End-stage renal failure | Failure of renal cortical gluconeogenesis |
| Excess alcohol | Enhanced insulin response to carbohydrate Inhibition of hepatic gluconeogenesis |
| After gastric surgery | Rapid gastric emptying, mismatch of food and insulin |
| Factitious hypoglycaemia | Surreptitious self-administration of insulin or sulphonylureas, often in a non-diabetic |

IGF-1, insulin-like growth factor: normally mainly produced by the liver, primarily a growth factor in physiological concentrations

scanning, scanning with radiolabelled somatostatin (some tumours express somatostatin receptors) and endoscopic ultrasound.

### Treatment

The treatment of choice is surgical excision of the tumour. Diazoxide, which inhibits insulin release from islet cells, is useful when the tumour is malignant, in patients in whom a tumour is very small and cannot be located, or in elderly patients with mild symptoms. Symptoms may also remit using a somatostatin analogue (octreotide or lanreotide).

## Disorders of lipid metabolism

(*K&C* p. 1104)

Fats are transported in the bloodstream as lipoprotein particles composed of lipids (principally triglycerides, cholesterol and cholesterol esters), phospholipids and proteins, called apoproteins. These proteins exert a stabilizing function and allow the particles to be recognized by receptors in the liver and peripheral tissues.

There are five principal types of lipoprotein particles:

- *Chylomicrons* are synthesized in the small intestine postprandially and serve to transport exogenous dietary fat (mainly triglycerides, small amounts of cholesterol) to the liver and peripheral tissues.
- *Very-low-density lipoproteins (VLDLs)* are synthesized and secreted by the liver and transport endogenous triglycerides (formed in the liver from plasma free fatty acids) to the periphery. In fat and muscle, triglycerides are removed from chylomicrons and VLDLs by the tissue enzyme lipoprotein lipase and the essential cofactor apoprotein C-II.
- *Intermediate-density lipoproteins (IDLs)*, derived from the peripheral breakdown of VLDLs, are transported back to the liver and metabolized to yield the cholesterol-rich particles – low-density lipoproteins (LDLs).
- *Low-density lipoproteins (LDLs)* deliver most cholesterol to the periphery and liver with subsequent binding to LDL receptors in these tissues.

- *High-density lipoproteins (HDLs)* transport cholesterol from peripheral tissues to the liver. HDL particles carry 20–30% of the total quantity of cholesterol in the blood.

The major clinical significance of hypercholesterolaemia (both total plasma and LDL concentration) is as a risk factor for atheroma and hence ischaemic heart disease. The risk is greatest in those with other risk factors, e.g. smoking and hypertension. There is a weak independent link between raised concentrations of (triglyceride-rich) VLDL particles and cardiovascular risk. More than half of all patients aged under 60 with angiographically confirmed coronary heart disease have a lipoprotein disorder. In addition, severe hypertriglyceridaemia (> 6 mmol/L) may induce acute pancreatitis and retinal vein thrombosis. In contrast, HDL particles, which transport cholesterol away from the periphery, appear to protect against atheroma.

## Measurement of plasma lipids

Most patients with hyperlipidaemia are asymptomatic, with no clinical signs, and they are discovered through routine screening (Table 14.8). A single fasting blood sample is necessary for the measurement of total plasma cholesterol, total triglyceride and HDL cholesterol levels. Specific diagnosis of the defect (see below) requires the

**Table 14.8**
Indications for measurement of plasma lipids

Coronary heart disease or other major atherosclerotic disease

Family history of coronary heart disease (especially below 50 years of age)

First-degree relative with a lipid disorder

Presence of a xanthoma

Presence of xanthelasma or corneal arcus before age 40 years

Obesity

Diabetes mellitus

Hypertension

Acute pancreatitis

Patients undergoing renal replacement therapy

**Table 14.9**
Causes of secondary hyperlipidaemia

Hypothyroidism

Poorly controlled diabetes mellitus

Obesity

Renal impairment

Nephrotic syndrome

Dysglobulinaemia

Hepatic dysfunction

Alcohol

Drugs: oral contraceptives in susceptible individuals, thiazide diuretics, corticosteroids

measurement of individual lipoproteins by electrophoresis, but this is not usually necessary. If a lipid disorder has been detected it is vital to carry out a clinical history, examination and simple special investigations (i.e. plasma glucose, urea and electrolytes, liver biochemistry and thyroid function tests) to detect the causes of secondary hyperlipidaemia (Table 14.9).

## The primary hyperlipidaemias (K&C p. 1107)

### Disorders of VLDL and chylomicrons – hypertriglyceridaemia alone

- Polygenic hypertriglyceridaemia accounts for most cases, in which there are many genes both acting together and interacting with environmental factors to produce a modest elevation in serum triglyceride levels.
- Familial hypertriglyceridaemia is inherited in an autosomal dominant fashion. The exact defect is not known and the only clinical feature is a history of pancreatitis or retinal vein thrombosis in some individuals.
- Lipoprotein lipase deficiency and apoprotein C-II deficiency are rare diseases which usually present in childhood with severe hypertriglyceridaemia complicated by pancreatitis, retinal vein thrombosis and eruptive xanthomas – crops of small yellow lipid deposits in the skin.

### Disorders of LDL – hypercholesterolaemia alone

- Familial hypercholesterolaemia is the result of underproduction of the LDL cholesterol receptor in the liver, which results in high plasma concentrations of LDL cholesterol. Heterozygotes may be asymptomatic or develop coronary artery disease in their 40s. Typical clinical features include tendon xanthomas (lipid nodules in the tendons, especially the extensor tendons of the fingers and the Achilles tendon) and xanthelasmas. Homozygotes have a total absence of LDL receptors in the liver. They have grossly elevated plasma cholesterol levels (> 16 mmol/L) and, without treatment, die in their teens from coronary artery disease.
- Mutations in the apoprotein B-100 gene result in a clinical picture resembling heterozygous familial hypercholesterolaemia. LDL particles normally bind to their clearance receptor in the liver through apoprotein B-100, and the mutation results in high LDL concentrations in the blood.
- Polygenic hypercholesterolaemia accounts for those patients with a raised serum cholesterol concentration, but without one of the monogenic disorders above. The precise nature of the polygenic variation in plasma cholesterol remains unknown.

### Combined hyperlipidaemia (hypercholesterolaemia and hyperlipidaemia)

Polygenic combined hyperlipidaemia and familial combined hyperlipidaemia account for the vast majority of patients in this group. A small minority is the result of the rare condition, remnant hyperlipidaemia.

### *Management of hyperlipidaemia* (K&C p. 1109)

The aim of treatment is to reduce serum cholesterol to less than 6.5 mmol/L. A serum triglyceride concentration below 2.0 mmol/L is normal; in the range 2.0–6.0 mmol/L no specific intervention will be needed. However, if there are other cardiovascular risk factors, particularly hypercholesterolaemia, the aim should be to reduce serum triglycerides into the normal range.

## Whom to treat

**Primary prevention**   In patients without clinically apparent vascular disease the need to measure blood cholesterol levels and treat if abnormal is determined by the patient's coronary heart disease risk factors. Risk of coronary events is not accurately predicted from cholesterol concentrations alone and methods that take into account factors such as smoking, hypertension and diabetes mellitus should be used to estimate risk. A guide to level of serum cholesterol at which drug treatment can reasonably be started is shown in Table 14.10.

**Secondary prevention**   Patients with clinical evidence of cardiovascular disease, e.g. those with a previous myocardial infarction, previous coronary revascularization, or those with angina, are at high risk of progressive heart disease. Hypercholesterolaemic patients should be started on a statin at lower serum cholesterol levels than for primary prevention (Table 14.10). Table 14.11 summarizes the drugs used in the management of hyperlipidaemia. They may be used singly or in combination.

## Guidelines to therapy

The initial treatment in all cases of hyperlipidaemia is dietary modification, but additional measures are usually necessary. Patients with familial hypercholesterolaemia will probably need drug treatment. Secondary hyperlipidaemia should be managed by treatment of the underlying condition wherever possible. In all patients, other treatable cardiovascular risk factors, including smoking, hypertension and excess weight should also be addressed in tandem with treatment of hyperlipidaemia.

### Lipid-lowering diet

- Dairy products and meat are the principal sources of fat in the diet. Chicken and poultry should be substituted for red meats and the food grilled rather than fried. Low-fat cheeses and skimmed milk should be substituted for the full-fat varieties.
- Polyunsaturated fats, e.g. corn and soya oil, should be used instead of saturated fats.

**Table 14.10**
Concentrations of cholesterol at which to consider drug treatment in the general population following failure of diet alone

| Clinical context | Total cholesterol (mmol/L) | LDL cholesterol (mmol/L) | HDL cholesterol (mmol/L) |
|---|---|---|---|
| **Secondary prevention** (known coronary artery disease) | >5.0 | >3.0 | >1.0 |
| **Primary prevention** | | | |
| Genetic lipid problem, or two of smoking, diabetes, hypertension | >6.5 | >3.8 | No study data |
| Asymptomatic men (positive family history) | >6.5 | >3.8 | No study data |
| Asymptomatic men (no family history) | >7.8 | >4.5 | No study data |

**Table 14.11**
Drugs used in the management of hyperlipidaemias (listed in the order in which they are usually selected for treatment)

| Hypertriglyceridaemia | Hypercholesterolaemia | Combined |
|---|---|---|
| Fibrates | Statins | Fibrates |
| Nicotinic acid | Fibrates | Nicotinic acid |
| Fish oil capsules (ω-3 marine triglycerides) | Bile acid-binding resins | |

- Reduction of cholesterol intake from liver, offal and fish roe.
- Increased intake of soluble fibres, e.g. pulses and legumes, which reduce circulating cholesterol.
- Avoid excess alcohol and obesity, both causes of secondary hyperlipidaemias.

### Lipid-lowering drugs

- HMG-CoA reductase inhibitors (statins), e.g. pravastatin, simvastatin, inhibit the enzyme hydroxymethylglutaryl-coenzyme A (HMG-CoA) reductase, an enzyme involved in cholesterol synthesis in the liver. They are more effective than other classes of drugs in lowering LDL cholesterol. Statins may cause myositis and hepatitis; liver biochemistry should be measured regularly during the first year of treatment.
- Fibrates, e.g. gemfibrozil and bezafibrate, are regarded as broad-spectrum lipid-modulating agents. They decrease serum triglycerides, raise HDL cholesterol and reduce LDL cholesterol concentrations. They are the drugs of first choice for treating hypertriglyceridaemia and are also used in patients with modest hypercholesterolaemia. The exact mechanism of action is not known. A rare but serious side-effect is muscle toxicity (myositis, rhabdomyolysis).
- Bile acid-binding resins, e.g. colestyramine and colestipol, bind bile acids in the intestine, preventing their reabsorption and thus lower the cholesterol pool. They reduce LDL cholesterol and have a synergistic

effect when given with an HMG-CoA reductase inhibitor.
- Fish-oils, rich in omega-3 marine triglycerides, reduce plasma triglycerides.
- Nicotinic acid reduces total and LDL cholesterol levels and can reduce triglyceride levels. It is not widely used because of side-effects.

# The porphyrias (K&C p. 1119)

The porphyrias form a rare heterogeneous group of inherited disorders of haem synthesis. This leads to an over-production of the intermediate compounds called porphyrins (Fig. 14.2). In porphyrias the excess production of porphyrins occurs within the liver (hepatic porphyria) or in the bone marrow (erythropoietic porphyria), but porphyrias can also be classified in terms of clinical presentation as acute or non-acute (Table 14.12). Acute porphyrias usually produce neuropsychiatric problems and are associated with excess production and urinary excretion of

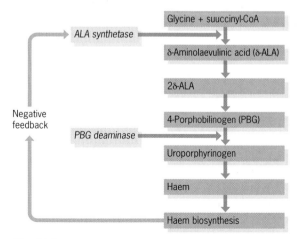

**Fig. 14.2 Pathways in porphyrin metabolism.**

**Table 14.12**
The classification of the porphyrias

|  | **Hepatic** | **Erythropoietic** |
| --- | --- | --- |
| Acute | Acute intermittent porphyria<br>Variegate porphyria<br>Hereditary coproporphyria |  |
| Non-acute | Porphyria cutanea tarda | Congenital porphyria<br>Erythropoietic<br>protoporphyria |

δ-aminolaevulinic acid (δ-ALA) and porphobilinogen. These metabolites are not increased in the non-acute porphyrias.

## Acute intermittent porphyria

This is an autosomal dominant disorder caused by a defect at the level of porphobilinogen deaminase. It is the commonest of the acute porphyrias. Presentation is in early adult life, and women are affected more than men.

### Clinical features

Abdominal pain, vomiting and constipation are the most common presenting features, occurring in 90% of patients (mimicking an acute abdomen, especially as there may be fever and leucocytosis). Additional features include polyneuropathy (especially motor), hypertension, tachycardia and neuropsychiatric disorder (fits, depression, anxiety and frank psychosis). The urine may turn red or brown on standing. Attacks may be precipitated by alcohol and a variety of drugs, especially those such as barbiturates, which are enzyme-inducing drugs and increase δ-ALA synthetase activity.

### Investigations

During an attack there may be a neutrophil leucocytosis, abnormal liver biochemistry and a raised urea.

The diagnosis is made during an attack by demonstrating increased urinary excretion of porphobilinogen. Erythrocyte porphobilinogen deaminase may be measured between attacks or, in some cases, urinary porphobilinogen remains high.

## Management

Abdominal pain is severe and may require opiate analgesia. A high carbohydrate intake (oral or intravenous glucose) must be maintained because this depresses δ-ALA synthetase activity. Haem arginate is a stable preparation of haem and is given intravenously during an acute attack. Haem inhibits ALA synthetase (Fig. 14.2) and hence reduces levels of the intermediate precursors.

## Other porphyrias

Variegate porphyria and hereditary coproporphyria present with features similar to those of acute intermittent porphyria, together with the cutaneous features of porphyria cutanea tarda. Porphyria cutanea tarda has a genetic predisposition and presents with a bullous eruption on exposure to light. The eruption heals with scarring. Most patients give a history of alcohol abuse.

The erythropoietic porphyrias are very rare and present with photosensitive skin lesions.

## Amyloidosis (K&C p. 1118)

This is a heterogeneous group of disorders characterized by extracellular deposition of an insoluble fibrillar protein called amyloid. Amyloidosis is acquired or hereditary, and may be localized or systemic. Clinical features are the result of amyloid deposits affecting the normal structure and function of the affected tissue. The diagnosis of amyloidosis is usually made with Congo red staining of a biopsy of affected tissues. In systemic amyloid a simple rectal biopsy may be used for histological diagnosis. Amyloid deposits stain red and show green fluorescence in polarized light. Scintigraphy using $^{123}$I-labelled serum amyloid P component is being increasingly employed for assessment.

The features of some systemic amyloid types are shown in Table 14.13.

Localized amyloid deposits occur in the brain of patients with Alzheimer's disease and in the joints of patients on long-term dialysis.

**Table 14.13**
Classification of the more common types of amyloid and amyloidosis

| Type | Fibril protein precursor | Clinical syndrome |
|---|---|---|
| AL | Monoclonal immunoglobulin light chains | Associated with myeloma, Waldenström's macroglobulinaemia and non-Hodgkin lymphoma. Presents with cardiac failure, nephrotic syndrome, carpal tunnel syndrome and macroglossia (large tongue) |
| ATTR (familial) | Abnormal transthyretin (plasma carrier protein) | Neuropathy and cardiomyopathy |
| AA | Protein A, a precursor of serum amyloid A (an acute phase reactant) | Occurs with chronic infections (e.g. TB), inflammation (e.g. rheumatoid arthritis) and malignancy (e.g. Hodgkin's disease). Presents with proteinuria and hepatosplenomegaly |

Amyloidosis

# Inborn errors of metabolism

Most of the inborn errors of metabolism are rare and tend to present early in childhood. They are described in detail in *Clinical Medicine* (*K&C* pp. 1114–1118).

---

**WEBSITES FOR PROFESSIONALS AND SUPPORT GROUPS FOR DIABETIC PATIENTS**

http://www.diabetes.org.uk
Diabetes UK (formerly the British Diabetic Association)

http://www.diabetic.org.uk
Diabetes Insight

http://www.jdf.org.uk
Juvenile Diabetes Foundation (UK)

---

## Common neurological symptoms

### Headache (K&C p. 1125)

Headache is a common complaint and does not usually indicate serious disease. In most patients presenting with headache there are no abnormal physical signs, so the diagnosis may depend entirely upon an accurate history. The causes of headache can be broadly divided depending on their onset and subsequent course (Table 15.1). The underlying causes of acute or subacute onset of headache are all potentially serious and require urgent investigation and assessment. In a patient with acute onset of headache the following features in the history suggest a subarachnoid haemorrhage (p. 672): onset over seconds or minutes, rapid onset with strenuous exercise, the 'worst ever' headache, absence of similar headaches in the past, a

**Table 15.1**
Causes of headache

**Acute severe (onset in minute or hours)**
Subarachnoid haemorrhage
Meningitis
Head injury
Migraine
Drugs, e.g. glyceryl trinitrate
Alcohol

**Subacute onset (onset in days to weeks)**
Intracranial mass lesion
Encephalitis
Meningitis
Giant cell arteritis
Sinusitis
Malignant hypertension

**Recurrent/chronic**
Migraine
Tension headache
Sinusitis
Cluster headaches

635

change in the level of consciousness. Neck stiffness and a positive Kerning's sign indicate meningeal irritation, which usually occurs because of bacterial or viral meningitis, or subarachnoid haemorrhage. Fever may also occur with these conditions. The history and physical examination are the keys to distinguishing serious from benign causes of headache in patients with chronic or recurrent headache; most are due to tension-type headache (p. 700) and do not require further investigation. Progressively worsening headaches, or chronic headaches that change in character, may be caused by raised intracranial pressure, e.g. due to a space-occupying lesion, and require imaging by CT scan or MRI. Other features which suggest raised intracranial pressure include headache upon waking in the morning that improves with sitting up, and headache associated with nausea and vomiting (which may also occur with migraine). Ataxia, neurological deficit, papilloedema and altered mental status also indicate a potentially serious underlying cause. Headache with generalized aches and pains in the elderly suggest giant cell arteritis (p. 702) and requires urgent treatment with steroids to prevent blindness.

# Dizziness, faints and 'funny turns'

(*K&C* p. 1125)

Episodes of transient disturbance of consciousness are common clinical problems (Table 15.2). Differentiation of seizures from other disorders often depends entirely on the medical history. An eye-witness account is invaluable.

## Dizziness and syncope

*Syncope* is the term used to describe a temporary impairment of consciousness caused by a reduction in cerebral blood flow. *Dizziness* (faintness) is the symptom that precedes syncope, and represents an incomplete form in which cerebral perfusion has not fallen sufficiently to cause loss of consciousness. Dizziness should be differentiated from *vertigo* (p. 657), which is an illusion of rotary movement resulting from disease of the inner ear, the eighth cranial nerve, or its central connections.

**Table 15.2**
Common causes of attacks of altered consciousness and falls in adults

Syncope
  'Simple faint'
  Cough
  Effort
  Micturition
  Carotid sinus

Cardiac arrhythmias

Postural hypotension

Epilepsy

Hypoglycaemia

Transient ischaemic attacks

Psychogenic attacks
  Panic attacks
  Hyperventilation

Narcolepsy and cataplexy

The most frequent cause of dizziness is vasovagal syncope (a simple faint), which occurs as a result of reflex bradycardia and peripheral and splanchnic vasodilatation. Fear, pain and prolonged standing are the principal causes. Fainting almost never occurs in the recumbent position. Rapid recovery from the attack and the absence of jerking movements or incontinence of urine suggest a faint as opposed to a fit. Syncope may occur after micturition in men (particularly at night), and when the venous return to the heart is obstructed by breath-holding and severe coughing. Carotid sinus syncope is thought to be the result of excessive sensitivity of the sinus to external pressure. It may occur in elderly patients who lose consciousness following pressure on the sinus (e.g. turning the head). Postural hypotension occurs on standing in those with impaired autonomic reflexes, e.g. elderly people, in autonomic neuropathy and with some drugs (phenothiazines, tricyclic antidepressants).

Narcolepsy is a rare disorder characterized by periods of irresistible sleep in inappropriate circumstances. Cataplexy is a related condition in which sudden loss of tone develops in the lower limbs, with preservation of consciousness.

Attacks are set off by sudden surprise or emotion (*K&C* p. 1181).

# Weakness and sensory loss (*K&C* p. 1143)

Skeletal muscle contraction is controlled by the motor axis of the central nervous system. Muscle weakness may be due to a defect or damage in one or more components of this system, i.e. the motor cortex, corticospinal tracts, anterior horn cells, spinal nerve roots, peripheral nerves, the neuromuscular junction and muscle fibres. It is necessary to determine whether there is true weakness rather than 'tiredness' or 'slowness', as in Parkinson's disease. The site of the lesion causing true muscle weakness is often identifiable from a detailed neurological examination. The distribution of weakness, the presence or absence of deep tendon reflexes, the plantar response (Table 15.3.) and related sensory defects are all helpful in localizing the lesion in the nervous system. Lesions that affect the upper motor neurone and peripheral nerve will also often involve the sensory system because of the proximity of sensory to motor nerves in these areas.

## The corticospinal tracts

***The upper motor neurone***  The corticospinal tracts originate from neurones of the motor cortex and terminate on the motor nuclei of the cranial nerves and the anterior horn cells. The clinically important pathways cross over in the medulla and pass to the contralateral halves of the spinal cord as the crossed lateral corticospinal tracts (Fig. 15.1), which then synapse with the anterior horn cells. This is known as the pyramidal system, disease of which results in upper motor neurone (UMN) lesions with characteristic clinical features (Table 15.3). Appropriate imaging studies of the central nervous system and spine such as MRI or CT scan may be necessary to identify the primary disease.

Two main patterns of clinical features occur in UMN disorders: hemiparesis and paraparesis:

- Hemiparesis means weakness of the limbs of one side, and is usually caused by a lesion within the brain or brainstem, e.g. a stroke.

**Table 15.3**
Comparison of the clinical features of upper and lower motor neurone lesions

| Upper motor neurone lesion* | Lower motor neurone lesion |
|---|---|
| Signs are on the opposite side to the lesion | Signs are on the same side as the lesion |
| No fasciculation | Fasciculation (visible contraction of single motor units) |
| No muscle wasting | Wasting |
| Spasticity ± clonus | Hypotonia |
| Weakness predominantly extensors in the arms, flexors in the legs | Weakness |
| Exaggerated tendon reflexes | Loss of tendon reflexes |
| Extensor plantar response | |
| Drift of the outstretched hand (downwards, medially with a tendency to pronate) | |

* Acute injury to the UMN can, however, be manifested by transient flaccid weakness and hyporeflexia

Common neurological symptoms

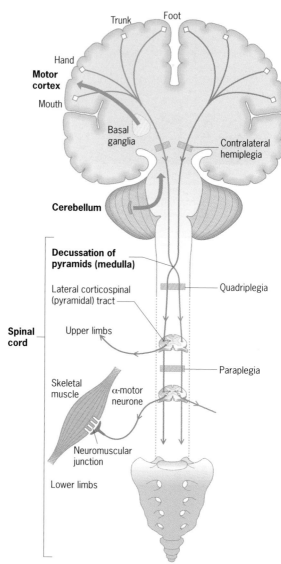

**Fig. 15.1 The crossed corticospinal ('pyramidal') tracts showing cortical representation of various parts of the body.** Lesions are shown on the right hand side of the figure.

- Paraparesis (weak legs) indicates bilateral damage to the corticospinal tracts and is most often caused by lesions in the spinal cord below T1 (p. 704). Tetraparesis (quadriplegic, weakness of the arms and legs) indicates high cervical cord damage, most commonly resulting from trauma.

***The lower motor neurone*** The lower motor neurone (LMN) is the motor pathway from the anterior horn cell or cranial nerve via a peripheral nerve to the motor endplate. Physical signs (Table 15.3) follow rapidly if the LMN is interrupted at any point in its course. Muscle disease may give a similar clinical picture, but reflexes are usually preserved.

LMN lesions are most commonly caused by the following:

- Anterior horn cell lesions, e.g. motor neurone disease, poliomyelitis
- Spinal root lesions, e.g. cervical and lumbar disc lesions
- Peripheral nerve lesions, e.g. trauma, compression or polyneuropathy.

The commonest disease of the neuromuscular junction is myasthenia gravis, which characteristically produces weakness of skeletal muscle and is rarely associated with wasting. Myopathies are discussed on page 714. Weakness of the proximal muscles, e.g. quadriceps, is typically seen with the various myopathies. Elevation of plasma muscle enzymes such as creatine kinase is highly suggestive of muscle diseases. Muscle biopsy may be necessary to determine the precise form of myopathy.

## Numbness (K&C p. 1149)

### The sensory system

The peripheral nerves carry all the modalities of sensation from nerve endings to the dorsal root ganglia and thence to the cord. These then ascend to the thalamus and cerebral cortex in two principal pathways (Fig. 15.2):

- Posterior columns, which carry sensory modalities for vibration, joint position sense (proprioception), two-point discrimination and light touch. These fibres

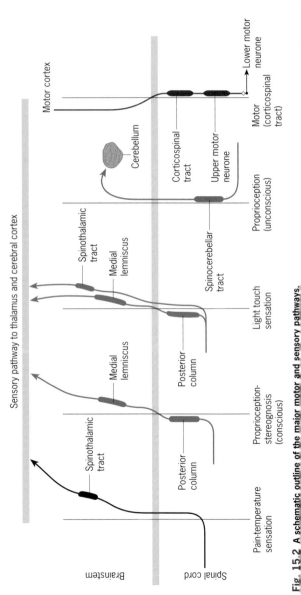

**Fig. 15.2 A schematic outline of the major motor and sensory pathways.**

ascend uncrossed to the gracile and cuneate nuclei in the medulla. Axons from the second-order neurones cross the midline to form the medial lemniscus and pass to the thalamus.

- Spinothalamic tracts, which carry sensations of pain and temperature. These fibres synapse in the dorsal horn of the cord, cross the midline and ascend as the spinothalamic tracts to the thalamus.

Paraesthesiae (pins and needles), numbness and pain are the principal symptoms of lesions of the sensory pathways below the level of the thalamus. The quality and distribution of the symptoms may suggest the site of the lesion.

*Peripheral nerve lesions*  Symptoms are felt in the distribution of the affected peripheral nerve, e.g. the ulnar or median nerve. Polyneuropathy is a subset of the peripheral nerve disorders characterized by bilateral symmetrical, distal sensory loss and burning (p. 711).

*Spinal root lesions*  Symptoms are referred to the dermatome supplied by that root, often with a tingling discomfort in that dermatome (Fig. 15.3). This is in contrast to lesions of sensory tracts within the central nervous system, which characteristically present as general defects in an extremity rather than specific dermatome defects.

*Spinal cord lesions*  Symptoms (e.g. loss of sensation) are usually evident below the level of the lesion. A lesion of the pain–temperature pathway (spinothalamic tract), whether within the brainstem or the spinal cord, will result in loss of pain–temperature sensation contralaterally, below the level of the lesion. A lesion at the spinal level of the pathway for proprioception will result in loss of these senses ipsilaterally below the level of the lesion. Dissociated sensory loss suggests a spinal cord lesion, for instance loss of pain–temperature sensation in the right leg and loss of proprioception in the left leg.

*Pontine lesions*  The pons lies above the decussation of the posterior columns. As the medial lemniscus and spinothalamic tracts are close together, pontine lesions

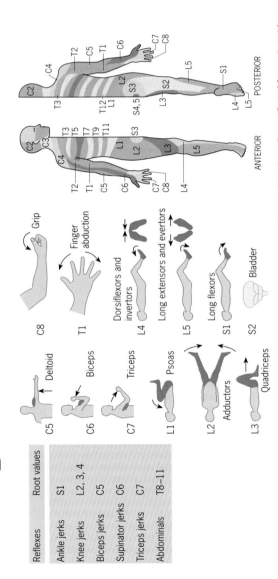

**Fig. 15.3 Simple scheme depicting motor and sensory innervation of arms and legs and root values for reflexes.** (Part of figure adapted from Parsons M (1993) A Colour Atlas of Clinical Neurology, London, Mosby Wolfe.)

| Reflexes | Root values |
| --- | --- |
| Ankle jerks | S1 |
| Knee jerks | L2, 3, 4 |
| Biceps jerks | C5 |
| Supinator jerks | C6 |
| Triceps jerks | C7 |
| Abdominals | T8–11 |

result in the loss of all forms of sensation on the side opposite the lesion.

**Thalamic lesions** A thalamic lesion is a rare cause of complete contralateral sensory loss. Spontaneous pain may also occur, most commonly as the result of a thalamic infarct.

**Cortical lesions** Sensory loss, neglect of one side of the body and subtle disorders of sensation may occur with lesions of the parietal cortex. Pain is not a feature of cortical lesions.

## Coordination of movement (K&C p. 1145)

The extrapyramidal system (p. 71) and the cerebellum coordinate movement. Disorders of these systems will not produce muscular weakness but may produce incoordination.

### The cerebellum

Each lateral lobe of the cerebellum is responsible for coordinating movement of the ipsilateral limb. The midline vermis is concerned with maintenance of axial (midline) balance and posture. Causes of cerebellar lesions are listed in Table 15.4.

A lesion within one cerebellar lobe causes one or all of the following:

- An ataxic gait with a broad base; the patient falters to the side of the lesion

**Table 15.4**
Some causes of cerebellar lesions

Multiple sclerosis

Space-occupying lesions
    Primary tumour, e.g. medulloblastoma
    Secondary tumour
    Abscess
    Haemorrhage

Chronic alcohol abuse

Anticonvulsant drugs

Non-metastatic manifestation of malignancy

- An 'intention tremor' (compare Parkinson's disease) with past-pointing
- Clumsy rapid alternating movements, e.g. tapping one hand on the back of the other (dysdiadochokinesis)
- Horizontal nystagmus with the fast component towards the side of the lesion (p. 658)
- Dysarthria, usually with bilateral lesions. The speech has a halting jerking quality – 'scanning speech'
- Titubation (rhythmic tremor of the head), hypotonia and depressed reflexes. There is no muscle weakness.

Lesions of the cerebellar vermis cause a characteristic ataxia of the trunk, so that the patient has difficulty sitting up or standing.

## The cranial nerves (K&C p. 1129)

The 12 cranial nerves and their nuclei are distributed approximately equally between the three brainstem segments (Fig. 15.4). The exceptions are the first and second

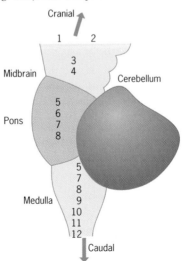

**Fig. 15.4** The location of the cranial nerves and their nuclei within the midbrain, pons and medulla as seen laterally.

cranial nerves (nerves I and II), whose neurones project to the cerebral cortex. In addition, the sensory nucleus of nerve V extends from the midbrain to the spinal cord, and the nuclei of nerves VII and VIII lie not only in the pons but also in the medulla.

# The olfactory nerve (first cranial nerve)

The olfactory nerve subserves the sense of smell. The most common cause of anosmia (loss of the sense of smell) is simply nasal congestion. Neurological causes include tumours on the floor of the anterior fossa and head injury.

# The optic nerve (second cranial nerve) and the visual system (K&C p. 1129)

The optic nerves enter the cranial cavity through the optic foramina and unite to form the optic chiasm, beyond which they are continued as the optic tracts. Fibres of the optic tract project to the visual cortex (via the lateral geniculate body) and the third nerve nucleus for pupillary light reflexes (Figs 15.5 and 15.6).

The assessment of optic nerve function includes measurement of visual acuity (using a Snellen test chart), colour vision (using Ishihara colour plates) and the visual fields (by confrontation and perimetry), and examination of the fundi with the ophthalmoscope. In addition the pupillary responses, mediated by both the optic and the oculomotor nerve (third cranial nerve), must be tested.

### Visual field defects

There are three main types of visual field defects (Fig. 15.5):

- Monocular, caused by damage to the eye or nerve
- Bitemporal, resulting from lesions at the chiasm
- Homonymous hemianopia, caused by lesions in the tract, radiation, or a lesion in the visual cortex.

*Optic nerve lesions* Unilateral visual loss, starting as a central or paracentral scotoma (an area of depressed vision within the visual field), is characteristic of optic nerve lesions. Complete destruction of one optic nerve results in blindness in that eye and loss of the pupillary light reflex (direct and consensual). Optic nerve lesions result from

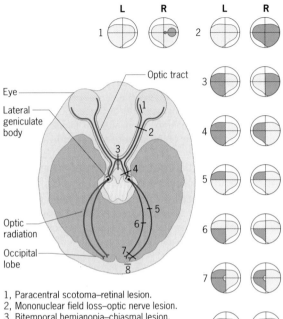

1, Paracentral scotoma–retinal lesion.
2, Mononuclear field loss–optic nerve lesion.
3, Bitemporal hemianopia–chiasmal lesion.
4, Homonymous hemianopia–optic tract lesion.
5, Homonymous quadrantanopia–temporal lesion.
6, Homonymous quadrantanopia–parietal lesion.
7, Homonymous hemianopia–occipital cortex or optic radiation.
8, Homonymous hemianopia–occipital pole lesion.
Dark blue = lesion; pale blue = normal field.

**Fig. 15.5 Diagram of the visual pathways demonstrating the main field defects.** At the optic chiasm (3), fibres derived from the nasal half of the retina (the temporal visual field) decussate, whereas the fibres from the temporal half of the retina remain uncrossed. Thus the right optic tract (4) is composed of fibres from the right half of each retina which 'see' the left half of both visual fields. Lesions of the retina (1) produce scotoma (small areas of visual loss) or quadrantanopia. Lesion at 2 produces blindness in the right eye with loss of direct light reflex. Lesion at 3 produces bitemporal hemianopia. Lesions at 4, 5 and 6 produce homonymous hemianopia with macular involvement. Lesions at 7 and 8 produce homonymous hemianopia with macular sparing. (Adapted from Swash (1989) Hutchison's Clinical Methods, 19th edn. London, Baillière Tindall.)

The optic nerve (second cranial nerve) and the visual system

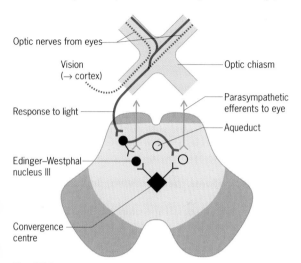

Optic nerves from eyes

Vision
(→ cortex)

Optic chiasm

Response to light

Parasympathetic
efferents to eye

Aqueduct

Edinger–Westphal
nucleus III

Convergence
centre

**Fig. 15.6 Midbrain control of response to light, accommodation and convergence.** Afferent impulses in the optic nerve are distributed bilaterally; thus when a light is shone in one eye both pupils will constrict (direct and consensual reflex). The reflex arc for the pupillary response to light is complete within the brainstem and thus the pupils of a patient rendered blind by damage to the occipital lobe will still react when illuminated.

demyelination (e.g. multiple sclerosis), nerve compression and occlusion of the retinal artery (e.g. in giant cell arteritis). Other causes include trauma, papilloedema, severe anaemia and drugs or toxins, e.g. ethambutol, quinine, tobacco and methyl alcohol.

**Defects of the optic chiasm** The most common cause of bitemporal hemianopia (i.e. blindness in the outer half of each visual field) is a pituitary adenoma, which compresses the decussating fibres from the nasal half of each eye. Other causes are craniopharyngioma and secondary neoplasm.

**Defects of the optic tract and radiation** Damage to the tracts or radiation, usually by tumour or a vascular accident, produces a homonymous hemianopia (blindness affecting either the right or the left half of each visual field) in one half of the visual field contralateral to the lesion.

**Defects of the occipital cortex** Homonymous hemianopic defects are caused by unilateral posterior cerebral artery infarction. The macular region may be spared in ischaemic lesions as a result of the dual blood supply to this area from the middle and posterior cerebral arteries. In contrast, injury to one occipital pole produces a bilateral macular (central) field defect.

## Optic disc oedema (papilloedema) and optic atrophy

The principal pathological appearances of the visible part of the nerve, the disc, are:

- Swelling (papilloedema)
- Pallor (optic atrophy).

**Papilloedema** Papilloedema produces few visual symptoms in the early stages. As disc oedema develops there is enlargement of the blind spot and blurring of vision. The exception is optic neuritis, in which there is early and severe visual loss. The common causes of papilloedema are:

- Raised intracranial pressure, e.g. from a tumour, an abscess or meningitis
- Retinal vein obstruction (thrombosis or compression)
- Optic neuritis (inflammation of the optic nerve, often caused by demyelination)
- Accelerated hypertension.

**Optic atrophy** Optic atrophy is the end result of many processes that damage the nerve (see Optic nerve lesions, above). The degree of visual loss depends upon the underlying cause.

## The pupils

The pupils constrict in response to bright light and convergence (when the centre of focus shifts from a distant to a near object). The parasympathetic efferents that control the constrictor muscle of the pupil arise in the Edinger–Westphal nucleus in the midbrain, and run with the oculomotor (third) nerve to the eye. The Edinger–Westphal nucleus receives afferents from the optic nerve (for the light reflex) and from the convergence centre in the midbrain (Fig. 15.6).

Sympathetic fibres which arise in the hypothalamus produce pupillary dilatation. They run from the hypothalamus through the brainstem and cervical cord and emerge from the spinal cord at T1. They then ascend in the neck as the cervical sympathetic chain, and travel with the carotid artery into the head.

The main causes of persistent pupillary dilatation are:

- A third cranial nerve palsy (see later).
- Antimuscarinic eyedrops (instilled to facilitate examination of the fundus).
- The myotonic pupil (Holmes–Adie pupil): this is a dilated pupil seen most commonly in young women. There is absent (or much delayed) reaction to light and convergence. It is of no pathological significance and may be associated with absent tendon reflexes.

The main causes of persistent pupillary constriction are:

- Parasympatheticomimetic eyedrops used in the treatment of glaucoma.
- Horner's syndrome, resulting from the interruption of sympathetic fibres to one eye. There is unilateral pupillary constriction, slight ptosis (sympathetic fibres innervate the levator palpebrae superioris), enophthalmos (backward displacement of the eyeball in the orbit) and loss of sweating on the ipsilateral side of the face. A lesion affecting any part of the sympathetic pathway to the eye results in a Horner's syndrome. Causes include diseases of the cervical cord, e.g. syringomyelia, involvement of the T1 root by apical lung cancer (Pancoast's tumour), and lesions in the neck, such as trauma, surgical resection or malignant lymph nodes.
- The Argyll Robertson pupil: this is the pupillary abnormality seen mainly in neurosyphilis and diabetes mellitus. There is a small irregular pupil which is fixed to light but which constricts on convergence.
- Opiate addiction.

# Cranial nerves III–XII

The cranial nerves III–XII may be damaged by lesions in the brainstem or during their intracranial and extracranial course. The causes are listed in Table 15.5. The site of a lesion may be suggested if clinical examination shows the involvement of other cranial nerves at that site, e.g. a seventh-nerve palsy, together with cerebellar signs and involvement of the fifth, sixth and eighth cranial nerves, suggests a lesion of the cerebellopontine angle, commonly a meningioma or acoustic neuroma. In contrast, an isolated seventh-nerve palsy in a patient with a parotid tumour suggests involvement during its extracranial course in the parotid.

## The ocular movements and the third, fourth and sixth cranial nerves (K&C p. 1134)

These three cranial nerves supply the six external ocular muscles which move the eye in the orbit (Fig. 15.7). The abducens nerve (sixth cranial nerve) supplies the lateral rectus muscle and the trochlear (fourth cranial nerve) supplies the superior oblique muscle. All the other extraocular muscles, the sphincter pupillae (parasympathetic fibres) and the levator palpebrae superioris are supplied by the oculomotor nerve (third cranial nerve). Normally the brainstem (with input from the cortex, cerebellum and vestibular nucleus) coordinates the functions of these three cranial nerves, so that eye movement is symmetrical (conjugate gaze). Thus *infranuclear (lower motor neurone)* lesions of the third, fourth and sixth cranial nerves lead to paralysis of individual muscles or muscle groups. *Supranuclear (upper*

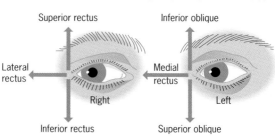

**Fig. 15.7 The action of the external ocular muscles.** (Adapted from Swash (1989) Hutchison's Clinical Methods. London, Baillière Tindall.)

**Table 15.5**
Some structural causes of lesions of cranial nerves III–XII

| Nerve | Brainstem (UMNL) | Intracranial course (LMNL) | Extracranial course (LMNL) |
|---|---|---|---|
| III<br>IV | Infarction<br>Tumour<br>MS | Posterior communicating artery aneurysm (III)<br>'Coning' of the temporal lobe (III)<br>Cavernous sinus lesions, e.g. internal carotid artery aneurysm | Orbital trauma |
| V<br>VI<br>VII<br>VIII | Infarction<br>Tumour<br>MS<br>MND | Cerebellopontine angle tumours<br>Cavernous sinus lesions (V and VI)<br>Petrous temporal bone lesions (VII and VIII) | Neoplastic infiltration of skull base<br>Parotid gland tumour (VII) |
| IX<br>X<br>XI<br>XII | Infarction<br>Tumour<br>MS<br>MND<br>Syringobulbia | Infiltrating nasopharyngeal carcinoma<br>Skull-base trauma | Tumours and trauma in the neck |

MS, multiple sclerosis; MND, motor neurone disease; UMNL, upper motor neurone lesion; LMNL, lower motor neurone lesion
The nerves may also be involved by any of the causes of mononeuritis multiplex (p. 709). Diabetes mellitus particularly affects the third and sixth nerves

*motor neurone*) lesions, e.g. brainstem involvement by multiple sclerosis, lead to paralysis of conjugate movements of the eyes.

A lesion of the oculomotor (third) nerve causes unilateral complete ptosis, the eye faces 'down and out', and the pupil is dilated and fixed to light and accommodation. This is the picture of a complete third-nerve palsy, of which the most common cause is a 'berry' aneurysm arising in the posterior communicating artery, which runs alongside the nerve. Frequently the lesion is partial, particularly in diabetes mellitus, when parasympathetic fibres are spared and the pupil reacts normally. Less common causes are listed in Table 15.5.

In a sixth-nerve lesion the eye cannot be abducted beyond the midline. The unopposed pull of the medial rectus muscle causes the eye to turn inward, thereby producing a squint (squint, or *strabismus*, is the appearance of the eyes when the visual axes do not meet at the point of fixation). Patients complain of diplopia or double vision, which worsens when they attempt to gaze to the side of the lesion.

Isolated lesions of the trochlear nerve are rare. The patient complains of diplopia when attempting to look down and away from the affected side.

Disordered ocular movements may also result from disease of the ocular muscles (e.g. muscular dystrophy, dystrophia myotonica) or of the neuromuscular junction (e.g. myasthenia gravis). In these conditions all the muscles tend to be affected equally, presenting a generalized restriction of eye movements.

## The trigeminal nerve (fifth cranial nerve)

(*K&C* p. 1136)

The trigeminal nerve, through its three divisions, supplies sensation to the face and scalp as far back as the vertex (Fig. 15.8). It also supplies the mucous membranes of the sinuses, the nose, mouth, tongue and teeth. The motor root travels with the mandibular division and supplies the muscles of mastication.

Diminution of the corneal reflex is often the first sign of a fifth-nerve lesion. A complete fifth-nerve lesion on one side causes unilateral sensory loss on the face, tongue and buccal

The facial nerve (seventh cranial nerve)

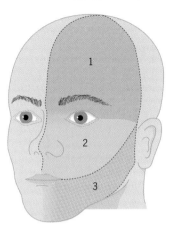

**Fig. 15.8** Cutaneous distribution of the trigeminal nerve.
1, ophthalmic or first division; 2, maxillary or second division;
3, mandibular or third division.

mucosa. The jaw deviates to the side of the lesion when the mouth is opened. A brisk jaw jerk is seen with upper motor neurone lesions, i.e. above the motor nucleus in the pons.

## The facial nerve (seventh cranial nerve)

(*K&C* p. 1137)

The facial nerve is largely motor in function, supplying the muscles of facial expression. It has, in addition, two major branches: the chorda tympani, which carries taste from the anterior two-thirds of the tongue, and the nerve to the stapedius muscle (this has a damping effect to protect the ear from loud noise). These two branches arise from the facial nerve during its intracranial course through the facial canal of the petrous temporal bone. Therefore, damage to the facial nerve in the temporal bone (e.g. Bell's palsy, trauma, herpes zoster, middle-ear infection) may be associated with undue sensitivity to sounds (hyperacusis) and loss of taste to the anterior two-thirds of the tongue.

### Lower motor neurone (LMN) lesions

A unilateral LMN lesion causes weakness of all the muscles of facial expression on the same side as the lesion.

The face, especially the angle of the mouth, falls and dribbling occurs from the corner of the mouth. There is weakness of frontalis, the eye will not close and the exposed cornea is at risk of ulceration. The most common cause of an LMN facial palsy is Bell's palsy (see below). Other structural causes are outlined in Table 15.5. In addition, the nerve may also be affected in polyneuritis (e.g. Guillain–Barré syndrome), when there may be bilateral involvement.

**Bell's palsy**  Bell's palsy is a common, acute, isolated facial nerve palsy that is probably the result of a viral infection that causes swelling of the nerve within the petrous temporal bone.

## Clinical features
There is lower motor neurone weakness of the facial muscles, sometimes with loss of taste on the anterior two-thirds of the tongue.

## Investigations
The diagnosis is clinical.

## Management
The eyelid must be closed to protect the cornea from ulceration (either adhesive tape or, in prolonged cases, surgery). Oral prednisolone reduces the proportion of patients with a severe deficit if given at the onset of symptoms.

## Prognosis
Most patients recover completely, although 15% are left with a severe permanent weakness.

**Ramsay Hunt syndrome**  This is herpes zoster (shingles) of the geniculate ganglion (the sensory ganglion for taste fibres) situated in the facial canal. There is an LMN facial palsy, with herpetic vesicles in the external auditory meatus and sometimes in the soft palate. Deafness may occur as a result of involvement of the eighth nerve in the facial canal. Treatment is with aciclovir.

## Upper motor neurone (UMN) lesions

An upper motor neurone lesion causes weakness of the lower part of the face on the side opposite the lesion. Upper facial muscles are spared because of the bilateral cortical innervation of neurones supplying the upper face. Wrinkling of the forehead (frontalis muscle) and eye closure are normal. The most common cause is a stroke, when there is an associated hemiparesis.

# The vestibulocochlear nerve (eighth cranial nerve) (K&C p. 1139)

The eighth cranial nerve has two components: cochlear and vestibular, subserving hearing and equilibrium, respectively. The clinical features of a cochlear nerve lesion are sensorineural deafness and tinnitus. The causes of a cochlear nerve lesion are outlined in Table 15.5; however, deafness is very rare in pontine lesions. Sensorineural deafness may also be the result of disease of the cochlea itself: Ménière's disease (see below), drugs (e.g. gentamicin) and presbyacusis (deafness of old age).

The main symptom of a vestibular nerve lesion is vertigo, which may be accompanied by vomiting. Nystagmus is the principal physical sign, often with ataxia (loss of balance).

## Vertigo

Vertigo is the definite illusion of movement – a sensation as if the external world were revolving around the patient. It results from disease of the inner ear, the eighth nerve or its central connections (Table 15.6).

**Table 15.6**
Principal causes of vertigo

| | |
|---|---|
| Labyrinth | Ménière's disease, vestibular neuronitis, benign positional vertigo |
| Eighth nerve | Cerebellopontine angle lesions, drugs (e.g. gentamicin) |
| Brainstem | Tumours, ischaemia/infarction, multiple sclerosis, migraine |
| Cerebellum | Acute cerebellar lesions |

### Nystagmus

Nystagmus is a rhythmic oscillation of the eyes, which must be sustained for more than a few beats to be significant. It is a sign of disease of either the ocular or the vestibular system and its connections. Nystagmus is described as either pendular or jerk.

***Pendular nystagmus*** A pendular movement of the eye occurs; there is no rapid phase. It occurs where there is poor visual fixation (i.e. long-standing severe visual impairment) or a congenital lesion.

***Jerk nystagmus*** Jerk nystagmus has a fast and a slow component to the rhythmic movement.

- Horizontal or rotary nystagmus may be either peripheral (middle ear) or central (brainstem and cerebellum) in origin. In peripheral lesions it is usually transient (minutes or hours); in central lesions it is long lasting (weeks, months or more).
- Vertical nystagmus is caused only by central lesions.

### Ménière's disease

Ménière's disease is a disorder of the inner ear in which there is dilatation of the membranous labyrinth because of the accumulation of endolymph. The aetiology is unknown and symptoms rarely start before middle age. It is characterized by recurrent attacks, lasting minutes to hours, of vertigo, tinnitus and deafness. Vomiting and nystagmus may accompany an attack. Ultimately deafness develops and the vertigo ceases. Betahistine, a histamine analogue, is useful in some cases. Recurrent severe attacks may require surgery (ultrasonic destruction of the labyrinth or vestibular nerve section).

### Vestibular neuronitis

Vestibular neuronitis is believed to be caused by a viral infection affecting the labyrinth. There is a sudden onset of severe vertigo, nystagmus and vomiting, but no deafness. The attack lasts several days or weeks, and treatment is symptomatic with vestibular sedatives (e.g. prochlorperazine).

**Benign positional vertigo**

Vertigo occurs with turning and moving. It may follow vestibular neuronitis, head injury or ear infection, and usually lasts for some months; treatment is with vestibular sedatives.

## Glossopharyngeal, vagus, accessory and hypoglossal nerves (ninth to 12th cranial nerves) (K&C p. 1139)

The lower four cranial nerves (ninth to 12th) which lie in the medulla (the 'bulb') are usually affected together; isolated lesions are rare. A *bulbar palsy* is a weakness of the lower motor neurone type of the muscles supplied by these cranial nerves. There is dysarthria, dysphagia and nasal regurgitation. The tongue is weak, wasted and fasciculating. The most common causes of a bulbar palsy are motor neurone disease (p. 708), syringobulbia (p. 706) and Guillain–Barré syndrome (p. 712). Poliomyelitis is now rare. *Pseudobulbar palsy* is an upper motor neurone weakness of the same muscle groups. There is also dysarthria, dysphagia and nasal regurgitation, but the tongue is small and spastic and there is no fasciculation. The jaw jerk is exaggerated and the patient is emotionally labile. In many patients there is a partial palsy with only some of these features. The most common cause of pseudobulbar palsy is a stroke, but it may also occur in motor neurone disease and multiple sclerosis.

## Unconsciousness and coma (K&C p. 1159)

The central reticular formation, which extends from the brainstem to the thalamus, influences the state of arousal. It consists of clusters of interconnected neurones throughout the brainstem, with projections to the spinal cord, the hypothalamus, the cerebellum and the cerebral cortex.

*Coma* is a state of unconsciousness from which the patient cannot be roused. A *stuporous* patient is sleepy but will respond to vigorous stimulation. The Glasgow Coma Scale (Table 15.7) is a simple grading system used to assess the level of consciousness. It is easy to perform and provides an objective assessment of the patient. Serial measurements

**Table 15.7**
Glasgow Coma Scale

| Category | Score |
| --- | --- |
| Eye opening | |
| Spontaneous | 4 |
| To speech | 3 |
| To pain | 2 |
| None | 1 |
| Best verbal response | |
| Orientated | 5 |
| Confused | 4 |
| Inappropriate | 3 |
| Incomprehensible | 2 |
| None | 1 |
| Best motor response | |
| Obeying commands | 6 |
| Localizing – use limb to resist a painful stimulus | 5 |
| Withdrawing | 4 |
| Flexing | 3 |
| Extending | 2 |
| None | 1 |

The scores in each category are added up to give an overall score, which may vary from 3 (in the deeply comatose patient) to 15

are particularly useful to monitor the conscious level and thus detect a deterioration which may indicate the need for further investigation or treatment.

## *Aetiology*

Altered consciousness is produced by three types of processes:

- Diffuse metabolic, toxic or neurological disturbance
- Brainstem lesions which damage the reticular formation
- Cortical and cerebellar lesions. These will only cause coma if there is raised intracranial pressure and secondary brainstem compression, i.e. an indirect effect.

The principal causes of coma and stupor are shown in Table 15.8. A common cause of coma in young adults is self-poisoning (p. 523).

**Table 15.8**
Causes of coma and stupor

| | |
|---|---|
| Toxins | Drug overdose, alcohol, anaesthetic gases, carbon monoxide poisoning |
| Metabolic | Hypo- or hyperglycaemia<br>Hypo- or hypercalcaemia – if severe<br>Hypo- or hypernatraemia – if severe<br>Hypoxic/ischaemic brain injury<br>Hypoadrenalism<br>Renal failure<br>Hepatic failure<br>Respiratory failure with $CO_2$ retention |
| Diffuse neurological disease | Subarachnoid haemorrhage<br>Hypertensive encephalopathy<br>Encephalitis, cerebral malaria |
| Brainstem lesions | Tumour<br>Haemorrhage/infarction<br>Demyelination, e.g. multiple sclerosis<br>Trauma<br>Wernicke–Korsakoff syndrome |
| Cortical/cerebellar lesions | Tumour<br>Haemorrhage/infarction<br>Abscess<br>Encephalitis |

## Assessment

**Immediate assessment,** which takes only seconds, is essential:

- Emergency resuscitation (p. 525).
- Clear the airway and intubate if ventilation is inadequate.
- Check the pulse; if absent and resuscitation is appropriate, perform cardiopulmonary resuscitation.
- Check for head injury and, if present, anticipate deterioration.

In all patients presenting in coma a history should be obtained from any witnesses and relatives (e.g. speed of onset of coma, diabetes, drug or alcohol abuse, past medical history and medication).

**Further assessment** The depth of coma should be noted (Table 15.7) and a full general examination carried out.

Clues to the cause of coma should be looked for, for example the smell of alcohol or ketones (in diabetic ketoacidosis) on the breath, needle-track marks in a drug abuser, or a Medic-Alert bracelet, as carried by some diabetic people and patients on steroid-replacement therapy. The neurological examination must include:

- The head and neck. The patient should be examined for evidence of trauma and neck stiffness (indicating meningitis or subarachnoid haemorrhage).
- The size of the pupils and their reaction to light must be recorded:
  - *A unilateral fixed dilated pupil* indicates herniation of the temporal lobe ('coning') through the tentorial hiatus and compression of the third cranial nerve (p. 652). This indicates the need for urgent neurosurgical intervention.
  - *Bilateral fixed dilated pupils* are a cardinal sign of brain death. They also occur in deep coma of any cause, but particularly coma caused by barbiturate intoxication or hypothermia.
  - *Pinpoint pupils* are seen with opiate overdose or with pontine lesions that interrupt the sympathetic pathways to the dilator muscle of the pupil.
  - *Midpoint pupils* that react to light are characteristic in coma of metabolic origin and coma caused by most CNS-depressant drugs.
- The fundi. These should be examined for papilloedema, which indicates raised intracranial pressure.
- Eye movements. *Conjugate lateral deviation of the eyes* indicates ipsilateral cerebral haemorrhage or infarction (the eyes look away from the paralysed limbs), or a contralateral pontine lesion (towards the paralysed limbs).

  Passive head rotation normally causes conjugate ocular deviation in the direction opposite to the induced head movement (doll's head reflex). This reflex is lost in very deep coma and is absent in brainstem lesions.
- Motor responses. Asymmetry of spontaneous limb movements, tone and reflexes indicates a unilateral

cerebral hemisphere or brainstem lesion. The plantar responses are often both extensor in coma of any cause.

## Investigations

In many cases the cause of coma will be evident from the history and examination and appropriate investigations should then be carried out. However, if the cause is still unclear further investigations will be necessary.

## Blood and urine tests

- Serum and urine for drug analysis, e.g. salicylates
- Serum for urea and electrolytes, liver biochemistry and calcium
- Blood glucose by immediate Stix testing and then formal laboratory testing
- Arterial blood gases
- Thyroid function tests and serum cortisol
- Blood cultures.

**Radiology** CT of the head may indicate an otherwise unsuspected mass lesion or intracranial haemorrhage.

**CSF examination** If a mass lesion is excluded on CT, lumbar puncture (p. 753) is performed if subarachnoid haemorrhage or meningoencephalitis is suspected.

## Management

The immediate management consists of treatment of the cause, careful nursing, meticulous attention to the airway and frequent observation to detect any change in vital function. Naloxone (p. 534) is given if opiate poisoning (pinpoint pupils, hypoventilation, drug addict) is suspected. Flumazenil (p. 533) is given if coma is a complication of benzodiazepines.

663

## Prognosis

The outlook depends upon the cause of coma. A cause must be established before decisions are made about withdrawing supportive care.

# Brain death

Brain death means the irreversible loss of the capacity for consciousness, combined with the irreversible loss of the capacity to breathe. Two independent senior medical opinions are required for the diagnosis to be made. The three main criteria for diagnosis are as follows:

- Irremediable structural brain damage. A disorder that can cause brainstem death, e.g. intracranial haemorrhage, must have been diagnosed with certainty. Patients with hypothermia, significant electrolyte imbalance or drug overdose are excluded, but may be reassessed when these are corrected.
- Absent motor responses to any stimulus. Spinal reflexes may be present.
- Absent brainstem function, demonstrated by:
  - Pupils fixed and unresponsive to light
  - Absent corneal, gag and cough reflexes
  - Absent doll's head reflex (p. 662)
  - Absent caloric responses: ice-cold water run into the external auditory meatus causes nystagmus when brainstem function is normal
  - Lack of spontaneous respiration.

In suitable cases, and provided the patient was carrying a donor card and/or the consent of relatives has been obtained, the organs of those in whom brainstem death has been established may be used for transplantation.

# Cerebrovascular disease (*K&C* p. 1163)

## Stroke

### Definitions (*K&C* p. 1163)

*Stroke* is a focal neurological deficit (e.g. hemiplegia) lasting longer than 24 hours which is the result of a vascular lesion. Onset is usually rapid. A completed stroke is when the neurological deficit has reached its maximum (usually within 6 hours).

**Stroke in evolution** is when the symptoms and signs are getting worse (usually within 24 hours of onset).

**A minor stroke** is one in which the patient recovers without a significant neurological deficit, usually within 1 week.

**Transient ischaemic attack** is a focal deficit lasting less than 24 hours and from which there is complete neurological recovery.

## Epidemiology

Stroke is the third most common cause of death in the UK and the most common cause of serious long-term physical disability in adults. The incidence rises steeply with age; it is uncommon in those under 40 years. It is slightly more common in men.

## Pathogenesis

A stroke is caused by cerebral infarction or cerebral haemorrhage. The clinical picture of 'stroke' may also be caused by a space-occupying lesion in the brain, e.g. a tumour or abscess, although the onset of symptoms and signs is usually much slower. In young adults one-fifth of strokes are caused by dissection of a major extracranial or intracranial artery, associated with trauma to, or manipulation of, the neck.

**Cerebral infarction (85% of strokes)** may be the result of:

- Thrombosis at the site of an atheromatous plaque in a major cerebral vessel or from small vessel disease deep within the brain
- Emboli arising from atheromatous plaques in the carotid/vertebrobasilar arteries, or from cardiac mural thrombi (e.g. following myocardial infarction), or from the left atrium in atrial fibrillation.

Rarely cerebral infarction is the result of severe hypotension (e.g. systolic blood pressure < 75 mmHg), vasculitis, meningovascular syphilis, or emboli from vegetations in infective endocarditis.

**Cerebral haemorrhage (15% of strokes)** In most cases this is the result of rupture of an intracranial microaneurysm (Charcot–Bouchard aneurysms) in a hypertensive patient.

## Risk factors

The major risk factors for thromboembolic stroke are those for atheroma, i.e. hypertension, diabetes mellitus, cigarette smoking and hyperlipidaemia. Others are obesity, oestrogen-containing oral contraceptives, excessive alcohol consumption and polycythaemia.

## Clinical features

The history and physical examination in all stroke patients must include a search for risk factors (see above) and source of emboli (? atrial fibrillation, valve lesion, carotid bruits in the neck).

In most patients symptoms and signs develop over a few minutes and reach maximum disability within 1–2 hours. Severe headache, vomiting and coma at onset are more common in cerebral haemorrhage than infarction but accurate differentiation requires CT or MR imaging.

The neurological deficit produced by the occlusion of a vessel may be predicted by a knowledge of neuroanatomy and vascular supply (Figs 15.1, 15.9). In practice it is less clear-cut because of collateral supply to brain areas.

***Cerebral hemisphere infarcts*** The most common stroke is the hemiplegia caused by infarction of the internal capsule (the narrow zone of motor and sensory fibres that converges on the brainstem from the cerebral cortex; Fig. 15.1) following occlusion of a branch of the middle cerebral artery. The signs are contralateral to the lesion: hemiplegia (arm > leg), hemisensory loss, upper motor neurone facial weakness and hemianopia. Initially the patient has a hypotonic hemiplegia with decreased reflexes; within days this develops into a spastic hemiplegia with increased reflexes and an extensor plantar response, i.e. an upper motor neurone lesion (Table 15.3). Weakness may recover gradually over days or months.

Occlusion of the main trunk of the middle cerebral artery produces contralateral hemiplegia, hemisensory loss and aphasia (if located in the dominant hemisphere). Lacunar infarcts are small infarcts that produce localized deficits, e.g. pure motor stroke, pure sensory stroke.

**(a)**

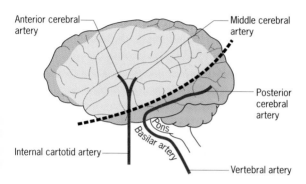

**(b)**

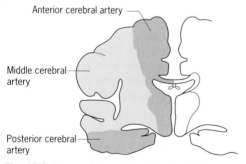

**Fig. 15.9 The arterial supply to the brain. (a)** The area above the dotted line is supplied by the internal carotid artery and the area below the line is supplied by the vertebral artery. **(b)** A coronal section through the brain. The anterior cerebral artery supplies the medial surface of the hemisphere and the middle cerebral artery supplies the lateral surface of the hemisphere, including the internal capsule.

667

***Brainstem infarction*** Brainstem infarction causes complex patterns of dysfunction depending on the sites involved:

- The lateral medullary syndrome, the most common of the brainstem vascular syndromes, is caused by occlusion of the posterior inferior cerebellar artery. It presents with sudden vomiting and vertigo, ipsilateral Horner's syndrome, facial numbness, cerebellar signs and palatal paralysis with a diminished gag reflex. On the side opposite the lesion there is loss of pain and temperature sensation.

- Coma as a result of involvement of the reticular formation.
- Pseudobulbar palsy (p. 659) is caused by lower brainstem infarction.

**Multi-infarct dementia** is a syndrome caused by multiple small cortical infarcts, resulting in generalized intellectual loss; there is a stepwise progression with each infarct. The final picture is of dementia, pseudobulbar palsy and a shuffling gait resembling Parkinson's disease.

## Management

Stroke is usually a straightforward clinical diagnosis. The management of acute stroke is summarized in Emergency Box 15.1. Patients with a large intracerebral haematoma causing deepening coma or patients with a cerebellar infarct or bleed causing hydrocephalus should be referred for immediate neurosurgical evaluation.

Further management of the stroke patient centres on identification and treatment of risk factors and rehabilitation to restore function. Optimal care is on a stroke rehabilitation unit where care is multidisciplinary involving doctors, nurses, physiotherapists, occupational therapists, speech and language therapists and social workers. Physiotherapy is particularly useful in the first few months in reducing spasticity, relieving contractures and teaching patients to use walking aids. Following recovery, the occupational therapist plays a valuable role in assessing the requirement for and arranging the provision of various aids and modifications in the home, such as stair rails, hoists, or wheelchairs. Patients and relatives may gain useful information and support from the UK Stroke Association (http://www.stroke.org.uk).

Carotid Doppler and duplex ultrasound scanning are indicated in patients with a cerebral infarct who may be

### Emergency Box 15.1

## Emergency management of acute stroke

### Investigations

- *CT (or MRI)* Demonstrates the site of the lesion; distinguishes between ischaemic/haemorrhagic stroke; identifies conditions mimicking stroke, e.g. cerebral tumour or abscess

  Neuroimaging is performed within 48 hours of admission, more urgently if thrombolysis is being considered, there is a recent history of head injury, the patient is taking warfarin or the conscious level is deteriorating

- *Blood glucose:* to exclude hyper- or hypoglycaemia
- *Urea and electrolytes*
- *Full blood count:* to identify polycythaemia
- *INR:* if taking warfarin
- *ESR:* raised in the few cases of endocarditis and vasculitis
- *ECG:* ? atrial fibrillation, myocardial infarction

### Treatment

- *Aspirin.* Aspirin 300 mg daily (orally, via nasogastric tube or rectally) started within 48 hours of acute ischaemic stroke reduces risk of subsequent death and disability.
- *Thrombolysis.* Intravenous tPA improves functional outcome if given within 3 hours of the onset of symptoms in acute ischaemic stroke. In the UK most patients would not reach hospital and have a CT scan within this time frame. The dose is 0.9 mg/kg over 60 min with 10% of dose within first minute. Contraindications to thrombolysis are listed on page 216.
- *Hypertension.* Treatment not indicated in all patients, as a reduction in arterial pressure may cause harmful decreases in local brain perfusion. Only treat if complications, e.g. heart failure, aortic dissection, or if BP very high.
- *Heparin.* Low-dose subcutaneous heparin in patients with acute ischaemic stroke and at high risk of DVT (p. 217).

### Supportive care

- *Stroke unit.* Dedicated stroke units improve outcome compared to management on a general ward.
- *Swallowing and feeding.* Dysphagia is common and may cause aspiration pneumonia and nutritional deficit. Formal assessment of swallowing by trained staff is essential. Feeding by fine-bore nasogastric tube or percutaneous gastrostomy may be necessary.
- *Unconscious patient.* Maintenance of hydration, frequent turning to avoid pressure sores and other measures (p. 663).

National Clinical Guidelines for Stroke (www.rcplondon.ac.uk/pubs/books/stroke)

669

suitable for carotid endarterectomy (p. 670), to look for carotid atheroma and stenosis. Magnetic resonance angiography or digital subtraction angiography should be performed if ultrasound suggests carotid stenosis. Detailed clotting studies and autoantibody screen to look for evidence of conditions associated with thrombophilia (Table 5.18) are indicated in younger patients with unexplained stroke. Echocardiography (in suspected cardioembolic stroke) and syphilis serology are performed in selected patients.

***Secondary prevention*** This involves advice and treatment to reverse risk factors (p. 666). Control of hypertension is the single most important factor in the prevention of stroke.

- Aspirin started for the treatment of acute ischaemic stroke should be continued indefinitely at 75 mg daily. Clopidrogel, a new antiplatelet agent is used in patients intolerant of aspirin.
- Long-term anticoagulation with warfarin is indicated in cerebral infarction when there is atrial fibrillation, with some valvular lesions (uninfected) or dilated cardiomyopathy.
- Internal carotid endarterectomy reduces the risk of recurrent stroke (by 75%) in patients who have had an infarct and who have internal carotid artery stenosis which narrows the arterial lumen by more than 70%. It is considered in patients with a non-disabling stroke who are likely to have some recoverable function.

## *Prognosis*

About one-quarter of patients will die in the first 2 years following a stroke; the prognosis is worse for bleeds than for infarction. Gradual improvement usually follows stroke although one-third of long-term survivors are permanently dependent on the help of others. About 10% of all patients will suffer a recurrent stroke within 1 year.

# Transient ischaemic attacks (K&C p. 1165)

Transient ischaemic attacks (TIAs) are less common than strokes but are an important predictive factor for stroke and myocardial infarction.

## Aetiology

TIAs are usually the result of passage of microemboli (which subsequently lyse) arising from atheromatous plaques or from cardiac mural thrombi. The risk factors and causes of TIAs are the same as those for thromboembolic stroke.

## Clinical features

There is a sudden loss of function in one region of the brain which, by definition, resolves in 24 hours. Symptoms and signs depend on the site of the brain involved (Table 15.9). The history and physical examination must include a search for risk factors and possible sources of emboli.

Amaurosis fugax is a sudden loss of vision in one eye as a result of the passage of emboli through the retinal arteries. Transient global amnesia is a condition in which there are sudden episodes of amnesia associated with confusion, probably caused by ischaemia in the posterior circulation.

The investigation and management of TIAs is similar to that of stroke. Aspirin (75 mg daily) reduces the incidence of subsequent stroke and is given to most patients.

**Table 15.9**
Features of TIAs in different arterial territories

| Carotid system | Vertebrobasilar system |
| --- | --- |
| Amaurosis fugax | Diplopia, vertigo, vomiting |
| Aphasia | Choking and dysarthria |
| Hemiparesis | Ataxia |
| Hemisensory loss | Hemisensory loss |
| Hemianopic visual loss | Hemianopic visual loss |
|  | Transient global amnesia |
|  | Loss of consciousness (rare) |

# Primary intracranial haemorrhage

(*K&C* p. 1171)

## Intracerebral haemorrhage

This is discussed under Stroke, above.

## Subarachnoid haemorrhage

The term 'subarachnoid haemorrhage' (SAH) describes spontaneous rather than traumatic arterial bleeding into the subarachnoid space.

### Incidence

SAH accounts for 5% of strokes and has an annual incidence of 6 per 100 000. The mean age of patients at presentation is 50 years.

### Aetiology

SAH is caused by rupture of:

- Saccular ('berry') aneurysms in 70% of cases. These are acquired lesions that are most commonly located at the branching points (Fig. 15.10) of the major arteries coursing through the subarachnoid space at the base of the brain (the circle of Willis).
- Congenital arteriovenous malformations in 10%.

In 20% of cases no lesion can be found.

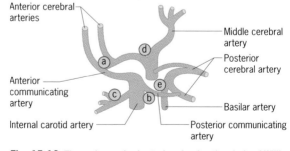

**Fig. 15.10 The main cerebral arteries showing the circle of Willis and the most common sites for berry aneurysms.** Frequency of occurrence, a–e (decreasing order). a, anterior communicating artery; b, origin of the posterior communicating artery; c, trifurcation of the middle cerebral artery; d, termination of the internal carotid artery; e, basilar artery.

## Clinical features

Most intracranial aneurysms remain asymptomatic until they rupture and cause a subarachnoid haemorrhage. Some, however, become symptomatic because of a mass effect, and the most common symptom is a painful third-nerve palsy (p. 652). The typical presentation of subarachnoid haemorrhage is the sudden onset of severe headache that reaches maximum intensity immediately or within minutes. It is often accompanied by nausea and vomiting, and sometimes loss of consciousness. On examination there may be signs of meningeal irritation (neck stiffness and a positive Kernig's sign), focal neurological signs and subhyaloid haemorrhages (between the retina and vitreous membrane) with or without papilloedema. Some patients have experienced small warning headaches a few days before the major bleed.

## Investigation

- CT scan shows subarachnoid or intraventricular blood in 95% of cases undergoing scanning within 24 hours of the haemorrhage.
- Lumbar puncture (LP) is indicated if there is a strong clinical suspicion of a subarachnoid haemorrhage but the CT scan is normal. It must be performed at least 6 hours after symptom onset. Xanthochromia (yellow discoloration detected by spectroscopy and caused by the breakdown of blood products) of the supernatant after centrifugation of the CSF is diagnostic of a subarachnoid haemorrhage.

Patients who are potentially fit for surgery, i.e. those not in a coma, should be referred urgently to a neurosurgical unit for cerebral angiography to establish the source and site of bleeding.

## Management

Immediate management consists of bed rest and supportive measures with cautious control of hypertension. Dexamethasone is often used to control cerebral oedema and is believed to stabilize the blood–brain barrier. Nimodipine, a calcium-channel blocker, is given by mouth (60 mg 4-hourly) or by intravenous infusion (1–2 mg per hour via a central line) to reduce cerebral artery spasm, an important cause of ischaemia and further neurological deterioration. Obliteration of the aneurysm by surgical clipping or insertion of a fine wire coil under radiological guidance prevents rebleeding.

### Prognosis

Approximately 50% of patients die suddenly or soon after the haemorrhage. A further 10–20% die in the early weeks in hospital from further bleeding. The outcome is variable in the survivors; some patients are left with major neurological deficits.

### Subdural haematoma

Subdural haematoma (SDH) occurs when blood accumulates in the subdural space following the rupture of a vein running from the hemisphere to the sagittal sinus. It is almost always the result of head injury, often minor, and the latent interval between injury and symptoms may be weeks or months. Elderly patients and alcoholics are particularly susceptible because they are accident prone and their atrophic brains make the connecting veins more susceptible to rupture. The main clinical symptoms are headache, drowsiness and confusion, which may fluctuate. The diagnosis is usually made on CT, and treatment is by surgical removal of the haematoma.

### Extradural haemorrhage

Extradural haematomas are caused by injuries that fracture the temporal bone and rupture the underlying middle meningeal artery. Clinically there is the picture of a head injury with a brief period of unconsciousness followed by a lucid interval of recovery. This is then followed by rapid deterioration with focal neurological signs and deterioration in conscious level if surgical drainage is not carried out.

## Epilepsy and other causes of loss of consciousness (K&C p. 1173)

## Epilepsy

A seizure is a convulsion or transient abnormal event resulting from a paroxysmal discharge of cerebral neurones. Epilepsy is the continuing tendency to have such seizures.

## Epidemiology

Epilepsy is a common condition, with 2% of the UK population having two or more seizures during their lives, and in 0.5% epilepsy is an active problem.

## Classification

Seizures are classified clinically as partial or generalized (Table 15.10). Partial seizures involve only a portion of the brain at their onset (e.g. temporal lobe), although these may later become generalized (secondarily generalized tonic–clonic seizures).

- *Tonic–clonic.* There is a sudden onset of a rigid tonic phase followed by a convulsion (clonic phase) in which the muscles jerk rhythmically. The episode lasts typically for seconds to minutes, may be associated with tongue biting and incontinence of urine, and is followed by a period of drowsiness or coma for several hours.
- *Typical absences (petit mal).* This is usually a disorder of childhood in which the child ceases activity, stares and pales for a few seconds only. It is characterized by 3-Hz spike and wave activity on the electroencephalogram (EEG).
- *Jacksonian (motor) seizures.* These simple partial seizures originate in the motor cortex and result in jerking movements, typically beginning in the corner

---

**Table 15.10**
The classification of epilepsy

**Generalized seizures**
Tonic–clonic (grand mal)
Absence seizures (petit mal)
Myoclonic seizures (rare form of epilepsy with involuntary muscle jerks)

**Partial seizures**
Simple partial seizures (no impairment of consciousness), e.g. Jacksonian seizures
Complex partial seizures (with impairment of consciousness), e.g. temporal lobe epilepsy

of the mouth or thumb and index finger, and spreading to involve the limbs on the opposite side of the epileptic focus. Paralysis of the involved limbs may follow for several hours (Todd's paralysis).

- *Temporal lobe seizures.* These complex partial seizures are associated with olfactory and visual hallucinations, feelings of unreality (jamais-vu) or undue familiarity (déjà-vu) with the surroundings.

### Precipitating factors
Flashing lights or a flickering television screen may provoke an attack in susceptible patients.

### Aetiology
No cause for epilepsy is found in over 75% of patients. About 30% of patients have a first-degree relative with epilepsy, although the exact mode of inheritance is unknown. Primary epilepsies are due to complex developmental abnormalities of neuronal control; there are abnormalities in synaptic connections and distribution and release of neurotransmitters. Epilepsy may occur secondary to head injury, brain surgery, cerebral tumours and infarction. Inflammatory conditions of the brain, such as encephalitis, chronic meningitis (e.g. TB) and cerebral abscess, may sometimes present initially with seizures. Drug overdose, alcohol withdrawal and metabolic disturbances, e.g. hypoglycaemia, hypoxia, hypocalcaemia and hyponatraemia, are other causes.

### Evaluation and investigation
There are three steps in the evaluation of a patient with possible epilepsy:

1. Confirm if the patient has epilepsy. The diagnosis is often made clinically; a detailed description of the attack from an eye-witness is invaluable. Disorders causing attacks of altered consciousness must be differentiated from epilepsy (Table 15.2).
2. Determine the patient's seizure type (see classification).
3. Identify any underlying cause for epilepsy.

- The electroencephalogram (EEG) is the single most useful test in the diagnosis of epilepsy, but the recording is frequently normal between attacks.

During a seizure the EEG is almost always abnormal and is shown typically by a cortical spike focus (e.g. in a temporal lobe) or by generalized spike and wave activity.

- CT or magnetic resonance imaging should be performed in all patients other than children to exclude an underlying lesion. Even in adults, however, the pick-up rate for treatable lesions is very low.

## Management

The emergency treatment is to ensure that patients harm themselves as little as possible and that the airway remains patent.

Drugs are indicated when there is a firm clinical diagnosis of recurrent seizures or a substantial risk of recurrence. Treatment is started with a single first-line antiepileptic drug (Table 15.11). The dose is increased until seizure control is achieved or tolerance exceeded. The therapeutic range of plasma drug concentrations has been established for some antiepileptic drugs and can be used together with the clinical response as a guide to dosing. Idiosyncratic side-effects (i.e. non-dose related), which tend to be more common than dose-related effects, are listed in Table 15.11. Intoxication with all anticonvulsants causes a syndrome of ataxia, nystagmus and dysarthria. Side-effects of chronic administration of phenytoin (gum hypertrophy, hypertrichosis,

**Table 15.11**
Recommended initial treatment depending on seizure type

| Seizure type | Drug | Major side-effects of drug treatment |
|---|---|---|
| Generalized tonic–clonic | Phenytoin | Rashes, blood dyscrasias, lymphadenopathy |
| | Carbamazepine | Rashes, leucopenia |
| | Sodium valproate | Anorexia, hair loss, liver damage |
| Generalized absence | Sodium valproate Ethosuximide | Rashes, blood dyscrasias, night terrors |
| Partial seizures | Carbamazepine Phenytoin Sodium valproate | |

677

osteomalacia and folate deficiency) are reduced by maintaining serum levels within the therapeutic range. Phenytoin is a potent hepatic enzyme inducer and will reduce the efficacy of the contraceptive pill. Second-line agents, e.g. vigabatrin, lamotrigine and gabapentin, are generally reserved for patients who are not controlled with maximally tolerated doses of first-line antiepileptics.

Gradual withdrawal of drugs should only be considered when the patient has been seizure-free for at least 2 years and is only achieved successfully in less than 50%. Many patients will have further fits, resulting in a threat to employment and driving (see below).

Neurosurgical treatment (e.g. amputation of the anterior temporal lobe) cures epilepsy in 50% of patients with poorly controlled epilepsy and a clearly defined focus of abnormal electrical activity (< 1% of all patients with epilepsy).

### Advice to patients

Patients should restrict their lives as little as possible but follow simple advice, e.g. avoid swimming alone, avoid dangerous sports, such as rock climbing, leave the door open when taking a bath. In the UK patients with epilepsy (whether on or off treatment) may drive a motor vehicle (but not a heavy goods or public service vehicle), provided that they have been seizure-free for 1 year or seizures have only occurred at night for the last 3 years. The British Epilepsy Association (http://www.epilepsy.org.uk) provides information about epilepsy for patients and relatives.

## Status epilepticus (K&C p. 1177)

Status epilepticus is a medical emergency which exists when two or more seizures follow each other without recovery of consciousness. When grand mal seizures follow one another, there is a risk of death from cardiorespiratory failure. Precipitating factors in a known epileptic include abruptly stopping antiepileptic treatment, intercurrent illness, alcohol abuse and poor compliance with therapy; 60% of all episodes occur in patients without any history of epilepsy. The initial treatment of generalized convulsive status epilepticus is with intravenous lorazepam or rectal diazepam (Emergency Box 15.2). Lorazepam may cause respiratory depression and hypotension, and facilities for

## Emergency Box 15.2

### Management and investigation of status epilepticus

#### General measures

- Secure the airway: remove false teeth and insert oropharyngeal tube
- Administer oxygen by nasal cannula or face mask
- Secure venous access: many anticonvulsants cause phlebitis, so choose a large vein
- Glucose, 50 mL of 50% intravenously (i.v.) if hypoglycaemia is a possibility
- Thiamine, 250 mg i.v. over 10 minutes, if nutrition poor or alcohol abuse suspected
- Cardiorespiratory monitoring and pulse oximetry. EEG monitoring in refractory status or diagnosis in doubt (? *pseudostatus*)

#### Control of seizures

*First line.* Lorazepam 4 mg i.v. at 2 mg/min, repeated after 20 min. Give rectal diazepam (10–20 mg) if intravenous access difficult.

*Second line.* If seizures continue, give phenytoin 15 mg/kg i.v. diluted to 10 mg/mL in 0.9% sodium chloride at a rate not exceeding 50 mg/min (average-sized adult 1000 mg over 20 min). Give a further bolus up to a total loading dose of 30 mg/kg if seizures persist. Maintenance dose 100 mg i.v. at intervals of 6–8 hours. Fosphenytoin, a prodrug of phenytoin, may be given faster and causes fewer infusion site reactions.

*Third line.* Phenobarbital 10 mg/kg at a rate not exceeding 100 mg/min and repeated at intervals of 6–8 hours if necessary. Intravenous clonazepam, paraldehyde and chlomethiazole are also used in refractory cases.

*Refractory status.* If seizures continue despite these measures, use tiopental or propofol general anaesthesia with assisted ventilation.

#### Investigations

- Urgent: blood glucose, serum electrolytes including calcium and magnesium
- Consider brain CT scan, lumbar puncture and blood cultures, depending on clinical circumstances. Serum anticonvulsant levels

resuscitation should be available. If lorazepam fails to control the seizures, an infusion of phenytoin or phenobarbital should be started. Rapid infusion of phenytoin may cause cardiac dysrhythmias, and ECG monitoring is necessary during the infusion. Paraldehyde, given rectally or by intramuscular injection, is occasionally used if intravenous access is difficult or where facilities for resuscitation are poor (it causes little respiratory depression). Once status is controlled, all of these drug treatments must be followed by regular anticonvulsant therapy to present subsequent fits. Intravenous treatment is withdrawn when anticonvulsant therapy is established.

## Extrapyramidal disease – Parkinson's disease and other movement disorders (K&C p. 1182)

The extrapyramidal system is a general term for the basal ganglia and their connections with other brain areas, particularly those concerned with movement. The overall function of this system is the initiation and modulation of movement. Clinically, extrapyramidal disorders are broadly classified into the akinetic–rigid syndromes, where there is loss of movement with increase in muscle tone, and dyskinesias, where there are added uncontrollable movements (Table 15.12). Parkinson's disease and essential tremor are the most common of these movement disorders.

## Akinetic–rigid syndromes

### Idiopathic Parkinson's disease (K&C p. 1182)

The clinical features of Parkinson's disease principally result from the depletion of dopamine-containing neurones in the substantia nigra of the basal ganglia and a relative excess of acetylcholine stimulation.

### Epidemiology

The disease usually presents in elderly people, the prevalence rising to 1 in 200 in those over 70.

> **Table 15.12**
> A classification of movement disorders
>
> **Akinetic–rigid syndromes**
> Idiopathic Parkinson's disease
> Drug-induced parkinsonism, e.g. phenothiazines
> MPTP-induced parkinsonism
> Postencephalitic parkinsonism
> 'Parkinsonism plus'
> Childhood akinetic–rigid syndromes, e.g. Wilson's disease and
> athetoid cerebral palsy
>
> **Dyskinesias**
> Benign essential tremor
> Chorea
> Hemiballismus
> Myoclonus
> Tic or habit spasms
> Torsion dystonias

MPTP, methylphenyltetrahydropyridine

## Aetiology

The cause of the disease is unknown. MPTP (methylphenyltetrahydropyridine, an impurity produced during illegal synthesis of opiates) produces severe and irreversible parkinsonism. Survivors of an encephalitis epidemic (encephalitis lethargica 1918–1930), which was presumed to be a viral disease, developed parkinsonism. There is no evidence, however, that idiopathic Parkinson's disease is caused by an environmental toxin or an infective agent, though interestingly the disease is less prevalent in tobacco smokers than in lifelong abstainers.

## Clinical features

There is a combination of tremor, rigidity and akinesia (slow movements), together with changes in posture. The features of Parkinson's disease may be unilateral initially, but the disease subsequently progresses to involve both sides of the body.

681

- *Tremor*. This is a characteristic 4–7 Hz resting tremor (cf. cerebellar disease), usually most obvious in the hands ('pill-rolling' of the thumb and fingers), improved by voluntary movement and made worse by anxiety.

- *Rigidity* refers to the increase in tone in the limbs and trunk. The limbs resist passive extension throughout movement (lead pipe rigidity, or cogwheel when combined with tremor), in contrast to the hypertonia of an upper motor neurone lesion (p. 638), where resistance falls away as the movement continues (clasp-knife).
- *Akinesia*. There is difficulty in initiating movement (starting to walk, or rising from a chair). The face is expressionless and unblinking and may give the appearance of depression. Speech is slow and monotonous. The writing becomes small (micrographia) and tends to tail off at the end of a line.
- *Postural changes*. A stoop is characteristic and the gait is shuffling, festinant and with poor arm swinging. The posture is sometimes called 'simian', to describe the forward flexion, immobility of the arms and lack of facial expression. Balance is poor, with a tendency to fall.

Other features include dribbling of saliva, dysphagia, constipation, depression and dementia in the later stages. There is gradual progression of the disease over 10–15 years, with death resulting most commonly from bronchopneumonia.

## Investigations

The diagnosis is clinical. Investigations for other akinetic–rigid syndromes are only necessary in an atypical case, e.g. a young patient.

## Management

682

**Levodopa** The treatment of choice is the dopamine precursor levodopa (L-dopa), in combination with a peripheral decarboxylase inhibitor, e.g. Madopar (L-dopa plus benserazide) or Sinemet (L-dopa plus carbidopa). This combined therapy reduces the peripheral side-effects, principally nausea, of L-dopa and its metabolites. Over the years, therapy may become less effective, even with increasing doses. Patients may also switch between periods of dopamine-induced dyskinesias (choreas and dystonic movements) and periods of immobility ('on–off' syndrome). This problem may be ameliorated by slow-release L-dopa; frequent small doses of L-dopa, or the addition of other antiparkinsonian drugs.

### Other treatments

- Bromocriptine, a dopamine agonist
- Selegiline – a type B monoamine oxidase inhibitor – inhibits the catabolism of dopamine in the brain
- Amantadine increases the synthesis and release of dopamine and has a weak antiparkinsonian effect
- Anticholinergic drugs, e.g. trihexyphenidyl (benzhexol), have most effect on tremor and little effect on akinesia. They often cause mental confusion.

**Additional treatment** Physiotherapy can improve gait and help to prevent falls. Selective serotonin reuptake inhibitors are the treatment of choice for depression. Surgery to transplant dopamine-producing cells (fetal or autologous adrenal medulla) has not produced significant clinical improvement. Information and support for patients and relatives is provided by the Parkinson's Disease Society (http://www.parkinsons.org.uk).

## Other akinetic–rigid syndromes

### Drug-induced parkinsonism (K&C p. 1185)
Reserpine, phenothiazines and butyrophenones block dopamine receptors and may induce a parkinsonian syndrome with slowness and rigidity, but usually with little tremor. These syndromes tend not to progress, they respond poorly to L-dopa, and the correct management is to stop the drug.

### 'Parkinsonism plus' (K&C p. 1186)
This describes rare disorders in which there is parkinsonism and evidence of a separate pathology. Progressive supranuclear palsy is the most common disorder and consists of axial rigidity, dementia and signs of parkinsonism, together with a striking inability to move the eyes vertically or laterally. There is a poor response to L-dopa.

Extrapyramidal disease

# Dyskinesias (*K&C* p. 1186)

## Benign essential tremor

This is usually a familial (autosomal dominant) tremor of the arms and head (titubation) which occurs most frequently in elderly people. Unlike the tremor of Parkinson's disease it is not usually present at rest, but is most obvious when the hands adopt a posture such as holding a glass or a spoon. It is made worse by anxiety and improved by alcohol and propranolol.

## Chorea

Chorea is a continuous flow of jerky, quasi-purposive movements, flitting from one part of the body to another. They may interfere with voluntary movements but cease during sleep. The causes of chorea are listed in Table 15.13. Treatment is with phenothiazines or tetrabenazine.

## Huntington's disease

Huntington's disease is a rare autosomal dominant condition with full penetrance. Expansion of CAG repeats in the Huntington's disease gene on chromosome 4 leads to production of mutant *huntingtin* protein. It is not known how the mutant protein causes disease. There is loss of neurones

---

**Table 15.13**
Causes of chorea

Huntington's disease

Sydenham's chorea (see Rheumatic fever)

Benign hereditary chorea in elderly people

Drug induced
    Phenytoin
    L-Dopa
    Alcohol

Systemic disease
    Thyrotoxicosis
    Systemic lupus erythematosus
    Pregnancy (chorea gravidarum)

Other CNS disease
    Stroke
    Trauma
    Tumour

within the basal ganglia, leading to depletion of GABA (γ-aminobutyric acid) and acetylcholine but sparing dopamine. Symptoms begin in middle age and there is then a relentlessly progressive course, with chorea and personality change preceding dementia and death. No treatment arrests the disease, and the management is symptomatic treatment of chorea and genetic counselling of family members.

## Hemiballismus

Hemiballismus (also called hemiballism) describes violent swinging movements of one side of the body, usually caused by infarction or haemorrhage in the contralateral subthalamic nucleus.

## Myoclonus

Myoclonus is the sudden, involuntary jerking of a single muscle or group of muscles. The most common example is benign essential myoclonus, which is the sudden jerking of a limb or the body on falling asleep. Myoclonus may also occur with epilepsy and some encephalopathies.

## Tics

Tics are brief, repeated stereotypical movements, usually involving the face and shoulders. Unlike other involuntary movements it is usually possible for the patient to control tics.

## Dystonias

Dystonias are prolonged spasms of muscle contraction. They may occasionally occur as a symptom of neurological disease, e.g. Wilson's disease, but are usually of unknown cause and occur without other neurological problems, e.g. blepharospasm (spasms of forced blinking) or spasmodic torticollis (the head is turned and held to one side or drawn backwards or forwards). The treatment of choice for many dystonias is the injection of minute amounts of botulinum toxin (which inhibits the release of acetylcholine from nerve endings) into the muscle. Acute dystonic reactions are seen with phenothiazines, butyrophenones and metoclopramide, and can occur after a single dose of the drug. Spasmodic torticollis, trismus and oculogyric crises (i.e.

685

episodes of sustained upward gaze) may occur. Acute dystonias respond promptly to an anticholinergic drug administered by intravenous or intramuscular injection, e.g. benzatropine (1–2 mg) or procyclidine (5 mg).

## Multiple sclerosis (*K&C* p. 1189)

Multiple sclerosis (MS) is a common disease of unknown cause in which there are multiple areas of demyelination within the brain and spinal cord. These are 'disseminated in time and place' (hence the old name 'disseminated sclerosis').

### Epidemiology

MS typically begins in early adulthood and the disease is more common in women. The prevalence varies widely (6 per 10 000 in England); it is rare in tropical countries.

### Aetiology

The aetiology is unknown; viruses and autoimmune mechanisms have been implicated. The disease is more common in family members, although there is no clear-cut pattern of inheritance.

### Pathology

The essential features are perivenular plaques of demyelination which have a predilection for the following sites within the brain and spinal cord:

- Optic nerves
- Periventricular white matter
- Brainstem and cerebellar connections
- Cervical spinal cord – corticospinal tracts and posterior columns.

The peripheral nerves are never affected.

### Clinical features

Symptoms are variable and characteristically evolve over a period of days, before resolving either partially or completely within weeks. Symptoms result from axonal demyelination, which leads to slowing or blockade of conduction. The regression of symptoms is attributed to the resolution of inflammatory oedema and to partial remyelination.

Inflammation of the optic nerve produces blurred vision and unilateral eye pain. A lesion in the optic nerve head produces disc swelling (optic neuritis) and pallor (optic atrophy) following the attack. When inflammation occurs in the optic nerve further away from the eye (retrobulbar neuritis) examination of the fundus is normal. Brainstem demyelination produces diplopia, vertigo, dysphagia and nystagmus. Sensory symptoms including numbness and pins and needles are common in MS and reflect spino-thalamic and posterior column lesions. Spastic paraparesis is the result of plaques of demyelination in the cervical or thoracic cord.

In some patients there will only be one or two attacks with little residual neurological deficit, and they remain very well for years. At the other extreme, in some patients an increasing neurological deficit accumulates and spastic tetraparesis, ataxia, brainstem signs, blindness, inconti-nence and dementia characterize the final stages. Death follows from recurrent urinary tract infection, uraemia and bronchopneumonia.

## Differential diagnosis

Initially individual plaques (e.g. in the optic nerve, brain-stem or cord) may cause diagnostic difficulty and must be distinguished from inflammatory, mass or vascular lesions. In young patients with a relapsing and remitting course the diagnosis is straightforward, as few other diseases produce this clinical picture.

## Investigations

- MRI of brain and spinal cord is the first-line investigation and shows plaques, particularly in the periventricular area and brainstem. Lesions are rarely visible on CT scanning.
- Electrophysiological tests. Visual, auditory and somatosensory evoked potentials may be prolonged, even in the absence of any past or present visual symptoms.
- CSF examination is usually unnecessary as the diagnosis is made with MRI or evoked potentials and a compatible clinical picture. Protein concentration and white cell count are raised. The IgG portion of the

total protein is increased and electrophoresis reveals oligoclonal bands, which indicate the production of immunoglobulin (to unknown antigens) within the CNS.

## Management

- Short courses of ACTH or corticosteroids (e.g. i.v. methylprednisolone 1000 mg/day for 3 days) may promote remission in relapse, but do not influence the outlook in the long term.
- Subcutaneous administration of β-interferon reduces the relapse rate by a third and may delay the time to severe debility. Treatment is prolonged, expensive and associated with side-effects, such as 'flu-like symptoms'.
- Physiotherapy and occupational therapy maintain the mobility of joints and muscle relaxants (e.g. baclofen, dantrolene and benzodiazepines) reduce the discomfort and pain of spasticity. Multidisciplinary team liaison between patient, carers, medical practitioners and therapists is essential for any patient with chronic disabling disease. Urinary catheterization is eventually needed for those with bladder involvement. The Multiple Sclerosis Society provides information and support for patients and relatives (http://www.mssociety.org.uk).

# Infective and inflammatory disease

(*K&C* p. 1191)

## Meningitis ND (*K&C* p. 1191)

Meningitis (inflammation of the meninges) can be caused by infection, drugs and contrast media, malignant cells and blood (following subarachnoid haemorrhage). The term is, however, usually reserved for inflammation caused by infective agents (Table 15.14).

### Clinical features

There is usually a rapid onset of severe headache, photophobia (intolerance of light) and vomiting with malaise, fever and rigors. Neck stiffness and Kernig's sign (inability

---

**Table 15.14**
Infective causes of meningitis in the UK

| | |
|---|---|
| Bacteria | *Neisseria meningitidis** |
| | *Streptococcus pneumoniae** |
| | *Haemophilus influenzae* (rare) |
| | *Staphylococcus aureus* |
| | *Listeria monocytogenes* |
| | Gram-negative bacilli |
| | *Mycobacterium tuberculosis*† |
| | *Treponema pallidum*† |
| | *Leptospira* spp. |
| Viruses | Enterovirus (echo, Coxsackie, polio) |
| | Mumps |
| | Herpes simplex virus |
| | HIV |
| | Epstein–Barr virus |
| Fungi | *Cryptococcus neoformans*† |
| | *Candida* spp. |

\* These organisms account for most cases of pyogenic meningitis in otherwise healthy adults
† May cause chronic meningitis with symptoms onset over weeks

---

to allow full extension of the knee when the hip is flexed 90°) are usually present. Consciousness is usually not impaired, although the patient may be delirious with a high fever. Papilloedema may occur. The presence of drowsiness, lateralizing signs and cranial nerve lesions indicates the existence of a complication, e.g. venous sinus thrombosis, severe cerebral oedema or cerebral abscess.

***Acute bacterial meningitis*** Most cases in adults are caused by meningococci. The organism is carried asymptomatically in the nasopharynx and spread from person to person by respiratory droplets or direct spread. Meningitis occurs after the organism invades the bloodstream from the nasopharynx, to reach the meninges. Characteristically there is a sudden onset of the disease with high fever, and a petechial/purpuric skin rash is often present. In patients with fulminant meningococcal septicaemia there are often large ecchymoses and gangrenous skin lesions.

Pneumococcus is the most common cause of meningitis in elderly people, and may complicate pneumonia or other respiratory tract infections. Direct spread of the organism may occur from an infected middle ear or via a skull fracture. The features of meningitis appear rapidly and the mortality rate may be as high as 30%.

**Viral meningitis** is usually a benign self-limiting condition lasting for about 4–10 days. There are no serious sequelae.

**Tuberculous meningitis** is often a chronic illness with vague symptoms of headache, lassitude, anorexia and vomiting. Signs of meningism may be absent or appear late in the course of the disease.

### Differential diagnosis
Conditions which can mimic meningitis include subarachnoid haemorrhage, migraine, viral encephalitis and cerebral malaria.

### Investigations
Suspected bacterial meningitis is a medical emergency with a high mortality rate and requires urgent investigation and treatment (Emergency Box 15.3).

### Notification
All cases of meningitis must (by law) be notified to the local Public Health Authority; this allows contact tracing and provides data for epidemiological studies.

### Meningococcal prophylaxis
Oral rifampicin is given to patients and close (usually household) contacts to eradicate nasopharyngeal carriage of the organism. A vaccine for meningococcal group C and *Haemophilus influenzae* is part of routine childhood UK immunization.

690

## Encephalitis (K&C p. 1194)
Encephalitis is inflammation of the brain parenchyma. It is caused by a wide variety of viruses and may also occur in bacterial and other infections. In certain groups (e.g. homosexuals, intravenous drug abusers) HIV infection and opportunistic organisms (e.g. *Toxoplasma gondii* in patients with full-blown AIDS) are important causes.

### Emergency Box 15.3

#### Investigation and treatment of suspected bacterial meningitis

**Note:** A petechial or ecchymotic skin rash suggests meningococcal infection and is an indication for **immediate** treatment with benzylpenicillin: 1200 mg by slow i.v. or i.m. injection in adults. If penicillin allergic, cefotaxime 1 g or chloramphenicol 25 mg/kg i.v.

**Investigations**

- *Lumbar puncture (LP)*. Urgent CSF microscopy, white cell count and differential, and analysis for protein and glucose concentration (Table 15.15). Ziehl–Nielsen (tuberculous) and Indian ink stain (cryptococcal infection) in immunocompromised or other at-risk individual.
- *Head CT scan*. Performed before LP only in patients who have clinical features that increase the likelihood of having intracranial mass lesions or increase in CSF pressure which would preclude LP: immunosuppression, bleeding tendency, focal neurological signs, papilloedema, loss of consciousness or seizure.
- *Other*. Blood cultures, blood glucose, viral and syphilis serology.

**Treatment**

**Note:** Antimicrobial therapy should not be delayed if there is a contraindication or inability to perform immediate LP

- Close liaison between clinician and microbiologist is essential
- Cefotaxime 2 g 6-hourly i.v. for the initial treatment of bacterial meningitis. Add ampicillin 2 g 4-hourly or co-trimoxazole if risk of *Listeria* (elderly, immunosuppressed)
- Subsequent treatment given depending on the results of Gram stain, culture and the antibiotic sensitivities of the organism (Table 15.16)
- Tuberculous meningitis is treated for at least 9 months with triple antituberculous therapy (p. 481)

691

## Acute viral encephalitis

A viral aetiology is often presumed, although not confirmed serologically or by culture. In the UK the common organisms are Echo, Coxsackie, mumps and herpes simplex viruses.

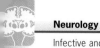

**Table 15.15**
Typical changes in the CSF in meningitis

|  | Normal | Pyogenic | Viral | Tuberculous |
|---|---|---|---|---|
| Appearance | Clear | Turbid/purulent | Clear/turbid | Turbid/viscous |
| Mononuclear cells/mm$^3$ | < 5 | < 50 | 10–100 | 100–300 |
| Polymorphs/mm$^3$ | Nil | 200–3000 | Nil | 0–200 |
| Protein (g/L) | 0.2–0.4 | 0.4–2.0 | 0.4–0.8 | 0.5–3.0 |
| Glucose (% blood glucose) | > 50 | < 50 | > 50 | < 30 |

NB: Malignant meningitis, e.g. with lymphoma, may give similar changes to TB

**Table 15.16**
Appropriate antibiotics in acute bacterial meningitis

| Organism | Antibiotic | Alternative |
| --- | --- | --- |
| Unknown pyogenic | Cefotaxime | Benzylpenicillin plus chloramphenicol |
| Meningococcus | Benzylpenicillin | Cefotaxime |
| Pneumococcus | Cefotaxime | Penicillin |
| Haemophilus | Cefotaxime | Chloramphenicol |

## Clinical features

Many of these infections cause a mild self-limiting illness with headache and drowsiness. Less commonly the illness is severe, with focal signs (e.g. hemiparesis, dysphasia), seizures and coma. Severe encephalitis, which has a mortality rate of about 20% even with treatment, is most commonly caused by herpes simplex virus (HSV-1).

## Investigations

- CSF analysis shows a moderate increase in mononuclear cells (5–500 cells/mm$^3$). Protein may also be increased.
- Viral serology of blood and CSF may identify the causative virus.
- HSV DNA detection by PCR has a sensitivity of 95% in early HSV encephalitis. It is recommended that a 0.5 ml sample of CSF be sent for HSV PCR in all suspected cases.
- CT may show areas of oedema.
- EEG often shows non-specific slow-wave activity.

## Treatment

Suspected herpes simplex encephalitis is immediately treated with intravenous aciclovir (10 mg/kg every 8 hours). If the patient is in a coma the prognosis is poor, whether or not treatment is given.

## Intracranial abscesses (K&C p. 1198)

An abscess may develop in the epidural, subdural or intracerebral sites. Epidural abscesses are uncommon; subdural abscess presents similarly to intracerebral abscess (see below).

# Cerebral abscess

Cerebral abscess may follow the direct spread of organisms from a skull fracture or a focus of infection in the paranasal sinuses or middle ear. Alternatively, haematogenous spread of infection may occur from the lung (e.g. bronchiectasis), heart (e.g. endocarditis) or bone (e.g. osteomyelitis). Frequently no cause is found. The most common organisms are streptococci, *Bacteroides* spp., staphylococci and enterobacteria. Infection with tubercle bacilli may result in chronic caseating granulomata (tuberculomas) presenting as intracranial mass lesions.

## Clinical features

Presenting features include fever, seizures, focal neurological signs, and symptoms and signs of raised intracranial pressure (p. 697).

## Investigations

CT or MRI will usually outline the abscess. Lumbar puncture is not performed if an abscess is suspected because of the danger of coning in the presence of raised intracranial pressure (p. 754).

## Management

Treatment involves a combination of intravenous antibiotics and surgical drainage.

# Neurosyphilis (K&C p. 1196)

Syphilis is described on page 40. Neurosyphilis occurs late in the course of untreated infection. It is now rarely seen in the UK because most cases of syphilis are recognized in the early stages and treated with penicillin. The different clinical syndromes (summarized in Table 15.17) may occur alone or in combination.

## Management

Treatment is with parenteral benzylpenicillin for 3 weeks, which may arrest (but not reverse) the neurological disease.

**Table 15.17**
The clinical syndromes of neurosyphilis

**Asymptomatic neurosyphilis**

Positive CSF serology without symptoms or signs

**Meningovascular syphilis**
3–4 years after primary infection

Subacute meningitis with cranial nerve palsies and papilloedema. Raised intracranial pressure and focal deficits caused by an expanding intracranial mass (gumma). Paraparesis caused by spinal meningovasculitis

**General paralysis of the insane**
10–15 years after primary infection

Progressive dementia
Brisk reflexes
Extensor plantar responses
Tremor

**Tabes dorsalis**
10–35 years after primary infection
(caused by demyelination in the dorsal roots)

Lightning pains: short, sharp, stabbing pains in the legs. Ataxia, loss of reflexes and sensory loss. Neuropathic joints (Charcot's joints), Argyll Robertson pupils (p. 651), ptosis and optic atrophy

# Creutzfeldt–Jakob disease (CJD)

(*K&C* p. 1197)

This is a progressive dementia, usually developing after 50 years of age, characterized pathologically by spongiform changes in the brain. It is one example of a prion (a protein-aceous infectious particle) disease and the pathology is similar to bovine spongiform encephalopathy (BSE) of cattle. The transmissible agent is resistant to many of the usual processes that destroy proteins. CJD occurs as a spor-adic form or an iatrogenic form as a result of contaminated material such as corneal grafts or human growth hormone. There is no known treatment and death is invariable, usually within 6 months of onset.

Variant CJD presents with neuropsychiatric symptoms, followed by ataxia and dementia, and affects a younger age group. The appearance of this variant has led to the specu-lation that there has been transmission from the animal to the human food chain, with infection from BSE-infected cattle to humans.

# Intracranial tumours (*K&C* p. 1198)

Primary intracranial tumours account for 10% of all neo-plasms, and about one-quarter of all intracranial tumours are metastatic. Primary intracranial tumours may be derived from the skull itself, from any of the structures lying within it, or from their tissue precursors. They may be malignant on histological investigation but rarely meta-stasize outside the brain. The most common intracranial tumours occurring in adults are listed in Table 15.18.

## Clinical features

The clinical features of a cerebral tumour are the result of the following:

- Progressive focal neurological deficit
- Raised intracranial pressure
- Focal or generalized epilepsy.

**Table 15.18**
Relative frequency of the most common intracranial tumours in adults

| Tumour | Relative frequency (%) |
|---|---|
| **Primary malignant**<br>Astrocytoma<br>Oligodendroglioma | 40 |
| **Benign**<br>Meningioma<br>Neurofibroma | 30 |
| **Metastases**<br>Bronchus<br>Breast<br>Stomach<br>Prostate<br>Thyroid<br>Kidney | 25 |

*Neurological deficit* is the result of a mass effect of the tumour and surrounding cerebral oedema. The deficit depends on the site of the tumour, e.g. a frontal lobe tumour will initially cause personality change, apathy and intellectual deterioration. Subsequent involvement of the frontal speech area and motor cortex produces expressive aphasia and hemiparesis. Rapidly growing tumours destroy cerebral tissue, and loss of function is an early feature.

*Raised intracranial pressure* produces headache, vomiting and papilloedema. The headache is typically most severe on waking and decreases as the patient stands up, thereby lowering intracranial pressure. It is made worse by coughing, straining and sneezing.

As the tumour grows there is downward displacement of the brain and pressure on the brainstem, causing drowsiness, which progresses eventually to respiratory depression, bradycardia, coma and death.

Distortion of normal structures at a distance from the growing tumour leads to focal neurological signs (false localizing signs). The most common are a third and sixth cranial nerve palsy (p. 654) resulting from stretching of the nerves by downward displacement of the temporal lobes.

**Epilepsy** Fits may be generalized or partial in nature. The site of origin of a partial seizure is frequently of value in localization.

## Differential diagnosis

The main differential is from other intracranial mass lesions (cerebral abscess, tuberculoma, subdural haematoma and intracranial haematoma) and a stroke, which may have an identical clinical presentation. Idiopathic intracranial hypertension presents with headache and papilloedema in young obese females. Neuroimaging is normal but at lumbar puncture shows there is raised CSF pressure.

## Investigations

- Radiology. CT with contrast enhancement is the investigation of choice when a tumour is suspected. MRI is of particular value in investigation of tumours of the posterior fossa and brainstem. Cerebral angiography is sometimes necessary to define the site or blood supply of a mass, particularly if surgery is planned. Plain skull X-rays are rarely of diagnostic value, with the exception of pituitary tumours.
- Other investigations. These include routine tests, e.g. chest X-ray if metastatic disease is suspected. Lumbar puncture and examination of the CSF is contraindicated in this situation because of danger of immediate herniation of the cerebellar tonsils, impaction within the foramen magnum and compression of the brainstem ('coning').

## Management

- Surgery. Surgical exploration, and either biopsy or removal of the mass, is usually carried out to ascertain its nature. Some benign tumours, e.g. meningiomas, can be removed in their entirety without unacceptable damage to surrounding structures.
- Radiotherapy is usually recommended for gliomas and radiosensitive metastases.
- Medical treatment. This is palliative to reduce the symptoms related to cerebral oedema and raised intracranial pressure. Dexamethasone (either orally or intravenously), a very potent corticosteroid, may

produce a dramatic improvement in symptoms. The prognosis is very poor in patients with malignant tumours, with only 50% surviving 1 year.

# Hydrocephalus (K&C p. 1201)

Hydrocephalus is a condition marked by an excessive amount of CSF within the cranium. CSF is produced in the cerebral ventricles and normally flows downward into the central canal of the spinal cord and then out into the subarachnoid space, from where it is reabsorbed. Hydrocephalus occurs when there is obstruction to the outflow of CSF; rarely it is the result of increased production of CSF.

## Aetiology

In children, hydrocephalus may be caused by a congenital malformation of the brain (e.g. Arnold–Chiari malformation), meningitis or haemorrhage causing obstruction to the flow of CSF. In adults hydrocephalus is caused by:

- A late presentation of a congenital malformation
- Cerebral tumours in the posterior fossa or brainstem which obstruct the aqueduct or fourth-ventricle outflow
- Subarachnoid haemorrhage, head injury and meningitis
- Normal-pressure hydrocephalus, in which there is dilatation of the cerebral ventricles without signs of raised intracranial pressure. It presents in elderly people with dementia, urinary incontinence and ataxia.

## Clinical features

The features are of headache, vomiting and papilloedema caused by raised intracranial pressure. There may be ataxia and bilateral pyramidal signs.

## Management

Treatment is by the surgical insertion of a shunt between the ventricles and the right atrium or peritoneum (ventriculoatrial or ventriculoperitoneal).

# Headache, migraine and facial pain
(*K&C* p. 1201)

## Tension headache (*K&C* p. 1201)

Tension headaches feel like pressure or tightness all around the head and there are no associated features of migraine (aura, nausea, photophobia). The precise pathophysiology is not known. Treatment consists of reassurance, simple analgesia such as paracetamol, and tricyclic antidepressants for patients with chronic headaches requiring daily analgesics.

## Migraine (*K&C* p. 1202)

Migraine is recurrent headache associated with both visual and gastrointestinal disturbance; in spite of the origin of the word, it does not invariably mean unilateral headache.

### Epidemiology

The prevalence of migraine is approximately 10%; some patients have a strong family history. Onset is usually before the age of 30 years.

### Pathogenesis

The cause of migraine remains controversial. The headache is due to vasodilatation or oedema of blood vessels, with stimulation of the nerve endings near affected extracranial meningeal arteries. Release of vaso-active substances such as nitric oxide are thought to play a role. Serotonin (5-hydroxytryptamine, 5-HT) also plays a role in the pathogenesis.

### Clinical features

The diagnosis of migraine is clinical. There are transient prodromal symptoms followed after 15–60 minutes by a throbbing headache which is often unilateral and accompanied by nausea, vomiting and photophobia. The headache may last for some days and is made worse by physical exertion. Prodromal symptoms are usually visual: scotomata, unilateral blindness, hemianopic field loss, flashes and fortification spectra. Other prodromal symptoms include aphasia, tingling, numbness and weakness of one side of the body. Migraine may also occur without these prodromal symptoms. The most common way in which a migraine attack resolves is through sleep.

## Differential diagnosis

The sudden onset of headache may be similar to meningitis or subarachnoid haemorrhage. The hemiplegic, visual and hemisensory symptoms must be distinguished from thromboembolic TIAs. In TIAs the maximum deficit is present immediately and headache is unusual (p. 671).

## Management

**General measures** Patients should avoid precipitating factors (chocolate, cheese, too much or too little sleep). Women taking the oral contraceptive pill may be helped by stopping the drug or changing the brand.

### Treatment of the acute attack

- Simple analgesia, e.g. paracetamol, and an antiemetic, e.g. metoclopramide, may be all that is necessary for many patients.
- Triptans, e.g. sumatriptan, naratriptan, zolmitriptan and rizatriptan, are 5-HT$_1$ agonists and constrict the cranial arteries. They are used in patients not responding to simple analgesia and may be given orally, by subcutaneous injection or intranasal spray.
- Ergotamine is less commonly used since the introduction of triptans. It may be given orally, rectally, intravenously or by nasal inhalation. Triptans and ergotamine are contraindicated in patients with ischaemic heart disease and peripheral vascular disease.

**Prophylaxis** Prophylaxis is indicated for frequent attacks (more than two per month) which do not respond rapidly to treatment. The options are:

- β-Blockers, e.g. propranolol
- Serotonin antagonists: pizotifen and methysergide
- Amitriptyline at night is sometimes helpful.

An occasional side-effect of methysergide is retroperitoneal fibrosis, which precludes its use for more than 6 months.

# Giant cell arteritis (cranial arteritis, temporal arteritis) (K&C p. 1203)

This is a granulomatous arteritis of unknown aetiology occurring chiefly in those over the age of 60 and affecting in particular the extradural arteries. Giant cell arteritis is closely related to polymyalgia rheumatica (p. 262) and these can occur in the same patient.

## Clinical features

There is headache, scalp tenderness (e.g. on combing the hair) and occasionally pain in the jaw and mouth which is characteristically worse on eating (jaw claudication). The superficial temporal artery may become tender, firm and pulseless. Visual loss caused by inflammation and occlusion of the ciliary and/or central retinal artery, occurs in 25% of untreated cases. Systemic features include weight loss, malaise and a low-grade fever.

## Investigations

- ESR is always elevated > 50 mm/h.
- Full blood count may show a normochromic, normocytic anaemia.
- Histology. A temporal artery biopsy, which can be performed under local anaesthetic, usually confirms the diagnosis. However, the granulomatous changes may be patchy and therefore missed.

## Management

High doses of steroids (oral prednisolone, initially 60–100 mg daily) should be started immediately in a patient with typical features, and a temporal artery biopsy obtained as soon as possible (the histological changes remain for up to a week after starting treatment). The steroid dose is gradually reduced, guided by symptoms and the ESR. Long-term steroids may be needed because the risk of visual loss persists.

# Facial pain (K&C p. 1203)

The face is richly supplied with pain-sensitive structures – the teeth, gums, sinuses, temporomandibular joints, jaws and eyes – disease of which causes facial pain. Trigeminal (fifth) nerve lesions (Table 15.5) may also present with facial pain, and this is suggested by the presence of trigeminal sensory or motor loss on physical examination.

# Cluster headaches (migrainous neuralgia)
(*K&C* p. 1203)
Cluster headaches are characterized by recurrent headaches that occur for weeks or months at a time followed by periods of remission. Men are affected more commonly than women with a peak age of onset of 20–50 years. There is a rapid onset of severe unilateral headache which often begins around the eye or temple. Cluster headaches are associated with ipsilateral lacrimation and redness of the eye, rhinorrhoea, and Horner' syndrome. Treatment of an acute attack is with triptans or inhalation of 100% oxygen. Lithium prevents attacks.

# Trigeminal neuralgia
Trigeminal neuralgia (tic douloureux) is a condition of unknown cause, seen most commonly in old age.

## Clinical features
Severe paroxysms of knife-like pain occur in one or more divisions of the trigeminal nerve (p. 655), although rarely in the ophthalmic division. Each paroxysm is stereotyped, brought on by stimulation of a specific 'trigger zone' in the face. The stimuli may be minimal, and include washing, shaving and eating. There are no objective physical signs and the diagnosis is based on the history.

## Management
The anticonvulsant carbamazepine suppresses attacks in most patients. If this fails, thermocoagulation of the trigeminal ganglion or section of the sensory division may be necessary.

## Differential diagnosis
Similar pain may occur with structural lesions involving the trigeminal nerve. These lesions are often accompanied by physical signs, e.g. a depressed corneal reflex.

---

# Diseases of the spinal cord (K&C p. 1205)

The spinal cord extends from C1 (its junction with the medulla) to the vertebral body of L1. The spinal canal below L1 is occupied by lumbar and sacral nerve roots, which group together to form the cauda equina and ultimately extend into the pelvis and thigh (Fig. 15.11). Paraplegia (weakness of both legs) is almost always caused by a spinal cord lesion, as opposed to hemiplegia (weakness of one side of the body), which is usually the result of a lesion in the brain.

## Spinal cord compression (K&C p. 1206)

### Clinical features

Patients present with back pain and spastic paraparesis: there is upper motor neurone weakness in the legs (Table 15.3) and sensory loss below the level of the lesion. Sometimes there is loss of sphincter control with urinary incontinence. There may be painless urinary retention and constipation in the later stages. The onset may be acute (hours to days) or chronic (weeks to months), depending on the cause.

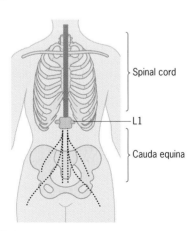

**Fig. 15.11 The spinal cord and cauda equina.** The cord extends from C1 (its junction with the medulla) to the vertebral body of L1. (From Parsons M (1993) A Colour Atlas of Clinical Neurology. London, Mosby Wolfe.)

## Aetiology

The causes of spinal cord compression are listed in Table 15.19; vertebral body neoplasms and disc and vertebral lesions are the commonest causes in developed countries. Spinal tuberculosis is a frequent cause in areas where TB is common, e.g. India, Asia and Africa.

## Investigations

Urgent investigation is essential in a patient with suspected cord compression, especially with acute or subacute onset, because irreversible paraplegia may follow if the cord is not decompressed.

- Spinal X-rays may show degenerative bone disease and destruction of vertebrae by infection or neoplasm.
- MRI identifies the cause and site of cord compression.

## Management

The treatment depends on the cause, but in most cases the initial treatment involves surgical decompression of the cord and stabilization of the spine. Dexamethasone improves outcome in patients with cord compression due to malignancy.

**Table 15.19**
Causes of spinal cord compression

| | |
|---|---|
| Vertebral body neoplasms | Metastases, e.g. from lung, breast, prostate<br>Myeloma<br>Lymphoma |
| Disc and vertebral lesions | Trauma<br>Chronic degenerative disease |
| Inflammatory | Epidural abscess<br>Tuberculosis (Pott's paraplegia) |
| Spinal cord neoplasms | Primary cord neoplasm, e.g. glioma, neurofibroma<br>Metastases |
| Rarities | Paget's disease, bone cysts, osteoporosis<br>Epidural haemorrhage, e.g. patients on warfarin |

### Differential diagnosis
The differential diagnosis is from intrinsic lesions of the cord causing paraparesis. Transverse myelitis (acute inflammation of the cord resulting from viral infection, syphilis or radiation therapy), anterior spinal artery occlusion and multiple sclerosis may present with a rapid onset of paraparesis. A more insidious onset occurs with motor neurone disease, subacute combined degeneration of the cord, and as a non-metastatic manifestation of malignancy. MRI should always be performed in a patient with a sensory or motor level.

Very rarely a parasagittal cortical lesion, e.g. meningioma, may cause paraplegia.

## Syringomyelia and syringobulbia
(*K&C* p. 1206)
Fluid-filled cavities within the spinal cord (myelia) and brainstem (bulbia) are the essential features of these conditions.

### Aetiology
The most frequent cause is blockage of CSF flow from the fourth ventricle in association with an Arnold–Chiari malformation (congenital herniation of the cerebellar tonsils through the foramen magnum). The normal pulsatile CSF pressure waves are transmitted to the delicate tissues of the cervical cord and brainstem, with secondary cavity formation. Hydrocephalus may also occur as a result of disturbed CSF flow.

### Clinical features
Patients usually present in the third or fourth decade with pain and sensory loss (pain and temperature) in the upper limbs. The clinical features are demonstrated in Figure 15.12.

### Investigation
MRI is the investigation of choice and demonstrates the intrinsic cavities.

### Treatment
Surgical decompression of the foramen magnum sometimes reduces the rate of deterioration.

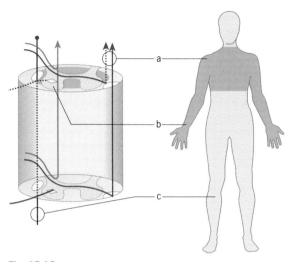

**Fig. 15.12 Production of physical signs in syringomyelia.** Expanding cavities distend the cord. Pain and temperature (a) fibres crossing at that level are destroyed, but sensory fibres in the posterior columns (other sensory modalities) and those that enter the spinothalamic tract at a lower level are spared. Sensory loss is therefore 'dissociated' and confined to the upper trunk and limbs. Further extension damages the anterior horn cells (b), the pyramidal tracts (c) and the medulla, causing wasting in the hands, a spastic paraplegia, nystagmus and a bulbar palsy. (From Parsons M (1993) A Colour Atlas of Clinical Neurology. London, Mosby Wolfe.)

## Friedreich's ataxia (K&C p. 1211)

Friedreich's ataxia is an autosomal recessive disorder and is the most common of the hereditary spinocerebellar degenerations. There is a progressive degeneration of the spinocerebellar tracts and cerebellum causing cerebellar ataxia, dysarthria and nystagmus. Degeneration of the corticospinal tracts causes weakness and an extensor plantar response. The tendon reflexes are absent as a result of peripheral nerve damage. Loss of the dorsal columns causes absent joint position and vibration sense. Other features are pes cavus, optic atrophy, cardiomyopathy, and death by middle age.

## Cauda equina lesion (K&C p. 1219)

Spinal damage at or distal to L1 (a common cause is central prolapse of an intervertebral disc at the lumbosacral junction) injures the cauda equina, which is formed by the lumbar and sacral nerve roots. This produces various mixtures of flaccid paralysis (compare spastic paralysis of a cord lesion above L1), sacral numbness, urinary retention and impotence.

## Management of the paraplegic patient
(*K&C* p. 1207)

The paraplegic patient requires skilled and prolonged nursing care. A pressure-relieving mattress and turning the patient every 2 hours will help to prevent pressure sores. Bladder catheterization (sometimes intermittent self-catheterization) is necessary to prevent urinary stasis and infection. Patients may need manual evacuation of faeces. This may become unnecessary as reflex emptying of the bladder and rectum develops. Passive physiotherapy helps to prevent contractures in paralysed limbs. Severe spasticity may be helped by dantrolene sodium, baclofen or diazepam. Many patients graduate to a wheelchair and maintain some degree of independence.

## Degenerative diseases (*K&C* p. 1208)

### Motor neurone disease (*K&C* p. 1208)

The symptoms of motor neurone disease (MND) are caused by a relentless and unexplained destruction of upper motor neurones and anterior horn cells in the brain and spinal cord, which is usually fatal within 3 years. Most die from respiratory failure as a result of bulbar palsy and pneumonia. It presents in middle age and is more common in men. Motor neurone injury is thought to reflect a complex interplay between genetic factors, oxidative stress, and imbalance of the glutamatergic excitatory control of motor neurones, which may result in damage to critical target proteins and organelles.

### Clinical features

Four clinical patterns may be identified at diagnosis; however, as the disease progresses most patients develop a mixed picture.

- *Progressive muscular atrophy* is a predominantly lower motor neurone lesion of the cord causing weakness, wasting and fasciculation in the hands and arms.
- *Amyotrophic lateral sclerosis* is a combination of disease of the lateral corticospinal tracts and anterior horn cells producing a progressive spastic tetraparesis or paraparesis with added lower motor neurone signs (wasting and fasciculation).
- *Progressive bulbar palsy* results from destruction of upper (pseudobulbar palsy) and lower (bulbar palsy) motor neurones in the lower cranial nerves. There is dysarthria, dysphagia with wasting, and fasciculation of the tongue.
- *Primary lateral sclerosis* is rare. There is a progressive tetraparesis.

There is no involvement of the sensory system or motor nerves to the eyes and sphincters in any of the clinical types.

### Investigations
The diagnosis is clinical. An EMG shows muscle denervation, but this is not a specific finding.

### Differential diagnosis
The differential diagnosis is a cervical spine lesion, which may present with upper and lower motor neurone signs in the arms and legs. It is often distinguished by the presence of sensory signs. Idiopathic multifocal motor neuropathy (Table 15.20) presents with weakness predominantly in the hands and profuse fasciculation.

| **Table 15.20** Causes of mononeuritis multiplex |
| --- |
| Diabetes mellitus |
| Leprosy (the most common cause world-wide) |
| Vasculitis |
| Sarcoidosis |
| Amyloidosis |
| Malignancy |
| Neurofibromatosis |
| HIV infection |
| Guillain–Barré syndrome |
| Idiopathic multifocal motor neuropathy |

### Management
The antiglutamate drug, riluzole, slows progression slightly. Ventilatory support and feeding via a PEG (p. 109) helps prolong survival for some months.

## Spinal muscular atrophies (K&C p. 1209)
This is a group of rare disorders which destroy the anterior horn cells of the spinal cord. Two forms present in adult life, causing a slowly progressive wasting and weakness of the limbs.

## Diseases of the peripheral nerves
(K&C p. 1211)

## Mononeuropathies (K&C p. 1212)
Mononeuropathy is a process affecting a single nerve, and multiple mononeuropathy (or mononeuritis multiplex) is a process affecting several or multiple nerves. Mononeuropathy may be the result of acute compression, particularly where the nerves are exposed anatomically (e.g. the common peroneal nerve at the head of the fibula), or entrapment, where the nerve passes through a relatively tight anatomical passage (e.g. the carpal tunnel). It may also be caused by direct damage, e.g. major trauma, surgery or penetrating injuries.

### Carpal tunnel syndrome
Carpal tunnel syndrome is the most common entrapment neuropathy. It results from pressure on the median nerve as it passes through the carpal tunnel.

### Aetiology
It is usually idiopathic but may be associated with hypothyroidism, diabetes mellitus, pregnancy, obesity, rheumatoid arthritis and acromegaly.

### Clinical features
The history is of pain and paraesthesiae in the hand, typically worse at night, when it may wake the patient. On examination there may be no physical signs or weakness

and wasting of the thenar muscles, and sensory loss of the palm and palmar aspects of the radial three and a half fingers. Tapping on the carpal tunnel may reproduce the pain (Tinnel's sign).

## Management

Treatment with nocturnal splints or local steroid injections gives temporary relief. Surgical decompression is the definitive treatment unless the condition is likely to resolve (e.g. with pregnancy, obesity).

Compression neuropathies may also affect the ulnar nerve (at the elbow), the radial nerve (caused by pressure against the humerus) and the common peroneal nerve (resulting from pressure at the head of the fibula).

## Mononeuritis multiplex

Mononeuritis multiplex often indicates a systemic disorder (Table 15.20); treatment is that of the underlying disease. Acute presentation is most commonly due to vasculitis when prompt treatment with steroids may prevent irreversible nerve damage.

## Polyneuropathy (K&C p. 1214)

Polyneuropathy describes a diffuse, usually symmetrical, disease process that may be acute or chronic and may involve motor, sensory and autonomic nerves, either alone or in combination. Sensory symptoms include numbness, tingling, 'pins and needles', pain in the extremities and unsteadiness on the feet. Numbness typically affects the distal arms and legs in a 'glove and stocking' distribution. Motor symptoms are usually those of weakness. Autonomic neuropathy causes postural hypotension, urinary retention, impotence, diarrhoea (or occasionally constipation), diminished sweating, impaired pupillary responses and cardiac arrhythmias.

Many varieties of neuropathy affect autonomic function to some degree, but occasionally autonomic features predominate. This occurs in diabetes mellitus, amyloidosis and the Guillain–Barré syndrome. A classification of polyneuropathy is given in Table 15.21. In Europe diabetes mellitus is the commonest cause. First-line investigations in a patient

**Table 15.21**
Classification of polyneuropathy

Idiopathic (the majority of cases)
Postinfective (Guillain–Barré syndrome)
Drugs: isoniazid, nitrofurantoin, metronidazole, vincristine
Toxins: excess alcohol, lead poisoning
Metabolic: diabetes mellitus, uraemia, amyloidosis
Vitamin deficiency: $B_1$, $B_6$, $B_{12}$
Non-metastatic manifestation of malignancy
HIV-associated polyneuropathy
Autonomic neuropathies
Neuropathies in connective tissue disease
Hereditary sensorimotor neuropathy

presenting with polyneuropathy include full blood count
and erythrocyte sedimentation rate, serum vitamin $B_{12}$, urea
and electrolytes and liver biochemistry.

## Peroneal muscular atrophy (K&C p. 1216)
Peroneal muscular atrophy (Charcot–Marie–Tooth disease)
is a common clinical syndrome in which there is distal limb
wasting and weakness that progress over many years,
mostly in the legs, with variable loss of sensation and
reflexes. In advanced cases the distal wasting below the
knees is so marked that the legs resemble 'inverted cham-
pagne bottles'. The most common form is inherited in an
autosomal dominant fashion.

## Postinfective polyneuropathy
## (Guillain–Barré syndrome) (K&C p. 1214)
Guillain-Barré syndrome is an acute inflammatory demyeli-
nating polyneuropathy characterized by progressive
muscle weakness and areflexia with recovery being the
rule. It is the most common acute neuropathy.

### Pathogenesis
It is thought to be caused by a cell-mediated immune
response directed at normal peripheral myelin, and this
may be provoked in some cases by preceding infection.

*Campylobacter jejuni* (p. 33) and cytomegalovirus (p. 15) are well-recognized causes.

## Clinical features

There is weakness and numbness (usually symmetrical) in the distal limbs which ascends over days or weeks. Disability ranges from mild to very severe, with involvement of the respiratory and facial muscles. Autonomic features, such as postural hypotension, ileus and bladder atony, are sometimes seen.

## Investigations

The diagnosis is established on clinical grounds and nerve conduction studies; these show slowing of motor conduction consistent with segmental demyelination. CSF protein is typically elevated, with a normal sugar and cell count.

## Differential diagnosis

Other causes of neuromuscular paralysis (botulism, poliomyelitis, primary muscle diseases, hypokalaemia) are rare and can usually be excluded on clinical grounds and investigation. MRI of the spine may be needed to exclude spinal cord compression.

## Management

Monitor:

1. Vital capacity 4-hourly, to recognize respiratory muscle weakness. A fall below 80% of predicted is an indication for transfer to ITU and possible mechanical ventilation.
2. ECG to document cardiac dysrhythmias associated with autonomic dysfunction.

713

Intravenous immune globulin and plasmapheresis improve outcome in severe disease. Supportive treatment includes heparin to prevent thrombosis, physiotherapy to prevent contractures and nasogastric or PEG feeding for patients with swallowing problems. Visiting and counselling services are offered by past patients through the Guillain–Barré Syndrome Support Group (http://www.gbs.org.uk).

# Vitamin deficiency neuropathies (K&C p. 1216)

## Thiamin (vitamin B₁)

Alcohol abuse is the most common cause of thiamin deficiency in the West. Presentation is with the Wernicke–Korsakoff syndrome (p. 537). Severe deficiency causes the clinical syndrome of beri-beri (polyneuropathy, Wernicke's encephalopathy and cardiac failure), rarely seen in western countries. Treatment is with intravenous or oral thiamine (50 mg daily).

## Pyridoxine (vitamin B₆)

Deficiency causes mainly a sensory neuropathy. It may be precipitated during isoniazid therapy (which complexes with pyridoxal phosphate) for tuberculosis in those who acetylate the drug slowly, and prophylactic pyridoxine (10 mg daily) is given with isoniazid.

## Vitamin B₁₂

Deficiency causes the syndrome of *subacute combined degeneration of the cord*. This comprises distal sensory loss (particularly the posterior column), absent ankle jerks (as a result of the neuropathy) and evidence of cord disease (exaggerated knee jerk reflexes, extensor plantar responses). Treatment is with intramuscular vitamin B₁₂ (p. 174), which reverses the peripheral nerve damage but has little effect on the CNS (cord and brain signs).

# Diseases of voluntary muscle

(K&C p. 1219)

## Myopathies

Weakness is the predominant feature of a myopathy. The myopathies are divided into those that are inherited (muscular dystrophies), inflammatory lesions (the most common is polymyositis, p. 260) and those associated with drugs, toxins and endocrine disease. The latter group usually produces weakness of the limb girdles (proximal myopathy), Table 15.22. However, severe hypokalaemia may produce a generalized flaccid weakness.

**Table 15.22**
Causes of a proximal myopathy

Prolonged high-dose steroid therapy
Cushing's syndrome
Thyrotoxicosis
Hypothyroidism (occasionally)
Osteomalacia
Hypokalaemia
Prolonged alcohol abuse
Other drugs, e.g. diamorphine, lithium, quinine, chloroquine

# Muscular dystrophies (K&C p. 1223)

Muscular dystrophies are an inherited group of progressive myopathic disorders resulting from defects in a number of genes needed for normal muscle function. The Duchenne and Becker muscular dystrophies are inherited as X-linked recessive traits caused by a mutation in the dystrophin gene on chromosome 21. Patients with Duchenne muscular dystrophy present in early childhood with weakness in the proximal muscles of the leg. There is progression to other muscle groups with severe disability and death in the late teens. There is no curative treatment. Patients with Becker muscle dystrophy present later and the degree of clinical involvement is milder. Other dystrophies present later in life and are summarized in Table 15.23.

**Table 15.23**
Limb girdle and facioscapulohumeral dystrophies

|  | **Limb girdle** | **Facioscapulohumeral** |
|---|---|---|
| Inheritance | Autosomal recessive | Autosomal dominant |
| Onset | 10–20 years | 10–40 years |
| Muscle affected | Shoulder and pelvic girdle | Face, shoulder and pelvic girdle |
| Progress | Severe disability in 20–25 years | Normal life expectancy |
| Pseudohypertrophy | Rare | Very rare |
| Serum CPK levels | Slightly raised | Slightly raised or normal |

CPK, creatine phosphokinase

Diseases of voluntary muscle

# Myasthenia gravis (*K&C* p. 1222)

Myasthenia gravis is an acquired condition characterized by weakness and fatiguability of proximal limb, ocular and bulbar muscles. The heart is not affected. It occurs most commonly in the third decade and is twice as common in women as in men.

## Aetiology

The cause is unknown. Serum IgG antibodies to acetylcholine receptors, in the postsynaptic membrane of the neuromuscular junction, cause receptor loss. Myasthenia gravis is associated with thymic hyperplasia in about 70% of patients under 40 years of age, and in about 10% a thymic tumour is found.

## Clinical features

Fatiguability is the most important feature, with the proximal limb muscles, extraocular muscles and muscles of mastication, speech and facial expression being most commonly involved. Fatigue can be demonstrated by ptosis on sustained upward gaze or asking the patient to sit with the arms outstretched and looking for a slow downward drift. The ocular muscles are the first to be involved in about 65% of patients, resulting in ptosis and complex ocular palsies.

## Investigations

- Acetylcholine receptor antibodies are specific for myasthenia gravis and are found in the serum in 90% of cases of generalized myasthenia gravis.
- The Tensilon test is positive. (Injection of 10 mg edrophonium, an anticholinesterase, results in rapid temporary improvement in weakness.)
- Nerve stimulation tests show a characteristic decrement in evoked potential following stimulation of the motor nerve.
- Mediastinal imaging with CT or MRI to look for a thymoma.

## Management

Anticholinesterases (pyridostigmine, neostigmine) form the mainstay of treatment and the dose is determined by the patient's response.

**In patients without thymoma** Anticholinesterase medication alone is given in mild disease. In patients under 45 with more severe disease thymectomy is usually indicated. This results in improvement in about 65% of cases. Immunosuppressive treatment with steroids and/or azathioprine should be considered in those who fail to respond to thymectomy.

**In patients with thymoma** Thymectomy is indicated in these patients because of the ability of the tumour to invade locally. It is unusual for myasthenia to improve following surgery, and immunosuppressive treatment is usually required.

## Myotonias (K&C p. 1223)

These conditions are characterized by myotonia (delayed muscle relaxation after contraction) which can be demonstrated by difficulty releasing the grasp after shaking hands. Patients tolerate general anaesthetics poorly. The two most common forms are dystrophia myotonica and myotonia congenita, described below.

## Dystrophia myotonica

Dystrophia myotonica is an autosomal dominant condition characterized by progressive distal muscle weakness with myotonia, ptosis, facial muscle weakness and wasting. Other features commonly present are cataracts, frontal baldness, cardiomyopathy, mild mental handicap, glucose intolerance and hypogonadism.

717

## Myotonia congenita

Myotonia congenita is also an autosomal dominant disorder characterized by mild isolated myotonia occurring in childhood and persisting throughout life. The myotonia is often accentuated by rest and cold.

# Dementia and delirium

## Delirium (toxic confusional state)

(K&C p. 1263)

Delirium is an acute or subacute condition in which impairment of consciousness is accompanied by abnormalities of perception and mood. Impairment of consciousness can vary in severity and often fluctuates (compare with dementia). Confusion is usually worse at night and may be accompanied by hallucinations, delusions, restlessness and aggression. Many diseases (Table 15.24) can be accompanied by delirium, particularly in the elderly. Infection and drugs are the most common causes.

### Management

Investigation and treatment of the underlying disease should be undertaken. General measures include with-

**Table 15.24**
Causes of delirium

| | |
|---|---|
| Systemic infection | |
| Drugs | Tricyclic antidepressants |
| | Benzodiazepines |
| | Opiates |
| | Anticonvulsants |
| Drug/alcohol withdrawal | |
| Metabolic disturbance | Hepatic failure |
| | Renal failure |
| | Disorders of electrolyte balance |
| | Hypoxia |
| | Hypoglycaemia |
| Vitamin deficiency | Vitamin $B_{12}$ |
| | Vitamin $B_1$ |
| | (Wernicke–Korsakoff syndrome) |
| Brain damage | Trauma |
| | Tumour |
| | Abscess |
| | Subarachnoid haemorrhage |

drawing all drugs where possible, rehydration, and adequate pain relief and sedation. The patient should be nursed in a quiet area of the ward. Sedation should only be used if the patient is at risk of self-injury or aggressive behaviour interferes with management. Benzodiazepines are usually the drugs of choice, although in severe delirium intramuscular haloperidol (2.5–5 mg) may be preferred. Management of alcohol withdrawal is summarized on page 538.

## Dementia (K&C p. 1264)

Dementia is characterized by a disturbance of multiple higher cortical functions, including memory, thinking, orientation, comprehension, calculation, learning capacity, language and judgement. Consciousness is not, however, clouded. Dementia affects about 10% of those aged 65 years and over, and 20% of those over 80. There are numerous causes of dementia (Table 15.25), although by far the most common is Alzheimer's disease, which accounts for 70%.

### Alzheimer's disease

Alzheimer's disease is a primary degenerative cerebral disease of unknown aetiology.

### *Clinical features*

There is an insidious onset with steady progression over years. Short-term memory loss is usually the most prominent early symptom, but subsequently there is slow

**Table 15.25**
Causes of dementia

Alzheimer's disease
Multiple cerebral infarction
Excess alcohol (Wernicke–Korsakoff syndrome)
Hypothyroidism
Intracranial mass: subdural haematoma, hydrocephalus
Chronic traumatic encephalopathy, e.g. punch drunkenness
Vitamin $B_{12}$ deficiency
Syphilis
Creutzfeldt–Jakob disease
Huntington's chorea
Late Parkinson's disease

disintegration of the personality and intellect, eventually affecting all aspects of cortical function. There are characteristic pathological features, which include neuronal reduction in several areas of the brain, neurofibrillary tangles, argentophile plaques, consisting largely of amyloid protein, and granulovacuolar bodies.

## Investigations

The presence of dementia is usually diagnosed clinically by a simple assessment of the mental state (Table 15.26). Exclusion of rare treatable causes of dementia (Table 15.25) should also be considered and blood taken for a full blood count, liver biochemistry, and measurement of vitamin $B_{12}$ and folate. A brain CT scan should be performed in younger patients or those with an atypical presentation. A social and family history will help to assess how vulnerable the person is in the community and what plans for support will need to be made.

## Management

In most cases there is no specific therapy although the associated anxiety and depression often need treatment. Attempts to therapeutically augment cholinergic activity have been based on the observations that there is impaired cortical cholinergic function as a result of reduced cerebral

---

**Table 15.26**
Simple clinical assessment of the mental state

Age
Time to nearest hour
Address for recall at the end of the test (house number and street name)
Year
Place – name of hospital
Recognition of 2 people (e.g. doctor, nurse)
Date of birth
Year of 1st World War
Name of present monarch
Count backwards 20 to 1

Each correct answer scores one mark. Healthy patients score > 8

production of choline acetyl transferase and a decrease in acetylcholine synthesis. Acetylcholinesterase inhibitors (donepezil, rivastigmine and galantamine) increase cholinergic transmission by inhibiting cholinesterase at the synaptic cleft. They have a modest benefit and slow intellectual deterioration in patients with mild to moderate Alzheimer's disease. Patients should be managed in the community as much as possible. A whole range of supportive interventions for both patient and carers is needed. Home care, day care, respite care and sitter services are all needed at various points during the progression of the disease. At some point long-term institutional care in a residential or nursing home may be required.

## Prognosis

The typical course is one of progressive decline. The average survival is 8–10 years.

## Vascular (multi-infarct) dementia

This is the second most common cause of dementia and can be distinguished by its history of onset, clinical features and subsequent course. Features that suggest the diagnosis include a stepwise deterioration with declines followed by short periods of stability. There is usually a history of transient ischaemic attacks, although the dementia may follow a succession of acute cerebrovascular accidents or, less commonly, a single major stroke. There may be other evidence of arteriopathy.

# 16 **Dermatology**

## Introduction

Skin diseases are extremely common, although their exact prevalence is unknown. There are over 1000 different entities described, but two-thirds of all cases are the result of fewer than 10 conditions. The most common include acne, eczema, psoriasis, warts and infections caused by bacteria (*K&C* p. 1274), fungi (*K&C* p. 1278) and viruses (*K&C* p. 1276). Some conditions may be part of normal development, e.g. acne; others may be inherited, e.g. Ehlers–Danlos syndrome; still others are part of a systemic disease, e.g. the rash of systemic lupus erythematosus.

Only the most common skin conditions will be described in the following sections.

## Common skin conditions

### Acne vulgaris (*K&C* p. 1292)

Acne vulgaris is a common condition affecting almost 90% of adolescents. It is thought to result from hyperactivity of the sebaceous glands leading to increased production of sebum with blockage of the follicular openings and the formation of comedones (blackheads), inflammatory papules, nodules and cysts. Normal skin bacteria, principally *Propionibacterium acnes*, within the blocked follicle are capable of producing pro-inflammatory mediators and lipolytic enzymes, which may be responsible for producing the clinical lesions.

### Clinical features

Non-inflammatory lesions include open and closed comedones. Closed comedones (whiteheads) are flesh-coloured papules with an apparently closed overlying surface. Open comedones (blackheads) appear as black plugs which distend the follicular orifice, the pigmentation being provided by oxidation of melanin pigment. These are often the forerunners of the more severe inflammatory lesions, such as papules, pustules, nodules and cysts. Other features that may be present include hypertrophic or keloidal scarring, and hyperpigmentation, which occurs predominantly in patients with darker complexions.

## Management

Acne should be actively treated to avoid unnecessary scarring and psychological distress. There are a variety of approaches to treatment, the choice of which depends on the severity of the disease.

### Topical treatments

- Local applications such as abrasives, astringents or exfoliatives are useful in mild disease.
- Tretinoin applied topically is useful in reversing abnormal follicular keratinization and reducing microcomedo formation. Clinical efficacy may take 3–4 months to become apparent.
- Antibiotics such as clindamycin and erythromycin applied topically are useful in mild to moderate inflammatory disease.
- Other agents, such as salicylic acid, benzoyl peroxide and, more recently, topical isotretinoin, are occasionally used.

### Systemic treatments

- Oral antibiotics, e.g. tetracycline or erythromycin, are indicated in those with moderate to severe disease, where topical treatment has failed, and those with involvement of the shoulders and back. Treatment over several months is often necessary.
- Isotretinoin (a vitamin A analogue given orally) is used in severe cystic disease that is unresponsive to other treatments. Although highly effective it is associated with several adverse effects. Most importantly this drug is highly teratogenic and is absolutely contraindicated during pregnancy. All women of childbearing age should be given the oral contraceptive pill during treatment with isotretinoin.
- Hormonal treatment with the oral contraceptive pill or an antiandrogen such as cyproterone acetate may be useful in women.

# Psoriasis (K&C p. 1287)

Psoriasis is a chronic hyperproliferative disorder character-ized by the presence of well-demarcated silvery-scaled plaques over extensor surfaces such as the elbows and knees, and in the scalp. It can affect any group with equal sex incidence, and occurs in about 2% of people in temper-ate zones.

## Aetiology

The cause of the condition is unknown, although genetic factors are felt to be important. It is associated with several HLA-specific antigens, particularly HLA-CW6. Trigger factors in genetically susceptible individuals include infec-tions (particularly streptococcal), local trauma, drugs such as lithium carbonate and β-blockers, and probably also stress.

## Clinical features

Several clinical patterns are recognized:

- Plaque psoriasis is the most common, occurring as well-demarcated, salmon-pink silvery scaling lesions on the extensor surfaces of the limbs, particularly the elbows and knees. Scalp involvement is common and is most often seen at the hair margin or over the occiput. Nail involvement, which can occur alone or in association with psoriasis elsewhere, is manifest as pitting and onycholysis (separation of the nail from the underlying vascular bed). The arthropathy associated with psoriasis is described on page 249.
- Flexural psoriasis presents as pinkish glazed lesions that are well demarcated and non-scaly. The groin, perianal and genital skin are most commonly involved.
- Pustular psoriasis most commonly affects the palms or soles. There are areas of well-demarcated scaling and erythema associated with white, yellow or green pustule formation. Identical features are seen as one of the cutaneous features of Reiter's syndrome (keratoderma blenorrhagica, p. 249).
- Erythrodermic psoriasis is a severe and potentially life-threatening condition. The trunk and limbs may be

involved by an almost universal scaling, sometimes associated with generalized pustule formation. This disease occurs classically following corticosteroid therapy.

## Management

The approach depends on the severity of the disease. As no treatment is universally effective, simple local treatment is used for mild disease, with systemic therapy reserved for severe or pustular psoriasis.

***Local therapy*** Topical steroids, dithranol (inhibits DNA synthesis), calcipotriol (topical vitamin $D_3$) and occasionally coal tar may all be useful for relatively mild disease, and are suitable for use on an outpatient basis.

### Systemic therapy

- Oral retinoic acid derivatives, e.g. acitretin or etretinate, are useful in severe erythrodermic or pustular psoriasis. Although effective, these agents are potentially toxic and also teratogenic. They should not therefore be used in women of childbearing ages.
- Low-dose oral methotrexate (7.5–20 mg once a week) can be highly effective, particularly in psoriatic arthritis. Other immunosuppressive agents, such as ciclosporin and tacrolimus, are sometimes useful in severe intractable disease, although toxicity often limits their long-term use.

***PUVA*** Psoralens (photosensitizing agents taken by mouth) and high-intensity ultraviolet A light (UVA) are usually highly effective for treating extensive psoriasis. Repeated treatments, however, carry the risk of UV-induced skin cancer.

## Eczema (*K&C* p. 1282)

Eczema is characterized by superficial skin inflammation with vesicles (when acute), redness, oedema, oozing, scaling and usually pruritus. The terms 'dermatitis' and 'eczema' are usually used interchangeably, as both conditions show similar inflammatory changes in the skin.

Eczema may arise from several different stimuli, but most commonly it is classified as:

- Endogenous (atopic)
- Exogenous due to allergy or chemical irritation.

## Atopic eczema

### Aetiology

The cause of this condition is not fully understood but there is a selective activation of TH2-type CD4 lymphocytes in the skin which drives the inflammatory process, resulting in a capacity to hyperreact to many environmental factors. There are high levels of serum IgE antibodies, although their significance in contributing to the pathogenesis is unclear. There is also a significant hereditary predisposition.

### Clinical features

The disease may start in the first few weeks of life with erythema, weeping, itching and scaling. In adults the flexures at the neck, elbow, wrist and knee are commonly involved.

### Management

The offending agents should be removed if possible. Regular use of emollients, such as aqueous cream or emulsifying ointments, is useful in hydrating the skin. Corticosteroid creams, e.g. 1% hydrocortisone, form the mainstay of treatment.

### Exogenous eczema (contact dermatitis)

In this condition there is acute or chronic skin inflammation, often sharply demarcated, produced by substances in contact with the skin. It may be caused by a primary chemical irritant, or may be the result of a type IV hypersensitivity reaction. Common chemical irritants are industrial solvents used in the workplace, or cleaning and detergent solutions used in the home. With allergic dermatitis there is sensitization of T lymphocytes over a period of time, which results in itching and dermatitis upon re-exposure to the antigen.

### Clinical features

An unusual pattern of rash with clear-cut demarcation or odd-shaped areas of erythema and scaling should arouse suspicion and, in combination with a careful history, should indicate a cause. Patch testing, where the suspected allergen is placed in contact with the skin, is often useful in identifying a suspected allergen.

### Management

Causative agents should be removed where possible. Steroid creams are useful for short periods in severe disease. Antipruritic agents are used for symptomatic relief of itching.

## Erythema nodosum (K&C p. 1297)

Erythema nodosum is an acute and sometimes recurrent paniculitis which produces painful nodules or plaques on the shins, with occasional spread to the thighs or arms. Adult females are most commonly affected. Histological features suggest that this is an immunological reaction with immune complex deposition within dermal vessels. In 50% of cases no obvious cause is found. Other causes are listed in Table 16.1.

**Table 16.1**
Some causes of erythema nodosum

| | |
|---|---|
| Drugs | Oral contraceptive pill |
| | Penicillin |
| | Sulphonamides |
| Systemic diseases | Sarcoidosis* |
| | Inflammatory bowel disease* |
| Infection | Bacteria and viruses* |
| |   Streptococcal* |
| |   Tuberculosis |
| |   Leprosy |
| |   Cat scratch disease |
| |   Tularaemia |
| |   *Chlamydia* spp. |
| |   Psittacosis |
| |   Lymphogranuloma venereum |
| | Fungal |
| |   Histoplasmosis |
| |   Coccidioidomycosis |
| |   Blastomycosis |
| Pregnancy | |

* The most common causes

## Clinical features

Painful nodules or plaques up to 5 cm in diameter appear in crops over 2 weeks, and slowly fade to leave bruising and staining of the skin. Systemic upset is common, with malaise, fever and arthralgia.

## Management

Symptoms should be treated with NSAIDs, light compression bandaging and bed rest. Recovery may take weeks, and recurrent attacks can occur. Dapsone, colchicine or oral prednisolone may be useful in resistant cases.

# Erythema multiforme (K&C p. 1297)

This is an acute self-limiting condition affecting the skin and mucosal surfaces which is probably related to the deposition of immune complexes. Children and young adults are most commonly affected. The disease is commonly associated with:

- Herpes simplex infection
- *Mycoplasma pneumoniae*
- Drugs, e.g. sulphonamides, sulphonylureas and barbiturates
- Connective tissue diseases.

## Clinical features

Symmetrically distributed erythematous papules occur most commonly on the back of the hands, the palms and the forearms. The lesions may show central pallor associated with oedema, bulla formation and peripheral erythema. Severe mucosal disease may predominate in, for example, infection with *Mycoplasma pneumoniae*. Eye changes include conjunctivitis, corneal ulceration and uveitis.

Toxic epidermal necrosis is a severe erythema multiforme with oral and genital ulceration and marked constitutional symptoms.

## Management

The disease is usually self-limiting although the Stevens–Johnson syndrome can be fatal. Offending drugs should be withdrawn and the underlying disease treated. In severe cases intravenous fluids and feeding may be required.

# Pyoderma gangrenosum *(K&C p. 1297)*

This condition presents with erythematous nodules or pustules which frequently ulcerate. The ulcers, which are often large, have a classical bluish black undermined edge and a purulent surface. The aetiology is unknown but it is associated with several conditions such as:

- Inflammatory bowel disease
- Rheumatoid arthritis
- Myeloma, lymphoma
- Primary biliary cirrhosis

### Management

The underlying condition should be treated appropriately. High-dose topical and/or oral steroids are used to prevent progressive ulceration. Other immunosuppressants such as ciclosporin are sometimes used.

# Other diseases affecting the skin

## Marfan's syndrome *(K&C p. 1311)*

Marfan's syndrome is an autosomal dominant disorder of collagen synthesis. Fragility of the skin may lead to bruising. The most obvious abnormalities are skeletal: tall stature, arm span greater than height, arachnodactyly (long spidery fingers), sternal depression, lax joints and a high arched palate. There is often upward dislocation of the lens as a result of weakness of the suspensory ligament. Cardiovascular complications (ascending aortic aneurysm formation, aortic dissection and aortic valve incompetence) are responsible for a greatly reduced life span.

## Ehlers–Danlos syndrome *(K&C p. 1311)*

Inherited defects of collagen lead to fragility and hyperelasticity of the skin, with easy bruising, 'paper-thin' scars and hypermobility of the joints. The walls of the aorta and gut are weak and may rarely rupture with catastrophic results.

# Neurofibromatosis (*K&C* p. 1210 & p. 1300)

Neurofibromatosis is an autosomal dominant disease with distinctive clinical features.

- Type 1 (von Recklinghausen's disease), with the abnormal gene on chromosome 17. Clinical features include multiple cutaneous neurofibromas, multiple 'café-au-lait' spots (light-brown macules of varying size), axillary freckling, scoliosis, and an increased incidence of a variety of neural tumours, e.g. meningioma, eighth-nerve tumours and gliomas.
- Type 2, with the abnormal gene on chromosome 22. Typically bilateral acoustic neuromas and other neural tumours occur.

# 17 Practical procedures

The purpose of this chapter is to describe some of the common practical procedures you may have to undertake as a house officer or, for a few of them, as a medical student. Before attempting them alone you should first perform them with a more experienced colleague. Because of space restrictions only a limited number of procedures have been listed and they are the ones that are carried out on a daily basis or which may have to be performed as an emergency. Elective procedures and those usually performed by more senior colleagues are not discussed.

## General principles for all procedures

A simple and concise explanation of the procedure must be given to the patient. In some cases, e.g. liver biopsy, it is usual to obtain written informed consent, which includes an explanation to the patient of the risks associated with the procedure. At the end of a procedure all needles, syringes and trocars should be disposed of in a sharps bin, and clinical waste, e.g. blood-soaked swabs, disposed of in appropriate disposal bags.

### Sterile procedures

Some procedures are performed under strict aseptic conditions to minimize the risks to the patient of introducing infection. The equipment and methods are similar in each case. The operator washes his or her hands thoroughly with a disinfecting agent such as povidone–iodine (Betadine) or chlorhexidine (Hibiscrub), and wears sterile gloves for the procedure. An assistant, who maintains a no-touch technique, helps to open dressing packs and gives needles and syringes to the operator. The operative field is cleaned with aqueous Betadine or 0.5% chlorhexidine in alcohol and the skin of the selected entry site is isolated with sterile towels.

# Local anaesthesia

A preparation of 1% lidocaine (lignocaine) is usually used for local anaesthesia. The maximum amount used in an adult should be less than 20 mL, although usually much less is necessary. After cleaning the skin a 25 gauge (orange) needle is inserted intradermally and a small bleb raised before infiltrating the deeper tissues with a 23 gauge (blue) needle. Before each injection the plunger of the syringe should be pulled back to ensure that a blood vessel has not been entered.

# Specific procedures

## Venepuncture

### *Equipment*

- Syringe (size will vary according to the amount of blood needed)
- 21 gauge (green) needle
- Tourniquet
- Alcohol swab
- Blood sample tubes as appropriate, label the sample tubes with the patient details after the blood is in them
- Gauze swabs or cotton wool balls.

Many hospitals now employ a vacutainer system where the tubes contain a vacuum and are attached to the needle while it is in the vein. This reduces the chances of a needlestick injury to the operator.

### *Methods*

The antecubital vein in the forearm is an ideal site and, if unsuccessful, more distal sites may be attempted. Palpate the vein to locate its position and make sure it is not an artery (which will pulsate). The tourniquet is applied proximally and the skin over the venepuncture site cleaned with a swab. Allow the skin to dry before proceeding. The skin over the vein is rendered tense with the operator's non-dominant hand, thus immobilizing the vein. The syringe with the needle attached is held in the dominant hand and the needle, with the bevel upwards, is passed at an angle of about 15° through the skin and pointed in the direction of blood flow. Loss of resistance is felt when the vein is entered and blood will appear at the end of the syringe. The required amount of blood is drawn slowly (to prevent both the vein collapsing and red cell haemolysis) up into the syringe. With a vacuum system blood will only appear when the sample tube is pushed onto the needle attachment inside the holder. At the end of the procedure the tourniquet is removed, a dry swab is applied to the venepuncture site and the needle removed from the vein while applying pressure on the swab. Using the non-touch needle-removing device on the sharps bin the needle is removed from the syringe before expelling the blood into the tubes. A butterfly cannula which can be left in situ is used for repeated sampling over a short time period, e.g. a glucose tolerance test.

### If you fail...

It is often easier to palpate a suitable vein than to see it. Vasodilatation may be achieved by exercising the arm (clenching and unclenching the fist), placing it in warm water or gently tapping over the vein. Try other sites, e.g. a vein in the foot.

## Setting up an intravenous (i.v.) cannula

### Indications

- Fluid replacement
- Administration of intravenous drugs (e.g. antibiotics)
- To ensure i.v. access in case of emergency (e.g. coronary care)
- Short-term feeding via a peripheral vein.

### Equipment

- Cannula. The size is determined by the type of fluid to be infused and the size and condition of the patient's veins
- Alcohol swab
- Adhesive tape
- Tourniquet
- 10 mL of 0.9% sodium chloride to flush the cannula
- Infusion fluid (if necessary) already run through a giving set. All i.v. fluids must be checked by a registered nurse. For some fluids, two nurses are

required to check the i.v. fluid. Syringe drivers or pumps are needed to control infusion rate of many solutions
- Sharps bin.

## Procedure

Read the protocol for taking venous blood as the methods are similar. Place the tourniquet around the upper arm and search carefully for a vein. Aim for a palpable vein, preferably away from joints and in the non-dominant arm. Place a towel or pad under the arm. Clean the skin with an alcohol swab and, if a large-bore cannula is being inserted (e.g. 14–16 gauge), anaesthetize the entry site with 2–3 mL of lidocaine (lignocaine) injected intradermally with a 25 gauge needle. Local anaesthetic cream is an alternative and must be applied at least 1 hour prior to the procedure. Once the cannula enters the vein, blood will flash back into the cannula. The cannula can then be advanced along the vein while gently withdrawing but not completely removing the trocar. Remove the tourniquet, occlude the tip of the cannula by pressing on the vein immediately above the end of the cannula with your finger. Remove the trocar and flush the cannula with 5–10 mL of 0.9% saline to ensure patency. Attach the plastic cap or giving set and ensure that the fluid is running adequately. Secure the cannula carefully with tape and dispose of sharps in sharps bin.

## Complications
- 'Tissuing' of drip
- Thrombophlebitis.

## If you fail...
- Come back and try later.
- Vasodilatation may be achieved by exercising the arm (clenching and unclenching the fist), placing it in warm water or gently tapping over the vein.
- Ask a colleague for help.
- Consider subcutaneous fluids: glucose and 0.9% saline, but not drugs, can be administered subcutaneously via a butterfly needle.

# Arterial sampling

## Indications
- Blood gas and acid–base analysis
- Very occasionally if blood cannot be obtained from a vein.

## Equipment
- Dedicated blood gas syringe or standard syringe with 2–3 mL of heparin
- 23 gauge needle
- Cotton-wool balls
- Alcohol swab
- Disposable gloves.

## Procedure
Note the concentration of any inspired oxygen the patient may be receiving. Decide on the site for arterial puncture: brachial, radial or femoral artery. The radial artery (non-dominant arm preferred) at the wrist is the best site for obtaining an arterial sample because it is near to the surface, relatively easy to palpate and stabilize, and usually has a good collateral supply from the ulnar artery. The brachial and femoral arteries do not have a good collateral supply. The femoral artery is more likely to be involved with atheroma, especially in the elderly. Clean the area with the alcohol swab and expel excess heparin from the blood gas syringe. Clean and anaesthetize the skin using local anaesthetic (p. 734). Palpate with three fingers over the course of the artery to determine the area of maximum pulsation. Insert the needle, bevel up, at about 45° to the skin. Once the artery is entered, blood will pulsate into the syringe. If no blood is obtained after the needle has been advanced an appropriate distance, withdraw the needle, exerting gentle traction on the plunger, as blood often enters on removal. If this is not successful the needle must be redirected. Once 1.5–2 mL of blood have been obtained, remove the needle and ask an assistant to apply firm pressure with the cotton wool to the puncture site for 5 minutes. Remove the needle from the syringe and expel any air bubbles. The syringe should be capped and sent for immediate analysis. (Table 17.1).

**Table 17.1**
Normal values for arterial blood gases

| | |
|---|---|
| pH | 7.35–7.45 |
| $P_{CO_2}$ | 4.3–6.0 kPa |
| $P_{O_2}$ | 10.5–14 kPa |
| Base excess | ± 2 mmol/L |
| $HCO_3$ | 22–26 mmol/L |
| $O_2$ saturation | 95–100% |

## Complications
- Arterial spasm and ischaemia
- Dislodgement of atheroma from femoral artery.

## If you fail...
Do not persist with several attempts but ask a colleague for help.

# Central venous cannulation

## Indications
- Measurement of central venous pressure (CVP)
- Infusion of substances irritant to small veins and tissues, e.g. dopamine
- Difficulty in obtaining peripheral venous access
- Administration of drugs during a cardiac arrest
- Modified central venous lines are used for administration of intravenous feeding, insertion of a Swan–Ganz catheter and temporary transvenous cardiac pacing.

## Contraindications
There are no absolute contraindications, but the cannula is placed away from an area of skin sepsis if possible.

## Equipment
- Materials for a sterile procedure performed under local anaesthetic (p. 733)
- Scalpel and blade
- Central line pack (e.g. Leader-Cath)

- Infusion fluid already run through a giving set, and a three-way tap
- CVP monitoring set if required.

## Method

The aim of central venous cannulation is to place the tip of the cannula in the right atrium or superior vena cava. This is usually achieved by percutaneous puncture of the right internal jugular or subclavian vein. The internal jugular vein is preferred in patients with respiratory disease (the risk of pneumothorax is less than with subclavian vein cannulation) or a bleeding tendency (bleeding can be more easily controlled by direct pressure in the neck if there is inadvertent arterial puncture).

This is a sterile procedure performed under local anaesthesia (p. 733). The patient is placed in a slightly head-down position and a small skin incision (see site, later) made with a scalpel blade in the anaesthetized skin. A needle, used to locate the vein, is attached to a saline-filled syringe and gentle aspiration is maintained as the needle is advanced through the skin and subcutaneous tissues towards the vein. Once in the vein the syringe is removed and the needle occluded with a finger to prevent air embolism. The flexible end of the guidewire is passed down the needle into the vein and the needle removed leaving the guidewire in place. The cannula is loaded on to the guidewire and slid into the vein, before the wire is removed leaving the cannula in position. The giving set is attached to the cannula, which is secured in position by a stitch and transparent adhesive dressing. A chest X-ray is taken as soon as possible after insertion to demonstrate the correct position of the cannula tip and exclude complications such as a pneumothorax.

When removing a central line, remember to place the patient in the head-down position and after removing the cannula press with a gauze pad for a few minutes to prevent bleeding and air embolus.

**Internal jugular vein puncture** The internal jugular vein runs behind the sternomastoid lateral to the carotid artery. The line of the carotid artery is located with the fingers of the left hand and the site of cannula insertion is chosen as a point at or just above an imaginary line drawn across the cricoid membrane; this avoids damage to structures in the root of the neck. With the right hand the needle is advanced just lateral to the fingers of the left hand and passed parallel to the midline at an angle of 45° to the skin.

**Subclavian vein puncture** The needle is inserted just below the midpoint of the clavicle and advanced along its posterior surface towards the suprasternal notch. The needle and syringe are kept parallel to the coronal plane at all times to avoid puncturing the pleura or subclavian artery.

## Complications
- Puncture of major arteries, pleura and thoracic duct
- Air and catheter embolism
- Catheter-related sepsis
- Venous thrombosis.

## If you fail...
Do not persist with several attempts but ask a senior colleague or anaesthetist for help.

# Measurement of central venous pressure
The CVP is the pressure in the right atrium and may be measured continuously using a pressure transducer, or intermittently using a manometer. A constant zero-reference level is essential for accurate measurement; either the mid-axillary line or the sternal angle is usually used. A mark should be made on the skin to indicate the level so that all subsequent readings are made from the same point. The normal value is between 0–4 and 3–7 $cmH_2O$, measured from the sternal angle and mid-axillary line, respectively, as the zero-reference points (Fig. 17.1).

740

1. With the three-way tap in position 'A' allow the 0.9% sodium chloride infusion to run rapidly for a few seconds to check that the line is patent.
2. Stop the infusion using the roller clamp and adjust the three-way tap on the manometer to position 'B'. Gradually open the roller clamp to allow fluid to fill

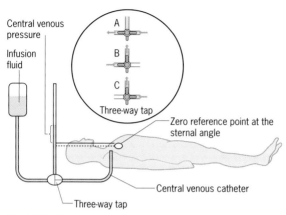

Central venous pressure

Infusion fluid

A

B

C

Three-way tap

Zero reference point at the sternal angle

Central venous catheter

Three-way tap

**Fig. 17.1 Measurement of central venous pressure using the mid-axillary line as a reference point.** (After Nicol M (2000) Essential Nursing Skills. St Louis, Mosby.)

the manometer column to about 5–10 cm. Close the roller clamp.

3. The manometer tube is connected to the patient by closing off the three-way tap to the infusion fluid (position 'C').

4. The meniscus in the manometer will drop steadily until it moves with respiration above and below a mean pressure. The pressure at the end of respiration is the CVP.

5. The infusion is reconnected to the patient via the three-way tap, thus isolating the manometer. Reset the infusion to the prescribed rate.

## Electrical cardioversion

Cardioversion is the delivery of energy that is synchronized to the QRS complex, whereas defibrillation is non-synchronized delivery of energy, i.e. the shock is delivered randomly during the cardiac cycle (see below).

### Indications

- Elective cardioversion
  - Atrial tachyarrhythmias

- Emergency cardioversion
  - Atrial tachyarrhythmias causing haemodynamic compromise, e.g. hypotension, pulmonary oedema
  - Ventricular tachycardia (VT)
  - Ventricular fibrillation (VF).

## Contraindications

Digitalis toxicity (relative contraindication) – induction of ventricular arrhythmias by cardioversion is more likely.

## Equipment

- Defibrillator
- Self-adhesive monitor–defibrillator pad electrodes
- Intravenous cannula in situ.

## Method

General anaesthesia is necessary in a conscious patient to induce amnesia and avoid the pain of the tetanic muscular contraction induced by the electric current through the thorax. Lay the patient flat. If in bed, remove pillows and the head of the bed. The two electrodes are placed in a position that will maximize transmyocardial current flow, and this is usually achieved by placing one at the apex of the heart and the other over the right second intercostal space. For all arrhythmias except VF the defibrillator should be enabled to deliver a synchronized shock, i.e. the shock is delivered on the R wave of the QRS complex. Failure to deliver a synchronized shock may induce VF. Energy selection in cardioversion is arrhythmia dependent (Table 17.2).

**Table 17.2**
Energy requirements for arrhythmias

| Arrhythmia | Initial shock energy (J) | Subsequent shocks (J) |
| --- | --- | --- |
| Supraventricular tachycardia | 100 | 200, 360, 360 |
| Atrial flutter | 50 | 100, 200, 300, 360 |
| Atrial fibrillation | 200 | 360, 360 |
| Ventricular arrhythmias | 200 | 200, 360 |

Before delivering the shock the operator must make sure that no-one, including him- or herself, has any contact with the patient either directly or indirectly, e.g. by touching the bed on which the patient is lying. The operator usually calls 'stand back' before delivering the shock.

## Complications
- Superficial burns to the skin
- Induction of arrhythmias
- Systemic embolization. This complication is more likely to occur in patients with AF who have not been anticoagulated prior to cardioversion (p. 379)
- Myocardial damage from excessive energy.

## If it fails...
Ensure the electrodes have been correctly placed. Consider a change of electrode position, e.g. anterior and posterior chest walls. Stop the procedure after a maximum of seven shocks in elective cardioversion. Consider chemical cardioversion with antiarrhythmic drugs.

A difficult decision is when to stop resuscitation and defibrillation efforts in a patient who is not responding. This depends on the patient, the circumstances of the arrest and how long the patient has had a non-perfusing cardiac rhythm. In general, if a patient arrests in hospital and resuscitation has not resulted in a perfusing cardiac rhythm after 30 minutes then further attempts are unlikely to be successful. The prognosis is poorer in patients who arrest outside hospital. There are exceptions: resuscitation is continued for longer in a hypothermic patient.

# Pleural aspiration

## Indications
- Diagnostic
    - To investigate the cause of a pleural effusion. A pleural biopsy is sometimes performed at the same time, as this increases the diagnostic yield
- Therapeutic
    - To drain large effusions for symptom relief
    - To instil therapeutic agents such as sclerosants.

## Equipment

- Materials for a sterile procedure performed under local anaesthesia (p. 733)
- Specimen containers
- For diagnostic tap: 20 mL syringe with 21 gauge needle
- For therapeutic tap:
  - 50 mL syringe with Luer-Lock fitting
  - Three-way tap
  - 14 gauge cannula
  - Receiver for fluid.

## Method

This is a sterile procedure performed with a local anaesthetic (p. 733). The patient should be sitting up and leaning over a suitably placed bed table with the arms folded in front of the body. The upper limit of the effusion posteriorly is determined from the chest X-ray and by percussion. The skin and subcutaneous tissues overlying the intercostal space at the chosen level are infiltrated with lidocaine (lignocaine) and the area anaesthetized down to the pleura. The needle is passed over the upper border of the rib to avoid damaging the subcostal neurovascular bundle. For a diagnostic tap 20 mL of fluid is aspirated, placed into appropriate containers and sent for microscopy and culture, cytology and protein concentration.

## If it fails …

If you cannot obtain any fluid try a different space, usually higher up. If fluid cannot be aspirated or only a small amount is obtained (e.g. with a loculated effusion) an ultrasound examination will identify whether fluid is actually present and, if so, the most promising site for aspiration can be marked.

744

## Complications

- Pneumothorax
- Pulmonary oedema; the risk is greatest with the rapid removal of large quantities of fluid (>1 litre)
- Damage to the neurovascular bundle which lies in the subcostal groove

- Infection
- Seeding of malignant cells along the tract with a malignant effusion.

## Chest drain insertion

### Indications
- Aspiration of air (pneumothorax)
- Aspiration of fluid (blood, effusions, pus).

### Equipment
- Materials for a sterile procedure performed under local anaesthetic (p. 733)
- Scalpel blade
- Chest drain
- Underwater-seal bottle and connecting tubing
- '0' or '1' silk or nylon suture
- Artery forceps
- Dressings.

### Procedure

This is a sterile procedure performed under local anaesthetic. The 4th–5th intercostal space in the mid-axillary line is preferred, although the second interspace in the mid-clavicular line can be used in an emergency. For the former approach the patient should be sitting up and leaning over a suitably placed bed table, with the arms folded in front of the body. A 28 French gauge or larger drain should be used for blood to minimize blockage. A 24 French gauge is adequate for air or low-viscosity effusions. The skin, underlying muscle and pleura should be infiltrated with 8–10 mL of 1% lidocaine (lignocaine), advancing over the upper border of the rib below to avoid the subcostal neurovascular bundle. Aspiration should be applied intermittently until the pleural cavity is entered and the presence of air or fluid confirmed. A 1 cm incision is made with the scalpel and a purse-string suture inserted loosely around the incision. Access to the pleural cavity through the intercostal muscles is obtained by blunt dissection using a pair of artery forceps, and the track widened to allow the passage of a finger. The length of tube required is measured and inserted, *without the use of the central trocar,* into the pleural cavity. The drain is connected to the underwater drainage system and secured with the purse-string suture and taped to the chest wall. The tube is then connected to the underwater drainage system and unclamped. If correctly placed, bubbling, drainage of fluid if present, and respiratory swing should be evident. The position of the tube and expansion of the lung are then checked with a chest X-ray. To remove the chest drain, ask the patient to exhale, remove the drain, and tighten the purse-string suture to close the incision.

### Complications
- Injury to the neurovascular bundle
- Re-expansion pulmonary oedema
- Infection.

## Nasogastric tube insertion
### Indications
- To drain gastric secretions, e.g. prior to surgery, acute pancreatitis or for bowel obstruction
- For enteral feeding (using a fine-bore tube).

### Equipment
- Nasogastric tube of appropriate size and type, e.g. large-bore (Ryles tube) for drainage of secretions
- Lidocaine (lignocaine) lubricating jelly
- Large-bore syringe
- Litmus paper
- Drainage bag
- Receiver or vomit bowl
- Adhesive tape.

### Procedure
Ask the patient to sit up if possible and protect the patient's clothing with a towel. Estimate the length of tube to be inserted by measuring the distance from the patient's nose to the tip of the earlobe and then to the xiphisternum and mark this distance on the tube. Ask the patient to clear the nasal passages by blowing the nose and select the best nostril. Lubricate the distal end of the tube with jelly and place into the nostril, advancing slowly along the floor of

the nostril to the nasopharynx. As the tube enters the pharynx, ask the patient to take a sip of water and to swallow as you advance the tube into the oesophagus. Once the tube has reached the measured distance and is thought to be in the stomach, aspirate fluid with the syringe and test for acid with litmus paper (blue to pink). In addition, insert 5–10 mL of air into the tube while a colleague listens over the stomach with a stethoscope to hear the air entering as a gurgling sound. It is not possible to aspirate through fine-bore feeding tubes, and therefore the correct position must be confirmed with a chest X-ray prior to commencing feeding. If a fine-bore tube has been used, remove the guidewire following X-ray. Remember to secure the tube to the nose with adhesive tape.

## Complications
- Aspiration
- Gastro-oesophageal reflux
- Local trauma to nose.

## If you fail...
- Try the other nostril
- Put tube in the refrigerator, which usually causes it to stiffen.

# Digital examination of the rectum

Place the patient in the left lateral position with the buttocks at the edge of the couch and ask the patient to curl up with the knees towards the chest. Wear a disposable glove on the right hand and separate the patient's buttocks with both hands. Examine the perineum and anus for inflammation, skin tags, external piles, fissures, fistulae and sinuses. If a prolapse is suspected ask the patient to bear down and look for the rectal mucosa or bowel appearing through the anus.

Put some lubricant on the index finger of the right hand and place the pulp of the finger flat on the anus. Introduce the finger into the anal canal by pushing gently in a slightly backwards direction. Extreme pain and spasm of the anal sphincter at this stage suggest an anal fissure, which may make further examination impossible. The lower end of the fissure, which is usually situated posteriorly, may be visible if the buttocks are gently separated. To examine the rectum, the finger is advanced and rotated through 180°C so that the pulp of the finger lies anteriorly. The walls of the rectum are normally smooth and soft, and any deviation, e.g. polyps, carcinoma, should be noted. Posteriorly the coccyx and sacrum can be felt through the rectal wall, and anteriorly the prostate gland in men and the cervix in women. The normal prostate gland is smooth and firm with a shallow midline groove separating two lateral lobes. A hard, irregular gland with loss of the median groove is characteristic of carcinoma.

After withdrawal, the examining finger should be inspected for blood and the colour of the faeces noted.

# Abdominal paracentesis

## Indications
- To investigate the cause of ascites
- Rapid relief of large-volume ascites.

## Equipment
- Materials for a sterile procedure performed under local anaesthetic (p. 733)
- For diagnostic tap: 20 mL syringe with 21 gauge needle
- For therapeutic tap
  - Large-bore (14 gauge) cannula with three-way tap
  - Collecting system and specimen containers
  - Intravenous giving set and plasma expander.

## Procedure
This is a sterile procedure performed under local anaesthesia (p. 733). Place the patient in a semirecumbent position and confirm the presence of ascites clinically.

Clean and anaesthetize the skin over the right flank. For a diagnostic tap, a standard 21 gauge (green) needle attached to a 20 mL syringe is introduced along the anaesthetized track to the peritoneal cavity and fluid aspirated and sent for white cell count, microscopy and culture, and measurement of protein and amylase. For therapeutic paracentesis a large-bore cannula is introduced in a similar fashion until fluid is aspirated. The stylet is then removed and a 50 mL syringe and collecting system is attached to the cannula via a three-way tap. Aspiration is continued until the desired volume of fluid is removed. If large-volume paracentesis is planned (> 3–4 L) an intravenous drip should be set up and albumin infused at a concentration of 8 g per litre of fluid removed. Following the procedure a simple dry dressing is applied.

## Complications
- Infection
- Ascitic fluid leak
- Puncture of intra-abdominal viscus
- Renal impairment and encephalopathy after large-volume paracentesis in patients with cirrhosis.

### If it fails...
Ask the radiologist to perform the procedure under ultra-sound control.

# Sengstaken tube insertion

## Indications
Variceal bleeding not controlled pharmacologically or by injection sclerotherapy.

## Equipment
- Sengstaken tube
- 50 mL syringe
- Radio-opaque contrast material (e.g. Omnipaque)
- Length of string
- 0.5 litre bag of saline or glucose
- Large collection bowl.

## Procedure
Familiarize yourself with the construction of the tube and identify the four ports: two for aspiration of the oesophagus and stomach, and two for inflation of the oesophageal and gastric balloons (Fig. 17.2). Check the capacity of both the gastric and the oesophageal balloon. With the patient on the left lateral side, insert the tube into the mouth and guide into the pharynx with the fingers. The tube should pass easily down the oesophagus. On entry into the

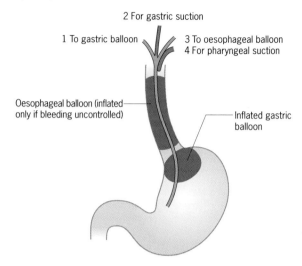

**Fig. 17.2** Diagram of a Sengstaken tube in situ.

stomach, blood is usually readily aspirated through the gastric aspiration port. Insert the tube as far as possible and inflate the gastric balloon with the appropriate volume of fluid (150–250 mL). Using a mixture of water and contrast material aids radiological confirmation of correct placement. The tube is then withdrawn until resistance at the gastro-oesophageal junction is felt. At this stage the 0.5 L bag of fluid is attached with string to the end of the tube and allowed to hang over the side of the bed, so that constant traction is applied to the balloon. It is not normally necessary to inflate the oesophageal balloon. The balloon should be left in place inflated for no longer than 24 hours to minimize the risk of pressure necrosis of the oesophagus.

## Complications
- Oesophageal rupture
- Pressure necrosis leading to oesophageal ulceration and stricture
- Aspiration leading to pneumonia.

# Urine collection and testing

Urine passed into a clean dry vessel is suitable for chemical tests. A mid-stream specimen of urine (MSU) collected into a sterile specimen pot is necessary for microscopy and culture. The urine should be analysed immediately or stored in a refrigerator to reduce the growth of contaminants.

## Urine testing

Commercially prepared paper strips are available to test for urine specific gravity, pH, protein, glucose, ketones, bilirubin, urobilinogen and blood. Usually one strip is impregnated with dyes specific for each test. It is important that the strips are kept in sealed, dry containers and the test areas not handled. The manufacturers' instructions must be followed exactly. The strip is dipped briefly into the urine and its edge then run against the rim of the container to remove excess fluid. The strip is held horizontally (to prevent urine running down the strip and mixing the dyes) and the colour changes read at exactly the times specified by the manufacturer. The colour changes are compared with the colour charts supplied on the outside of the strip containers.

# Bladder catheterization (urethral)

## Indications

- Relief of urinary retention
- To monitor urinary output in the critically ill
- Urinary incontinence
- Collection of an uncontaminated urine specimen for bacteriological analysis.

## Equipment

- Sterile catheter pack (usually prepacked, containing kidney dish, dressing towels, gallipot for sterile saline and gauze swabs)
- Sterile lidocaine (lignocaine) gel with nozzle
- Sterile 0.9% sodium chloride for cleaning
- 12–14 gauge catheter (usually Foley type)
- Sterile gloves

- 20 mL syringe with sterile water
- Catheter bag with stand/holder
- Disposable waterproof absorbent pad.

## Procedure

Place the patient in a supine, slightly reclining position. Women should have their knees flexed and the thighs apart. Remove the bedclothes to expose the genital area and place the disposable pad beneath the buttocks. Wash your hands and open the catheter pack, ensuring that principles of asepsis are maintained throughout. Open the catheter, but do not remove it from its internal wrapping, and place it on the sterile receiver on the trolley. Wash your hands and put on the sterile gloves. Place sterile dressing towels onto the bed area between the patient's legs and over the thighs. In men tear a hole in the centre of the towel and allow the penis to protrude through. In the female use one gloved hand to cleanse the urethral meatus with saline while holding the labia apart with the other. Use a new gauze swab for each stroke and clean from the front towards the anus. In the male the foreskin, if present, should be retracted in order to cleanse the meatus. Apply sterile lidocaine (lignocaine) gel to the tip of the catheter and into the urethra in men. Place a kidney dish between the legs in readiness. Insert the catheter into the urethra, holding the penis perpendicular to the body. Gradually advance the catheter out of its wrapper and into the urethra. Gentle pressure is required to advance the catheter into the bladder, at which point urine should flow into the kidney dish. Any resistance should prompt withdrawal and reinsertion. The catheter should be inserted almost to the side arm before inflating the balloon with the volume of sterile water indicated on the catheter. The catheter is then withdrawn to lie at the bladder neck and connected to the catheter drainage bag. Reposition the foreskin in uncircumcised men, and record the volume of urine drained.

## Complications

- Infection
- Urethral trauma and stricture formation.

## If you fail...

Do not make repeated attempts in the male, as damage to the longer urethra can occur. Ask advice of surgeons/urologists for consideration of a suprapubic approach through the abdominal wall, directly into the bladder.

# Lumbar puncture

## Indications

- To obtain a sample of CSF for detection of infection, blood, malignant cells or abnormal proteins
- Administration of chemotherapeutic drugs.

A brain CT or MRI scan should be performed before LP in patients who have clinical features that increase the likelihood of having intracranial mass lesions or increase in CSF pressure which would preclude LP: immunosuppression, bleeding tendency, focal neurological signs, papilloedema, loss of consciousness or seizure.

## Equipment

- Materials for a sterile procedure performed under local anaesthetic (p. 733)
- 23–24 gauge spinal needle
- Manometer
- Three separate numbered sterile collection bottles.

## Procedure

This is a sterile procedure performed under local anaesthetic. Position the patient on the left side on the edge of the bed with the knees curled up to the chest. Identify the L3–L4 interspace by palpating the anterior superior iliac spine and marking the interspace perpendicularly below it. Having cleansed and anaesthetized the skin, insert the spinal needle in the interspace with the stylet in place, aiming for the umbilicus. Resistance is usually felt at the spinal ligaments and again at the dura. The stylet can then be removed, at which stage clear colourless fluid should emerge. The manometer is then attached to measure pressure (normally 80–180 mmH$_2$O). Fluid is collected into the three separate numbered bottles. A decreasing concentration of red blood cells from bottles 1 to 3 indicates a traumatic tap, rather than blood in the CSF. Fluid should be sent for microscopy and culture, protein, and glucose concentration with a simultaneous plasma glucose sample. Additional investigations may be appropriate depending on the suspected diagnosis. The patient should lie flat for 12 hours after the procedure to avoid a headache that may develop.

### Complications
- Post-procedure headache
- Infection
- Herniation of the brainstem through the foramen magnum ('coning').

### If you fail...
Try with the patient sitting upright on the edge of the bed (CSF pressure cannot be measured in this position).

## Procedures after death

## Diagnosis of death
When asked to confirm a patient's death it is important to see the body and to confirm the identity of the patient with the nursing staff.

Confirmation of death involves the demonstration of:
- Fixed and dilated pupils
- Absent carotid pulse
- No breath sounds over 1 minute
- No heart sounds over 1 minute
- No response to painful stimuli, e.g. pressing firmly on the sternum.

Record these details in the notes, giving the time and date of confirmation of death, and sign your name clearly.

## Death certification and referral to the Coroner
A death certificate is usually completed on the day following death. It is signed by a doctor who attended the deceased in his or her last illness, and that doctor must have

seen the patient both within 14 days before death and after death. Although there is no legal requirement for a doctor to inform the Coroner of a death (this is the legal responsibility of the Registrar of Deaths), it is usual to inform the Coroner of a death under particular circumstances. These include:

- Uncertain cause of death
- The patient has not been seen by the doctor within 14 days before death
- The death was suspicious
- Death occurred within 24 hours of admission to hospital without a firm diagnosis being made
- Deaths due to accidents, injuries, suicide, neglect, poisoning or drug or alcohol overdose
- Death of persons in legal custody
- Death related to medical treatment or within 24 hours of an anaesthetic.

## Cremation forms

If the patient is to be cremated you will be asked to complete form B, the Certificate of Medical Attendance of the cremation form. You must have attended the patient within 14 days prior to death and you must see the patient after death (ensuring that there are no pacemaker implants in the body); make certain that the cause of death on the cremation form is identical to that on the death certificate.

# Examination questions

## Infectious diseases and tropical medicine

1. Discuss the management of an otherwise healthy 32-year-old man who has just been found to be HIV positive.
2. What are the early symptoms and signs of rubella? Write short notes on its prevention.
3. How would you investigate and treat a young male patient presenting with urethral discharge?
4. Write short notes on diarrhoea 1 week after return from the Far East.
5. Describe briefly the intestinal infections produced by:
   (a) *Campylobacter* sp.
   (b) *Yersinia* sp.
   (c) *Clostridium difficile*.
6. A 1-year-old boy has been unwell for 6 hours, temperature 40.5°C with eight petechial spots on the trunk and legs. He is drowsy, with systolic blood pressure of 45 mmHg.
   (a) What is the probable diagnosis?
   (b) What immediate treatment would you give?
   (c) What treatment would you give the rest of the family?
   (d) Can the disease be prevented in this age group?
   (e) What complications would you examine for at an outpatient visit 6 weeks later?

## Answers

1. Most patients are found to be positive on antibody testing. Before any patient is tested for evidence of HIV infection he or she must be advised by a trained counsellor about the implications of a positive test. Some patients will require this information to be discussed again when they are subsequently found

to have a positive test. They must be told that the result is confidential and will only be known by those staff involved with the care. A risk history must be established (e.g. intravenous drug abuse, sexual history) and advice given about avoiding transmission to others (i.e. non-penetrative sex, no sharing of needles). This patient is said to be healthy, but a full physical examination must be carried out to look for evidence of AIDS. A full list of those diseases that indicate AIDS in an HIV-positive patient is given in Table 2.10.

The natural history of the disease must be discussed (see p. 52). Baseline investigations include FBC, CD4 count and HIV RNA to assess viral load. The mainstay of treatment is antiretroviral therapy. Examples of these drugs and indications for their use are given on page 50.

2. The clinical features of rubella are discussed on page 12. Prevention is active (live attenuated rubella vaccine given with mumps and measles (MMR) as a single dose at between 12 and 18 months of age) or passive (human immunoglobulin reduces symptoms but does not reduce teratogenic effects).

3. This is discussed on pages 39–40.

4. This is traveller's diarrhoea and the causes are listed in Table 2.8. This question does not say whether this is bloody diarrhoea (dysentery), but the presence of blood narrows the differential diagnosis. Most cases are self-limiting but antibiotics may be necessary for severe infections. Ciprofloxacin covers most of these organisms. Metronidazole is given for amoebiasis or giardiasis. Antibiotics are also required for treatment of dysentery which is due to infection with *Shigella* spp., *Entamoeba histolytica*, *Campylobacter* spp., *Salmonella* spp. or enteroinvasive *E. coli*.

5. (a) The only campylobacter producing intestinal infection is *Campylobacter jejuni*. *Campylobacter* and *Salmonella* species account for most cases of food poisoning (poultry is the main source of infection in both). Campylobacter infection produces a prodromal febrile infection lasting 1–4 days, followed by a diarrhoeal phase which

may last 1–2 weeks. Severe abdominal pains often accompany the diarrhoea, which may be bloodstained. Septicaemia may occur, but rarely death. Sigmoidoscopy may show an acute colitis resembling ulcerative colitis. Diagnosis is made by microscopy (seen as motile rods) and culture of faeces. Infection is usually self-limiting; antibiotic treatment with erythromycin is given to those with systemic symptoms. Complications include cholecystitis, pancreatitis and reactive arthritis.

(b) There are three main *Yersinia* species in humans, all of which are uncommon in Britain. *Y. pseudotuberculosis* and *Y. enterocolitica* cause diarrhoea, terminal ileitis and mesenteric adenitis (may be confused with appendicitis). Diagnosis is usually by serology, demonstrating a rise in antibody titre on paired samples. The illness is usually self-limiting, but tetracycline may be helpful for treating a severe infection. The third species, *Y. pestis*, causes plague.

(c) *Clostridium difficile* produces pseudomembranous colitis, which is an uncommon complication of antibiotic therapy. *C. difficile* is present in the colon of some healthy individuals, and colitis has been attributed to the selection of drug-resistant *C. difficile* that proliferates in the colon and produces a necrotizing toxin. Diagnosis is by demonstration of the toxin in stool and by typical sigmoidoscopic appearances (pseudomembranous on an erythematous background). Treatment is with oral metronidazole 400 mg three times daily or oral vancomycin 250 mg four times daily for up to 10 days.

6. The temperature and hypotension indicate septicaemic shock. The petechial spots suggest this is caused by infection with *Neisseria meningitidis* (not all of these infections produce meningitis).

(a) Fulminant meningococcaemia is a severe life-threatening illness with a rapidly progressive downhill course.

(b) The initial treatment is intravenous benzylpenicillin, which must be started immediately the diagnosis is clinically suspected. The management of suspected bacterial meningitis is outlined in Emergency Box 15.3.

(c) Family contacts should receive prophylaxis with rifampicin 600 mg twice daily for 2 days.

(d) A vaccine for meningococcal group C and *Haemophilus influenzae* is available and is part of routine childhood immunization in the UK.

(e) A small number of patients develop chronic complications, e.g. arthritis, vasculitis and pericarditis, which may be due to immune complex disease.

---

# Gastroenterology

1. State the causes of bloody diarrhoea. What are the most common infectious causes and what specific antibacterial therapy is available to treat them?

2. Write short notes on the management of massive haematemesis.

3. A 30-year-old man presents with a 10-week history of discomfort in the right iliac fossa. He has also noticed some weight loss. The ESR is raised (50 mm/h). What are the likely causes? What imaging tests might be appropriate?

4. A 23-year-old beautician, who is otherwise well, gives a 5-year history of alternating morning diarrhoea, constipation, flatulence and left lower quadrant abdominal pain. What is the most likely diagnosis and how would you manage the problem?

5. A man of 30 presents with a 3-month history of difficulty in swallowing. What features of the history and clinical examination would help in making a diagnosis?

6. How would you investigate and manage a 44-year-old patient found to have a lesser curve gastric ulcer on a barium meal examination?

7. A 45-year-old man presents with a 6-month history of loose, pale, bulky offensive stools associated with

mild abdominal discomfort. Discuss the differential diagnosis and your approach to investigation and treatment.

## Answers

1. Bloody diarrhoea strongly suggests colonic disease. The common causes are inflammatory bowel disease and infections, although colon cancer (usually blood mixed in with the stools, not frank diarrhoea) and acute intestinal ischaemia should be borne in mind. The infectious causes of bloody diarrhoea include *Campylobacter jejuni*, *Shigella* sp. (bacillary dysentery), *Entamoeba histolytica* (amoebic dysentery, occurring in the tropics), some types of *Escherichia coli* and, rarely, *Salmonella* sp. and *Clostridium difficile*. Ciprofloxacin will cover the common organisms except *Entamoeba histolytica*, which is treated with metronidazole.

2. Massive haematemesis is usually the result of bleeding from varices or large peptic ulcers. Patients are usually shocked on presentation and must be aggressively resuscitated, initially with plasma expanders (p. 508) and subsequently with whole blood. After adequate resuscitation the source of bleeding is localized at gastroscopy; further management depends on the cause (p. 73). A stepwise approach to management is outlined in Emergency Box 3.1.

3. In a young person right iliac fossa discomfort associated with weight loss and a raised ESR strongly suggests Crohn's disease (p. 85). An appendix mass must be considered, although the history is long. In immigrants, ileocaecal tuberculosis should be considered (p. 81). Amoebiasis may sometimes cause right iliac fossa pain, usually with the formation of an 'amoeboma', and this should be considered in travellers from the tropics. Imaging is with abdominal ultrasonography and small-bowel barium follow-through. Colonoscopy with direct visualization of the ileum may also be indicated.

4. These features, particularly in a young, otherwise healthy female, are very suggestive of irritable bowel syndrome. The approach to management is outlined on page 102.

5. The causes of dysphagia are listed on page 57. Progressive dysphagia associated with weight loss is suggestive of malignancy, although this would be unusual in a young man. A preceding history of heartburn suggests reflux with a complicating peptic stricture. Chest pain, regurgitation and dysphagia for liquids points to a motility disorder such as achalasia. Oesophageal candidiasis or cytomegalovirus infection may cause dysphagia in patients with AIDS.

6. The investigation and management of gastric ulceration is described on pages 67–8. Benign gastric ulcers may appear radiologically similar to gastric cancer, and therefore endoscopy with multiple biopsies is usually recommended. Ulcers associated with *Helicobacter pylori* infection are treated by eradicating *H. pylori* (p. 66). Ulcers that are *H. pylori* negative, e.g. those associated with aspirin or NSAID ingestion, are treated with proton pump inhibitors such as omeprazole or lansoprazole. Patients with gastric ulcers should be re-endoscoped following treatment to ensure healing. An ulcer that is resistant to treatment raises the question of malignancy (initial biopsies may be negative because of sampling error), and repeat biopsies must be taken. Remember that NSAIDs are an important cause of gastric ulceration, so these should be withdrawn if possible.

7. These features are strongly suggestive of malabsorption, which usually results from either chronic pancreatic insufficiency (p. 161) or disease of the small intestine. A careful history may elucidate the cause (? family history, ?travel abroad, ?heavy alcohol consumption). Initial screening tests would include the measurement of stool fat and stool weight, and blood tests including FBC, serum $B_{12}$ and red cell folate, serum anti-endomysial antibodies and liver biochemistry. Small intestinal causes of malabsorption are discussed on pages 76–81. Assessment of pancreatic structure and function is dealt with on page 162.

# Liver, biliary tract and pancreatic diseases

1. A 50-year-old woman complains of itching, passing dark urine and pale stools, and is deeply jaundiced. What causes should be considered in the first instance and how would you investigate these?

2. A 36-year-old woman presents with a 4-day history of painless jaundice. There is no previous history of medical illness and, apart from marked jaundice, there are no abnormal physical signs. Initial investigations show:
   - Hb 11.5 g/dL, WCC 36 × 10⁹/L, MCV 106 fL, platelets 41 × 10⁹/L
   - Serum sodium 129 mmol/L, potassium 2 mmol/L, urea 1.4 mmol/L
   - Serum bilirubin 190 mmol/L, alkaline phosphatase 350 U/L, ALT 108 U/L, γ-GT 250 U/L.

   Hepatitis B and A antibody titres are not elevated. Serum vitamin B$_{12}$ and folate are normal.

   What is the probable diagnosis and what further tests would be useful? What is the initial management?

Other questions relate to the management of complications that may develop in chronic liver disease.

3. Discuss the immediate and subsequent management of a patient with haematemesis caused by oesophageal varices.

4. Describe the factors underlying the formation of ascites. Describe the principles of management when the ascites results from chronic liver disease.

## Answers

1. The jaundice is associated with pruritus, dark urine and pale stools, and is therefore cholestatic. The next step is to establish whether this is intrahepatic or extrahepatic. The causes are listed in Table 4.1. Information obtained from a detailed clinical history

763

and physical examination may well point to one of these as the probable cause; ultrasound examination of the gall bladder, biliary tree and pancreas is the initial key investigation (Fig. 4.2).

2. The most probable diagnosis is alcoholic hepatitis superimposed on a background of chronic alcoholic liver disease (even in the absence of physical signs). The raised MCV (with a normal vitamin $B_{12}$ and folate), very high γ-GT and thrombocytopenia all suggest alcohol abuse. The very high WCC is typical of alcoholic hepatitis. The sodium is probably low because of inability to excrete a free water load and dilutional hyponatraemia (p. 295). Further investigations and initial management are discussed on page 148. In addition, thiamine must be given to prevent Wernicke's encephalopathy (p. 537).

3. The answers to this question are discussed on pages 136 and 137, respectively.

4. The aetiology and management of ascites associated with chronic liver disease is discussed on page 138.

# Diseases of the blood and haematological malignancies

1. Discuss the causes of hypochromic/microcytic anaemia.

2. You are asked to assess a 25-year-old woman who is found to have a low haemoglobin at her first antenatal booking clinic. There are no physical abnormalities. The values are as follows: Hb 10.7 g/dL, MCV 64 fL, WBC $7.2 \times 10^9$/L, platelets $202 \times 10^9$/L. What diagnoses do you consider and what simple investigations would you request in the first instance? Why are they important?

3. A 36-year-old woman complains of being easily tired over 6 months, and her stools have become more frequent. An FBC shows a Hb of 8 g/dL, MCV 110 fL. Describe your investigations and treatment.

4. A 65-year-old woman comes to see you complaining of severe headaches for several weeks, and of now

having lost vision in one eye. Initial investigations show: Hb 10.5 g/dL, WBC 8.0 × 10⁹/L, ESR 90 mm/h.

(a) What features would you pay attention to in the physical examination?
(b) What is the probable diagnosis?
(c) What further diagnostic investigation would you arrange?
(d) What treatment would you give?
(e) What possible complications of this treatment would concern you in a patient of this age?

5. Discuss the diagnostic considerations in investigating an adult presenting with non-accidental bruising.

6. Discuss the investigation and management of a 50-year-old man found to have a raised haematocrit (packed cell volume or PCV) on routine blood count.

7. Discuss the causes and investigation of persistent enlargement of the cervical lymph nodes in a man aged 25 years.

8. A 60-year-old woman with repeated sore throats has a blood count carried out by her general practitioner who seeks your advice. Investigations reveal: Hb 9.1 g/dL, WBC 2.0 × 10⁹/L, platelets 80 × 10⁹/L. What does it show and what causes should you consider?

# Answers

1. The causes of hypochromic/microcytic anaemia are discussed on pages 167–8. Iron deficiency is the most common cause.

2. This woman has a mild microcytic anaemia. The most probable causes are thalassaemia trait (particularly with the very low MCV) and iron deficiency anaemia. Iron requirements increase during pregnancy (2 mg/day) as a result of transfer of iron to the fetus and an increased red cell mass. These processes occur largely in the second trimester, and therefore it is likely that she was iron deficient before pregnancy (if this is the cause of the anaemia). In a young woman the most probable cause of iron deficiency is heavy menstrual blood loss (suggested by frequent periods, the passage of clots and frequent changes of pads/tampons). Investigations are Hb electrophoresis and iron studies (p. 170).

3. Anaemia with an MCV >100 fL is most probably the result of vitamin $B_{12}$ or folate deficiency. The frequent stools suggest gastrointestinal disease. Taking these two together, the most likely diagnosis is small bowel disease, either Crohn's or coeliac disease (pp. 84 and 76). Initial investigations are the measurement of serum vitamin $B_{12}$, red cell folate, anti-endomysial antibodies, small bowel barium follow-through and distal duodenal biopsies. There may also be malabsorption of iron, and iron deficiency must be excluded (p. 170). Treatment is that of the underlying disease and the replacement of haematinics (pp. 174 and 176).

4. The most probable diagnosis is giant cell arteritis (p. 702) causing central retinal artery occlusion and anaemia of chronic disease. Examine the temporal arteries, the eyes (milky-white fundus as a result of oedema) and look for systemic features of disease (fever, weight loss). The diagnosis and treatment are discussed on page 702. Complications of steroid treatment are: osteoporosis and fractures, diabetes mellitus, hypertension, depression, psychosis and risk of peptic ulceration, particularly when taken together with NSAIDs.

5. The causes and investigation of a bleeding disorder are discussed on pages 206–7. Bruising suggests a platelet or vascular problem. Inherited clotting factor deficiency usually presents with mucosal bleeding, bleeding after surgery and haemarthroses. The probable cause may be suggested after thorough history and examination (e.g. female or male patient, age, family history, concomitant disease, drugs, alcohol).

6. This is polycythaemia and is discussed on page 194.

7. Persistent enlargement of a group of nodes makes most infections unlikely. In a young man this is most probably the result of Hodgkin's disease, leukaemia, or possibly TB. Non-Hodgkin's lymphoma is uncommon in a young person. If there are risk factors, HIV infection (usually generalized lymphadenopathy) must be considered. Initial investigations include FBC and blood film, ESR, and

lymph node biopsy for histological examination. Further investigation, which includes chest X-ray, CT scan of chest and abdomen, bone marrow examination and HIV test, would depend partly on initial results.

8. This elderly woman has pancytopenia, the causes of which are listed in Table 5.7. The probable cause may be suggested by a detailed history (particularly drugs) and physical examination. A bone marrow trephine biopsy is the key investigation.

# Rheumatology

1. Describe a typical attack of gout. How would you confirm the diagnosis and treat the patient?

2. Write short notes on the investigation and treatment of an acute arthritis of one ankle in a man aged 50 years.

3. A 45-year-old woman with a long-standing history of rheumatoid arthritis presents with a 6-month history of increasing dyspnoea. She does not experience orthopnoea. The venous pressure is not elevated and her heart sounds are normal. Her electrocardiogram is normal. Blood gases on air show an arterial $Po_2$ 7.7 kPa, venous $Pco_2$ 4.9 kPa, pH 7.45.
   (a) What is the probable diagnosis?
   (b) What other physical signs would you look for?
   (c) What other investigations would be helpful and what would you expect the results to show?

4. Write short notes on the causes of tetany in a 23-year-old woman.

5. A woman of 55 presents with backache which proves to be osteoporotic in origin. What features would lead to this diagnosis, what are the predisposing factors and how would you treat her?

6. A 60-year-old woman with a long history of alcohol abuse presents because she can no longer climb stairs or rise from chairs. She has recently begun treatment with NSAIDs given by her general practitioner for presumed osteoarthritis of both hips. Biochemical investigations reveal the following data: serum

sodium 142 mmol/L, potassium 4.2 mmol/L,
chloride 102 mmol/L, urea 8 mmol/L, creatinine
60 mmol/L, corrected calcium 2.2 mmol/L,
phosphate 0.5 mmol/L, alkaline phosphatase
1000 U/L. Discuss these results. What do you
consider to be the most probable diagnosis? Describe
appropriate investigations to support your diagnosis
and discuss what might be the best treatment.

## Answers

1. A typical attack of gout is described on page 266.
   The diagnosis is confirmed by joint aspiration. The
   serum uric acid is measured, but may be normal in
   an acute attack. X-rays are rarely helpful; they are
   normal in the early stages, but in chronic disease
   there may be periarticular erosions. Treatment is
   (a) of the acute attack, (b) general advice, and
   (c) consideration of long-term therapy if there have
   been many previous attacks or evidence of chronic
   gouty tophi on physical examination (p. 268).
2. The causes and immediate investigation of a large joint
   monoarthritis are discussed on pages 235 and 251.
   Subsequent tests would depend on the findings on
   joint aspiration, and may include X-ray of the joint and
   the measurement of serum uric acid concentration.
3. The probable diagnosis is fibrosing alveolitis, a rare
   complication of rheumatoid arthritis. Less probably it
   is drug induced (rare side-effects of gold and
   methotrexate). She has type I respiratory failure
   (p. 515). Physical signs to look for are central cyanosis,
   clubbing, reduced chest expansion and end-expiratory
   crackles at the lung bases. Investigations to confirm
   the diagnosis are listed on page 487.
4. In a 23-year-old, presumably otherwise healthy,
   woman the most probable cause is respiratory
   alkalosis secondary to hyperventilation. Alkalosis
   causes tetany by reducing ionization of calcium salts
   (ionized calcium is physiologically active). Other
   causes of tetany – hypocalcaemia (p. 588),
   hypokalaemia (p. 298) and hypomagnesaemia (p. 300)
   – are much less likely, but must be considered.

5. Backache occurs in osteoporosis as a result of vertebral collapse or a crush fracture (not osteoporosis per se), which is seen on a plain X-ray. Bone densitometry (DXA) is used to confirm the diagnosis of osteoporosis and measure the response to treatment. The predisposing factors are listed on page 279; of these, the most important is early menopause. The treatment is analgesia in the short term and, in the long term, elimination of risk factors where possible, maintenance of calcium intake, hormone replacement therapy, and bisphosphonates (p. 279).

6. There is a borderline low serum calcium, a very low serum phosphate and markedly raised alkaline phosphatase. The diagnosis is probably osteomalacia (resulting from vitamin D deficiency), causing a proximal myopathy. Against this is the very high alkaline phosphatase, which is usually only moderately raised in osteomalacia. The myopathy may be the result of alcohol, but this does not explain the very high alkaline phosphatase. The serum urea is raised and the creatinine is at the lower end of the normal range. This picture is seen with dehydration or a gastrointestinal bleed (possibly related to ingestion of NSAIDs).

# Water and electrolytes

1. A 39-year-old woman is admitted to a hospital with a 3-week history of nausea, vomiting and weakness following a chest infection. She has a past history of depression and hypothyroidism, for which she was taking thyroxine. On examination she is dehydrated, drowsy and pigmented, with a blood pressure of 70/40 mmHg. She is oliguric and investigation shows: haemoglobin 14.9 g/dL, white blood cells 7.4 × $10^9$/L, urea 22.8 mmol/L, creatinine 290 mmol/L, sodium 118 mmol/L, potassium 5.7 mmol/L, bicarbonate 23 mmol/L, thyroxine 29.6 mmol/L, free $T_4$ 4.5 pmol/L, TSH >50 mU/L.

    (a) What are the probable diagnoses and their cause?

    (b) What further investigations are indicated?

    (c) What is the initial treatment?

2. Write short notes on potassium deficiency.

3. What are the possible causes of a low plasma sodium concentration and how may they be distinguished? What clinical effects may be attributable to this abnormality?

## Answers

1. (a) This presentation is typical of an Addisonian crisis precipitated by the chest infection. The patient is markedly hypotensive and dehydrated on clinical examination. The raised urea and creatinine are compatible with dehydration and prerenal acute renal failure (p. 341). The serum sodium is very low and, in combination with the clinical findings, suggests that the cause is salt and water loss (p. 290), from either the kidney or the gastrointestinal tract. The combination of pigmented skin, a history of probable autoimmune disease (the most common cause of hypothyroidism is autoimmune) and hyperkalaemia suggests Addison's disease (p. 573) resulting from autoimmune adrenal destruction. The thyroid function tests show evidence of hypothyroidism (low thyroxine, low T4 and raised TSH).

    (b) Blood glucose (to look for hypoglycaemia), random plasma cortisol and ACTH, chest X-ray, blood cultures, serum adrenal autoantibodies.

    (c) The immediate and subsequent management of an Addisonian crisis is given in Emergency Box 13.3.

2. Potassium deficiency (which implies total body depletion) is not the same as hypokalaemia (which means a low serum concentration and may be caused by deficiency or redistribution into cells). Depletion occurs with excess losses or inadequate intake (rare) and the causes are listed in Table 7.7.

3. The causes, investigation and symptoms of hyponatraemia are discussed on pages 293–296. Management of hyponatraemia resulting from water excess is given in Emergency Box 7.1.

## Renal disease

Three topics occur commonly and with almost equal frequency. These are chronic renal failure, the causes and management of acute renal failure, and the causes of proteinuria and the nephrotic syndrome.

1. What are the clinical features of 'end-stage' renal failure, and how may it be treated?
2. What clinical and other evidence would lead you to suspect the diagnosis of chronic renal failure in a 50-year-old man? How would you determine the cause of renal failure?
3. In a patient presenting with a plasma creatinine of 500 μmol/L, which of the following features would suggest that the renal failure is chronic, rather than acute?
   (a) Reduced renal size detected by ultrasonography.
   (b) A urine sodium concentration of less than 10 mmol/L.
   (c) Elevated serum alkaline phosphatase and subperiosteal erosions on X-ray of the hands.
   (d) A haemoglobin of 14 g/L.
   (e) The presence of ureteric obstruction on renal ultrasonography.
   (f) Evidence of polyneuropathy.
4. List the causes of renal failure resulting from poor perfusion of the kidneys. What are the clinical and laboratory features?
5. What factors contribute to the development of acute renal failure in a patient with multiple injuries following a road traffic accident? Outline your management during the first 24–48 hours.
6. You have been asked to see a 45-year-old man with a creatinine of 530 μmol/L whose urinary output has fallen to 150 mL over 24 hours. Discuss the

differential diagnosis and your approach to
investigation.
7. A 50-year-old man presents with bilateral ankle
swelling and is found to have a serum albumin of
28 g/L. Discuss the differential diagnosis in terms of
history, possible physical findings and further
helpful investigations.

Other questions are:
8. Describe how patients with glomerulonephritis may
present.
9. Discuss the presentation and management of
recurrent urinary tract infection in women.

## Answers
1. The clinical features and treatment of end-stage renal
failure are discussed on pages 348–351.
2. A patient presenting with any of the complications
discussed on page 350 would lead you to suspect
chronic renal failure (CRF), but the usual ways in
which patients present are with hypertension,
nocturia and polyuria, or with symptoms of anaemia.
The investigations for renal failure are discussed on
page 348. A renal biopsy is performed in patients
with normal-sized kidneys. Small kidneys are
technically difficult to biopsy, histological
investigations are hard to interpret, and at this late
stage the prognosis would not be influenced by
treatment of the underlying condition.
3. (a), (c) and (f) suggest chronic renal failure. The urine
sodium concentration is very low, and this may occur
with prerenal acute renal failure (when the kidney is
conserving sodium) and with chronic renal failure
when the concentrating ability of the kidney is lost
and large amounts of dilute urine are produced. The
normal Hb is in favour of acute renal failure.
4. This is discussed on page 341. Poor perfusion of the
kidneys is usually caused by hypovolaemia; other
causes include pump failure (cardiogenic shock) or
shock resulting from a pulmonary embolism. The
clinical and laboratory features are described on
pages 341 and 342.

5. The most probable cause is poor renal perfusion secondary to hypovolaemia from blood loss. Other causes include rhabdomyolysis (extensive crush injury to muscle leads to the release of myoglobin, which is directly toxic to renal tubular cells), ruptured urethra (suspect with severe pelvic fractures and anuria) and later septicaemia and drugs (e.g. gentamicin). Initial management is to correct hypovolaemia with whole blood (measurement of central venous pressure will guide replacement) followed by a bolus of furosemide (frusemide) (p. 343) if the patient remains oliguric. If urine output does not increase and urethral rupture is excluded as the cause of oliguria, then treatment is as for established acute tubular necrosis (p. 347). The investigations must include measurement of the muscle enzyme creatinine phosphokinase.

6. The short history of oliguria and decline of renal function suggests acute renal failure. The aetiology and investigations are discussed on pages 344–5.

7. Hypoalbuminaemia is caused by decreased synthesis (liver disease) or increased loss from the kidneys or, rarely, the gut (protein-losing enteropathy). The main differential is between liver disease and nephrotic syndrome. Important points in the history are risk factors for chronic liver disease (e.g. alcohol, intravenous drug abuse) and diseases that may be associated with nephrotic syndrome (e.g. diabetes, chronic infections and amyloidosis, drugs). Signs of chronic liver disease must be looked for on physical examination. Initial investigations are liver biochemistry and measurement of urinary protein excretion.

8. This is discussed on page 318.

9. This is discussed on pages 327.

# Cardiovascular disease

1. What simple screening tests are justified in a 45-year-old man presenting with hypertension? What are the

causes of secondary hypertension, and how could your investigations demonstrate them?

2. A 55-year-old man presents with retrosternal chest pain radiating to the left arm and jaw. The character of the pain is suggestive of myocardial ischaemia.

   (a) What additional features in the clinical history would suggest that the pain is angina rather than myocardial infarction?

   (b) What features in the history would suggest that this is unstable angina?

   (c) Describe the management of a patient with unstable angina.

3. A 28-year-old married man with a family history of ischaemic heart disease presents with exertional chest pain. Discuss the investigation and management.

4. (a) How would you try to differentiate acute pericarditis from acute myocardial infarction clinically?

   (b) Pericarditis may be a complication of myocardial infarction. When after the infarction does it typically occur?

   (c) What are the most common causes of acute pericarditis in the UK?

5. A 60-year-old woman presents with breathlessness and clinical features of mild heart failure. She is found to have atrial fibrillation with an uncontrolled ventricular response (130 beats/min).

   (a) Give four possible causes for the atrial fibrillation.

   (b) Name three drugs that may be used to control the ventricular response.

   (c) What investigations would you order?

6. A 44-year-old woman is admitted to hospital with malaise and fever. She has felt unwell for 6 months. Examination shows pallor, an apical pansystolic murmur and splenomegaly. A blood count sent by the general practitioner shows a haemoglobin of 8.4 g/dL, WBC $7.2 \times 10^9$/L and platelets $394 \times 10^9$/L.

   (a) What investigations are required?

   (b) How might treatment be monitored?

7. (a) Discuss the clinical features of an acute attack of left ventricular failure.
   (b) Name three physical findings that would be of most value in distinguishing it from other causes of severe shortness of breath.

8. What are the key points to the management of acute pulmonary oedema?

9. A 50-year-old man complains of a painful red swollen calf.
   (a) What factors may be responsible?
   (b) How would you discriminate between the causes?

10. A 61-year-old man is admitted following a year's history of dizziness on exertion, culminating in a black-out while cutting the lawn. On admission he has a slow rising pulse and a systolic ejection murmur. There is no history of angina.
    (a) What is the likely diagnosis?
    (b) How would you estimate its clinical severity?
    (c) What is the most probable pathology?
    (d) What is the treatment?

# Answers

1. If the history or physical examination does not suggest a secondary cause for hypertension the screening tests in a middle-aged man are a chest X-ray, serum urea, creatinine and electrolytes, and Stix testing of the urine to look for protein and blood. The secondary causes of hypertension are listed on page 436 and the relevance of these investigations is discussed on page 437. An ECG is also performed to look for end-organ damage (left ventricular hypertrophy), which is an indication for early treatment rather than observation in a patient with mild hypertension.

2. (a) The pain of angina is usually less severe than that of myocardial infarction. Classic angina comes on with exercise and is relieved by rest, and the pain is usually not accompanied by other symptoms such as sweating, nausea or vomiting. The pain of myocardial infarction may come on at rest, is persistent and may last several hours, and is often accompanied by sweating, nausea and vomiting.

(b) Unstable angina is angina of recent onset (less than 1 month), worsening angina or angina at rest.

(c) This is discussed on page 402.

3. The nature of the chest pain and the positive family history suggest a diagnosis of angina resulting from ischaemic heart disease. He is very young and every effort should be made to confirm the diagnosis, identify risk factors and determine the extent and site of coronary artery stenosis. A resting ECG, and usually an exercise ECG, is performed (p. 367). Risk factors (p. 397) are identified from the history, physical examination and measurement of serum cholesterol and blood glucose; every effort must be made to correct abnormalities. In younger people (< 50 years) coronary angiography is often performed to document the site and extent of coronary artery stenosis, which will guide future management. In patients with left main stem or multivessel disease, coronary artery bypass grafting is of clear prognostic benefit compared to medical therapy. Treatment is medical (p. 400) in the first instance in the absence of these lesions. His siblings and children should also be screened for risk factors, e.g. familial hypercholesterolaemia.

4. (a) Acute pericarditis and myocardial infarction are discussed on pages 433 and 403. They can usually be differentiated on the basis of the nature, the site and radiation of the pain, and the presence of associated symptoms and signs (e.g. nausea, vomiting, breathlessness, pericardial rub on auscultation).

   (b) Pericarditis is common in the first few days, particularly in anterior wall infarction. Post-myocardial infarction syndrome (Dressler's syndrome) is much less common. It occurs weeks or months after an acute myocardial infarction and consists of pericarditis, fever and a pericardial effusion. It is caused by an autoimmune response to damaged cardiac tissue.

   (c) Coxsackie viral infection and myocardial infarction.

5. The causes of atrial fibrillation are listed on page 377. In an elderly woman the probable causes are

ischaemic heart disease, mitral valve disease,
thyrotoxicosis and cardiomyopathy. The drugs
usually used to control the ventricular rate are those
that slow conduction through the AV node: digoxin,
β-blockers and verapamil. Digoxin is the only one
not to have a negative inotropic action, and can thus
be used in heart failure. Investigations are an ECG
(which will show fibrillation and may show evidence
of ischaemia or mitral valve disease, Fig. 9.7b), a
chest X-ray (which will confirm the clinical diagnosis
of heart failure and may show evidence of mitral
valve disease, Fig. 9.14), an echocardiogram, and
thyroid function tests.

6. This combination of clinical signs suggests infective
endocarditis affecting the mitral valve. Investigations
are discussed on page 424. Treatment is monitored
clinically (patient well-being, temperature charts,
evidence of heart failure) and by regular blood counts,
ESR and echocardiography. Antibiotic doses are
adjusted according to bacteriological studies
(minimum bactericidal concentration) and gentamicin
levels (to ensure therapeutic levels are obtained but
without toxic levels likely to cause side-effects).

7. (a) Clinical features of acute left ventricular failure
are listed on page 395.
   (b) A gallop rhythm, widespread crackles and
pulsus alternans differentiate pulmonary oedema
from other causes of acute shortness of breath
(listed in Table 10.2). In pulsus alternans the
arterial pressure alternates between high and
low systolic peaks. Its presence indicates severe
left ventricular failure.

8. The key points to the management of pulmonary
oedema are listed in Emergency Box 9.2.

9. (a) The differential diagnosis of a swollen calf
includes deep venous thrombosis (DVT),
cellulitis or a ruptured Baker's cyst. Oedema in
heart failure or hypoalbuminaemia also causes a
swollen calf, but this is usually bilateral. A
Baker's cyst (popliteal cyst) is a synovial cyst in
the popliteal fossa which sometimes occurs in
patients with a knee effusion. Rupture of the cyst

produces sudden and severe pain, swelling and tenderness of the upper calf.

(b) The diagnosis of a ruptured Baker's cyst is often missed and treated inappropriately with anticoagulants. An ultrasound will distinguish a ruptured cyst from a DVT.

10. (a) The history and examination are typical of aortic stenosis (p. 418). As in this case, presentation is usually in the sixth decade.

(b) The presence of symptoms indicates at least moderately severe aortic stenosis. A longer ejection systolic murmur, clinical and ECG evidence of left ventricular hypertrophy all indicate more severe stenosis. The severity may be more accurately assessed by Doppler echocardiography.

(c) The most likely pathology is a calcified bicuspid aortic valve.

(d) Treatment in a symptomatic patient is valve replacement.

# Respiratory disease

1. A 17-year-old girl presents to Accident and Emergency with an acute exacerbation of asthma.
   (a) What features on clinical examination would suggest a severe attack of asthma?
   (b) How would your findings influence the management of this patient?

2. A 45-year-old woman develops breathlessness and wheezing following a cold. What features would you seek to support a diagnosis of asthma?

3. Describe your approach to the investigation and management of pneumonia in a 50-year-old ventilation engineer.

4. (a) What are the main causes of haemoptysis?
   (b) How would you investigate a patient with this complaint?

5. (a) List the conditions which you consider most likely to account for acute shortness of breath in a 50-year-old man.

(b) What are the most important physical signs for each condition?

(c) Which initial investigation is likely to be most helpful, together with the clinical history and examination, in distinguishing between these causes?

6. Discuss your management of a 25-year-old man presenting with acute right pleural pain, in whom the X-ray shows air in the pleural cavity and a completely collapsed right lung.

7. A 28-year-old previously healthy Caucasian female presents with a persistent dry cough for 4 weeks. She has also recently developed a nodular rash on her legs. She does not smoke and works in an office. Physical examination reveals coarse crackles at both lung bases and a rash on her legs. A chest X-ray shows prominent bilateral hilar lymphadenopathy and reticulonodular infiltrates in both lung fields.

(a) What is the most likely diagnosis?

(b) What is the most likely cause of the rash on the legs?

(c) If a lung biopsy was obtained, what would you expect it to show?

8. A 35-year-old woman is admitted as an emergency with acute onset of shortness of breath and central chest pain. She was recently discharged from hospital after a cholecystectomy. On examination she is obese, pale, sweating, pulse 120/min and BP 80/50. The JVP is raised by 4 cm and there is a left parasternal heave. She smokes 30 cigarettes per day and takes the combined oral contraceptive pill.

(a) What is the most likely diagnosis?

(b) In this patient, what are the risk factors for the presumed diagnosis?

(c) What is the immediate treatment of this condition?

## Answers

1. (a) Features of a severe attack of asthma are:
   - Inability to complete a sentence in one breath
   - Pulse > 110 beats/min
   - Respirations ≥ 25 breaths/min

- PEFR 30–50% of predicted value or 30–50% of patient's best.

There are additional clinical features which suggest that the attack is life-threatening, and these are listed on page 469.

(b) Acute severe asthma is a medical emergency and an indication for urgent treatment. The management is discussed in Emergency Box 10.1.

2. The classic triad of symptoms associated with asthma consists of cough, shortness of breath, and wheezing. However, one or more of these symptoms may be absent and they are not specific for asthma. A history of intermittent, seasonal waxing and waning of symptoms; nocturnal episodes; exacerbation of symptoms on exposure to stimuli such as exercise, cold air, allergens, air pollutants and with upper respiratory tract infections argues for the diagnosis of asthma.

3. The causes of pneumonia in a healthy adult are listed on page 472. Pneumonia in a ventilation engineer may be the result of any of the causes of community-acquired pneumonia, but he is particularly at risk of infection with *Legionella* sp. The initial treatment must cover this organism, and investigations performed must look particularly for evidence of this infection (p. 476). Additional treatment includes oxygen therapy to correct hypoxaemia and treatment of complications, e.g. acute renal failure, hyponatraemia.

4. The causes of haemoptysis and its investigation are on page 446.

5. (a) Acute means onset over hours. The most probable causes are pneumonia, pulmonary oedema and asthma (particularly with a past history). Dyspnoea due to a pneumothorax or pulmonary embolism usually comes on over minutes. Associated symptoms and signs may provide clues to the diagnosis, e.g. retrosternal chest pain with myocardial infarction and cardiac failure, fever, cough and sputum with pneumonia, and wheezing with asthma. Pulmonary embolism may occur, particularly in a patient with risk factors (p. 426).

(b) A patient with pulmonary oedema is acutely breathless, wheezy (cardiac asthma) and may cough up frothy blood-tinged sputum. The patient may be sweating profusely, and on auscultation there is a gallop rhythm and wheezes and crackles are heard throughout the chest. Pneumonia and pulmonary embolism may produce pleuritic chest pain and a pleuritic rub may be present. The patient with pneumonia will probably have a temperature. The clinical features of pneumothorax and pulmonary embolism are described on pages 501 and 426, and vary according to the size of the pneumothorax or embolism.

(c) The most useful investigation in the first instance is a chest X-ray.

6. The chest X-ray appearances describe a pneumothorax. The initial treatment in a patient with complete collapse is aspiration with insertion of a chest drain (p. 745) if this is unsuccessful.

7. (a) There are many causes of hilar lymphadenopathy. However, the clinical history together with the bilateral hilar enlargement suggest sarcoidosis.

(b) Erythema nodosum.

(c) Lymphocytes, macrophages and sometimes fibrosis. Non-caseating granulomas are the key histopathological feature of sarcoidosis and are found in lymph nodes and in a lymphatic distribution in the lung.

8. (a) The history and examination findings are suggestive of a massive pulmonary embolism with acute right heart strain. A similar clinical picture may also be seen with a right ventricular infarct, but she has a number of risk factors which are more in favour of pulmonary embolism.

(b) Recent surgery, smoking, obesity and the combined oral contraceptive pill.

(c) 100% oxygen and pain relief with diamorphine. This patient has a massive embolism with hypotension and right heart strain (raised JVP and right ventricular heave) and you should

781

consider giving thrombolysis. She may also
require intravenous fluids to try to raise the
filling pressure of the right ventricle, thereby
increasing cardiac output. Treatment with
heparin and subsequently warfarin should also
be given to reduce the chance of further emboli.
The management of a pulmonary embolism is
summarized in Emergency Box 9.4.

# Intensive care medicine

1. A man aged 55 years who underwent right
   hemicolectomy for carcinoma of the caecum 4 days
   ago has developed acute circulatory failure ('shock'),
   with an arterial pressure of 65/40 mmHg and heart
   rate of 120/min.
   (a) List the probable causes of this occurrence.
   (b) Indicate the clinical features that would aid you
       in distinguishing between them, and outline
       your initial management of the situation.
2. Write short notes on the management of cardiogenic
   shock.
3. Compare the clinical manifestations of acute
   haemorrhagic, acute cardiogenic and acute bacterial
   (septicaemic) shock.

## Answers

1. The two most likely causes are sepsis or a massive
   pulmonary embolism. Less likely are gastrointestinal
   haemorrhage and a perioperative myocardial
   infarction complicated by cardiogenic shock. The
   clinical features of each of these conditions are
   discussed on pages 508, 426 and 507, respectively.
   Management involves:
   • Emergency resuscitation with 60% oxygen, large-
     bore intravenous cannulae and administration of
     colloid.
   • Make a diagnosis: temperature charts and
     physical examination will often reveal the cause.
     Consider: ECG, blood gases, chest X-ray.

- Further treatment depends on the response to fluids and the likely cause.
2. Cardiogenic shock is an extreme form of cardiac failure ('pump failure'), often secondary to a myocardial infarction in which there has been extensive damage to the left ventricular muscle. The mortality rate is 90%. Management therefore involves admission to the ICU, oxygen therapy, relief of pain and intensive monitoring (Emergency Box 11.1), including a Swan–Ganz catheter. Dobutamine is given for its inotropic action (Table 11.2). If PCWP is below 18 mmHg fluid is cautiously infused so as to optimize the filling pressures of the heart. Vasodilators are sometimes given (p. 510).
3. This is discussed on pages 507–8.

# Poisoning, drug and alcohol abuse

1. After a disagreement with her boyfriend, a 20-year-old woman was seen to ingest 50 tablets of aspirin (i.e. 15 g total) and was brought to hospital 4 hours later. You find her alert and complaining of mild tinnitus only. The salicylate concentration in a blood sample taken in the Accident and Emergency department is within the therapeutic range. She wishes to return home and regrets the whole incident; in particular, she assures you that she has no suicidal intent. Briefly outline the major points of management.
2. A girl aged 17 is admitted after a suicide attempt with a single drug. Initial blood gases were: $P_aO_2$ 13.7 kPa, $P_aCO_2$ 3.7 kPa, pH 7.49.
   (a) What is the metabolic abnormality?
   (b) What drug has this woman probably taken?
   (c) What acid–base changes may occur later?
   (d) When she has recovered, what features would alert you to the risk of a further life-threatening suicide attempt?
3. Outline the effects and management of paracetamol poisoning.

4. (a) Outline the various physical disorders that may occur as a result of excessive alcohol consumption.
   (b) What features in a routine haematological screen would lead you to suspect alcohol abuse?

# Answers

1. Ingestion of 10–20 g of aspirin may produce severe toxicity. This case represents a very serious overdose and serum levels are within the normal range because intestinal absorption is still taking place (see p. 529). Initial management involves administration of intravenous fluids to correct dehydration and initiate a diuresis; further management depends on the salicylate concentration in a repeat blood sample taken 6 hours after drug ingestion (p. 529). More than one drug is often taken in overdose cases, and this should be sought from the history and measurement of plasma paracetamol levels. Several points suggest that the overdose is not a serious suicide attempt (Table 12.2) and psychiatric referral is probably not necessary.

2. (a) The patient has a respiratory alkalosis.
   (b) Aspirin.
   (c) Respiratory alkalosis is due to direct stimulation of the respiratory centre by salicylates. Initially renal excretion of bicarbonate will bring the pH towards normal, producing some compensation of the alkalosis. Subsequently a combined respiratory and metabolic acidosis develops because:

   - Hypotension and dehydration impair renal function with retention of organic acids.
   - Salicylates interfere with carbohydrate, fat and protein metabolism, as well as with oxidative phosphorylation. This gives rise to increased lactate, pyruvate and ketone bodies, all of which contribute to the acidosis.
   - Salicylate and its metabolites are acidic and further enhance the metabolic acidosis.
   - Severe overdose produces depression of the respiratory centre and a respiratory acidosis.

   (d) Risk factors for suicide are listed in Table 12.2.

3. This is discussed on pages 530–1.
4. (a) The physical complications of alcohol abuse are discussed on page 536.
   (b) Macrocytosis and, less commonly, thrombocytopenia are seen with alcohol abuse.

# Endocrinology

1. An otherwise healthy 36-year-old woman presents with 8 months of feeling anxious and tremulous. On examination her pulse is 115 per minute, BP 155/90 and there is a moderately enlarged, non-tender, non-nodular thyroid and hyperreflexia.
   (a) What is your clinical diagnosis?
   (b) What tests would you order? What would you expect the results to be?
   (c) What are the main treatment options for this patient?

2. A 29-year-old man presents with 5 days of pain and tenderness over the thyroid gland. He feels jittery but otherwise well. On examination, he is afebrile, pulse 120 per minute, BP 140/90. His thyroid is enlarged and diffusely tender, with no evidence of nodules.
   (a) What is your clinical diagnosis and how would you confirm it?
   (b) How would you treat this patient?
   (c) What is his prognosis?

3. (a) What are the clinical features of myxoedema?
   (b) How would you confirm or refute the diagnosis?

4. An 85-year-old woman is found lying on the floor of her unheated flat; hypothermia is suspected.
   (a) How would you confirm the diagnosis?
   (b) What abnormality might there be on ECG?
   (c) What would be your management?

5. A 64-year-old smoker presents with haemoptysis and a 4-week history of proximal muscle weakness. On examination he is noted to have a plethoric complexion, hypertension, abdominal striae and skin bruising. The chest X-ray shows a mass in the right lower zone. The plasma potassium is 2.9 mmol/L and blood glucose 16 mmol/L.

(a) What diagnosis do you suspect?

(b) How would you confirm the endocrine abnormality?

6. A 72-year-old woman with known breast cancer presents with dehydration, confusion and vomiting. Her corrected serum calcium is 3.8 mmol/L. Discuss your approach to management.

## Answers

1. (a) Hyperthyroidism which, clinically and epidemiologically, is likely to be Graves' disease.

   (b) Serum TSH will be low, often undetectable. Serum $T_4$ and $T_3$ will be high. Serum microsomal and thyroglobulin antibodies will be present in the serum in most cases of Graves' disease.

   (c) Antithyroid drugs given for about 2 years in the hope that the disease remits on its own. These include:

   - Carbimazole, most often used in the UK
   - Methimazole, the active metabolite of carbimazole, used in the USA
   - Propylthiouracil, occasionally used.

   β-blockers for symptomatic relief, but they do not alter the course of the disease.

   Radioiodine is more commonly preferred for definitive treatment of Graves' disease, surgery is particularly suited to patients with large goitres which are unlikely to remit after medical treatment.

2. (a) The presence of diffuse swelling and tenderness of the thyroid gland, together with the history of pain, suggests de Quervain's thyroiditis. Inflammation of the gland leads to the release of preformed hormone. The serum TSH would be low. A radioactive iodine uptake scan would show reduced uptake by the thyroid because the gland is not actively synthesizing thyroid hormone. This test is not routinely performed, but in other cases of hyperthyroidism there would be increased uptake.

   (b) The disease is generally mild and limited to a few weeks, so definitive therapy is rarely needed. β-Blockers are used for symptomatic relief. Patients may become transiently hypothyroid during recovery.

(c) Spontaneous remission in a few weeks.

3. (a) The symptoms and signs of myxoedema are listed on page 563.

(b) Almost all cases of hypothyroidism are the result of disease of the thyroid gland; much less commonly it is caused by hypothalamic–pituitary disease. In primary hypothyroidism measurement of serum TSH (which will be high because of loss of feedback inhibition of secretion by $T_4$) and free $T_4$ (which will be low) will confirm the diagnosis.

4. (a) The diagnosis and management of hypothermia are discussed on page 595–6. Hypothermia is diagnosed when the core (rectal) temperature is $< 35°C$ measured with a low-reading rectal thermometer.

(b) The ECG abnormalities are 'J' waves (pathognomonic of hypothermia), a tachycardia with a bradycardia developing at temperatures $< 32°C$. At very low temperatures there may be ventricular arrhythmias.

(c) The treatment is described on page 596.

5. The history of haemoptysis in a smoker with an abnormal chest X-ray is highly suggestive of bronchial carcinoma. The proximal muscle weakness, hypertension, striae, bruising, hypokalaemia and high blood sugar suggest Cushing's syndrome, which is most likely due to ectopic ACTH production by a small-cell lung cancer. A low-dose dexamethasone suppression test and measurement of serum ACTH will confirm the diagnosis.

6. Severe hypercalcaemia such as this is a medical emergency and almost certainly related to malignancy. Management is discussed in Emergency Box 13.4. Other causes of hypercalcaemia are listed in Table 13.16.

# Diabetes mellitus and other disorders of metabolism

1. A 45-year-old West Indian woman weighing 95 kg and 160 cm (5 feet 4 inches) tall is found, on routine examination, to have glycosuria without ketonuria, and a random blood glucose of 17 mmol/L.
   (a) What is the diagnosis?
   (b) What type do you suspect?
   (c) What is the initial management?

2. A man of 56 has been diabetic since the age of 20. He now complains of bilateral ankle swelling.
   (a) What is the differential diagnosis?
   (b) How would you investigate and manage this patient?

3. An 18-year-old man who is a known diabetic is admitted as an emergency. His parents say that he has become unwell over the last 3 days, with vomiting and confusion. Laboratory investigations reveal a blood glucose 36 mmol/L, serum sodium 147 mmol/L, urea 12 mmol/L, potassium 5.0 mmol/L and arterial blood pH 7.1.
   (a) What is the diagnosis?
   (b) Considering the serum potassium concentration, is his total body potassium high, low or normal?
   (c) Outline your initial treatment of this patient.

4. A 20-year-old woman complains of being very thirsty and passing large quantities of urine.
   (a) What are the likely causes?
   (b) How would you establish the diagnosis?

5. (a) What are the features of an attack of hypoglycaemia? Suggest the mechanism of each manifestation.
   (b) What causes of a series of proven attacks ought to be considered?

6. A 37-year-old man presents for an evaluation because his brother recently died of coronary disease in his early 40s. The patient's father also has a history of elevated cholesterol and early coronary disease. The patient denies smoking cigarettes and has eliminated high-fat dairy products, most red meat

and alcohol from his diet. There is no history of hypertension and physical examination is unremarkable. Measurement of plasma lipids shows a triglyceride of 1.5 mmoL, total cholesterol 9.0 mmol/L, LDL-cholesterol 6.8 mmol/L, HDL-cholesterol 1.5 mmol/L.

   (a) What lipid abnormality do you suspect?
   (b) What other tests would you perform?
   (c) What drug therapy would you prescribe in order to lower the cholesterol?

7. Describe the changes on serum cholesterol of changes in:
   (a) dietary saturated fat
   (b) dietary unsaturated fat
   (c) dietary cholesterol
   (d) sugar.

## Answers

1. (a) The random blood sugar confirms the presence of diabetes mellitus.
   (b) Her age, obesity (body mass index > 30) and absence of symptoms or ketosis suggest that this is type 2 diabetes mellitus.
   (c) Initial management involves patient education and weight reduction, achieved with a 1000–1600 kcal diet planned in conjunction with a dietician. Diabetic complications must be sought by physical examination, blood tests and urinalysis (p. 616). Oral hypoglycaemics (p. 614) are necessary if blood glucose remains high in spite of weight loss having been achieved.

2. (a) The most probable causes of leg oedema in this patient are complications resulting from long-standing diabetes, i.e. nephrotic syndrome (p. 322) or heart failure (secondary to ischaemic heart disease).
   (b) These will be distinguished by physical examination, chest X-ray, urinalysis and measurement of the serum albumin. Further management depends on the cause and is described on pages 324 and 391.

3. (a) This is diabetic ketoacidosis, as shown by the high blood glucose and acidosis. This is the typical hyperglycaemic emergency of the young diabetic.

   (b) The serum potassium concentration is a poor indicator of total body potassium because most potassium is intracellular. Total body potassium is low with diabetic ketoacidosis because of increased potassium excretion in the urine and loss in the vomit.

   (c) The initial treatment is with intravenous saline, soluble insulin and potassium supplements (p. 611).

4. (a) Frequency of micturition must not be confused with polyuria (usually > 3 L/day); a 24-hour urine output chart is helpful if there is doubt.

   (b) The first and most simple test to perform is a random blood sugar, which will be high if polyuria is secondary to diabetes mellitus. Other causes are primary or hysterical polydipsia (a relatively common cause of polyuria and polydipsia in young women), cranial diabetes insipidus (CDI), nephrogenic DI (p. 582) and chronic renal failure. A full history and examination must include a drug history (e.g. lithium causes nephrogenic DI). Investigations, other than a blood glucose, include serum osmolality, urine osmolality, serum urea, electrolytes and calcium. A water deprivation test may be necessary (p. 584).

5. (a) Symptoms are the result of secretion of counter-regulatory hormones (catecholamines cause hunger, sweating, pallor and tachycardia) and neuroglycopenia (e.g. confusion, drowsiness, fits and eventually coma).

   (b) The causes of hypoglycaemia are listed on page 622. In an otherwise healthy person (e.g. in the absence of cancer, severe liver or renal failure), the most likely causes of recurrent hypoglycaemia are drugs, factitious hypoglycaemia, alcoholic binges and insulinoma. Often the cause will be apparent from the history, physical examination and measurement of blood glucose and plasma insulin during a hypoglycaemic episode. A supervised fast with measurement of glucose and insulin may be needed (p. 621).

6. (a) The patient may have monogenic familial hypercholesterolaemia caused by a defect in the LDL receptor gene (p. 625), or he may have a polygenic predisposition to elevated LDL-cholesterol. The distinction is not clinically important.

   (b) It is important to identify causes of secondary hyperlipidaemia. Screening for diabetes mellitus (with a fasting blood glucose) and hypothyroidism (with a serum TSH) should be performed.

   (c) Drugs of choice are the HMG-CoA reductase inhibitors and fibrates.

7. Serum cholesterol is mainly derived from endogenous synthesis and thus any dietary modification will have only a moderate effect. Hypercholesterolaemia is reduced by restricting the intake of cholesterol and saturated fat (both found in animal fat) and replacing with vegetable fat (containing unsaturated fats). Carbohydrate restriction reduces serum triglyceride levels.

# Neurology

1. A lady of 70 wakes one morning with weakness in the right arm and some difficulty in speaking. The symptoms are present the following day and her family bring her to the Accident and Emergency department.
   (a) What are the likely causes?
   (b) How would you manage this patient?
   (c) What information would you give to the patient and relatives?

2. A man of 65 suddenly develops weakness and numbness of the left arm, which gradually passes off after 15 minutes.
   (a) What are the likely causes?
   (b) How might they be investigated?

3. A 16-year-old girl presents with a 1-day history of severe headache with fever, nausea, vomiting, muscle and joint pains. Over the last 6 hours she had become disorientated and developed a rash. Findings on examination were pulse 125/minute, BP 95/55, temperature 39.5°C. Petechiae and purpura were present on the hands and legs.
   (a) What is your clinical diagnosis?
   (b) What is your immediate management?
   (c) Despite treatment she deteriorated rapidly and developed a widespread haemorrhagic rash, BP 70/40, disseminated intravascular coagulation (DIC) and anuria. What is this condition called?

4. A 40-year-old known alcoholic is brought into Accident and Emergency unconscious and smelling of alcohol.
   (a) What are the most likely causes of coma in this patient?
   (b) Describe your management?

5. (a) List the potentially treatable or reversible causes of apparent dementia.
   (b) What features of the history and clinical findings might arouse your suspicions?

6. A 34-year-old homosexual man with a previous episode of *P. carinii* pneumonia first noted 1 week previous to admission poor control of his left hand, and would walk to his left. He also noticed difficulty in remembering events, understanding what was read, and dressing apraxia. He had also had early morning headaches. On examination he was afebrile, he had oral thrush, and fundal examination showed white exudates. He had a left-sided weakness, left homonymous hemianopia and left-sided neglect.
   (a) Do you think this patient has AIDS?
   (b) The history and examination is suggestive of a space-occupying lesion. Where is it situated?
   (c) A brain CT scan shows a ring-enhancing lesion with surrounding oedema and some compression of the adjacent ventricle. What is your differential diagnosis in this patient?

7. A 23-year-old woman was admitted through Accident and Emergency with a 2-day history of

symmetrical leg weakness and paraesthesiae. Later she was unable to sit up in bed and reported difficulty in coughing and stiffness of the face.

   (a) What is the most likely diagnosis?

   (b) What confirmatory tests would you obtain?

   (c) What is the most common antecedent infection to this condition?

   (d) What is the management of this condition?

8. Give three common causes of ptosis and mention the associated features in each case.

9. What are the features of Horner's syndrome? Briefly describe the anatomical pathways involved. What underlying causes may be responsible?

10. A 30-year-old Asian is admitted with headache and neck stiffness. CSF findings: pressure 23 mmH$_2$O, red blood cells 0, white cells 290 × 10$^6$/L (lymphocytes 82%, monocytes 10%, neutrophils 8%), protein 2 g/L, glucose 1.8 mmol/L, blood glucose 6 mmol/L.

   (a) What are the abnormalities?

   (b) What is the diagnosis?

## Answers

1. (a) The history is of sudden onset of right-sided weakness and dysphasia, which is almost certainly due to a vascular lesion (i.e. stroke). The causes of stroke are discussed on page 665; in a woman of this age it is most likely to be due to thrombosis at the site of atheromatous degeneration in the middle cerebral artery (p. 667).

   (b) The investigations and treatment of stroke are discussed on pages 668–9. A brain CT scan will differentiate between infarction and haemorrhage. Aspirin is given to patients with infarction to reduce the risk of further attacks.

   (c) The family must be told that some recovery of function is expected. Any recovery of speech is likely to be within the first few days.

2. (a) This is a transient ischaemic attack (TIA), probably in the territory of the right middle cerebral artery.

   (b) The causes and investigation of a TIA are listed on page 671.

3. (a) Meningitis. The petechial skin rash suggests meningococcal meningitis.

   (b) Immediate intravenous benzylpenicillin should be given. In the presence of a typical skin rash lumbar puncture is not usually necessary and the organism is found on blood cultures. A CT scan should be performed if there is any suspicion of an intracranial mass lesion. Emergency management of suspected meningitis is outlined in Emergency Box 15.3 on p. 691.

   (c) The rapid downhill course is suggestive of fulminant meningococcaemia (Waterhouse–Friderichsen syndrome). Haemorrhage into the adrenal glands may or may not be present.

4. (a) Coma must never be ascribed to excess alcohol until a thorough history (from relatives, ambulance staff), physical examination and investigation have ruled out other causes. The most likely causes (Table 15.8) in this case are alcohol, drug overdose (with alcohol as a second agent), hypoglycaemia, intracerebral haemorrhage, infarction and Wernicke–Korsakoff syndrome (p. 537).

   (b) The initial management consists of emergency resuscitation to stabilize the patient (p. 525). Intravenous glucose and thiamine (see later) are given. Further assessment (p. 661) and investigations (p. 663) are performed to find the cause of coma. Further management consists of treatment of the underlying cause and care of the unconscious patient (p. 663).

5. The causes of dementia are listed in Table 15.25. Treatable causes include hypothyroidism, vitamin $B_{12}$ deficiency, uraemia, hepatic failure, operable cerebral tumour, subdural haematoma and normal pressure hydrocephalus (p. 699). Depression may produce a clinical picture that is indistinguishable from dementia (pseudodementia) and resolves with treatment. Neurosyphilis (p. 694) and Wernicke–Korsakoff syndrome (p. 537) may cause

dementia; treatment should always be given, as the disease process may be arrested but rarely reversed. Young age, focal neurological signs, a history of head injury and evidence of anaemia or hypothyroidism should arouse suspicion that this is not Alzheimer's disease (the usual cause of dementia).

6.  (a) The history of *P. carinii* pneumonia and oral thrush occurring in a gay man suggests AIDS.

    (b) Right parietal lobe.

    (c) Ring-enhancing lesions in HIV-infected patients may be caused by *Toxoplasma gondii*, bacteria or lymphoma. Ring enhancement is non-specific and indicates increased vascularity. This patient in fact had a brain abscess caused by infection with *T. gondii* due to reactivation of a previous infection.

7.  (a) The distal weakness progressing proximally is the typical picture of Guillain–Barré syndrome (GBS, acute inflammatory polyneuropathy) (p. 712), the commonest cause of acute generalized muscle weakness.

    (b) The diagnosis is made clinically, by nerve conduction studies and examination of the CSF obtained at lumbar puncture (p. 713).

    (c) *Campylobacter jejuni* is a major cause of antecedent infection in GBS patients, and may be associated with a more severe form that tends to be exclusively motor.

    (d) The management is:
    - *General.* The monitoring and general treatment of these patients is discussed on page 713. In this particular case the difficulty in coughing suggests involvement of the respiratory muscles, and ventilation may well be necessary.
    - *Specific.* All patients with any but the mildest deficit should have either plasma exchange or intravenous immune globulin, started as early as possible. Which one is given will often depend on local preference and circumstances.

8. The causes of ptosis are third-nerve lesions (usually complete unilateral ptosis with other eye signs, p. 652), sympathetic paralysis (partial unilateral ptosis with other features of Horner's syndrome, p. 651), myopathy (partial bilateral), congenital (present since birth, usually partial, no other neurological signs) and syphilis (tabes dorsalis, p. 695).

9. The features and causes of Horner's syndrome are described on page 651.

10. (a) There is a CSF lymphocytosis, reduced glucose (in the absence of hypoglycaemia), markedly raised protein and raised CSF pressure. A raised CSF protein occurs with any inflammatory lesion of the CNS. A reduced CSF glucose occurs with bacterial or tuberculous meningitis, and rarely with viral and fungal infections and malignancy. The CSF lymphocytosis is against bacterial meningitis unless it has been partially treated.

    (b) The findings are most likely to be due to tuberculous meningitis, which is particularly common in Asians.

---

## Dermatology

1. What are the features and common causes of erythema nodosum? How would you investigate a patient with this condition?

2. Write short notes on the management of psoriasis.

## Answers

1. The causes and clinical features of erythema nodosum are listed on page 728. Sarcoidosis and inflammatory bowel disease are the most common causes in the UK. A history of recent antibiotic ingestion, oral contraceptives or alteration in bowel habit should be sought. Basic investigations should include a full blood count, ESR and chest X-ray. Further investigations will depend on the history and associated clinical findings. For instance, in a patient who also has diarrhoea it would be reasonable to

perform a small bowel barium follow-through examination to look for Crohn's disease. In a patient who is otherwise well and with a single attack, further investigation may be unnecessary.

2. The management of psoriasis is outlined on page 726.

# Dictionary of terms

There are excellent on-line medical dictionaries with definitions for thousands of medical words and conditions. Sites for two of them are:

http://www.medterms.com
http://cancerweb.ncl.ac.uk/omd/

**Adenoma** A benign epithelial neoplasm in which the cells form recognizable glandular structures or in which they are clearly derived from glandular epithelium.

**Adjuvant** Term applied to chemotherapy or hormone therapy given after local treatment, in tumours where dissemination is undetectable but can be assumed to have occurred. If effective, it should lead to an increase in cure rate or overall disease-free survival.

**Aerobic** In microbiology refers to growing, living or occurring in the presence of molecular oxygen. Bacteria that require oxygen to survive (aerobic bacteria).

**Afterload** The load against which the cardiac muscle exerts its contractile force, i.e. the peripheral vascular tree.

**Agonist** A drug that has affinity for and in some way activates a receptor when it occupies it.

**Allogeneic transplantation** When another individual acts as the donor.

**Anaerobic** Lacking molecular oxygen. Growing, living or occurring in the absence of molecular oxygen, pertaining to an anaerobe.

**Angiography** A radiographic technique where a radio-opaque contrast material is injected into a blood vessel for the purpose of identifying its anatomy on X-ray.

**Annular lesions**   Lesions occurring in rings.

**Antibody**   An immunoglobulin molecule that has a specific amino acid sequence by virtue of which it interacts only with the antigen that induced its synthesis in cells of the lymphoid series (especially plasma cells), or with antigen closely related to it.

**Antigen**   Any substance, organism or foreign material recognized by the immune system as being 'non-self', which will provoke the production of a specific antibody.

**Antineutrophil cytoplasmic antibodies (ANCAs)**   These are detected on fixed human neutrophils. There are two types:

- Antibodies directed against proteinase 3 (PR3-ANCA), formerly called cytoplasmic or cANCA. Present in 90% of patients with Wegener's granulomatosis.
- Antibodies directed against myeloperoxidase, formerly called perinuclear or pANCA. Present in 60% of some other vasculitides, such as microscopic polyangiitis and Churg–Strauss syndrome. Also found in inflammatory bowel disease and rheumatological disease which is not associated with a vasculitis.

**Antinuclear antibodies (ANA)**   Represent a wide spectrum of autoantibodies. They are non-specific and may occur at low titre (e.g. 1:10) in healthy individuals.

**Antioxidant**   An enzyme or other organic substance that has the ability to counteract the damaging effects of oxygen in tissues. It has been suggested that anti-oxidant vitamins such as Vitamin E may provide protection against certain diseases, including atherosclerosis.

**Aphasia (dysphasia)**   A disturbance of the ability to use language, whether in speaking, writing or comprehending. It is caused by left frontoparietal lesions, often a stroke.

- Broca's aphasia (expressive aphasia) is due to a lesion in the left frontal lobe. There is reduced fluency of speech, with comprehension relatively preserved. The patient knows what he/she wants to say but cannot get the words out.

- Wernicke's aphasia (receptive aphasia) is due to a left temporoparietal lesion. The patient speaks fluently but words are put together in the wrong order, and in the most severe forms the patient speaks complete rubbish with the insertion of non-existent words. Comprehension is severely impaired.
- Global aphasia is due to widespread damage to the areas concerned with speech. The patient shows combined expressive and receptive dysphasia.

**Alopecia**   Hair loss from areas where it is normally present.

**Antagonist**   A drug that binds to a cell receptor and does not activate it.

**Apoptosis**   Programmed cell death, as signalled by the nuclei in normally functioning cells when age or state of cell health dictates.

**Apraxia**   Loss of the ability to carry out familiar purposeful movements in the absence of paralysis or other motor or sensory impairment.

**Ataxia**   is due to failure of coordination of complex muscular movements despite intact individual movements and sensation.

**Atrophy**   Thinning (e.g. of the skin).

**Autoantibody**   An antibody that reacts with an antigen which is a normal component of the body.

**Autologous**   When the patient acts as his or her own source of cells.

**Autosomal dominant**   Requires only one affected parent to have the trait to pass it on to offspring.

**Autosomal recessive**   Mutation carried on an autosome (i.e. a chromosome not involved in sex determination) that is deleterious only in homozygotes (identical alleles of the gene are carried). Both affected parents must have the trait to pass it on to their offspring.

**Behçet's disease**  A rare multisystem chronic recurrent disease characterized by recurrent ulceration in the mouth and genitalia, iritis, uveitis, arthritis, superficial thrombophlebitis and major vascular thrombosis (usually venous). Often treated with immunosuppressive therapy (corticosteroids, chlorambucil).

**Bone marrow**  is obtained for examination by aspiration from the anterior iliac crest or sternum. In many cases a trephine biopsy (removal of a core of bone marrow tissue) is also necessary.

**Bronchoalveolar lavage**  At bronchoscopy a lung segment is washed with saline and the fluid retrieved for cell analysis.

**Bulla**  A large vesicle.

**Bursa**  A closed fluid-filled sac lined with synovium that functions to facilitate movement and reduce friction between tissues of the body. Bursitis is inflammation of a bursa.

**Carcinoma**  A malignant neoplasm arising from epithelium.

**Cardiac catheterization**  The passage of a small catheter through a peripheral vein (study of right-sided heart structures) or artery (for study of left-sided heart structures) into the heart, permitting the securing of blood samples, measurement of intracardiac pressures and determination of cardiac anomalies.

**Cardiac nuclear imaging**  uses radiotracers (injected intravenously) which diffuse freely into myocardial tissue or attach to red blood cells.

- Thallium-201 is taken up by cardiac myocytes. Ischaemic areas (produced by exercising the patient) with reduced tracer uptake are seen as 'cold spots' when imaged with a γ camera.
- Technetium-99m is used to label red blood cells and produce images of the left ventricle during systole and diastole.

**Caseating**   Developing a necrotic centre.

**CD (cluster differentiation) antigens**   Antigens on the cell surface that can be detected by immune reagents and which are associated with the differentiation of a particular cell type or types. Many cells can be identified by their possession of a unique set of differentiation antigens, e.g. CD4, CD8.

**Cheyne–Stoke respiration**   An abnormal breathing pattern in which there are periods of rapid breathing alternating with periods of no breathing or slow breathing.

**Chronotropic**   Positively chronotropic means to increase the rate of contraction of the heart; negatively chronotropic is the opposite.

**Clone**   A population of identical cells or organisms that are derived from a single cell or ancestor and contain identical DNA molecules.

**Clubbing**   Broadening or thickening of the tips of the fingers and toes with increased lengthwise curvature of the nail and a decrease in the angle normally seen between cuticle and fingernail. Causes include congenital, respiratory (lung cancer, tuberculosis, bronchiectasis, lung abscess or empyema, lung fibrosis), cardiac (bacterial endocarditis, cyanotic congenital heart disease), and rarely gastrointestinal (Crohn's disease, cirrhosis).

**Congenital**   Something that is present at birth. It may or may not be genetic (inherited).

**Constructional apraxia**   Inability to copy simple drawings: often seen in hepatic encephalopathy, when the patient is unable to copy a five-pointed star.

**Contraindication**   Any condition, especially a disease or current treatment, which renders some particular line of treatment undesirable.

**C-reactive protein (CRP)**   is synthesized in the liver and produced during the acute-phase response. It is quick and easy to measure and is replacing measurement of the ESR in some centres.

**Crust**  Dried exudate on the skin.

**Cryoglobulins**  Immunoglobulins that precipitate when cold or during exercise. They may be monoclonal or polyclonal, e.g. mixed essential cryoglobulinaemia, and result in a cutaneous vasculitis or occasionally a multisystem disorder.

**Cryptogenic**  A disease of obscure or unknown origin.

**CT scan (computed tomography)**  CT combines the use of X-rays with computerized analysis of the images to assimilate multiple X-ray images into a two-dimensional cross-sectional image. With helical or spiral CT scanning, computer interpolation allows reconstruction of standard transverse scans or images in any preferred plane. CT angiography uses X-rays to visualize blood flow in arterial vessels throughout the body.

**Cytokines**  Soluble messenger molecules which enable the immune system to communicate through its different compartments. Cytokines are made by many cells, such as lymphocytes (lymphokines) and other white cells (interleukins). Examples of cytokines, other than interleukins, include tumour necrosis factor (TNF), interferons and granulocyte colony-stimulating factor (G-CSF).

**Distal**  A term of comparison meaning farther from a point of reference; it is the opposite of proximal.

**Dysarthria**  Disordered articulation. Any lesion that produces paralysis, slowing or incoordination of the muscles of articulation, or local discomfort, will cause dysarthria. Examples are upper and lower motor lesions of the lower cranial nerves, cerebellar lesions, Parkinson's disease and local lesions in the mouth, larynx, pharynx and tongue.

**Dysplasia**  Abnormal cell growth or maturation of cells.

**Ecchymoses**  Bruises > 3 mm in diameter.

**Echocardiography**  Non-invasive method of recording the position and motion of the structures of the heart by echo obtained from beams of ultrasonic waves directed through the chest wall.

- Transoesophageal echo uses miniaturized transducers incorporated into special endoscopes. It allows better visualization of some structures and pathology, e.g. aortic dissection, prosthetic valve endocarditis.
- Doppler echocardiography uses the Doppler principle (in this case, the frequency of ultrasonic waves reflected from blood cells is related to their velocity and direction of flow) to identify and assess the severity of valve lesions.

**Ectopic**  Located away from its normal position, such as an ectopic pregnancy.

**Ejection fraction**  The fraction of the ventricular end-diastolic volume that is ejected during cardiac systole. It is usually equal to about 60%.

**Electroencephalogram (EEG)**  Electrodes applied to the patient's scalp pick up small changes in electrical potential which, after amplification, are recorded on paper or displayed on a video monitor. It is used in the investigation of epilepsy and diffuse brain disorders.

**Electromyography (EMG)**  A needle electrode is inserted percutaneously into voluntary muscle. Amplified action potentials are recorded on an oscilloscope. Normal resting muscle shows no activity, and during increasing muscle contractions progressively larger numbers of motor units are recruited. EMG is useful in the diagnosis of primary muscle disease (myopathies and dystrophies, individual motor unit potentials are small) and of lower motor neurone lesions (denervation, spontaneous activity appears at rest).

**Empirical**  Based on experience. Empirical treatment refers to treatment given to an individual that is based on the experience of the physician in treating previous patients with a similar presentation. It is not completely 'scientific' treatment.

**End-diastolic volume**  The volume of blood in the ventricle at the end of diastole.

**Endemic**  Present in a community at all times.

**Endogenous**  Related to or produced by the body.

**Enzyme-linked immunosorbent (ELISA) assay**  A serologic test used for the detection of particular antibodies or antigens in the blood. ELISA technology links a measurable enzyme to either an antigen or antibody. In this way it can then measure the presence of an antibody or an antigen in the bloodstream.

**Eosinophilia**  (normal range 0.04–0.44 × 10⁹/L, 1–6% of total white cells) occurs in asthma and allergic disorders, parasitic infections (e.g. *Ascaris*), skin disorders (urticaria, pemphigus and eczema), malignancy and the hypereosinophilic syndrome (restrictive cardiomyopathy, hepatosplenomegaly and very high eosinophil count).

**Epidemic**  An outbreak of a disease affecting a large number of individuals in a community at the same time. The number of people affected is in excess of the expected.

**Epidemiology**  The study of the distribution and determinants of health-related states and events in populations.

**Epitope**  That part of an antigenic molecule to which an antibody or T-cell receptor responds.

**ERCP**  Endoscopic retrograde cholangiopancreatography. The ampulla of Vater is cannulated, and after injection of radio-opaque contrast medium the pancreatic and common bile ducts (CBD) can be visualized. The sphincter of Oddi may be cut (sphincterotomy) to facilitate the removal of stones and insertion of stents.

**Erythema**  Redness.

**Erythrocyte sedimentation rate (ESR)**  The rate of fall of red cells in a column of blood; a measure of the acute-phase response. The speed is mainly determined by the concentration of large proteins, e.g. fibrinogen.

The ESR is higher in women and rises with age. It is raised in a wide variety of systemic inflammatory and neoplastic diseases. The highest values (>100 mm/h) are found in chronic infections (e.g. TB), myeloma, connective tissue disorders and cancer.

**Erythroderma**  Widespread redness of the skin, with scaling.

**Euthanasia**  The illegal act of killing someone painlessly, especially to relieve suffering from an incurable disease.

**Excoriation**  Linear marks caused by scratching.

**Excretion urography**  (intravenous urography (IVU) or intravenous pyelography (IVP). Serial radiographs are taken of the kidney and the full length of the abdomen, following intravenous injection of contrast, usually an organic iodine-containing medium.

**Exogenous**  Developed or originated outside of the body.

**Extractable nuclear antigens (ENA)**  Nuclear components that are soluble in saline. Examples are Sm, Ro, La and ribonucleoprotein (RNP) antigen. The presence of serum anti-Sm antibodies is highly specific for SLE. Anti-Ro (SS-A) and anti-La (SS-B) occur in patients with Sjögren's syndrome and in some patients with SLE.

**Exudate**  Fluid rich in protein and cells which has leaked from blood vessels and deposited in tissues.

**Factitious**  Artificial, self-induced.

**Familial Mediterranean fever**  Inherited disorder more common in those of Mediterranean descent. Recurrent episodes of abdominal pain (due to peritoneal inflammation), fever and arthritis.

**Fissure**  A cleft, groove or slit, e.g. an anal fissure is an ulcer in the anal canal.

**Fistula**  A tunnel or abnormal passage connecting two epithelial surfaces, frequently designated according to the organs or parts with which it communicates, e.g. a vesicocolic fistula connects the bladder to the colon.

**Gaucher's disease** Inherited (autosomal recessive) disorder of lipid metabolism caused by a deficiency of the enzyme β-glucocerebrosidase. Clinical features include hepatosplenomegaly and sometimes neurological dysfunction.

**Generic drugs** Non-proprietary drugs. They should usually be used when prescribing in preference to proprietary titles.

**Glomerular filtration rate (GFR)** This is the most widely used test of renal function. In routine clinical practice the most reliable index of GFR is measurement of endogenous creatinine clearance, which is calculated from a 24-hour urine collection and measurement of a single serum creatinine value during the 24 hours.

**Histocompatibility antigens** Genetically determined isoantigens present on the membranes of nucleated cells. They incite an immune response when grafted on to genetically disparate individuals, and thus determine the compatibility of cells in transplantation.

**Howell–Jolly bodies** DNA remnants in peripheral RBCs seen postsplenectomy, in leukaemia and megaloblastic anaemia.

**Human leucocyte antigens (HLA)** Human histocompatibility antigens determined by a region on chromosome 6. There are several genetic loci, each having multiple alleles, designated HLA-A, HLA-B, HLA-C, HLA-DP, -DQ and -DR. The susceptibility to some diseases is associated with certain HLA alleles (e.g. HLA-B27 in 95% of patients with ankylosing spondylitis), although their exact role in aetiology is unclear.

**Hyperplasia** The abnormal multiplication or increase in the number of normal cells in normal arrangement in a tissue.

**Hypertrophy** The enlargement or overgrowth of an organ or part due to an increase in size of its constituent cells.

**Iatrogenic**  Induced inadvertently by medical treatment or procedures, or activity of attending physician.

**Idiopathic**  Of unknown cause.

**Idiosyncratic**  Relates to idiosyncrasy – an abnormal susceptibility to a drug or other agent which is peculiar to the individual.

**Incidence**  An expression of the rate at which a certain event occurs as the number of new cases of a specific disease occurring during a certain period.

**Inotropic**  Positively inotropic means increasing the force of cardiac muscle contraction.

**In vitro**  Outside of the body in an artificial environment such as a test tube.

**In vivo**  Within the body.

**Left shift**  Immature white cells appear in the peripheral blood, e.g. with infection.

**Leucocytosis**  An increase in the total circulating white cells ($> 11 \times 10^9/L$).

**Leucoerythroblastic reaction**  Immature red and white cells appearing in the peripheral blood. It occurs in marrow infiltration (e.g. malignancy), myeloid leukaemia and severe anaemia.

**Leucopenia**  A decrease in the total circulating white cells ($< 4.0 \times 10^9/L$).

**Leukaemoid reaction**  A reactive but excessive leucocytosis characterized by the presence of immature cells in the peripheral blood.

**Kawasaki disease**  An acute febrile illness (lasting more than 5 days) of unknown aetiology that occurs mainly in children. Features include damage to the coronary arteries which is reduced by treatment with aspirin and intravenous γ-globulin.

**Macule**  A flat circumscribed area of discoloration.

**Maculopapule**  A raised and discoloured circumscribed lesion.

**Magnetic resonance imaging (MRI)**  uses the body's natural magnetic properties to produce detailed images from any part of the body. It does not involve radiation. Pacemakers, metallic clips, metal valves and joint prostheses can be dangerous in MRI scanners because of potential movement within a magnetic field.

**Marfan's syndrome**  Autosomal dominant connective tissue disorder associated with mutations in the fibrillin 1 gene on chromosome 15. Up to one-third are new mutations. Clinical features include tall stature, long thin digits (arachnodactly), high arched palate, hypermobile joints, lens subluxation, incompetence of aortic and mitral valves, aortic dissection and spontaneous pneumothorax.

**Metaplasia**  A change in the type of cells in a tissue to a form which is not normal for that tissue.

**Micturating cystoscopy**  Used mainly for the evaluation of vesicoureteric reflux in children. Contrast medium is instilled into the bladder via a catheter, and the ureters and kidneys are then screened during micturition.

**Monocytosis**  (normal range 0.04–0.44 × $10^9$/L, 1–6% of total white cells) occurs in chronic bacterial infections (e.g. TB), myelodysplasia and malignancy, particularly chronic myelomonocytic leukaemia.

**National Institute for Clinical Excellence (NICE)**  This is part of the National Health Service (NHS) in the UK and its role is to provide patients, health professionals and the public with authoritative, robust and reliable guidance on current 'best practice'.

**ND**  Notifiable disease.

**Necrosis**  Morphological changes indicative of cell death and caused by the progressive degradative action of enzymes; it may affect groups of cells or part of a structure or an organ.

**Neutropenia**   (normal range $2–7.5 \times 10^9/L$, 40–75% of total white cells). Causes include racial (in black Africans), viral infection, severe bacterial infection, megaloblastic anaemia, pancytopenia and drugs (marrow aplasia or immune destruction).

**Neutrophil leucocytosis**   Occurs in bacterial infection, tissue necrosis, inflammation, corticosteroid therapy, myeloproliferative disease, leukaemoid reaction, leucoerythroblastic anaemia, acute haemorrhage and haemolysis.

**Nodule**   A circumscribed large palpable mass >1 cm in diameter.

**Normoblasts**   Immature nucleated red blood cells (RBCs) seen in the peripheral blood with a leucoerthyro-blastic reaction and severe anaemia.

**Oligoarticular**   Affecting a limited number of joints.

**Oncogene**   Gene coding for proteins which are either growth factors, growth factor receptors, secondary messengers or DNA-binding proteins. Mutation of the gene promotes abnormal cell growth.

**Osmolality**   The concentration of osmotically active particles in solution expressed in terms of osmoles of solute per kilogram of solvent.

**Osmolarity**   The concentration of osmotically active particles expressed in terms of osmoles of solute per litre of solution.

**Pancytopenia**   Deficiency of all cell elements of the blood.

**Papule**   A circumscribed raised palpable area.

**Pathognomonic**   A symptom or sign that, when present, points unmistakably to the presence of a certain definite disease.

**Persistent vegetative state**   A condition of life without consciousness or will as a result of brain damage.

**Petechiae**   Bruises <3 mm in diameter.

**Phenotype**   The appearance and function of an organism as a result of its genotype and its environment.

**Plaque**   A disc-shaped lesion; can result from coalescence of papules.

**Polychromasia**   Blue tinge to red blood cells in the blood film caused by the presence of young red cells.

**Polymerase chain reaction (PCR)**   Technique for rapid detection and analysis of DNA and, by a modification of the method, RNA. Using oligo-nucleotide primers and DNA polymerase, minute amounts of genomic DNA can be amplified over a million times into measurable quantities.

**Prevalence**   Total number of cases of a disease in existence at a certain time in a designated area.

**Prognosis**   A forecast as to the probable outcome of an attack or disease.

**Promyelocytes, myelocytes and metamyelocytes**   Immature white cells seen in the peripheral blood in leucoerythroblastic anaemia.

**Prophylaxis**   Prevention of disease.

**Proximal**   A term of comparison meaning nearer or closer to a point of reference; for example, proximal myopathy is weakness of muscles nearest to the trunk, e.g. quadriceps.

**Purpura**   Extravasation of blood into the skin; does not blanch on pressure.

**Pustule**   A pus-filled blister.

**Radioimmunoassay (RIA)**   Any system for testing antigen–antibody reactions in which use is made of radioactive labelling of antigen or antibody to detect the extent of the reaction.

### Renal scintigraphy

- Static scanning is performed after an intravenous injection of technetium-99m-labelled dimercaptosuccinic

acid ($^{99m}$Tc-DMSA), which is taken up by the kidneys. It allows an assessment of the function of each kidney
- Dynamic scanning is performed after an intravenous injection of technetium-99m-labelled diethylenetriaminepentaacetic acid ($^{99m}$Tc-DTPA), which is taken up by the kidneys and excreted into the collecting systems, ureter and bladder. It allows assessment of renal blood flow, estimation of GFR and assessment of obstructive uropathy.

**Retrograde pyelography** Following cystoscopy a catheter is placed in the ureteral orifice and contrast injected. It is used to investigate lesions of the lower ureter and to define the lower level of ureteral obstruction shown on ultrasound or antegrade studies.

**Rhabdomyolysis** The destruction of skeletal muscle cells. May be due to electrical injury, alcoholism, injury, drug side-effects or toxins.

**Rheumatoid factors (RhF)** Autoantibodies found in the serum, usually of the IgM class, which are directed against the Fc portion of human IgG. They are found in high titre in 70% of patients with rheumatoid arthritis. They may also be detected in other auto-immune rheumatic diseases, autoimmune hepatitis, chronic infections, and in elderly people at low titres.

**Scales** Dried flakes of dead skin.

**Serum** The cell-free portion of blood from which fibrinogen has been separated in the process of clotting. Serum is the supernatant obtained by high-speed centrifugation of whole blood collected in a plain tube.

**Sinus** A blind track opening onto the skin or a mucous surface.

**Syndrome** A set of signs or a series of events occurring together that point to a single condition as the cause.

**Target cells** ('Mexican hat cells') Red blood cells with central staining surrounded by a ring of pallor and an outer ring of staining. They occur in thalassaemia, sickle cell disease and liver disease.

**Telangiectasia**   A visible, dilated blood vessel creating small focal red lesions in skin, mucous membranes or gut.

**TNM classification** (tumour, node, metastasis)   Staging system for many cancers. T is the extent of primary tumour, N is the involvement of lymph nodes and M indicates the presence or absence of metastases. For instance T0–T4 indicates increasing local tumour spread.

**Transudate**   A plasma-derived fluid that accumulates in tissues/cavities as a result of venous and capillary pressure.

**Tumour suppressor genes**   Genes whose protein products induce the repair or self-destruction (apoptosis) of cells containing damaged DNA. Unlike oncogenes, they restrict undue cell proliferation.

**Turner's syndrome**   Females with chromosome 45X instead of the normal female chromosomes, 46XX. Growth failure, gonadal dysgenesis, widely spaced nipples, webbed neck, cardiac abnormalities, intelligence usually normal.

**Vesicle**   A small, visible, fluid-filled blister.

**Weal**   A transiently raised reddened area associated with scratching.

**Xenotransplantation**   Transplantation of organs or tissues between different species.

**Zoonosis**   Transmission of a disease from an animal or non-human species to humans. The reservoir for the disease is not human.

# Index

**Notes**
Page references in **bold** refer to
major discussions.

## A

abacavir 51
  AIDS 50
abacteriuric frequency **328**
abciximab
  acute coronary syndrome 402
  arterial thrombosis 215
ABC system 384
abdomen, acute **102–106**
abdominal aortic aneurysms **440**
abdominal pain 53, **102–106**
  acute intermittent porphyria
    631
abdominal paracentesis 748–749
ABO blood groups **201–204**
abscesses
  Bartholin's 39
  cerebral **694**
  intracranial **693–694**
  liver see liver abscesses
  lung 477–478
absences, typical 675
acamprosate 539
acanthosis nigricans 496
acarbose 606
accessory nerve (eleventh cranial)
    659
accommodation 649
ACE inhibitors see angiotensin
    converting enzyme (ACE)
    inhibitors
acetaminophen see paracetamol
    (acetaminophen)
acetylcholine receptor antibodies
    715–716
acetylcholinesterase inhibitors
    721
N-acetylcysteine (NAC)
    530–531
achalasia **60–61**
Achilles tendinitis 247

aciclovir
  meningitis 693
  Ramsay Hunt syndrome 656
  viral infections 13, 14, 47
acid–base disorders **302–308**
acidophil adenomas 545
acidosis
  blood gas changes 304
  chronic renal failure 351–352
  lactic **305**
  metabolic see metabolic acidosis
  renal tubular see renal tubular
    acidosis
  respiratory 303
  uraemic 307–308
acitretin 726
acne vulgaris **723–724**
acquired haemolytic anaemias
    **189–193**
acquired immunodeficiency
    syndrome see AIDS
acromegaly **559–561**
  secondary hypertension 436
activated charcoal
  aspirin overdose 529
  poisoning 526
activated partial thromboplastin
    time (APTT) 208
acute abdomen **102–106**
acute coronary syndromes (ACS)
    399, **402**
acute disturbances of
    haemodynamic function see
    shock
acute exacerbation of COPD
    455–456
acute intermittent porphyria
    **631–632**
acute lung injury (ALI) **520–521**
acute lymphoblastic leukaemia
    (ALL) **222–223**, **224–225**
acute myelogenous leukaemia
    (AML) **222–225**
acute physiology and chronic
    health inquiry score
    (APACHE) 505
  pancreatitis 160

acute promyelocytic leukaemia (APML) 224
acute respiratory distress syndrome (ARDS) 507, **520–521**
acute sequestration crisis 186
acute seroconversion syndrome 43
acute tumour lysis syndrome (ATLS) 223
Addisonian crisis 574
  emergency management 576
Addison's disease 562, **573–575**, 770
  dilutional hyponatraemia 295
adenoma 799
  acidophil 545
  adrenal glands 579, 592
  basophil 545
  hepatic 153
  pituitary gland 557, 580
  toxic 565
adenoma–carcinoma sequence 95
adenomatous polyps **94**
adenosine 380
adjuvant 799
adrenal glands
  adenomas 579, 592
  carcinomas 579
  diseases/disorders **573–581**
  incidental tumours 581
adrenaline *see* epinephrine
adrenocorticotrophin (ACTH) 541, 542, 546
  Cushing's syndrome 580
  gout 267
  hypoadrenalism 577
  multiple sclerosis 688
  release 573
$\beta_2$-adrenoreceptor agonists *see* $\beta_2$-adrenoreceptor agonists *(under beta)*
$\alpha_1$-adrenoreceptor antagonists 439
  benign prostatic hypertrophy 359
  chronic cardiac failure 394
$\beta$-adrenoreceptor antagonists *see* $\beta$-blockers
adult polycystic renal disease (APCD) **356**
advanced life support 384
aerobic, definition 799
afterload 799

agonist, definition 799
AIDS **45–50**, 795
  bacterial infections 48–49
  diagnosis 45, 50
  diarrhoea 100
  fungal infections 48
  protozoal infections 46–47
  sclerosing cholangitis 158
  viral infections 47–48
  *see also* HIV infection
airway remodelling 464
akinesia 682
akinetic-rigid syndromes 680–683
alabaster skin 547–548
alanine aminotransferase (ALT) 115
albendazole 36, 38
albumin 201
  volume replacement therapy 510
alcohol
  hypertension 440
  liver disease **148–149**
  overdose 534
  units 536
alcohol abuse **536–539**, 578, 785, 794
  acute intermittent porphyria 631
  examination questions 783–785
  unconsciousness 661–662
  withdrawal 538–539
alcoholic cirrhosis **149**
alcoholic hepatitis 148, 764
alcoholic liver diseases **148–149**
aldosterone 591, 592
alendronate 279–280
alfacalcidol 589
alkaline phosphatase
  liver disease 115
  lumbar back pain 269
  lung carcinoma 497
  osteomalacia 277
  Paget's disease 282
alkalosis
  blood gas changes 304
  metabolic 308
  respiratory *see* respiratory alkalosis
alkylating agents 233, 234
allergens 464–465
allergic bronchopulmonary aspergillosis 465

allergic rhinitis   449
allergies   463
allogeneic transplantation   799
allogenic bone marrow
        transplantation   231–232
allopurinol   267
alopecia   801
$\alpha_1$-antitrypsin deficiency   **147,**
        453
alpha-fetoprotein (AFP)
    cirrhosis   134
    hepatocellular carcinoma   153
alpha-interferon (IFN-$\alpha$) *see*
        interferon alpha (IFN-$\alpha$)
alprostadil   551
alteplase   215
Alzheimer's disease   **719–721,**
        795
    amyloid deposits   632
amantadine   683
amaurosis fugax   671
ambulatory blood pressure
        monitoring   435
amenorrhoea   **553–555**
    hyperprolactinaemia   557
    polycystic ovary syndrome
        556
amfetamine abuse   535
amiloride   289
    chronic cardiac failure   392
aminoaciduria   313
    renal tubular acidosis   307
aminoglutethimide   580
aminoglycosides   327
$\delta$-aminolaevulinic acid ($\delta$-ALA)
        630–631
aminophylline   469
5-aminosalicylic acid   89
aminotransferases   115
amiodarone
    adverse effects   565
    atrial fibrillation   409
    in cardiac arrest management
        385
    hypertrophic cardiomyopathy
        432
    junctional tachycardias   381
    ventricular ectopic beats   382
    ventricular fibrillation   409
    ventricular tachycardia   382
amitriptyline   701
amlodipine
    angina   401
    chronic cardiac failure   394
    hypertension   439

ammonia   140
amoebiasis   **25, 27–28,** 758, 761
amoebic colitis   27
amoebic dysentery   27
amoebic liver abscess   27,
        **151–152**
amoxicillin
    *H. pylori* infection   66
    Lyme disease   16
    pneumonia   474
    salmonella arthritis   252
    typhoid fever   25
    urinary tract infections   327
amphetamine abuse   535
amphotericin B   48
amprenavir   51
Amsterdam criteria   97
amyloid glomerulonephritis   323
amyloidosis   **632–633**
amyotrophic lateral sclerosis   709
amyotrophy, diabetic   618
anaemias   **165–193,** 765–766
    acute renal failure   344
    alcohol abuse   538
    aplastic   **177–178**
    of chronic disease   **170–171**
    chronic renal failure   348, 351
    classification   167, 168
    haemolytic *see* haemolytic
        anaemias
    inflammatory bowel disease
        85, 87
    iron deficiency   170
    leukaemias   222
    macrocytic   168, **171–176**
    megaloblastic   **171–172**
    microcytic   **167–171,** 765
    mouth ulcers   55
    pernicious   **172–175**
    rheumatoid arthritis   243
    sickle-cell *see* sickle cell disease
    sideroblastic   **171**
    systemic sclerosis   258
anaerobic, definition   799
anaesthesia, local   734
analgesic nephropathy   329
analgesics
    acute intermittent porphyria
        632
    headache   700
    migraine   701
    osteoarthritis   239
    pneumonia   474
    psoriatic arthritis   250
    pulmonary oedema   396

A

analgesics (*contd*)
  renal stone disease   336
  spondylolisthesis   274–275
  tubulointerstitial nephritis
       328–329
anaphylactic shock   506, 507, **508,**
       510, 513
  blood transfusions   203
  emergency management   514
*Ancylostoma duodenale* infections
       35
androgen deficiency   549
angina   **398–402,** 775–776
  acute coronary syndromes   **402**
  anaemia   166
  aortic stenosis   419
  cardiac syndrome X   399
  decubitus   399
  hypertrophic cardiomyopathy
       432
  Prinzmetal's   399
  unstable   399, **402,** 776
  variant   399
angiodysplasia   74
angiography   799
  angina   400
  aortic stenosis   420
  pulmonary embolism   427–428
  radionuclide   391
  unilateral renal disease   331
angioplasty
  angina   **401–402**
  myocardial infarction   408
angiotensin   591
angiotensin converting enzyme
       (ACE)   591
  coronary artery disease   398
  granulomatous lung disease
       485
angiotensin converting enzyme
       (ACE) inhibitors
  acute renal failure   341
  adverse effects   393, 439
  bilateral renal disease   330
  chronic cardiac failure   393,
       394
  chronic renal failure   351
  diabetic nephropathy   616
  hypertension   437, 438–439
  myocardial infarction   408
  unilateral renal disease   331
angiotensin II (AII) type 1
       receptor antagonists
  chronic cardiac failure   393
  hypertension   439

angiotensinogen   591
anion gap
  high   306
  low   307
ankylosing spondylitis (AS)
       **246–248**
  enteropathic arthritis   250
  juvenile   265
  neck pain   275
annular lesions   800
anorexia   479
anorexia nervosa   **111**
  amenorrhoea   554
anosmia   647
antacids   59
antagonist, definition   801
anterior horn cell lesions   641
anterior spinal artery occlusion
       705
anti-androgen agents   557
anti-arrhythmic drugs
  atrial fibrillation   379–380
  atrial flutter   378
  chronic cardiac failure   394
  classification   379
  sinus bradycardia   373
  sinus node dysfunction   374
antibiotics
  acne vulgaris   725
  acute exacerbation of COPD
       456
  bronchiectasis   458
  cholecystitis   156
  diverticular disease   92
  empyema   478
  infective endocarditis   424
  influenza   451
  meningitis   693
  pharyngitis   450
  portosystemic encephalopathy
       141–142
  Reiter's syndrome   249
  septic arthritis   251
  septicemia   11
  septic shock   513
  traveller's diarrhoea   31, 758
  typhoid fever   25
  urinary tract infections   327
antibody   800
anticholinergic bronchodilators
       466
anticholinergic drugs
  dystonias   686
  incontinence   362
  myasthenia gravis   717

anticholinergic drugs   (contd)
Parkinson's disease   683
anticoagulation treatment
**214–219**
atrial fibrillation   379–380
deep vein thrombosis (DVT)
441–442
mitral valve prolapse   418
pulmonary embolism   429
stroke   670
antidiuretic hormone (ADH)
287, 542, 543, 547
impaired secretion   582–583
inappropriate secretion
**581–582**
see also vasopressin, synthetic
antiemetics   701
anti-epileptic drugs   677–678
adverse effects   677–678
withdrawal   678
antigen   800
antiglomerular basement
membrane antibodies   317
antihistamines   449
antihypertensive drugs
chronic renal failure   351
hypertension   438–439
anti-inflammatory drugs
adverse effects   288
asthma   469
see also non-steroidal anti-
inflammatory drugs
(NSAIDs)
antilymphocyte globulin
aplastic anaemia   178
renal transplantation   355
antimitochondrial antibodies
142
antimuscarinic eyedrops   651
antineutrophil cytoplasmic
antibodies (ANCA)   264,
486, 487, 800
c-ANCA and p-ANCA   800
antinuclear antibodies (ANAs)
800
overlap syndrome   261
Sjögren's syndrome   261
systemic lupus erythematosus
254
systemic sclerosis   258
antioxidants   108, 800
antiphospholipid syndrome
**256–257**
antipruritic agents   728
antipyretic agents   22

antiretroviral therapy   50, 51
effects on HIV infection   44
antithrombin   206
antithyroid drugs
hyperthyroidism   567
thyroid crisis   568
$\alpha_1$-antitrypsin deficiency   **147,**
453
antituberculous drugs   481–482
adverse effects   482
anuria   311
aortic aneurysms   **440**
aortic dissection   440
aortic regurgitation   **419–420**
rheumatic fever   411
aortic stenosis   **418–419,** 778
exercise ECG   372
aortography   420
apathetic thyrotoxicosis   566
aphasia   671, 800–801
types   800–801
aplastic anaemia   **177–178**
aplastic crisis   186
apoprotein B-100 mutations   626
apoprotein C-II deficiency   625
apoptosis   801
appendicitis, acute   **104–105**
apraxia   801
constructional   141, 803
apudomas   164
arachnodactyly   730
Argyll Robertson pupil   651
Arnold–Chiari malformation
699, 706
arrhythmias see cardiac
arrhythmias
arrhythmogenic right ventricular
cardiomyopathy   **433**
arterial blood gases see blood
gases
arterial disease   **440–442**
arterial sampling   737–738
arterial thrombosis   **214–216**
arthralgia   235, 729
arthritis   **237–253,** 768
children   265
enteropathic   **250**
gonococcal   **252**
hereditary haemochromatosis
144
infective   **250–253**
juvenile chronic   265
meningococcal   **252**
psoriatic   **249–250**
reactive   **249**

**A**

arthritis (*contd*)
  Reiter's syndrome  248
  rheumatoid *see* rheumatoid
      arthritis (RA)
  salmonella  **252–253**
  septic *see* septic arthritis
  tuberculous  **252**
arthritis mutilans  243, 249
arthropathy, neuropathic  617
asbestosis  491–492, 493
*Ascaris lumbricoides* infections  34,
    35
ascites  **138–140**, 764
  constrictive pericarditis  435
  portal hypertension  136
aspartate aminotranspeptidase
    (AST)  115
  myocardial infarction  405
*Aspergillus fumigatus*  449
  AIDS  48
  asthma  463, 465
aspiration pneumonia  476–477
aspirin
  angina  400, 401–402
  antiphospholipid syndrome
      257
  arterial thrombosis  215
  asthma  464
  atrial fibrillation  380
  de Quervain's thyroiditis  565
  gastrointestinal bleeding  72
  gastropathy  64
  influenza  451
  myocardial infarction  406, 408
  overdose  528–529, 784
  peptic ulcers  67
  rheumatic fever  412
  stroke  669, 670
  transient ischaemic attacks
      671
asterixis  141
asthma  **461–471**, 779–780
  chronic  468
  cough  444
  lung function tests  448
  management  466–469
  wheeze  446
asthma, acute severe  **469–471**,
    780
  emergency management  470
ataxia  657, 801
  alcohol abuse  537
  anticonvulsant drugs  677
  cerebellar lesions  645
  with headache  636

atenolol  400–401
atheroma  397
  renal artery stenosis  331
atherosclerosis  614
atlantoaxial subluxation  242, 243
atopic eczema  727
atopic glossitis  **55**
atopy  463
atrial arrhythmias  **376–381**
  hypertrophic cardiomyopathy
      432
  myocardial infarction  409
atrial ectopic beats  377–378
atrial fibrillation (AF)  **379–380**,
    776–777
  electrical cardioversion  742
  hyperthyroidism  566
  mitral stenosis  414
  myocardial infarction  409
atrial flutter  **378**
  electrical cardioversion  742
atrial natriuretic peptides (ANPs)
    287
  cardiac failure  388
atrial pacing  381
atrial tachyarrhythmias  374–375
atrioventricular block  **374–376**
atrioventricular (AV) node  371
atrophic hypothyroidism
    561–562
atrophy  801
atropine
  sinus bradycardia  373, 409
  sinus tachycardia  409
Auer rods  222
auranofin
  adverse effects  245
  rheumatoid arthritis  244
Austin Flint murmur  421
autoantibodies  801
  antinuclear *see* antinuclear
      antibodies
  mitochondria  142
  rheumatoid arthritis  242
  systemic sclerosis  258
autoimmune diseases
  diabetes mellitus association
      600
  Graves' disease  565
  haemolytic anaemias  **189–192**,
      202
  hepatitis  **131–132**
  hypothyroidism  561–562
  primary biliary cirrhosis  143
  renal tubular acidosis  307

autoimmune thrombocytopenic purpura (AITP) **210–211**
autologous, definition 801
autologous bone marrow transplantation 232
autonomic neuropathy 618
autosomal dominant, definition 801
autosomal recessive, definition 801
azathioprine
  adverse effects 245
  autoimmune haemolytic anaemia 192
  autoimmune thrombocytopenic purpura 211
  Behçet's syndrome 265
  Churg–Strauss syndrome 265
  cryptogenic fibrosing alveolitis 488
  Cushing's syndrome 580–581
  polymyositis 260
  Reiter's syndrome 249
  renal transplantation 355
  rheumatoid arthritis 244
  systemic lupus erythematosus 256
azithromycin
  pneumonia 474
  tuberculosis 481

# B

bacillary dysentery **28**
bacille Calmette–Guérin (BCG) 482
*Bacillus cereus* infections 32
back pain **269–272**
baclofen 708
bacteraemia 9
bacterial gastroenteritis 30–33
bacterial meningitis 689–690
  emergency management 691
bacterial overgrowth **79–80**
bacterial peritonitis 140
bacteriuria 315
  Stix tests 312
*Bacteroides* infections 694
Baker's cyst 777–778
balloon tamponade
  aortic stenosis 420
  mitral stenosis 415
  variceal haemorrhage 137
barotrauma 519

Barrett's oesophagus 60, 62
Bartholin's abscess 39
basic life support 384–385
basophil adenomas 545
BCG vaccine 482
*BCR-ABL*
  chronic myeloid leukaemia 225
  leukaemias 220
Becker muscular dystrophy **715**
beclometasone dipropionate 466, 469
Behçet's disease **264–265,** 802
  genital ulcers 40
  mouth ulcers 55
Bell's palsy **656**
Bence-Jones protein 233
bendroflumethiazide (bendrofluazide) 289
  chronic cardiac failure 392
  hypertension 437
benign essential tremor 684
benign positional vertigo 659
benign prostatic hypertrophy 309, **359**
  overflow incontinence 363
benzatropine 686
benzodiazepines
  delirium 719
  overdose 533
benzylpenicillin
  infective endocarditis 424
  meningitis 693
  neurosyphilis 694
beri-beri **714**
Bernard–Soulier disease 205, 209
'berry' aneurysms 672
β₂-adrenoreceptor agonists
  acute asthma 471
  asthma 466
β-blockers
  adverse effects 438
  angina 400–401
  asthma 464
  chronic cardiac failure 394
  hypertension 437
  hyperthyroidism 567
  hypertrophic cardiomyopathy 432
  junctional tachycardias 381
  migraine 701
  mitral valve prolapse 418
  myocardial infarction 408
  overdose 533
  sinus bradycardia 373
  sinus tachycardia 373

B

betahistine 658
bezafibrate 629
bicarbonate 303
biguanides 605
bilateral adrenal hyperplasia 592
bilateral diaphragmatic weakness 503
bilateral hilar lymphadenopathy 484, 485, 781
bilateral renal disease 330
bile acid-binding resins 629–630
bilharzia 37
biliary pain (colic) 154–155
biliary tract diseases 153–158
  examination questions 763–764
  see also liver diseases/disorders
bilirubin
  jaundice 116–117
  liver disease 115
bird fancier's lung 490
birthweight, low 440
bisoprolol 394
bisphosphonates
  hypercalcaemia 587
  osteoporosis 279–280
  Paget's disease 282
bitemporal hemianopia 545, 648, 649
bitemporal visual defects 647
Björk–Shiley valve 413
blackheads 723
Blackwater fever 21
bladder
  catheterization 751–753
  physiology 362
  tumours 358
bladder stones 334
bleeding disorders 204–214
  classification 207
  investigation 207–209
bleeding gums 56
bleeding time 208
bleomycin 501
blepharospasm 685
'block-and-replace' regimen 567
blood chemistry
  asthma 466
  cardiac failure 390
  hypertension 437
  myocardial infarction 405
  pancreatitis 159
  values 166

blood coagulation 204–206
  cascade 204–206
  disorders 203–214
  limitation 206–207
blood count
  pneumonia 473
  rheumatic fever 412
blood cultures
  infective endocarditis 424
  pneumonia 473
blood flukes 37
blood gases 304, 448
  acute asthma 471
  COPD 454
  cryptogenic fibrosing alveolitis 488
  normal values 738
  pneumonia 474
  pulmonary embolism 427
  pulmonary oedema 396
  respiratory failure 516
blood glucose 599
  see also glycaemic control
blood groups 201–204
blood pressure
  control 616
  endocrinology 590–595
  shock 513
blood products 200–204
blood sampling 737–738
blood transfusions 200–204
  checking procedure 202
  decreased extracellular volume 291
  thalassaemias 184
bloody diarrhoea 31, 761
blue bloaters 452, 454
body fluid compartments 283–287
body mass index (BMI) 108
Boerhaave's syndrome 63
bone densitometry
  coeliac disease 78
  osteoporosis 279
bone disease 275–281
  chronic renal failure 349
bone marrow 802
bone marrow transplantation 231–232
  aplastic anaemia 178
  chronic myeloid leukaemia 225
  myelodysplasia 199
bone metabolism 276
bone remodelling 275

bone scans
  back pain 272
  Paget's disease 282
bone tuberculosis 481
Bornholm disease 498
*Borrelia burgdorferi* infection 15–16
Bouchard nodes 238
Boutonnière deformity 242
bovine spongiform
        encephalopathy (BSE) 696
bowel disorders, functional
        **100–102**
bradycardias 373, **374–376**
  acute asthma 471
  sinus *see* sinus bradycardia
brain death **664**
brainstem infarction 667–668
brain surgery 676
breath tests 79–80
brittle diabetes **621**
Broca's aphasia 800–801
bromocriptine
  acromegaly 560
  hyperprolactinaemia 558
  Parkinson's disease 683
bronchial carcinoma **492–498**,
        787
bronchiectasis 446, **457–459**
  cerebral abscess 694
bronchitis
  acute **452**
  chronic 452
bronchoalveolar lavage 802
bronchodilators
  asthma 466
  bronchiectasis 458
  COPD 455
bronchoscopy 802
Bruce protocol 372
bruises 805
Budd–Chiari syndrome **149–150**
  antiphospholipid syndrome
        257
budesonide 466, 469
bulbar palsy 659
bulla 802
bumetanide 289
  chronic cardiac failure 392
bundle of His 371
  disturbances 376
buprenorphine 534
*Burkholderia cepacia* infection 461
Burkitt's lymphoma 231
burns 290, 291
bursa 802

bursitis 241, 802
busulfan 197
butyrophenones 683, 685

# C

C3d (complement) 191
'cafe-au-lait' spots 731
Calcinosis, Raynaud's
        phenomenon, oEsophgeal
        involvement, Sclerodactyly,
        Telangiectasia (CREST)
        258
calcipotriol 726
calcium
  homeostasis **584–589**
  metabolism 276
  supplements 279
calcium-channel blockers (calcium
        antagonists)
  adverse effects 401, 439
  angina 401
  chronic cardiac failure
        393–394
  hypertension 437, 439
  oesophageal spasm 61
  pulmonary hypertension 426
  subarachnoid haemorrhage
        673–674
calcium gluconate 589
calcium oxalate 332–333
calculi
  hypercalcaemia 586
  renal **332–337**
  salivary glands 56
  staghorn 334
*Campylobacter* infections 758,
        761, 795
  food poisoning 33, 758–759
  Guillain–Barré syndrome
        712–713
  Reiter's syndrome 248
cancers *see individual cancers*
candesartan 439
*Candida albicans* infections *see*
        candidiasis
candidiasis 34, 310, 762
  AIDS 48
  diabetes mellitus 619
  infective endocarditis 423
  oesophagus 57
cannabis 535
cannula, intravenous 735–736
capnography 516–517

capreomycin 481
captopril
  chronic cardiac failure 393
  hypertension 438–439
carbamazepine
  diabetic neuropathy 618
  epilepsy 677
  postherpetic neuralgia 14
  trigeminal neuralgia 703
carbimazole
  hyperthyroidism 567
  thyroid crisis 568
carbon monoxide poisoning 532, 534
carboxyhaemoglobin 532, 534
carcinoid syndrome **82–83**
carcinomas 802
  *see also individual carcinomas*
cardiac arrest **383–385**
  emergency management 384–385
cardiac arrhythmias 365, **372–385, 376–385**
  alcohol abuse 537
  atrial *see* atrial arrhythmias
  electrical cardioversion 742
  emergency management 384–385
  hypokalaemia 299
  intraventricular conduction disturbances 376
  myocarditis 430
  sinus 373
  ventricular *see* ventricular arrhythmias
  *see also* bradycardias; tachycardias
cardiac catheterization 391, 802
cardiac failure **386–397**
  acute 389
  anaemia 167
  biventricular 386, 389
  chronic 391–395
  increased extracellular volume 287
  left 386, 389
  myocardial infarction 410
  rheumatic fever 411
  right 386, 389
  summary of treatment 394
cardiac nuclear imaging 802
cardiac output 515
cardiac syndrome X 399
cardiac transplantation 395
  restrictive cardiomyopathy 433

cardiogenic shock **396–397, 507–508,** 783
cardiomyopathy **430–433**
  alcohol abuse 537
  arrhythmogenic right ventricular **433**
  chronic renal failure 350
  dilated **430–431**
  hereditary haemochromatosis 144
  hypertrophic **431–432**
  procedure 777
  restrictive **432–433**
cardiovascular disease **365–442**
  chronic renal failure 350
  examination questions 773–778
  *see also* heart disease
cardiovascular syphilis 41
cardioversion 741–743
β-carotene 108
carotid sinus syncope 637
carotid stenosis 670
carpal tunnel syndrome **710–711**
  rheumatoid arthritis 243
carpopedal spasm 589
carvedilol 394
caseating, definition 803
cataplexy 637–638
cataracts 616
catecholamines 610
catheterization **751–753**
cauda equina 704, **707–708**
CD4 lymphocytes 50
CD (cluster differentiation) antigens 803
cefaclor 478
cefotaxime
  cholecystitis 156
  meningitis 693
  septicemia 11
cefuroxime
  acute pyelonephritis 327
  empyema 478
  pancreatitis 160
  septic shock 513
celecoxib 239–240
central oedema 611
central pontine myelinolysis 296
central venous cannulation 738–740
central venous pressure (CVP)
  measurement 740–741
  shock 513–514
cephalosporins 16

cerebellum
  alcohol abuse 537
  lesions **645–646**
cerebral abscesses **694**
cerebral arteries 667, 672
cerebral dysfunction, metabolic
      acidosis 305
cerebral haemorrhage 665–666
cerebral infarcts 187, 665, 666,
      670
cerebral malaria 21
cerebral tumours 676, 699
cerebrospinal fluid (CSF)
  meningitis 692, 693
  multiple sclerosis 687–688
  unconsciousness 663
cerebrovascular disease
      **664–674**
  see also stroke
cestode infections 35–36
cetirizine 449
CFTR gene 459–460
Chagas' disease 93
charcoal, activated 526
Charcot–Bouchard aneurysms
      665
Charcot–Marie–Tooth disease
      **712**
Charcot's joints 617, 618
Charcot's triad 156
chemotherapeutic agents
  adverse effects 221
  leukaemia 221
  lung carcinoma 497
  non-Hodgkin's lymphoma
      229–230
chest drain insertion 745–746
chest leads 367, 368
chest pain
  acute pericarditis 433
  causes 366
  heart disease **365**
  mitral valve prolapse 418
  myocardial infarction 403
  pulmonary embolism 426
  pulmonary hypertension
      425
  respiratory disease 446
  rheumatic fever 411
  see also angina
Cheyne–Stoke respiration 803
chickenpox **13–14**
Chlamydia infections 34, 39, 40,
      310, 475
  infective endocarditis 423

chlorambucil
  chronic lymphocytic leukaemia
      226
  non-Hodgkin's lymphoma 230
chloramphenicol 177
chloroquine 22, 23
cholecystectomy 156
cholecystitis
  acute **155–156**
  chronic **156**
cholelithiasis **156–157**
cholera **29–30**
cholera toxin 29
cholestatic jaundice **118–120**
cholesterol
  coronary artery disease 398
  transport 623–624
cholestyramine 629–630
chondrocalcinosis 269
CHOP 230
chorea 684
Christmas disease 212
chromophobe, adenomas 545
chromophobe adenomas 545
chronic lymphocytic leukaemia
      (CLL) **226–227**
chronic myeloid leukaemia (CML)
      **225–226**
chronic obstructive pulmonary
      disease (COPD) **452–456**
  acute exacerbation 455–456
  cor pulmonale 429
  lung function tests 448
  pneumothorax 501
chronotropic, definition 803
Churg–Strauss syndrome **265,**
      486, 800
Chvostek's sign 589
chylomicrons 623
  diseases/disorders **624–625**
chylothorax 498–499
ciclosporin
  aplastic anaemia 178
  Behçet's syndrome 265
  liver transplantation 149
  nephrotic syndrome 324
  psoriasis 726
  psoriatic arthritis 250
  pyoderma gangrenosum 730
  renal transplantation 355
  ulcerative colitis 90
cimetidine 557
ciprofloxacin
  acute pyelonephritis 327
  diverticular disease 92

C

ciprofloxacin (*contd*)
  gonorrhoea 40
  shigellosis 28
  traveller's diarrhoea 31, 758
  tuberculosis 481
  typhoid fever 25
circadian rhythms 573
circle of Willis 672
cirrhosis 132–135, **142–149**
  alcoholic **148**
  ascites 138–139
  increased extracellular volume 288
  micronodular/macronodular 132
  primary biliary **142–143**
  secondary biliary **144**
clarithromycin
  *H. pylori* infection 66
  pneumonia 475
  tuberculosis 481
claudication, intermittent 166
clindamycin 725
clomifene 557
clone 803
*Clonorchis sinensis* infections 37
clopidogrel
  angina 401–402
  arterial thrombosis 215
  stroke 670
*Clostridium* infections 759, 761
  food poisoning 32
clubbing 803
  cystic fibrosis 460
  infective endocarditis 423
  lung carcinoma 495
cluster headaches **703**
coagulation *see* blood coagulation
coal tar 726
coal worker's pneumoconiosis 491
cocaine abuse 535
codeine abuse 534
coeliac disease **76–78**
  mouth ulcers 55
colchicine
  erythema nodosum 729
  gout 267
cold, common **448–449**
cold antibodies 189, 190, 192
cold sores 13
'cold turkey' 534
colectomy with ileorectal anastomosis 90
colestipol 629–630

colestyramine 629–630
colitis 47
  amoebic 27
  ischaemic 74, **93**
  ulcerative *see* ulcerative colitis (UC)
collagen vascular disease 7
colloids 509–510
colonic pseudobstruction, chronic 106
colon polyps **93–94**
colorectal cancer **94–97**
  inflammatory bowel disease 91
  sporadic **95–97**
colorectal disorders **92–97**
coma **659–663**, 668
comedones 723
common bile duct stones **156–157**
common cold **448–449**
complement 317
compliance, tuberculosis 481–482
computed tomography (CT) 804
  Alzheimer's disease 720
  aortic aneurysm 440
  constrictive pericarditis 435
  cryptogenic fibrosing alveolitis 488
  epilepsy 677
  headache 636
  liver disease 116
  meningitis 693
  neurological disease 638
  pancreatic cancer 163
  pulmonary embolism 427
  renal cell carcinoma 357
  spinal stenosis 275
  stroke 666, 669
  subarachnoid haemorrhage 673
  subdural haematoma 674
  unilateral renal disease 331
  urinary tract obstruction 339
condylomata lata 41
confrontation 647
congenital, definition 803
congenital hyperbilirubinaemia **118**
congenital hypertrophy of the retinal epithelium 94
congenital rubella syndrome 12
congenital syphilis 41
conjunctivitis 248

connective tissue disease
**253–265**
Conn's syndrome 592
 secondary hypertension 436
constipation **54, 92–93**
 acute intermittent porphyria
 631
constrictive pericarditis **434–435**
constructional apraxia 141, 803
contact dermatitis 726–727
continuous ambulatory peritoneal
 dialysis (CAPD) 354
continuous positive airway
 pressure (CPAP)
 obstructive sleep apnoea 457
 respiratory failure 517
contraindication, definition 803
contralateral hemiplegia 640
convergence 649
Cooley's anaemia 182
Coomb's test 189, 191, 192
coordination **645–646**
COPD see chronic obstructive
 pulmonary disease (COPD)
copper excretion 146
co-proxamol poisoning 532
corneal reflex 664
coronary artery bypass grafting
 (CABG) 401, **402**
coronary artery disease (CAD)
 397–398
 see also angina; myocardial
 infarction (MI)
Coroner referral 754–755
cor pulmonale
 chronic **429**
 granulomatous lung disease
 484
cortical lesions 645
corticospinal tracts 638–641, 640
corticosteroids
 acute pericarditis 433
 adverse effects 577
 alcoholic hepatitis 148
 asthma 466, 469
 atopic eczema 727
 COPD 455
 giant cell arteritis 263
 gout 266
 inflammatory bowel disease
 89
 mouth ulcers 55
 multiple sclerosis 688
 polymyalgia rheumatica 263
 psoriatic arthritis 250

pyrophosphate arthropathy
 269
 Reiter's syndrome 249
 renal transplantation 355
 rheumatoid arthritis 245
 systemic lupus erythematosus
 256
 see also prednisolone; steroids
corticotrophin-releasing hormone
 (CRH) 542, 573
 test 580
cortisol 610
coryza, acute **448–449**
costochondritis 366
co-trimoxazole
 paratyphoid 25
 Pneumocystis infections 48
 Whipple's disease 80
cough
 asthma 465, 780
 COPD 453–454
 pneumonia 471
 respiratory disease 443–444
cough reflex 664
COX-1 inhibitors 239
COX-2 specific inhibitors 288
 gout 266
 osteoarthritis 239–240
 rheumatoid arthritis 244
 systemic lupus erythematosus
 256
Coxiella burnetii infections
 infective endocarditis 423
 pneumonia 472
Coxsackie virus infections 498,
 776
 acute pericarditis 433
 meningitis 691, 693
 mouth ulcers 55
 myocarditis 430
'crack' 535
cranial arteritis (giant cell arteritis)
 **262–263**, 649, **701**, 766
cranial diabetes insipidus (CDI)
 582–583, 790
cranial nerves **647–659**
 lesions 652–654
 see also individual nerves
craniopharyngioma 649
C-reactive protein (CRP) 803
 ankylosing spondylitis 247
 rheumatoid arthritis 242
creatine kinase (CK) 405
creatinine clearance 321
 chronic renal failure 352

C

cremation forms 755
CREST syndrome 258
Creutzfeldt–Jakob disease **696**
   blood transfusions 203
Criglar–Najar syndrome 118
Crohn's disease 81, **84–91**, 761,
   766
   anaemia 170
   enteral nutrition 109
   enteropathic arthritis 250
croup 450
crust (dried exudate on skin)
   804
cryoglobulins 804
cryoprecipitate 201
Cryptococcus infections 48
cryptogenic, definition 804
cryptogenic fibrosing alveolitis
   (CFA) **487–488**
cryptosporidosis 47
crystal deposition diseases
   **265–269**
crystalloids 510
CT scan see computed
   tomography (CT)
Cullen's sign 159
Curling's ulcer 64
Cushing's disease 578
Cushing's syndrome 544, 545,
   **577–581**, 787
   secondary hypertension 436
cyclophosphamide
   autoimmune haemolytic
     anaemia 192
   Churg–Strauss syndrome 265
   cryptogenic fibrosing alveolitis
     488
   multiple myeloma 233
   nephrotic syndrome 324
   non-Hodgkin's lymphoma 230
   systemic lupus erythematosus
     256
cyproheptadine 83
cyproterone acetate 557
cyst(s)
   Baker's 777–778
   popliteal 777–778
   renal **355–357**
   synovial 777–778
cysteine stones 334
   prevention 336
cystic fibrosis (CF) **459–461**
   bronchiectasis 457, 460
   management 462
cystic renal disease **355–357**

cystinuria 334
cystitis 310, 326, 327
cystoscopy 339
   micturating 810
cytarabine 224
cytokines 804
cytomegalovirus (CMV) infection
   15
   AIDS 47
   Guillain–Barré syndrome
     712–713
cytotoxins 26

# D

dactylitis 187
Dane particle 124
dantrolene 708
dapsone
   erythema nodosum 729
   *Pneumocystis* infections 48
daunorubicin 224
D-dimers 427
death certification 754–755
decongestants 449
decubitus angina 399
deep vein thrombosis (DVT)
   441–442, 777–778
   antiphospholipid syndrome
     257
   pulmonary embolism 426
   see also venous
     thromboembolism
defibrillators 382
degenerative diseases **708–710**
deliberate self-harm 523–534,
   784–785
delirium **718–719**
delirium tremens 538–539
   emergency management 538
dementia **719–721**, 794–795
   alcohol abuse 537
   multi-infarct 668
Dengue fever **24**
depression 794–795
de Quervains thyroiditis **565**,
   786–787
dermatitis see eczema
dermatitis herpetiformis **78**
dermatology **723–731**
   examination questions
     796–797
dermatomyositis **260–261**
desmopressin 583–584

dexamethasone
  intracranial tumours 698–699
  spinal cord compression 705
  subarachnoid haemorrhage
      673
  thyroid crisis 568
dexamethasone suppression test
      544
  Cushing's syndrome 579, 580
dextrans 510
diabetes insipidus 310, **582–584**
diabetes mellitus **599–622**
  brittle **621**
  CAD 398
  chronic pancreatitis 161
  complications **614–619**
  cystic fibrosis 460
  examination questions
      788–791
  eye disease **614–616**
  foot complications **618–619**
  gestational 620
  glycosuria 313
  kidney disease **616–617**
  metabolic emergencies
      **608–614**
  microalbuminuria 313
  myocardial infarction 406, 408
  pancreatic cancer 163
  pregnancy **620**
  renal failure (chronic) 340,
      **347–352**, 772
  surgery **619**
  type 1 600, 601
  type 2 600, 601
diabetic amyotrophy 618
diabetic eye disease **614–616**
diabetic ketoacidosis 306, 602,
      **609–611**, 613, 790
  emergency management 612
  hypokalaemia 299
  unconsciousness 661–662
diabetic mononeuropathy 618
diabetic nephropathy **616–617**
diabetic neuropathy **617–618**
diabetic retinopathy **614–616**
dialysis **352–355**
  acute renal failure 346
  chronic renal failure 352
  poisoning 527
diamorphine abuse 534
diaphragma sellae 546
diaphragm diseases **502–504**
diarrhoea 54, 76, **97–100**
  bloody 31, 761

cholera 29
  osmotic **98**
  secretory **98**
  shigellosis 28
diazepam
  delirium tremens 538–539
  paraplegia 708
diazoxide 623
didanosine 51
diet
  acute intermittent porphyria
      632
  chronic renal failure 351
  diabetes mellitus 604
  hyperlipidaemia 627, 629
  hypertension 437
  low-protein 142, 351
dietary requirements **106–107**
diethylenetriaminepentaacetic
      acid, technetium-99m-
      labelled ($^{99m}$Tc-DTPA)
      813
diffuse oesophageal spasm **61**
diffuse parenchymal lung
      diseases (DPLDs) **483–489**
diffuse systemic sclerosis 258
digitalis 373
digital rectal examination 359,
      747–748
digoxin
  atrial fibrillation 409
  chronic cardiac failure 394
  toxicity 299
dilated cardiomyopathy (DCM)
      **430–431**
diloxanide furoate 28
diltiazem
  angina 401
  chronic cardiac failure 393
dilutional hyponatraemia
      **295–296**
dimercaptosuccinic acid,
      technetium-99m-labelled
      ($^{99m}$Tc-DMSA) 813
dimethylchlorotetracycline 583
diplopia 654
dipyridamole 215
discoid lupus 254, 256
disc prolapse see intervertebral
      disc disease
disease-modifying anti-rheumatic
      drugs (DMARDs)
      244–245
disopyramide 381, 382
dissecting aortic aneurysm 440

**D**

disseminated intravascular
      coagulation (DIC)
      **213–214**
   leukaemias  224
distal, definition  804
distal interphalangeal joints (DIJ)
      238
distal renal tube acidosis  307
diuretics  289
   adverse effects  295, 308, 392
   ascites  139
   chronic cardiac failure  392,
      394
   hypertension  437
   increased extracellular volume
      289
   loop  392
   potassium-sparing  289, 392
   pulmonary oedema  396
   renal tubular acidosis  306
   thiazides *see* thiazide diuretics
diverticular disease  **92**
   gastrointestinal bleeding  74
dizziness  **636–638**
dobutamine
   chronic cardiac failure  394
   shock  510, 512
doll's head reflex  664
domperidone  59
donepezil  721
dopamine  542
   chronic cardiac failure  394
   shock  510, 512
dopexamine  512
Doppler principle  805
Dormia basket  157
dorsum sellae  546
double vision  654
doxazosin  439
doxorubicin
   non-Hodgkin's lymphoma  230
   Waldenströms
         macroglobulinaemia
         234
doxycycline  16
Dressler's syndrome  410, 776
driving, epilepsy  678
drug abuse  **534–539**
   examination questions
      783–785
   hyperthermia  597
   pneumonia  472
drug hypersensitivity  7
drug-induced haemolytic
      anaemias  **192**

drugs, generic  808
dry pleurisy  **498**
dual energy X-ray absorptiometry
      (DXA)  279
Dubin–Johnson syndrome  118
Duchenne muscular dystrophy
      **715**
Duckett Jones criteria  412
Duffy blood groups  201
Dukes' grading  95
duodenal disorders  **63–71**
duodenal ulcers  66
dysarthria  804
   anticonvulsant drugs  677
   bulbar palsy  659
   cerebellar lesions  646
dysdiadochokinesis  646
dysentery
   amoebic  27
   bacillary  **28**
dyshormonogenesis  562
dyskinesias  **684–686**
dyspepsia  53
   aortic regurgitation  420
   functional  101
   management  **69**
dysphagia  53, **56–57,** 762
   bulbar palsy  659
   CMV infection  47
dysphasia  800–801
dysplasia, definition  804
dyspnoea  **444,** 780–781
   exertional  414
   granulomatous lung disease
      484
   heart disease  **365**
   hypertrophic cardiomyopathy
      432
   paroxysmal nocturnal  365
   pneumonia  471
   pulmonary embolism  426
   pulmonary hypertension  425
dystonias  685–686
dystrophia myotonica  **717**
   visual defects  654
dysuria  309, **310, 328**
   urinary tract infections  326

## E

Eaton–Lambert syndrome  496
ecchymoses, superficial  208, 804
*Echinococcus granulosus* infections
      38

echocardiography 804
  aortic regurgitation 420
  aortic stenosis 420
  cardiac failure 390
  dilated cardiomyopathy 431
  Doppler 805
  hypertrophic cardiomyopathy 432
  infective endocarditis 424
  mitral regurgitation 417
  mitral stenosis 415
  pericardial tamponade 434
  pulmonary hypertension 425
  restrictive cardiomyopathy 432
  transoesophageal 805
Echo virus infection 691, 692
ecstasy
  abuse 535
  hyperthermia 597
ectopic, definition 805
eczema **726–728**
  atopic 727
  exogenous 727–728
Edinger–Westphal nucleus III 649, 650–651
efavirenz 51
Ehlers–Danlos syndrome 723, **730**
ejection fraction 805
electrical cardioversion 741–743
electrocardiography (ECG) **367–372**, 805
  acute pericarditis 433
  angina 399
  aortic regurgitation 420
  aortic stenosis 420
  atrial fibrillation 379
  atrial flutter 378
  atrioventricular block 374–376
  cardiac failure 390
  chest leads 367, 368
  definitions 368–372
  dilated cardiomyopathy 431
  exercise *see* exercise electrocardiography
  Guillain–Barré syndrome 713
  hypertension 437
  hypertrophic cardiomyopathy 432
  infective endocarditis 424
  limb leads 367, 369
  mitral regurgitation 417
  mitral stenosis 415
  myocardial infarction 403–405

  pericardial tamponade 434
  pulmonary embolism 427
  pulmonary hypertension 425
  pulmonary oedema 396
  restrictive cardiomyopathy 432
  torsades de pointes 383
  ventricular tachycardia 382
  waveform 368–372
  Wolff–Parkinson–White syndrome 381
  *see also individual waveforms*
electroencephalography (EEG)
  epilepsy 676–677
  meningitis 693
electrolyte disorders **283–308**
  examination questions 769–771
electromyography (EMG) 260, 805
electrophysiological tests 687
eleventh cranial nerve 659
ELISA (enzyme-linked immunosorbent assay) 806
elliptocytosis, hereditary 181
embolism, pulmonary *see* pulmonary embolism (PE)
embolization 423
emollients 727
emphysema 452
  surgical 519
empirical, definition 805
'empty sella' syndrome 548
empyemas 476, 477–478, 498–499
enalapril
  chronic cardiac failure 393
  hypertension 438–439
encephalitis **690–693**
  epilepsy 676
end-diastolic volume 806
endemic, definition 806
endobronchial irradiation 497
endocarditis, infective *see* infective endocarditis
endocrine diseases **544–597**
  secondary hypertension 436
  symptoms **544–549**
endocrinology **541–597**
  blood pressure **590–595**
  examination questions 785–787
endogenous, definition 806
endomysial (EMA) antibodies 78

E

endoscopic gastroplasty   59
endoscopic laser therapy   497
endoscopic retrograde
       cholangiopancreatography
       (ERCP)   806
   bile duct stones   157
   cholestatic jaundice   119
   gallstones   155
   liver disease   116
enophthalmos   651
enoxaparin   218
enoximone   512
*Entamoeba histolytica* infections
       25, **27–28**
   liver abscesses   151–152
enteral nutrition   **109**
   inflammatory bowel disease
       89–90
   pancreatitis   160
enteric fever   **24**
enterobacteria   694
*Enterobius vermicularis* infections
       34, 36
*Enterococcus faecalis* infections
   infective endocarditis   422
   septicaemia   9
enterocolitis   **25**
enteropathic arthritis   **250**
enteropathy, gluten-sensitive *see*
       coeliac disease
enteropathy, protein-losing
       **81–82**
enterotoxigenic *Escherichia coli*
       31
enterotoxins   26
enthesitis   247
enzyme-linked immunosorbent
       assay (ELISA)   806
eosinophilia   806
epidemic, definition   806
epidemic myalgia   498
epidemiology   806
epididymitis   39
epilepsy   **674–680**
   alcohol abuse   537
   classification   675
   intracranial tumours   698
   *see also* seizures
epinephrine
   glucose homeostasis   599
   shock   511
epitope, definition   806
Epstein–Barr virus (EBV) infection
       15
   AIDS   47

eptifibatide   215
ERCP *see* endoscopic retrograde
       cholangiopancreatography
       (ERCP)
erectile impotence   551
ergotamine   701
erythema   806
erythema marginatum   411
erythema migrans   15–16
erythema multiforme   **729**
   mycoplasmal pneumonia   475
erythema nodosum   485,
       **728–729,** 796–797
erythematous macropapular rash
       24
erythrocyte sedimentation rate
       (ESR)   806
   ankylosing spondylitis   247
   giant cell arteritis   702
   normal values   166
   osteoarthritis   239
   polymyositis   260
   Reiter's syndrome   248
   rheumatoid arthritis   242
   systemic lupus erythematosus
       254
   systemic sclerosis   258
erythroderma   807
erythrodermic psoriasis   725–726
erythromycin
   acne vulgaris   725
   *Chlamydia* infections   475
   empyema   478
   leptospirosis   17
   NGU   40
   pneumonia   474, 475
   septic arthritis   251
erythropoietic porphyria   630
erythropoietin   351
*Escherichia coli* infections   758
   liver abscesses   151
   septicaemia   9
*Escherichia coli* O157:H7 infections
       32
esomeprazole   59
essential hypertension   435–436
essential mixed
       cryoglobulinaemia   129
essential thrombocythaemia   197
etanercept   244–245
ethambutol
   adverse effects   482
   tuberculosis   481
ethosuximide   677
etidronate   279–280

etretinate 726
euthanasia 807
excoriation 807
excretion urography (intravenous urography, IVU) 807
  renal cell carcinoma 357
  renal stone disease 335
  urinary tract infections 327
  urinary tract obstruction 339
exercise
  coronary artery disease 398
  hypertension 437
  osteoporosis 279
exercise electrocardiography 372
  angina 399
exertional dyspnoea 414
exertional syncope 419
exogenous, definition 807
exogenous eczema 727–728
exophthalmos 569
expressive aphasia 800–801
extracellular fluid distribution 285–286
extracellular volume abnormalities 287–291
extracorporeal shock wave lithotripsy (ESWL) 336
extractable nuclear antigens (ENA) 807
extradural haematomas 674
extrapyramidal disease 680–688
extrarenal volume receptors 287
extrinsic allergic alveolitis 489, 490
exudate 807
eye disease, diabetes 614–616
eyedrops 651
eye tests 647

**F**

facial nerve (seventh cranial) 655–657
facial pain 702–703
factitious, definition 807
factor VII 205–206
factor VIII
  haemophilia A 211–212
  von Willdebrand disease 213
factor IX 205–206
factor X 205–206
famciclovir 14
familial adenomatous polyps (FAP) 94

familial hypercholesterolaemia 626
familial hypertriglyceridaemia 625
familial Mediterranean fever 807
Fanconi's syndrome 209, 313
fansidar 22
farmer's lung 489, 490
*Fasciola hepatica* infections 37
fasting
  diabetes mellitus 602
  hypoglycaemia 621, 623
fatty liver 148
fatty liver of pregnancy, acute 152
Felty's syndrome 243
female hypogonadism 553–555
ferritin 169
  anaemias 170
ferrous sulphate 170
fetor hepaticus 140–141
fever
  erythema nodosum 729
  headache 636
  tropical infections 17, 18
  of unknown origin 7–9
fibrates 629
fibrillation, ventricular 383
fibrin degradation products (FDPs) 207, 213
fibrinolytic system 207
fibromuscular hyperplasia 331
fibrosing alveolitis 768
fibrosis, pulmonary 487–489
fibrositis 275
finasteride
  benign prostatic hypertrophy 359
  hirsutism 557
finger-prick testing 608
first cranial nerve 647
fish oils 630
fissure 807
fistula 807
flashing lights 676
flatulence 53
flecainide 381, 382
flexural psoriasis 725
flucloxacillin
  bronchiectasis 458
  pneumonia 474
  septic arthritis 251
fluconazole 48

F

fludrocortisone
  Addison's disease 574
  renal tubular acidosis 306
flumazenil 663
5-fluorouracil 96
fluticasone propionate 466, 469
folate **175**
  deficiency **175–176**
  sickle cell disease 188
folinic acid 46
follicle-stimulating hormone
    (FSH) 542, 545, 546
  amenorrhoea 554
  menopause 552–553
  secretion 549
food poisoning **30–33**
forced expiratory volume (FEV)
    **448**
  asthma 465
  COPD 454
forced vital capacity (FVC) 448
  COPD 454
foreign bodies, inhalation
    451–452
formoterol 466
foscarnet 47
fourth cranial nerve **652–654**
fresh frozen plasma (FFP) 201
Friedreich's ataxia **707**
fructosamine 608
fulminant hepatic failure
    **130–131**
fulminant meningococcaemia 794
functional bowel disorders
    **100–102**
fundoplication 59
furosemide 289
  acute renal failure 343
  ascites 139
  chronic cardiac failure 392
  hypertension 437
  increased extracellular volume
    289
  syndrome of inappropriate
    ADH secretion 583

## G

gabapentin 618, 678
gag reflex 664
galactorrhoea 557
galantamine 721
gallstones **153–158**
ganciclovir 47

*Gardnerella vaginalis* infections 310
gastric cancer **69–70**
gastric lavage 529
gastric outlet obstruction 68–69
gastrinomas 164
gastritis **63–64**
gastroenteritis **30–33**
  pathogenic mechanisms 26
gastroenterology **53–106**
  examination questions 760–762
gastrointestinal bleeding **71–75**
  emergency management 73
  portal hypertension **135–138**
gastrointestinal disease
  alcohol abuse 537–538
  hypomagnesaemia 300
  stomach *see* stomach disorders
  symptoms 53–54
gastro-oesophageal reflux disease
    (GORD) **58–60**
gastropathy **63–64**
Gaucher's disease 808
Gelofusin 510
gemcitabine 497
gemfibrozil 629
generic drugs 808
genetic screening 461
genital ulcers **40**
  sexually transmitted infections
    34
gentamicin
  acute pyelonephritis 327
  infective endocarditis 424
  septicemia 11
  septic shock 513
geographical tongue **55–56**
gestational diabetes 620
giant cell arteritis **262–263**, 649,
    **701**, 766
giardiasis **30**
gigantism 558
Gilbert's syndrome 118
  liver function tests 115
gingivitis 55
  acute ulcerative 56
Glasgow Coma Scale 659–660
glaucoma 651
  diabetes mellitus 616
glibenclamide 604–605
global aphasia 801
glomerular basement membrane
    (GBM) 315
glomerular filtration rate (GFR)
    310, 315, 317, 808
  acute renal failure 341

glomerulonephritis **315–325**
  amyloid  323
  causes  320
  characterization  319
  investigations  321
  membranous  322
  minimal change  322–323
  poststreptococcal  318, 320
  secondary hypertension  436
glomerulus structure  315–317
glossitis  173
glossopharyngeal nerve (ninth
    cranial)  659
glucagon  599
  diabetic ketoacidosis  610
glucagonomas  164
glucocorticoid axis  **573–581**
glucocorticoid deficiency  549
glucose homeostasis  599
  *see also* glycaemic control
glucose-6-phosphate
    dehydrogenase (G6PD)
    deficiency  **188–189**
glucose tolerance test  602, 603
  acromegaly  559
α-glucosidase inhibitors  606
γ-glutamyl transpeptidase
  alcohol abuse  536
  liver disease  115–116
gluten  76–77
glycaemic control  603
  measurement  607–608
glyceryl trinitrate  400
glycogen  599
glycoprotein gp120  43
glycoprotein IIb/IIIA (GPIIb/IIIa)
    receptor  205
  inhibitors  402
glycosuria  313, 314
  renal tubular acidosis  307
glycosylated haemoglobin  608
glycosylphosphatidylinositol
    (GPI) anchor  193
goitre  **570–571**
  toxic multinodular  565, **565**
gonadotrophin deficiency  547
gonadotrophin-releasing hormone
    (GnRH)  542, 549
  deficiency  555
gonococcal arthritis  **252**
gonorrhoea  **39–40**, 310
Goodpasture's syndrome  317,
    355, 446
gout  **265–268**, 768
  management  266

Graham–Steell murmur  422
Gram-negative organisms
  cystic fibrosis  460
  septicaemia  9
Gram-positive organisms,
    septicaemia  9
Gram stain
  pleural effusion  499
  sputum  447
granuloma annulare  619
granulomatosis, pulmonary
    **486–487**
granulomatous lung disease
    **483–486**
Graves' disease  **565**, 786
  eye complications  569
  symptoms  570
Grey Turner's sign  159
growth axis  **558–561**
growth factors  237
growth hormone (GH)
    542, 545
  acromegaly  560
  deficiency  547, 558
  diseases/disorders  **558–561**
  hypopituitarism  548
Guillain–Barré syndrome  659,
    **712–713**, 795
  diaphragm involvement  503
gum bleeding  56
gumma  41
gynaecomastia  **551–552**

## H

$H_2$-receptor antagonists  59
Haemaccel  510
haem arginate  632
haemarthroses  208
haematemesis  71, 761
haematological diseases
    **165–234**
  alcohol abuse  538
  examination questions
    764–767
haematomas  **674**
haematuria  309, **313–314**
  acute nephritic syndrome
    320
  bladder tumours  358
  glomerulonephritis  318
  hypertension  437
  infective endocarditis  424
  microscopic  17

haematuria (*contd*)
  renal cell carcinoma  357
  Stix tests  311–312
  urinary tract infections  326
haemochromatosis (HH)
      144–146
haemodialysis  353
  aspirin overdose  529
haemofiltration  353–354
haemoglobin  165–166
  abnormalities  **181–188**
  glycosylated  608
haemoglobin S  185
haemoglobinuria  179
haemolysis
  autoimmune  202
  microangiopathic  193
  pre-eclamptic toxaemia  152
haemolytic anaemias  **178–193**
  acquired  **189–193**
  autoimmune  **189–192**
  drug-induced  **192**
  inherited  **180–189**
  mechanical  **193**
  mycoplasmal pneumonia  475
  non-immune  **193**
haemolytic jaundice  **117–118**
haemophilia A  **211–212**
haemophilia B  212
*Haemophilus influenzae* infection
      449, 450, 760
  AIDS  49
  bronchiectasis  458
  cystic fibrosis  460
  pneumonia  475
haemopoiesis  165
haemoptysis  **446**, 780, 787
  pulmonary embolism  426
haemorrhage
  cerebral  665–666, 794
  intracranial  **672–674**
  subarachnoid  **672–674**, 699
  variceal  136, 137–138
haemosiderin  179
haemostasis  **204–206**
haemothorax  498
hairy leukoplakia  55
haloperidol  719
hamartomatous polyps  **94**
Hamman–Rich syndrome  487
haptoglobins  179, 180
Hashimoto's thyroiditis  562
hay fever  449
HDL (high-density lipoproteins)
      624

headache  **635–636, 700–703**
  hydrocephalus  699
  intracranial tumours  697
  migraine  **700–701**
  subarachnoid haemorrhage
      673
head injury  676
heart
  anatomy  371
  conduction system  371
  *see also entries beginning cardiac*
heart block  410
heartburn  **53**, 57, 762
  gastro-oesophageal reflux
      disease  58
heart disease  537
  ischaemic  **397–412**, 776, 777
  pulmonary  **425–429**
  rheumatic  412
  symptoms  **365–372**
  valvular  **412–425**
heart failure *see cardiac failure*
heart murmurs
  infective endocarditis  423
  rheumatic fever  411
heart rate  368
Heberden's nodes  238
Heimlich manoeuvre  451–452
*Helicobacter pylori* infection  64,
      **65–69**, 762
Heller's cardiomyotomy  61
helminthic infections  34, **35–38**
  gastroenteritis  31
hemianopia
  bitemporal  545, 648, 649
  homonymous  647, 648,
      649–650
hemiballismus  685
hemiparesis  638
  transient ischaemic attacks
      671
hemiplegia  704
Henoch–Schönlein purpura  **264**
heparin
  acute coronary syndrome  402
  deep vein thrombosis  442
  stroke  669
  venous thromboembolism
      217, 219
hepatic adenomas  153
hepatic encephalopathy  130–131
hepatic porphyria  630
hepatitis  **120–142**
  acute  121
  alcoholic  **148**, 764

hepatitis *(contd)*
  autoimmune **131–132**
  chronic 121
  fulminant 123
  granulomatous lung disease
      484
  viral **120–131**
hepatitis A virus (HAV) infection
    **121–123**
hepatitis B surface antigen
    (HBsAG) 124–125, 263
hepatitis B virus (HBV) infection
    **123–129**
  hepatocellular carcinoma 152
hepatitis C virus (HCV) infection
    **129–130**
  hepatocellular carcinoma 152
hepatitis D infection **129**
hepatitis E virus (HEV) infection
    122, **130**
hepatocellular carcinoma (HCC)
    **152–153**
hepatolenticular degeneration *see*
    Wilson's disease
hepatomegaly
  constrictive pericarditis 435
  typhoid fever 24
hepatorenal syndrome 131
hepatosplenomegaly
  autoimmune hepatitis 132
  granulomatous lung disease
      484
  Hodgkin's disease 227
  leptospirosis 17
hereditary coproporphyria 631,
    632
hereditary elliptocytosis 181
hereditary haemochromatosis
    (HH) **144–146**
hereditary non-polyposis
    colorectal cancer (HNPCC)
    **97**
hereditary spherocytosis
    **180–181**
heroin abuse 534
herpes simplex virus (HSV)
    infection 13, **13**
  AIDS 47
  erythema multiforme 729
  meningitis 690, 693
  mouth ulcers 55
  sexually transmitted infections
      39
herpes viruses **13–15**
  AIDS 47

herpes zoster virus infection
    **13–14**
  mouth ulcers 55
hiatus hernia **61–62**
high-density lipoproteins (HDLs)
    624
highly active antiviral treatment
    (HAART) 45–46, 48, 52
Hirschsprung's disease 93
hirsutism **555–557**
His–Purkinje system 371
histamine bronchial provocation
    tests 465–466
histocompatibility antigens 808
HIV infection **42–45,** 757–758,
    766–767, 795
  antiretroviral therapy effects
      44
  diagnosis 49–50
  direct effects 46
  pyrexia of unknown origin 8
  *see also* AIDS
HLA antigens 808
  psoriasis 725
  spondarthritides 246
  systemic lupus erythematosus
      254
HMG-CoA reductase inhibitors
    (statins) 627, 629
Hodgkin's disease **227–229,**
    766–767
  staging classification 229
Holmes–Adie pupil 651
homocysteine 398
homonymous hemianopia 647,
    648, 649–650
homonymous quadrantanopia
    648
honeycomb lung 487
hookworm infections 35
horizontal nystagmus 646, 658
hormonal therapy 725
hormone replacement therapy
    (HRT)
  menopause 553
  osteoporosis 280
Horner's syndrome 492, 651,
    668, 796
  cluster headaches 703
house-dust mite allergy 463, 464
Howell–Jolly bodies 808
Howell–Jolly body 808
5-HT$_1$ agonists 701
human leucocyte antigens (HLA)
    *see* HLA antigens

human papilloma virus (HPV)
    infections  47–48
humidifier fever  490
Huntington's disease  684–685
hyaline casts  315
hydatid disease  38
hydralazine  254
hydramnios  620
hydrocephalus  546, **699**, 706
hydrocortisone
    Addison's disease  574
    hypopituitarism  548
hydrotherapy  239
hydroxycarbamide (hydroxyurea)
    chronic myeloid leukaemia
        225
    myelofibrosis  198
    sickle cell disease  188
    thrombocythaemia  197
hydroxychloroquine
    adverse effects  245
    rheumatoid arthritis  244
    systemic lupus erythematosus
        256
hydroxycobalamin  174
5-hydroxyindoleacetic acid (5-
    HIAA)  83
hyperacusis  655
hyperaldosteronism
    metabolic alkalosis  308
    primary  592
hyperbilirubinaemia  115
    congenital  **118**
hypercalcaemia  **585–588**, 787
    emergency management  587
    granulomatous lung disease
        484
    kidney stone disease  333
    multiple myeloma  233
hypercalciuria
    kidney stone disease  332–333
    prevention  336
hypercholesterolaemia  624, **626**,
    791
    drug treatment  629
    monogenic familial  791
hypereosinophilic syndrome  806
hypergammaglobulinaemia  131
hyperglycaemia  600
hyperkalaemia  **299–300**
    blood transfusions  203
    causes  300
    ECG changes  302
    emergency management  301
    renal tubular acidosis  306

hyperlipidaemia  **625–630**
    coronary artery disease  398
    diabetes mellitus  603
    nephrotic syndrome  323
    polycystic ovary syndrome
        555
    primary prevention  627, 628
    secondary prevention  627
hypermagnesaemia  **301**
hypernatraemia  **296–297**
    emergency management  296
hyperoxaluria  333
hyperparathyroidism  **585–588**
    chronic renal failure  349
    peptic ulcers  67, 68
hyperphosphataemia  351
hyperpigmentation  724
    Addison's disease  574
hyperplasia, definition  808
hyperprolactinaemia  546, 547,
    **557–558**
    acromegaly  560
    amenorrhoea  554
hyperpyrexia  **596–597**
    thyroid crisis  568
hypersplenism  **199–200**
hypertension  775
    acute intermittent porphyria
        631
    acute nephritic syndrome  320
    control in stroke  670
    coronary artery disease  398
    diabetes mellitus  603
    endocrine causes  590
    essential  435–436
    exercise ECG  372
    grading  437
    management  438–439
    polycystic ovary syndrome
        555
    pulmonary  **425–426**
    renal involvement  **330–332**
    secondary  440
    systemic  **435–43**
hyperthermia  **596–597**
hyperthyroidism  **565–568**, 786
hypertriglyceridaemia  **625**
    drug treatment  629
hypertrophic cardiomyopathy
    **431–432**
hypertrophic scarring  724
hypertrophy, definition  808
hyperuricaemia  266, 267
    renal stone disease  333
hyperventilation  305

hyperviscosity 233
hypervolaemia 293
hypoadrenalism
  primary **573–575**
  secondary **576–577**
hypoalbuminaemia 773
  increased extracellular volume 288
  nephrotic syndrome 322
hypocalcaemia **588–589**, 768
  blood transfusions 203
hypoglossal nerve (twelfth cranial) 659
hypoglycaemia **608–613**, 790–791, 794
hypogonadism
  female **553–555**
  male **549–551**
hypokalaemia **298–299**, 768, 770
  causes 298
  Conn's syndrome 437
  hypertension 437
  hypomagnesaemia in 299, 301
  myopathies 714
  renal tubular acidosis 306–307
  torsades de pointes 383
hypomagnesaemia **300–301**, 768
  hypokalaemia 299, 301
  torsades de pointes 383
hyponatraemia **293–296**, 771
  diagnosis 294
  dilutional **295–296**
  hypovolaemic **294–295**
  salt loss **294–295**
  syndrome of inappropriate ADH secretion 582–583
  water loss **295–296**
hypoparathyroidism **588–589**
hyporeninaemic hypoaldosteronism 306
hypotension
  decreased extracellular volume 290
  metabolic acidosis 305
  oliguria 311
  pericardial tamponade 434
  postural 636
hypothalamic–pituitary–testicular axis 549–550
hypothalamic–pituitary–thyroid feedback system 543

hypothalamus **541–544**
  anatomy 546
  hormone release 542
  see also pituitary
hypothermia **595–596**
  blood transfusions 203
hypothyroidism **561–564**, 787
  amenorrhoea 554
  atrophic 561–562
  autoimmune 561–562
  dilutional hyponatraemia 295
  hypothermia 596
  iatrogenic 562
  management 597
hypotonia 646
hypoventilation 515
hypovolaemia 287, 293, 772–773
  acute renal failure 341
  management 293
  oliguria 311
hypovolaemic hyponatraemia **294–295**
hypovolaemic shock 506, **507**
hypoxia 520

# I

iatrogenic, definition 809
iatrogenic hypothyroidism 562
ibuprofen 239–240
icterus see jaundice
idiopathic, definition 809
idiosyncratic, definition 809
ileoanal anastomosis 90
imipenem 160
immune complexes
  glomerulonephritis 317
  infective endocarditis 423
immunization, active see vaccination
immunization, passive 128–129
immunoglobulin 201
immunoglobulin A nephropathy 317
immunosuppressive therapy
  aplastic anaemia 178
  asthma 469
  autoimmune haemolytic anaemia 192
  autoimmune thrombocytopenic purpura 211
  Behçet's syndrome 265
  Cushing's syndrome 580–581
  nephrotic syndrome 324

immunosuppressive therapy
(contd)
polymyositis 260
psoriasis 726
pyoderma gangrenosum 730
renal transplantation 355
systemic lupus erythematosus
256
implantable
cardioverter–defibrillator
(ICD) 394
impotence 551
inborn errors of metabolism 634
incidence 809
incontinence, urinary 362–363
indigestion 53
see also heartburn
indinavir 51
AIDS 52
infarctions 665–668
cerebral 665
infectious diseases 17–30
examination questions
757–760
infectious mononucleosis 15
infective endocarditis 422–425,
777
anaemia 170
cerebral abscess 694
inflammatory bowel disease (IBD)
84–91
and cancer 91
emergency management 89
mouth ulcers 55
pyoderma gangrenosum 730
systemic symptoms 87
inflammatory mediators
inflammatory bowel disease 84
osteoarthritis 237
septicaemia 7
syphilis 42
infliximab 90
influenza 450–451
infranuclear lesions 652, 654
inhalation of foreign bodies
451–452
inhalers 466–467
inotropic, definition 809
inotropic agents 809
chronic cardiac failure 394
shock 510, 511–512
insulin
analogues 606
in diabetes mellitus 603–604,
606–608

prolonged-action 607
resistance 555
soluble 606
insulin-dependent diabetes
mellitus (IDDM) see
diabetes mellitus
insulinomas 621–623
intensive care medicine 505–521
examination questions
782–783
'intention tremor' 646
β-interferon 688
interferon alpha (IFN-α)
hepatitis virus infection 127,
130
renal cell carcinoma 358
thrombocythaemia 197
interleukin-2 358
interleukins 358, 463, 804
intermediate-density lipoproteins
(IDLs) 623
intermittent mandatory
ventilation (IMV) 518
intermittent peritoneal dialysis
354
intermittent positive-pressure
ventilation (IPPV) 518,
519
internal carotid endarterectomy
670
internal defibrillator 432
internal jugular vein puncture
739–740
international normalized ratio
(INR)
atrial fibrillation 380
coagulation disorders 208
paracetamol overdose 529
stroke 669
thromboembolism 219
interstitial fluid 283
intervertebral disc disease
272–275
acute 274
intestinal amoebiasis 27
intestinal ischaemia, chronic 82
intestinal obstruction 105–106
intestinal resection 80
intra-aortic counterpulsation
(IACP) 513
intracellular fluid 283
intracerebral haemorrhage
665–666, 794
intracoronary stents 401
intracranial abscesses 693–694

intracranial haemorrhage **672–674**
intracranial pressure, raised 636, 697
intracranial tumours **696–699**
intrarenal volume receptors 287
intravenous cannula 735–736
intravenous fluids 292
  administration 291, 293
intravenous pyelography (IVP) *see* excretion urography (intravenous urography, IVU)
intravenous urography (IVU) *see* excretion urography (intravenous urography, IVU)
in vitro, definition 809
in vivo, definition 809
iodine, radioactive 567
iodine deficiency 562
ipratropium bromide 466
ipsilateral lacrimation 703
irebesartan 439
iron deficiency 167, 169–170
iron stores 167
irritable bowel syndrome (IBS) **101–102,** 761
ischaemic colitis **93**
  gastrointestinal bleeding 74
ischaemic heart disease **397–412,** 776, 777
Ishihara colour plates 647
isoniazid
  adverse effects 482
  tuberculosis 81, 481, 482–483
isophane insulins 607
isoprenaline 511
isotretinoin 725
itraconazole 448

**J**

Jacksonian seizures 675–676
Janeway lesions 423
Jarisch–Herxheimer reaction 42, 696
jaundice (icterus) **116–120,** 763–764
  autoimmune hepatitis 132
  leptospirosis 17
  pregnancy 152
  vitamin $B_{12}$ deficiency 173
jejunal mucosal biopsy 77

jerk nystagmus 658
jugular vein puncture 739–740
jugular venous pressure 323
junctional tachycardias **380–381**
juvenile ankylosing spondylitis 265
juvenile chronic arthritis 265
juvenile rheumatoid arthritis 265

**K**

Kallmann's syndrome 548
Kaposi's sarcoma 49
Kartagener's syndrome 458
Kawasaki's disease 262, 809
Kayser–Fleischer rings 146
Kell blood groups 201
keloidal scarring 724
keratoconjunctivitis sicca 261
keratoderma blenorrhagica 725
Kerley B lines 390, 395
Kernig's sign 636
  meningitis 688–689
  subarachnoid haemorrhage 673
ketoconazole 580
Ketostix 608
kidney
  anatomy 315–317
  diseases *see* renal disease
  physiology 309
  transplantation **355**
Kimmelstiel–Wilson lesion 616
kinin systems 318
*Klebsiella pneumoniae* infections 477
Klinefelter's syndrome 550
koilonychia 169
Korsakoff's syndrome 537
Kussmaul's sign
  acute renal failure 344
  constrictive pericarditis 435
  diabetic ketoacidosis 610
  pericardial tamponade 434
kyphosis 247

**L**

lactic acidosis **305,** 605, **614**
lactic dehydrogenase (LDH)
  myocardial infarction 405
  pleural effusion 499

lactulose 141
lamivudine 51
  AIDS 52
  hepatitis B virus infection 127
lamotrigine 678
lanreotide
  acromegaly 560
  hypoglycaemia 623
lansoprazole 59
laryngotracheobronchitis, acute **450**
lateral medullary syndrome 668
laxatives
  adverse effects 301
  portosystemic encephalopathy 141
LDLs *see* low-density lipoproteins (LDLs)
lead pipe rigidity 682
leflunomide 244–245
left bundle branch 371
  disturbances 376
left shift, definition 809
left ventricular hypertrophy 775
  ECG 370–371
*Legionella pneumophila* infections 472, **476,** 780
legionellosis 472, **476,** 780
Legionnaire's disease 472, **476,** 780
leptospirosis **16–17**
leucocytosis 809
  neutrophil 811
leucoerythroblastic reaction 809
leucopenia 171, 809
leucovorin 46
leukaemias **219–227**
  acute **222–225**
  chronic **225–227**
  classification 219–220, 223
  treatment 221–223
leukaemoid reaction 809
leukoplakia **55**
leukotriene receptor antagonists (LTRA) 469
levamisole
  colon cancer 96
  helminthic infections 35
levodopa 682–683
libido loss 551
lichen planus 129
lidocaine
  ventricular fibrillation 409
  ventricular tachycardia 382, 409

life support
  advanced 384
  basic 384–385
limb leads 367, 369
limited systemic sclerosis 257–258
lipid-lowering therapy **627–630**
  angina 400
lipids
  diseases/disorders **623–630**
  measurement **624–625**
  plasma 623–630
lipohypertrophy 619
lipoprotein lipase deficiency 625
lipoproteins 623–624
lisinopril
  chronic cardiac failure 393
  hypertension 438–439
listeriosis 31
lithotripsy 157
liver abscesses **150–152**
  amoebic 27, **151–152**
  pyogenic **150–151**
liver diseases/disorders **113–153**
  abscesses *see* liver abscesses
  adenomas 153
  alcoholic **148–149**
  alcoholic hepatitis **148,** 764
  blood coagulation 214
  chronic 128, 129, 764
  damage 530–531, 532
  encephalopathy 130–131
  examination questions 763–764
  *Fasciola hepatica* infections 37
  fatty liver **148**
  fatty liver of pregnancy 152
  fulminant hepatic failure **130–131**
  hepatitis *see* hepatitis
  hepatocellular carcinoma **152–153**
  hepatomegaly *see* hepatomegaly
  non-alcoholic fatty liver disease 148
  paracetamol toxicity **530–531,** 532
  porphyria 630
  recurrent intrahepatic cholestasis 152
  symptoms **113–114**
  tumours **152–153**
  *see also* biliary tract diseases
liver flukes 37

liver function tests (LFTs)
**114–116**
 alcoholic cirrhosis 149
 alcoholic hepatitis 148
 bile duct stones 157
 cholecystitis 156
 cirrhosis 133–134
 fatty liver 148
 hepatitis A 123
 hepatocellular carcinoma 153
 hereditary haemochromatosis
  145
 liver abscesses 151
 pneumonia 473
 primary biliary cirrhosis 143
liver transplantation **149**
local anaesthesia 734
long QT syndrome 383
loop diuretics 289
 chronic cardiac failure 392
 hypertension 437
 increased extracellular volume
  289
Looser's zones 277
loperamide 31
lorazepam 678, 680
losartan
 chronic cardiac failure 393
 hypertension 439
low back pain 271
low-density lipoproteins (LDLs)
  623
 diseases/disorders **626**
lower motor neurone (LMN)
  lesions 641
 facial nerve 655–656
 optic nerve 652, 654
 upper motor neurone lesion
  comparison 639
lower oesophageal sphincter 58
low-molecular weight heparins
  218
lumbago 274
lumbar back pain **269,** 270, 272
lumbar puncture
 intracranial tumours 698
 procedure 753–754
 subarachnoid haemorrhage 673
lung abscesses 477–478
lung carcinomas **492–498**
lung function tests **447–448**
 asthma 465
 COPD 454
 cryptogenic fibrosing alveolitis
  488

extrinsic allergic alveolitis 489
granulomatous lung disease
  485
lung injury, acute 395, **520–521**
lupus nephritis 318
lutenizing hormone (LH) 542,
  545, 546
 amenorrhoea 554
 menopause 553
 secretion 549
lutenizing hormone-releasing
  hormone (LHRH) 542,
  549, 555
Lyme borreliosis **15–16**
lymphadenopathy
 bilateral hilar 484, 485, 781
 Graves' disease 565
 rheumatoid arthritis 243
lymphocytosis 796
lymphomas **227–231**
 Burkitt's 231
 MALT 231
 pyoderma gangrenosum 730
 small intestine 83
 see also Hodgkin's disease; non-
  Hodgkin's lymphoma
  (NHL)
lysergic acid diethylamine (LSD)
 abuse 535
lysergide abuse 535

**M**

macrocytic anaemia 168,
  **171–176**
macrocytosis 176
macronodular cirrhosis 132
macrosomia 620
macular oedema 615
macule 809
maculopapule 809
maculopathy 615
magnesium homeostasis 284
 disorders **300–301**
magnetic resonance angiography
 stroke 670
 unilateral renal disease 331
magnetic resonance
  cholangiopancreatography
  (MRCP)
 bile duct stones 157
 cholestatic jaundice 119
 gallstones 155
 liver disease 116

magnetic resonance imaging (MRI) 810
  acromegaly 560
  aortic aneurysm 440
  back pain 272
  epilepsy 677
  Guillain–Barré syndrome 713
  headache 636
  intervertebral disc disease 274
  lung carcinoma 495
  multiple sclerosis 687
  neurological disease 638
  osteoarthritis 239
  polymyositis 260
  pulmonary embolism 427
  renal cell carcinoma 357
  spinal stenosis 275
  stroke 666, 669
  syringomyelia 706
malabsorption 762
  causes 76
  osteomalacia 275
malaria **19–25**
malarone 22, 24
male hypogonadism **549–551**
malignant hyperpyrexia 596
Mallory–Weiss syndrome 72
malnourishment 108–109
MALT lymphoma 231
malt worker's lung 490
Mantoux test 479, 480, 481
march haemoglobinuria 193
Marfan's syndrome **730**, 810
  mitral valve prolapse 417
MDMA abuse 535
mean corpuscular haemoglobin (MCH) 166
mean corpuscular haemoglobin concentration (MCHC) 166
mean corpuscular volume (MCV) 166
measles **11**
  bronchiectasis 457
  Crohn's disease 84
measles mumps and rubella (MMR) vaccine 11
mebendazole 35, 36
mechanical haemolytic anaemias 193
mechanical shock **508**
Meckel's diverticulum **82**
meconium ileus equivalent (MIE) syndrome 460
mediastinoscopy 497

medroxyprogesterone 358
medullary sponge kidney **357**
mefloquine 22, 23–24
megacolon **93**
megaloblastic anaemia **171–172**
Meig's syndrome 139
melaena 71–72
melphalan 233
membranoproliferative glomerulonephritis 129
membranous glomerulonephritis 322
MEN 1 and 2 (multiple endocrine neoplasia) **593–595**, 621
Mendelson's syndrome 477
Ménétrièr's disease 81–82
Ménière's disease 657, **658**
meningitis **688–690**, 794
  AIDS 48
  bacterial see bacterial meningitis
  epilepsy 676
  hydrocephalus 699
  tuberculous 481
meningococcal arthritis **252**
meningococci 689
meningoencephalitis
  Lyme disease 16
  *Mycoplasma* pneumonia 475
menopause **552–553**
  osteoporosis 279
menstruation 168, 170
6-mercaptopurine 89–90
metabolic acidosis **305–308**
  causes 307
metabolic alkalosis 308
metalloproteinases 237
metamyelocytes 812
metaplasia, definition 810
metformin 605, 606
methacholine bronchial provocation tests 465–466
methadone 534
methaemalbumin 179
methotrexate
  adverse effects 245
  ankylosing spondylitis 248
  asthma 469
  Crohn's disease 90
  polymyositis 260
  psoriasis 726
  psoriatic arthritis 250
  rheumatoid arthritis 244
methylcellulose eyedrops 569

3,4-methylenedioxy-
    methamphetamine (MDMA)
  abuse 535
  hyperthermia 597
methylphenyltetrahydropyridine
    (MPTP) 681
methylsergide 701
metoclopramide
  adverse effects 557, 685
  gastro-oesophageal reflux
      disease 59
  migraine 701
metolazone 392
metoprolol
  angina 400–401
  chronic cardiac failure 394
metronidazole
  amoebiasis 28
  Crohn's disease 90
  diverticular disease 92
  empyema 478
  giardiasis 30
  H. pylori infection 66
  liver abscesses 152
  periodontal disorders 56
  portosystemic encephalopathy
      142
  traveller's diarrhoea 758
metyrapone 580
'Mexican hat cells' 814
mexiletine 382
microalbuminuria 313
  diabetic nephropathy 616
microangiopathic haemolysis
    193
microcytic anaemia **167–171**,
    765
$β_2$-microglobin-related
    amyloidosis 350
micrographia 682
micronodular cirrhosis 132
microscopic colitis 88
microscopic haematuria 17
microscopic polyangiitis **264**,
    486, 800
microscopy, glomerulonephritis
    318, 319
Microsporidia infections 47
micturating cystoscopy 810
micturition frequency 309, 326
mid-stream urine specimen
    (MSU) 326
migraine **700–701**
Mikulicz syndrome 56
miliary tuberculosis 478–479

minimal change
    glomerulonephritis
    322–323
mitral regurgitation **416–417**
  mitral valve prolapse 418
  rheumatic fever 411
mitral stenosis **413–416**
mitral valve prolapse **417–418**,
    777
Mobitz blocks 374–375
monoclonal gammopathy of
    undetermined significance
    **234**
monocular visual defects 647,
    648
monocytosis 810
monogenic familial
    hypercholesterolaemia
    791
mononeuritis multiplex 709,
    **711**
mononeuropathies **710–711**
  diabetic 618
montelukast 469
morning stiffness 235
  ankylosing spondylitis 246
motor neurone disease (MND)
    641, 659, **708–710**
  diaphragm involvement 503
motor pathways 642, 644
mouth ulcers
  infective 55
  non-infective 54–55
mucosa-associated lymphoid tissue
    (MALT) lymphoma 231
multidrug resistance, tuberculosis
    481
multi-infarct dementia 668, **721**
multiple endocrine neoplasia
    (MEN) **593–595**, 621
multiple myeloma **232–233**
  pyoderma gangrenosum 730
multiple organ dysfunction
    syndrome (MODS) 507
multiple organ failure (MOF)
    507
multiple sclerosis (MS) **686–688**,
    705
  eye defects 649
mumps **11–12**
  meningitis 690, 693
Murphy's sign 156
muscle contractions 805
muscle weakness **638–641**
  polymyositis 260

**M**

muscular dystrophy **715**
  diaphragm involvement 503
  visual defects 654
musculoskeletal problems
**235–281**
myasthenia gravis 641, **716–717**
  Graves' disease 565
*Mycobacterium avium-intracellulaire*
  infection 49
*Mycobacterium tuberculosis*
  infection *see* tuberculosis
mycophenolate mofetil 355
*Mycoplasma pneumoniae* infections
475
  erythema multiforme 729
mycosis fungoides 231
myeloablative therapy **231–232**
myelocytes 812
myelodysplasia 194, **198–199**
myelofibrosis, primary **197–198**
myelography 274
myeloproliferative disorders
**193–199**
myelosclerosis **197–198**
myocardial contractility 510
myocardial disease **430**
myocardial infarction (MI)
**403–411,** 776
  acute pericarditis 433
  emergency management 407
  exercise ECG 372
  without ST segment elevation
402
myocarditis **430**
  Lyme disease 16
  *Mycoplasma* pneumonia 475
myoclonus 685
myopathies **714**
  alcohol abuse 537
  polymyositis 260
  proximal 276
myotonia congenita **717–718**
myotonias **717–718**
myotonic pupil 651
myxoedema 542, 787
  madness 564
  pretibial 565–566
myxoedema coma **564**
  emergency management 564

naratriptan 701
narcolepsy 637
nasogastric tube insertion
746–747
nasopharyngitis 444
National Institute for Clinical
  Excellence (NICE) 810
nausea
  with headache 636
  migraine 700–701
  *see also* vomiting
*Necator americanus* infections 35
neck pain **275**
neck stiffness 688
necrobiosis lipoidica
  diabeticorum 619
necrosis, definition 810
*Neisseria gonorrhoeae* infections
34, 39–40
*Neisseria meningitidis* infections
759–760
nelfinavir 51
nematode infection 35–36
neostigmine 717
nephrectomy 357–358
nephritic syndrome, acute **319,
320**
nephritis, tubulointerstitial *see*
  tubulointerstitial nephritis
nephrocalcinosis **337**
  renal tubular acidosis 307
nephrogenic diabetes insipidus
  (NDI) 582–583, 790
nephrotic syndrome **322–325,**
773, 789
  glomerulonephritis 318
neural tube defects 176
neuroendocrine system, shock
506
neurofibromatosis **731**
neuroleptic malignant syndrome
597
neurology **635–721**
  alcohol abuse 537
  examination questions
791–796
neuronitis, vestibular **658**
neuropathy
  chronic renal failure 349–350
  diabetes mellitus **617–618**
neurosyphilis 41, **694–696,**
794–795
neurotoxins 26
neutropenia, definition 811
neutrophil leucocytosis 811

# N

*N*-acetylcysteine (NAC) 530–531
naloxone 663

nevirapine   51
nicorandil   401
nicotinic acid   630
nifedipine
    angina   401
    chronic cardiac failure   393
    hypertension   439
    Raynaud's disease   441
nimodipine   673
ninth cranial nerve   659
Nissen fundoplication   59
nitrates
    adverse effects   401
    angina   401
    pulmonary oedema   396
nitric oxide   520
nitrofurantoin   327
nitroprusside   394
nocturia   **310**
    diabetes insipidus   582–583
    tubulointerstitial nephritis   329
nodules   811
non-alcoholic fatty liver disease
        (NAFLD)   148
non-gonococcal urethritis (NGU)
        **40**
non-Hodgkin's lymphoma (NHL)
        **229–230**, 766–767
    AIDS   49
    small intestine   83
non-immune haemolytic
        anaemias   **193**
non-insulin dependent diabetes
        mellitus (NIDDM) *see*
        diabetes mellitus
non-invasive positive-pressure
        ventilation (NIPPV)
    acute exacerbation of COPD
        456
    respiratory failure   517–518
non-ketotic hyperosmolar state
        **611, 613**
non-nucleoside reverse
        transcriptase inhibitors
        50, 51
non-small cell lung cancer   497
non-steroidal anti-inflammatory
        drugs (NSAIDs)
    acute pericarditis   433
    acute renal failure   341
    adverse effects   240, 288, 328
    ankylosing spondylitis   248
    asthma   464
    erythema nodosum   729
    gastrointestinal bleeding   72

gastropathy   64
gout   266
intervertebral disc disease
        274
osteoarthritis   239–240
overdose   533
peptic ulcers   67
pericarditis   410
psoriatic arthritis   250
pyrophosphate arthropathy
        269
Reiter's syndrome   249
renal stone disease   336
rheumatoid arthritis   244
septic arthritis   251
systemic lupus erythematosus
        256
tubulointerstitial nephritis
        328–329
norepinephrine   510, 511
normoblasts   811
notifiable diseases   481
nucleoside analogues   51
nucleoside reverse transcriptase
        inhibitors   50
nucleotide analogues   51
numbness   **641–645**
nutcracker oesophagus   61
nutrition   **106–111**
nutritional support   **108–111**
    monitoring   110–111
nystagmus   657, **658**
    anticonvulsant drugs   677
    horizontal   646

# O

obesity   **111**
    coronary artery disease   398
    diabetes mellitus   603
    diabetes mellitus type 2   600
    hypertension   440
obstruction, intestinal   **105–106**
obstructive sleep apnoea (OSA)
        **456–457**
occipital cortex defects   650
occupational therapy   688
octreotide
    acromegaly   560
    carcinoid syndrome   83
    hypoglycaemia   623
    variceal haemorrhage   137
ocular movements   652–654
oculogyric crisis   685–686

oculomotor nerve (third cranial)
652, **652–654**
  intracranial tumours 697
odynophagia (painful
  swallowing) 56, 57
oedema 285–286
  acute nephritic syndrome 320
  central 611
  cerebral 297
  macular 615
  nephrotic syndrome 322
  pulmonary see pulmonary
    oedema
oesophageal adenocarcinomas
  62
oesophageal disorders **56–57**
  functional 101
  perforation 63
  tumours 62–63
  ulceration 47
oesophagitis 537
oesophagoscopy
  achalasia 60
  gastro-oesophageal reflux
    disease 58
oestrogens 552
  adverse effects 557
  amenorrhoea 554
  deficiency 278, 553–555
  hirsutism 557
  menopause 553
Ogilvie's syndrome 106
olfactory nerve (first cranial) 647
oligoarticular, definition 811
oligomenorrhoea 553–554
  hyperprolactinaemia 557
  polycystic ovary syndrome
    556
oliguria 309, **310–311**
  acute nephritic syndrome 320
  acute renal failure 344
omeprazole
  gastro-oesophageal reflux
    disease 59
  H. pylori infection 66
oncogenes 811
  colorectal cancer 95
  multiple endocrine neoplasia
    595
onycholysis 725
ophthalmia neonatorum 40
ophthalmopathy 565
ophthalmoplegia 569
opioids
  abuse 534, 651

  overdose 534, 663
  pulmonary oedema 396
  renal stone disease 336
Opisthorchis infections 37
optic atrophy **650**
  multiple sclerosis 687
optic chiasma 546
optic disc oedema **650**
optic nerve (second cranial)
  647–651
  lesions 647–649
  visual pathways 648
optic neuritis 687
oral diseases **54–56**
oral hairy leukoplakia 47
oral rehydration solutions (ORS)
  291
  cholera 29
  traveller's diarrhoea 31
oral white patches **55**
orchidectomy 361
orlistat 111
orthopnea 444
  aortic regurgitation 420
  heart disease **365**
Osler's nodes 423
osmolality 811
osmolarity 283, 285, 811
  hypernatraemia 297
osmotic demyelination syndrome
  296
osmotic diarrhoea **98**
osteoarthritis (OA) **237–240**
  secondary 237
osteoblasts 275
osteoclasts 275
  viral infection 280
osteomalacia **276–278**, 769
osteomyelitis 694
osteoporosis **278–280**, 769
  menopause 553
  steroid-induced 263
overflow incontinence 363
overlap syndrome **261**
overnight oximetry 457
oximetry, overnight 457
oxitropium bromide 466
oxybutynin 362
oxygen therapy
  COPD 455
  obstructive sleep apnoea 457
  pneumonia 474
  respiratory failure 517–519
oxytetracycline 40
oxytocin 542, 543, 547

# P

Pabrinex 537
pacemakers 374
packed cell volume (PCV) 166
packed red cells 200
Paget's disease **280–281**
pain *see specific type*
palmar erythema 131–132
palpitations **365**
palsy, bulbar 659
palsy, pseudo-bulbar 668
Pancoast's tumour 492, 651
pancreatic diseases **158–164**
  carcinoma **162–163**
  endocrine tumours **164**
  examination questions
    763–764
pancreatitis **158–162**
  acute **158–161**
  alcohol abuse 537
  chronic **161–162**
  hypertriglyceridaemia 625
pancreolauryl test 162
pancytopenia 178, 767, 811
panhypopituitarism 547
pannus 241
panproctocolectomy with
  ileostomy 90
pansinusitis 460
pantoprazole 59
papaverine 551
papilloedema 649, **650**
  hydrocephalus 699
  intracranial tumours 697
papovavirus infections 47–48
papule 811
paracentesis 139–140
paracetamol (acetaminophen)
  headache 700
  hepatotoxicity **530–531**, 532
  migraine 701
  osteoarthritis 239–240
  overdose *see* paracetamol
    overdose
paracetamol overdose 130,
  **529–532**
  emergency management
    530
paraesthesiae 643
paraldehyde 680
para-oesophageal hiatus hernia
  61
paraparesis 641

paraplegia 640, 704
  management 708
paraproteinaemias **232–234**
parasympathetic eyedrops 651
parathyroidectomy 585, 588
parathyroid gland
  diseases/disorders
    **584–589**
parathyroid hormone (PTH)
  bone metabolism 275
  chronic renal failure 349
paratyphoid fever **25**
parkinsonism, drug-induced
  683
'Parkinsonism plus' 673
Parkinson's disease **680–683**
parotid gland tumours 56
paroxysmal nocturnal dyspnoea
  444
  heart disease 365
paroxysmal nocturnal
  haemoglobinuria (PNH)
  193
patch testing 728
pathognomonic, definition 811
Patterson–Brown–Kelly syndrome
  169
Paul–Bunnell reaction 15
peak expiratory flow rate (PEFR)
  **448**
  asthma 465
  COPD 454
pegvisomant 560
pelvic floor exercises 362
pendular nystagmus 658
penicillamine
  adverse effects 245
  rheumatoid arthritis 244
  Wilson's disease 147
penicillin
  adverse effects 328
  infective arthritis 252
  leptospirosis 17
  rheumatic fever 412
  tubulointerstitial nephritis
    328
'pen injector' 607
pentamidine 48
peptic ulcer disease **66–69**, 762
  gastrointestinal bleeding 72
  *H. pylori* infections 65
percutaneous endoscopic
  gastrostomy (PEG) 109
percutaneous nephrolithotomy
  336

P

percutaneous transhepatic
      cholangiopancreatography
      (PTC)
   cholestatic jaundice   119
   liver disease   116
perennial rhinitis   449
perforated ulcers   68
pericardial disease   **433–435**
pericardial effusion   **434**
pericardial tamponade   **434**
pericardiocentesis   434
pericarditis   776
   acute   **433**
   acute renal failure   344–345
   constrictive   **434–435**
   myocardial infarction   410
   myocarditis   430
   rheumatoid arthritis   243
perimetry   647
perinuclear antineutrophil
      cytoplasmic antibodies
      (pANCA)
   microscopic polyangiitis   264
   pulmonary vasculitis   486,
      487
periodontal disorders   56
peripheral nerve diseases
      **710–714**
peripheral nerve lesions   643
peritoneal dialysis   354
peritonitis
   acute   **105,** 106
   bacterial   140
pernicious anaemia   **172–175**
   Graves' disease   565
peroneal muscular atrophy   **712**
persistent vegetative state   811
petechiae   208, 811
Peutz–Jegher syndrome   83
phaeochromocytoma   **593**
   secondary hypertension   436
pharyngitis, acute   **450**
phenobarbital   680
phenothiazines
   adverse effects   557, 597, 683,
      685
   overdose   533
phenotype, definition   812
phenoxybenzamine   593
phentolamine   551
phenytoin
   adverse effects   677–678
   epilepsy   677
   postherpetic neuralgia   14
   status epilepticus   680

Philadelphia chromosome
   chronic myeloid leukaemia
      225
   leukaemias   220
   myelofibrosis   198
phosphaturia   313
photophobia   700–701
physiotherapy
   bronchiectasis   458
   intervertebral disc disease
      274
   multiple sclerosis   688
   osteoarthritis   239
   paraplegia   708
   Parkinson's disease   683
pink puffers   452, 454
pioglitazone   606
piperacillin   11
pitting   286
pituitary apoplexy   548
pituitary gland   **541–544**
   adenomas   557, 580
   anatomy   542, 546
   tumours   **545–546**
   *see also* hypothalamus
plantar fasciitis   247
plaque (skin)   812
plaque psoriasis   725
plasma   283
plasmapheresis   234
plasmin   207
plasminogen   207
*Plasmodium* infections   **19–25**
platelets
   blood coagulation   205
   concentrates   201
   count   197, 208
   defects   **209–211**
pleural aspiration   743–745
pleural diseases   **498–502**
pleural effusion   **498–499, 501**
   causes   500
   rheumatoid arthritis   243
   *Staphylococcus aureus*
      pneumonia   476
pleurisy
   dry   **498**
   pneumonia   471
Plummer's disease   **565**
pneumococcal antigen   474
pneumococci   689–690
pneumoconiosis   491
*Pneumocystis carinii* infections
      476
   AIDS   48, 795

pneumonia **471–478**, 780
  aetiology 472
  aspiration 476–477
  diagnosis 473
pneumothorax **501–502**, 519, 781
  emergency management 503
  *Staphylococcus aureus*
    pneumonia 476
  tension 501
poisoning **523–534**
  emergency resuscitation
    525–526
  examination questions
    783–785
  management 525–528
poliomyelitis 641
polyangiitis, microscopic **264**,
    486, 800
polyarteritis nodosa **263–264**
polyarthritis
  rheumatic fever 411
  symmetrical 249
polychromasia 812
polycystic ovary syndrome
    (PCOS) 554, **555–557**
polycythaemia **194–197**, 766
polycythaemia vera **195–196**
polydipsia 310, 790
polygenic hypercholesterolaemia
    626
polygenic hypertriglyceridaemia
    625
polymerase chain reaction (PCR)
    812
polymyalgia rheumatica
    **262–263**
  anaemia 170
polymyositis **260–261**
polyneuritis 656
polyneuropathy 641, 643,
    **711–713**
  acute intermittent porphyria
    631
  alcohol abuse 537
  Lyme disease 16
  postinfective *see* Guillain–Barré
    syndrome
polyp(s)
  adenomatous **94**
  colon **93–94**
polyposis syndrome **93–94**
polysomnography 457
polyunsaturated fats 627
polyuria 309, **310**
  acute renal failure 344

diabetes insipidus 582–583
diabetes mellitus 602
tubulointerstitial nephritis 329
pontine lesions 643, 645
popliteal cysts 777–778
porphyria cutanea tarda 631, 632
porphyrias **630–633**
portal hypertension **135–138**
  *see also* gastrointestinal bleeding
portosystemic encephalopathy
    (PSE) **140–142**
positive end-expiratory pressure
    (PEEP) 518
posterior clinoid 546
postherpetic neuralgia (PHN) 14
postinfective polyneuropathy *see*
    Guillain–Barré syndrome
post nasal drip 444
post-phlebitic syndrome 216
post-transfusion purpura 204
postural changes, Parkinson's
    disease 682
postural hypotension 636, 711
  chronic renal failure 350
  decreased extracellular volume
    290
postural proteinuria 312
potassium homeostasis 284
  disorders **297–300**, 770
potassium-sparing diuretics 392
pravastatin 629
praziquantel 37, 38
prazosin 394
prednisolone
  asthma 466, 471
  autoimmune haemolytic
    anaemia 192
  autoimmune hepatitis 132
  autoimmune thrombocytopenic
    purpura 211
  Bell's palsy 656
  chronic lymphocytic leukaemia
    226
  Churg–Strauss syndrome 265
  cryptogenic fibrosing alveolitis
    488
  de Quervains thyroiditis 565
  erythema nodosum 729
  extrinsic allergic alveolitis 489
  giant cell arteritis 702
  granulomatous lung disease
    486
  leukaemia 224
  nephrotic syndrome 324
  non-Hodgkin's lymphoma 230

P

prednisolone (*contd*)
  polymyositis 260
  rhinitis 449
  systemic lupus erythematosus
    256
  tubulointerstitial nephritis
    328–329
pre-eclampsia
  diabetes mellitus 620
  secondary hypertension 436
pre-eclamptic toxaemia 152
pregnancy
  acute pyelonephritis 327–328
  diabetes mellitus **620**
  jaundice 152
  urinary tract infections
    327–328
pre-proliferative retinopathy 615
presbycusis 657
pressure–flow studies 339
pretibial myxoedema 565–566
prevalence 812
primaquine 22
primary biliary cirrhosis (PBC)
  **142–143**
  pyoderma gangrenosum 730
  Sjögren's syndrome 261
primary hyperaldosteronism
  **592**
primary hyperparathyroidism
  585
primary lateral sclerosis 709
primary myelofibrosis **197–198**
primary polycythaemia **195–196**
primary sclerosing cholangitis
  (PSC) **157–158**
primary thrombocythaemia 197
PR interval
  atrioventricular block 374–375
  ECG 371
Prinzmetal's angina 399
probenecid
  gout 267
  typhoid fever 25
procainamide 254
procaine benzylpenicillin 42
procedures **733–755**
procyclidine 686
progesterone 552
prognosis 812
progressive bulbar palsy 709
progressive massive fibrosis
  (PMF) 492
progressive muscular atrophy
  709

progressive supranuclear palsy
  683
pro-inflammatory cytokines 240
prolactin 542, 545
  amenorrhoea 554
prolactinoma 557
proliferative retinopathy 615
promyelocytes 812
propranolol
  phaeochromocytoma 593
  thyroid crisis 568
  variceal haemorrhage 137
prophylaxis, definition 812
*Propionibacterium acnes* 723
proprioception 641, 643
prostacyclins
  acute respiratory distress
    syndrome 520
  pulmonary hypertension 426
prostatectomy 360
prostate gland
  carcinoma **360–361**
  diseases **359–361**
  enlargement *see* benign
    prostatic hypertrophy
prostate-specific antigen (PSA)
  back pain 272
  benign prostatic hypertrophy
    359
  prostate gland carcinoma
    360
prostatitis 39
prosthetic heart valves **413**
  haemolytic anaemia 193
  mitral regurgitation 417
protamine insulins 607
protease inhibitors 50, 51
protein C 207
protein-losing enteropathy
  **81–82**
protein S 207
proteinuria **312–313**
  acute nephritic syndrome
    320
  diabetic nephropathy 616
  glomerulonephritis 318
  hypertension 437
  nephrotic syndrome 322
  Stix tests 311–312
prothrombin 205
prothrombin time (PT)
  cholestatic jaundice 120
  coagulation disorders 208
  liver disease 114
  paracetamol overdose 529

proton pump inhibitors (PPIs)
  *H. pylori* infection 66
  peptic ulcer disease 74
  peptic ulcers 68
proximal, definition 812
proximal renal tube acidosis
    306–307
pruritus 114
  primary biliary cirrhosis 142
pseudo-bulbar palsy 659, 668
pseudo-Cushing's syndrome 578
pseudodementia 794
pseudogout **268–269**
pseudohyponatraemia 293
*Pseudomonas aeruginosa* infections
  bronchiectasis 458
  cystic fibrosis 460
  pneumonia 476
  septicaemia 9
psittacosis 472
psoralens 726
psoriasis **725–726,** 797
psoriatic arthritis **249–250**
psychiatric assessments, self-harm
    527–528
psychiatric diseases, alcohol
    abuse 538
ptosis 796
  Horner's syndrome 651
pulmonary artery wedge pressure
    (PAWP) 514–515
pulmonary embolism (PE)
    **426–429,** 781–782, 782–783
  emergency management 428
pulmonary fibrosis **487–489**
pulmonary granulomatosis
    **486–487**
pulmonary heart disease **425–429**
pulmonary hypertension
    **425–426**
pulmonary oedema **395–396,**
    777, 781
  emergency management 396
  mitral regurgitation 416
  myocardial infarction 410
  non-cardiogenic (acute lung
    injury) 395, **520–521**
pulmonary regurgitation 421
pulmonary stenosis 421
pulmonary valve disease
    **421–422**
pulmonary vasculitis **486–487**
pulse oximetry 516
pupils **650–651**
  unconsciousness 662

purpura, post-transfusion 204,
    812
pustular psoriasis 725
pustules 812
P wave
  atrial fibrillation 379
  ECG 368–369
pyelography
  intravenous *see* excretion
       urography (intravenous
       urography, IVU)
  retrograde 813
pyelonephritis, acute 326, 327
  pregnancy 327–328
pyoderma gangrenosum **730**
pyogenic liver abscesses
    **150–151**
pyrantel pamoate 36
pyrazinamide
  adverse effects 482
  tuberculosis 81, 481
pyrexia 471
pyrexia of unknown origin (PUO)
    **7–9**
pyridostigmine 717
pyridoxine 481
  deficiency **714**
pyrimethamine 46
pyrophosphate arthropathy
    (pseudogout) **268–269**

**Q**

Q fever (*Coxiella burnetii* infection)
  423, 472
QRS complex
  ECG 369–370
  intraventricular conduction
      disturbances 375
  junctional tachycardias 380
QT interval 383
quadrantanopia, homonymous
    648
quadriplegia 640, 641
quinapril 393
quinine 22
quinolone antibiotics 25
Q wave 369, 370

**R**

radiofrequency ablation 381
radioimmunoassay (RIA) 812

radiology
  acute respiratory distress syndrome 520
  ankylosing spondylitis 247–248
  aortic aneurysm 440
  aortic regurgitation 420
  aortic stenosis 420
  asthma 466
  back pain 272
  bronchiectasis 458
  cardiac failure 389–390
  constrictive pericarditis 435
  COPD 454
  cryptogenic fibrosing alveolitis 487
  dilated cardiomyopathy (DCM) 431
  extrinsic allergic alveolitis 489
  granulomatous lung disease 484
  hypertension 437
  infective endocarditis 424
  intervertebral disc disease 274
  intracranial tumours 698
  lung carcinoma 495
  mitral regurgitation 417
  mitral stenosis 415
  osteoarthritis 239
  osteomalacia 277
  osteoporosis 279
  Paget's disease 282
  pancreatitis 159, 162
  pericardial tamponade 434
  pleural effusion 499
  pneumonia 474
  psoriatic arthritis 250
  pulmonary embolism 427
  pulmonary hypertension 425
  pulmonary oedema 395
  pyrophosphate arthropathy 269
  renal failure 345
  renal stone disease 335
  respiratory disease **447**
  restrictive cardiomyopathy 432
  rheumatoid arthritis 242
  systemic sclerosis 258
  tuberculosis 479
  unconsciousness 663
radionuclide angiography 391
radionuclide lung scan 427
radiotherapy
  acromegaly 560
  Cushing's syndrome 580
  hyperprolactinaemia 558
  intracranial tumours 698
  leukaemias 221–222
  lung carcinoma 497
  non-Hodgkin's lymphoma 230
raloxifene 280
ramipril 438–439
Ramsay Hunt syndrome 656, **656**
ranitidine 59
rapid urease test 65
rashes, polymyositis 260
RAST test 449
Raynaud's disease **440–441**
Raynaud's phenomena **440–441**
  polymyositis 260
  systemic sclerosis 257
reactive arthritis **249**
receptive aphasia 801
recurrent intrahepatic cholestasis 152
red cell concentrates 200
red cell count (RCC) 166
5α-reductase inhibitors
  benign prostatic hypertrophy 359
  hirsutism 557
re-entry circuits 376–377
reflexes 644
reflux, gastro-oesophageal **58–60**
reflux nephropathy 436
Regional Poisons Centre 525
regurgitation, pulmonary 421
Reiter's syndrome **248–249**, 725
  mouth ulcers 55
remnant hyperlipidaemia 626
renal arteriography 331
renal artery stenosis 331
  secondary hypertension 436
renal cell carcinoma **357–358**
renal disease 309–636
  bilateral **330**
  cysts **355–357**
  examination questions 771–773
  infective lesions 617
  ischaemic lesions 616–617
  osteomalacia 275
  proximal tubule defects 313
  secondary hypertension 436
  stones **332–337**
  tumours **357–358**
  unilateral 331–332

renal failure **340–352**
  acute *see* renal failure, acute
  chronic 340, **347–352,** 772
  glomerulonephritis 318
  hypercalcaemia 586
  multiple myeloma 233
renal failure, acute **340–347,** 773
  emergency management 347
  nephrotic syndrome 325
  vs chronic renal failure 350
renal hypertension **330–332**
renal osteodystrophy 349
renal replacement therapy
    **352–355**
renal scintigraphy 812
renal stone disease **332–337**
renal transplantation 355
renal tubular acidosis 306–307,
    313
  type 1 307
  type 2 306–307
  type 4 306
renin 590, 591
renin–angiotensin system
    **590–591**
  cardiac failure 388
  shock 505–506
repaglinide 606
reproduction **549–558**
  female **552–558**
  male **549–552**
reserpine 683
residual volume (RV) 448
respiratory acidosis 303
respiratory alkalosis 305, 768
  aspirin overdose 528, 784
respiratory diseases/disorders
    **443–504**
  acidosis 303
  acute respiratory distress
      syndrome 507, **520–521**
  alkalosis *see* respiratory
      alkalosis
  allergic bronchopulmonary
      aspergillosis 465
  COPD *see* chronic obstructive
      pulmonary disease
      (COPD)
  diaphragm **502–503**
  examination questions
      778–782
  failure **515–519**
  investigations **447–448**
  lower tract **452–460**
  lung carcinomas **492–497**

lung parenchyma **483–489**
  metastases 498
  occupational **489–491**
  pleura **498–502**
  pulmonary oedema *see*
      pulmonary oedema
  symptoms 443–446
  upper tract **448–452**
respiratory support **517–519**
restenosis 401
restrictive cardiomyopathy
    **432–433**
resuscitation 661
reteplase 215
reticulocyte count 165
retinal ischaemia 187
retinoic acid 726
retinopathy, diabetic **614–616**
retinosis 47
*Ret* proto-oncogene 595
retrograde pyelography 813
retrovirus 42, 43
rhabdomyolysis 773, 813
rhesus blood groups 201–202
rheumatic fever 411–412
rheumatic heart disease, chronic
    412
rheumatic valvular disease,
    chronic 412
rheumatoid arthritis (RA)
    **240–246**
  juvenile 265
  neck pain 275
  pyoderma gangrenosum 730
  Sjögren's syndrome 261
  vasculitis 262
rheumatoid factors (RhF) 241,
    813
rheumatoid nodules 241
rheumatology **235–281**
  examination questions
      767–769
rhinitis 444, **449**
rhinorrhoea 703
ribavirin 130
rifampicin
  adverse effects 482
  meningitis 690
  tuberculosis 81, 481
rifaximin 142
right bundle branch 376
right ventricular hypertrophy
    371
rigidity 682
riluzole 710

R

ring sideroblasts 171
risedronate 279–280
ritonavir 51
rivastigmine 721
rizatriptan 701
rofecoxib 239–240
rosiglitazone 606
rotary nystagmus 658
Roth's spots 423
Rotor syndrome 118
roundworm infections 35–36
rubella **12,** 758
'rugger jersey spine' 349
R wave 369, 370

# S

saccular aneurysms 672
SAD PERSONS scale 527
salbutamol 466
salivary gland disorders **56**
salmeterol 466
salmonella arthritis **252–253**
*Salmonella* infections 25, 758,
    761
  enteric fever 24, 254
  food poisoning 32
  Reiter's syndrome 248
salpingitis 39
saquinavir 51
sarcoidosis 56, 796–797
  extrapulmonary features 485
  granulomatous lung disease
      483
scales 813
Schilling test 173–174
Schirmer test 261–262
schistosomiasis 37
Schumm's test 179
sciatica 274
sclerodactyly 257–258
scleroderma *see* systemic sclerosis
    (scleroderma)
sclerosis, systemic *see* systemic
    sclerosis (scleroderma)
sclerotherapy 73, 136
scotoma 647, 648, 649
seasonal rhinitis 449
secondarily generated
    tonic–clonic seizures 675
secondary hyperparathyroidism
    585
secondary osteoarthritis (OA)
    237

secondary polycythaemia
    196–197
secretory diarrhoea **98**
seizures 675–676
  tonic–clonic *see* tonic–clonic
      seizures
  *see also* epilepsy
selective oestrogen-receptor
    modulators (SERMs) 280
selective serotonin reuptake
    inhibitors (SSRIs) 683
selegiline 683
sella turcica 546
Sengstaken–Blakemore tube
  gastrointestinal bleeding 73
  insertion 749–750
  variceal haemorrhage 137
sensory loss **637–641**
sensory pathways 641–643, 644
sepsis 9
  nephrotic syndrome 325
septicaemia **9–10**
septic arthritis **250–251**
  emergency management 251
septic shock 506, **508,** 510, 513,
    759–760
serology, pneumonia 474
serotonin 700
serotonin antagonists 701
serum 813
seventh cranial nerve **655–657**
sexually transmitted infections
    (STIs) **34–42**
Sézary syndrome 231
Sheehan's syndrome 548
*Shigella* infections **28,** 761
  food poisoning 33
  Reiter's syndrome 248
  traveller's diarrhoea 758
shingles **14**
shock **505–515**
  anaphylactic *see* anaphylactic
      shock
  cardiogenic **396–397,** 783
  emergency management 509
  mechanical **508**
  septic **508,** 510, 513, 759–760
Sicca syndrome 261–262
sickle cell disease **185–188**
  complications 187
  emergency management 187
sick sinus syndrome **374**
sideroblastic anaemia **171**
sildenafil citrate 551
silver wiring 437

simvastatin 629
sinoatrial block 374
sino-atrial node, dysfunction **374**
sino-atrial (SA) node 371
sinus (blind track opening on
    skin) 813
sinus arrest 374
sinus arrhythmias 373
sinus bradycardia 373
    myocardial infarction 409
sinusitis 444, **449**
sinus tachycardia 373
    myocardial infarction 409
sixth cranial nerve **652–654**
    intracranial tumours 697
Sjögren's syndrome **261–262**
    secondary 243
skin, diabetes mellitus 619
skin-prick testing 449
    asthma 466
sleep apnoea 456–457
sliding hiatus hernia 61
small intestine disorders **75–83**
    adenocarcinomas 83
    benign tumours **83**
    carcinoid tumours **82–83**
    malignant tumours **82–83**
smoking
    cessation 454
    COPD 453
    coronary artery disease 398
    Crohn's disease 84
    hyperlipidaemia 629
    lung cancer 492
Snellen test chart 647
sodium aurothiomalate 245
sodium cromoglicate 469
sodium homeostasis 284
    disorders **291–297,** 771
    normal values 285
    regulation 286–287
sodium retention 288
sodium urate crystals 265
sodium valproate 677
solitary toxic nodule **565**
solvent abuse 535–536
somatostatin 542
somatostatin analogues
    acromegaly 560
    hypoglycaemia 623
    see also octreotide
spasmodic torticollis 685–686
sphenoid sinus 546
spherocytosis, hereditary
    **180–181**

sphincterotomy 157, 363
spider naevae 132
spinal cord 704
spinal cord diseases/disorders
    **704–708**
    compression 275, **704–706**
    root lesions 641, 643
    tuberculosis 705
spinal muscular atrophies 710
spinal root lesions 641, 643
spinal stenosis **275**
spinal tuberculosis 705
spinothalamic tracts 6473
spironolactone 289
    ascites 139
    chronic cardiac failure 392,
        394
    hirsutism 557
spleen **199–200**
splenectomy **200**
    autoimmune thrombocytopenic
        purpura 211
    hereditary spherocytosis
        **180–181**
    myelofibrosis 198
splenic atrophy 187
splenomegaly **199–200**
    Graves' disease 565
    infective endocarditis 423
    typhoid fever 24
spondarthritides **246–250**
spondylolisthesis **274–275**
sprue, tropical **78–79**
sputum sampling 447
    bronchiectasis 458
    pneumonia 473
    tuberculosis 479
squamous cell carcinoma 55, 62
squint 654
St. Jude valve 413
St. Vitus dance 411
staghorn calculi 334
*Staphylococcus aureus* infection,
        pneumonia complications
        477
*Staphylococcus* infections 450, 694
    bronchiectasis 458
    cystic fibrosis 460
    food poisoning 32
    infective endocarditis 423
    pneumonia 472, 475–476, 477
    septicaemia 9
    septic arthritis 250–251
Starling curve 387, 388
Starr–Edwards valve 413

statins   627, 629
status epilepticus   **678–680**
   emergency management   679
stavudine   51
steatorrhoea   **54,** 76
   chronic pancreatitis   161
   cystic fibrosis   460
   primary biliary cirrhosis   143
stenosis, pulmonary   421
stenosis, spinal   **275**
sterile procedures   733
Sternberg–Reed cells   227
steroids   **575–576**
   adverse effects   575–576, 577,
      766
   asthma   466
   autoimmune haemolytic
      anaemia   192
   Behçet's syndrome   265
   bronchiectasis   458
   Cushing's syndrome   580–581
   discoid lupus   256
   exogenous eczema   728
   giant cell arteritis   702
   nephrotic syndrome   324
   neurosyphilis   696
   psoriasis   726
   pyoderma gangrenosum   730
   rhinitis   449
   thyroid eye disease   569
   *see also* corticosteroids
Stix tests   310, **311–314,** 751
   acute renal failure   345
   glycaemic control   608
   hypertension   437
   urinary tract infections   326
'stocking and glove' neuropathy
   617, 711
Stokes–Adams attacks   375
stomach disorders   **63–71**
   benign tumours   71
   malignant tumours   **69–70**
strabismus   654
streptococci   694
*Streptococcus* infections   449, 450
   AIDS   49
   glomerulonephritis   318, 320
   group A infections, rheumatic
      fever   411–412
   infective endocarditis   422
   liver abscesses   151
streptokinase
   arterial thrombosis   215
   myocardial infarction   406
streptomycin   481

stress incontinence   362
Stretta procedure   59
stroke   **664–670,** 793
   emergency management   669
*Strongyloides stercoralis* infections
   35
ST segment
   depression   372
   ECG   371–372
   elevation   371–372
subacute combined degeneration
   of the cord   714
subacute (bacterial) endocarditis
   (SBE)   422
subacute sclerosing
   panencephalitis   11
subarachnoid haemorrhage
   **672–674**
   hydrocephalus   699
subclavian vein puncture   740
subdural haematoma   **674**
suicide   523–534
sulfadiazine   46
sulfasalazine
   adverse effects   245
   ankylosing spondylitis   248
   Reiter's syndrome   249
   rheumatoid arthritis   244
sulfonamides   729
sulfonylureas   604–605
sumatriptan   701
sunlight   254
superficial ecchymoses   208
superficial thrombophlebitis   441
supranuclear lesions   652, 654
supraventricular tachycardias
   373
   electrical cardioversion   742
surgery
   acromegaly   560
   Cushing's syndrome   580
   diabetes mellitus   **619**
   hyperprolactinaemia   558
   hyperthyroidism   567
   hypoglycaemia   623
   intervertebral disc disease   274
   intracranial tumours   698
   lung carcinoma   497
   osteoarthritis   240
   phaeochromocytoma   593
   renal cell carcinoma   357–358
   unilateral renal disease   331
swallowing, painful   56, 57
Swan–Ganz catheter   514–515,
   783

Swan neck deformity   242
S wave   370
sweat testing   460–461
Sydenham's chorea   411
sympathetic nervous system
   387–388
sympathoadrenal shock   505–506
synacthen test   574, 575, 577
syncope   **636–638**
   exertional   419
   heart disease   **367**
   hypertrophic cardiomyopathy
      432
   pulmonary embolism   426
   pulmonary hypertension   425
syndrome of inappropriate ADH
      secretion (SIADH)
      **581–582**, 813
   dilutional hyponatraemia   295
syngeneic bone marrow
      transplantation   232
synovial cysts   777–778
synovitis   268
syphilis   **40–42**
syringobulbia   659, **706**
syringomyelia   651, **706–707**
systemic hypertension   **435–439**
systemic inflammatory response
      syndrome (SIRS)   505
systemic lupus erythematosus
      (SLE)   **253–256**, 723
   acute nephritic syndrome   318
   clinical features   254–255
   management   256
   mouth ulcers   55
   renal tubular acidosis   307
   Sjögren's syndrome   261
   vasculitis   262
systemic sclerosis (scleroderma)
      61, **257–260**
   diffuse   258
   limited   257–258

**T**

tachyarrhythmias   374
   atrial   374–375
tachy–brady syndrome   374
tachycardias   365, 373, **376–381**
   acute asthma   469
   acute intermittent porphyria
      631
   decreased extracellular volume
      290

pericardial tamponade   434
   pulmonary embolism   426
   sinus see sinus tachycardia
   supraventricular   373
   thyroid crisis   568
   ventricular   373, **382–383**
tachypnoea
   acute respiratory distress
      syndrome   520
   extrinsic allergic alveolitis   489
   pulmonary embolism   426
tacrolimus
   psoriasis   726
   renal transplantation   355
*Taenia* infections   34, 38
tamsulosin   359
tapeworms   34, 38
target cells   813
technetium-99m   802
telangiectasia   258, 814
temperature regulation disorders
      **595–597**
temporal arteritis (giant cell
      arteritis)   **262–263**, 649,
      **701, 766**
temporal lobe seizures   676
tendon xanthomas   626
tenofovir   51
tenosynovitis   265
Tensilon test   **716**
tension headache   **700–701**
tension pneumothorax   501
terbutaline   466
terlipressin   137
tertiary hyperparathyroidism   585
testicular cancer   **361**
testosterone   542
tetany   589
tetracosactide test   574, 575, 577
tetracycline
   acne vulgaris   725
   *Chlamydia* infections   475
   cholera   30
   malaria   22
   pleural effusion   501
   sprue   79
tetraparesis   641
thalamic lesions   645
thalassaemias   **182, 184**
thallium-201   802
thiamin deficiency   **714**
thiazide diuretics   289
   adverse effects   438
   chronic cardiac failure   392
   hypertension   437

thiazolidinediones 606
third cranial nerve **652–654**
  intracranial tumours 697
third nerve nucleus 647
thirst axis **581–584**
thoracic aortic aneurysms **440**
threadworm infections 36
thrombin 205–206
thrombin time (TT) 208
thrombocythaemia 197
thrombocytopenia **209–211**
  alcohol abuse 538
  blood transfusions 204
  causes 209
  leukaemias 222
  megaloblastic anaemia 171
thromboembolism
  atrial fibrillation 380
  mitral regurgitation 416–417
  myocardial infarction 410
  sinus node dysfunction 374
thrombolytic therapy
  arterial thrombosis 215–216
  deep vein thrombosis (DVT)
      442
  myocardial infarction 406
  stroke 669
thrombophilia 670
thrombophlebitis, superficial
      441
thrombosis **214–219**
  arterial **214–216**
  venous **216–219**
thymectomy 717
thymic hyperplasia 715
thymomas 716–717
thyroid
  acropachy 566
  carcinoma **571–573**
  diseases/disorders **561–573**
thyroid crisis **568–569**
  emergency management 568
thyroidectomy 567
thyroid eye disease **569**
thyroid function tests 561
  goitre 571
thyroiditis factitia 565
thyroid replacement therapy 548
thyroid-stimulating hormone
      (TSH) 541, 542, 543–544,
      546
thyrotoxicosis 777
  thyroid crisis 568
thyrotrophin-releasing hormone
      (TRH) 542, 543–544

thyroxine ($T_4$) 542, 543
  hypopituitarism 548
  hypothyroidism 563–564
  secretion 561
thyroxine-binding globulin (TBG)
      561
tiabendazole 35, 37
tic douloureux **703**
ticlopidine 215
tics 685
Tinnel's sign 711
tirofiban 215
tissue factor (TF) 205–206
tissue transglutaminase (tTG)
      antibodies 78
tissue-type plasminogen activator
      (tPA)
  arterial thrombosis 215
  myocardial infarction 406
titubation 684
  cerebellar lesions 646
TNM classification 814
Todd's paralysis 677
tolbutamide 605
tonic–clonic seizures 672
  secondary 675
tophaceous urate deposits 266
tophi 265
torsades de pointes 383
total lung capacity (TLC) 448
total parenteral nutrition (TPN)
      **109–110**
toxic adenoma 565
toxic confusional state **718–719**
toxic epidermal necrosis 40,
      729
toxic multinodular goitre 565,
      **565**
toxic shock syndrome 10
*Toxocara canis* infections 36
toxoplasmosis 15
  AIDS 46–47, 795
tracheitis 450
transbronchial biopsy 485
transbronchial stenting 497
transfer coefficient ($K_{CO}$) 448
transfer factor ($T_{CO}$) 448
transferrin 167, 169
transient ischaemic attack (TIA)
      665, **671**, 793
transjugular hepatic
      portosystemic shunt (TIPS)
      73
  ascites 140
  variceal haemorrhage 137

transplantation
  allogeneic 799
  heart 395
  kidney **355**
transudate 814
transurethral resection of the
      prostate (TURP) 359
transverse myelitis 706
traveller's diarrhoea **31, 34,** 758
  giardiasis 30
trematode infection 35–36
tremor 681
*Treponema pallidum*
      haemagglutination assay
      (TPHA) 41
*Treponema pallidum* infections
    40–42
tretinoin 725
triamterene 392
*Trichinella spiralis* infections 36
*Trichomonas vaginalis* infections
    34
*Trichuris trichiura* infections 36
tricuspid regurgitation 421
tricuspid stenosis 421
tricuspid valve disease
    **421–422**
tricyclic antidepressants
  diabetic neuropathy 618
  headache 700
  overdose 533
trigeminal nerve (fifth cranial)
    **654–655**
trigeminal neuralgia **703**
trihexyphenidyl 683
triiodothyronine (T₃) 543
  secretion 561
trimethoprim
  *Pneumocystis* infections 48
  urinary tract infections 327
triptans 701
trismus 685–686
tropical infections **17–30**
  examination questions
    727–760
  incubation periods 18
  investigations 19
tropical sprue **78–79**
troponin I 405
troponin T 405
Trousseau's sign 589
TSH 541, 542, 543–544, 546
tuberculosis 446, **478–483**
  AIDS 48–49, 478
  anaemia 170

diabetes mellitus 619
  intestinal complications **81**
  lymph node 481
  miliary 478–479
  spinal 705
  terminal ileitis 88
  urinary tract 328
tuberculous arthritis **252**
tuberculous meningitis 481, 690,
    796
tubulointerstitial nephritis
    **328–329**
  acute 328–329
  chronic 329
tumours *see individual tumours*
tumour suppressor genes 814
Turner's syndrome 814
T waves 371
twelfth cranial nerve 659
type 1 diabetes mellitus *see*
    diabetes mellitus
type 2 diabetes mellitus *see*
    diabetes mellitus
typhoid fever **24–25**
typical absences 675

# U

ulcer(s)
  Curling's 64
  duodenal 66
  genital 34, **40**
  mouth 54–55
  peptic *see* peptic ulcer disease
ulcerative colitis (UC) **84–91**
  enteropathic arthritis 250
ulcerative gingivitis, acute 56
ulnar deviation 242
ultrasonography
  aortic aneurysm 440
  deep vein thrombosis (DVT)
    441
  liver disease 116
  lung carcinoma 497
  pancreatic cancer 163
  pulmonary embolism 427
  renal cell carcinoma 357
  stroke 668, 670
  testicular cancer 361
  urinary tract obstruction 339
unconsciousness **659–663**
unilateral posterior cerebral
    infarction 650
unilateral renal disease 331–332

unstable angina (UA)  399, **402,**
        776
    exercise ECG  372
upper motor neurone (UMN)
        lesions  638, 640
    facial nerve  657
    lower motor neurone lesion
        comparison  639
    optic nerve  652, 654
uraemia  320
uraemic acidosis  307–308
urea breath test  65–66
ureteric stones  334
urethral catheterization  751–753
urethral discharge  34
urethral stones  334
urethral syndrome  **328**
urethritis  **39,** 310
    Reiter's syndrome  248
uretography  339
urge incontinence  362
uric acid  266
uric acid stones  333
    prevention  336
urinary calculi  **332–337**
urinary tract infections (UTIs)
        309, **325–328**
    bacteriuria  315
    causative organisms  325
    cellular infiltrates  314
    diabetes mellitus  619
    pregnancy  327–328
urinary tract obstruction
        **338–340**
urine
    alkalinization  527, 529
    collection  751
    microscopy  **314–315**
    pH  311
    testing  608, 751
urography, excretion/intravenous
        see excretion urography
        (intravenous urography,
        IVU)
urolithiasis  **332–337**
urothelial tumours  **358**
ursodeoxycholic acid  143
urticaria  203

influenza  451
meningitis  690
sickle cell disease  188
tropical infections  18
tuberculosis  482
typhoid fever  25
vaginal discharge  34
vagus nerve (tenth cranial)  659
Valsalva manoeuvre  380
valsartan  439
valvotomy  413
valvular heart disease  **412–425**
vancomycin  424
variant angina  399
variant CJD  696
variceal band ligation  136
variceal haemorrhage  136,
        137–138
varicella  **13–14**
    AIDS  47
variegate porphyria  631, 632
vascular cell adhesion molecule-1
        (VCAM-1)  240–241
vascular dementia  **721**
vasculitis  106, **262**
    classification  262
    pulmonary  **486–487**
vasoconstriction  290
vasodilation  507
vasodilator therapy
    chronic cardiac failure  **392–394**
    shock  510, 512
vaso-occlusion  186
vasopressin see antidiuretic
        hormone (ADH)
vasopressin, synthetic
    haemophilia A  212
    von Willdebrand disease  **213**
    see also antidiuretic hormone
        (ADH)
vasovagal syncope  637
Vaughan Williams classification
        379
venepuncture  734–735
Venereal Disease Research
        Laboratory (VDRL) test
        41–42
venesection  145
venography  441
venous disease  **441–442**
venous thromboembolism
        **216–219**
    nephrotic syndrome  324
    see also deep vein thrombosis
        (DVT)

# V

vaccination
    COPD  455
    hepatitis B virus  123, 128

ventilation–perfusion scan   427
ventricular arrhythmias   **382–385**
  electrical cardioversion   742
  hypertrophic cardiomyopathy
    432
  myocardial infarction   409–410
ventricular dilatation   388
ventricular ectopic beats   382
ventricular fibrillation   383
  myocardial infarction   409
ventricular hypertrophy   370–371
ventricular tachyarrhythmias
  432
ventricular tachycardias   373,
  **382–383,** 409
Venturi mask
  acute exacerbation of COPD
    455
  respiratory failure   517
verapamil
  hypertrophic cardiomyopathy
    432
  junctional tachycardias   381
vertical nystagmus   658
vertical transmission   123
vertigo   636, **657**
  benign positional   659
vertiginocochlear nerve (eighth
  cranial)   **657–659**
*Vibrio cholerae* infection   29–30
vigabatrin   678
villous atrophy   77
Vincent's infection   56
vincristine
  leukaemia   224
  non-Hodgkin's lymphoma   230
vipomas   164
viral encephalitis   691, 693
viral gastroenteritis   30–33
viral load   49–50
viral meningitis   690
Virchow's node   70
virilization   **555–557**
visual cortex   647
visual field defects   647–650
vitamin B$_1$ deficiency   **714**
vitamin B$_6$ deficiency   108, **714**
vitamin B$_{12}$   **172**
  deficiency   **172–175, 714,** 766
vitamin D
  bone metabolism   275

metabolism   277
  supplements   279, 351
vitamin deficiencies   107–108,
  **172–175,** 276, **714,** 766
  neuropathies   714
  *see also individual vitamins*
vitamin E   108
vitamin K
  deficiency   214
  dependent enzymes
    205–206
  malabsorption   120
  supplement   529
vitiligo
  Addison's disease   574
  diabetes mellitus   619
  Graves' disease   565
VLDLs *see* very-low-density
  lipoproteins (VLDLs)
volume replacement   508–510
vomiting   **53–54**
  acute intermittent porphyria
    631
  with headache   636
  hydrocephalus   699
  intracranial tumours   697
  metabolic alkalosis   308
  migraine   700–701
  poisoning   527
von Recklinghausen's disease
  **731**
von Willdebrand disease   205,
  **212–213**
von Willdebrand factor   205
*V/Q* scan   427
V/scan (ventilation–perfusion
  scan)   427

very-low-density lipoproteins
  (VLDLs)   623, 624
  diseases/disorders   **624–625**
vesicle   814
vestibulocochlear nerve (eighth

# W

Waldenstroms
  macroglobulinaemia
  **234**
warfarin
  pulmonary hypertension   426
  stroke   670
  thromboembolism   410
  venous thromboembolism
    217, 218
warm antibodies   189, 190
water deprivation test   583–584
water homeostasis   **283–308**
  examination questions
    769–771

water homeostasis (*contd*)
  normal values   285
  regulation   287
Waterhouse–Friderichsen
      syndrome   10, 794
weal   814
Wegener's granulomatosis   446,
      486
  glomerulonephritis   317
Weil's disease   17
Wenckebach's phenomenon
      374–375
Wernicke–Korsakoff syndrome
      714, 794–795
Wernicke's aphasia   801
Wernicke's encephalopathy (WE)
      537, 764
wheeze   444, 446
  asthma   465, 780
Whipple's disease   **80**
whipworm infections   36
white cell count (WCC), normal
      values   166
whiteheads   723
whole blood   200
  volume replacement therapy
      508–509
whole bowel irrigation   526
whooping cough   457
Wilson's disease   **146–147**
  dystonias   685
Wiskott–Aldrich syndrome
      209
Wolff–Parkinson–White
      syndrome   380–381
World Health Organization
      (WHO), leukaemia
      classification   223

## X

xamoterol   394
xanthochromia   673
xanthomas
  hypertriglyceridaemia   625
  tendon   626
xenograft, heart valves   413
xenotransplantation   814
xerostomia   56, 261
47, XXY   550

## Y

*Yersinia* infections   759
  Reiter's syndrome   248
  terminal ileitis   88

## Z

zafirlukast   469
zalcitabine   51
zidovudine   51
  AIDS   52
Ziehl–Nielsen stain
  pleural effusion   499
  sputum   447
  tuberculosis   479
zinc insulins   607
Zollinger–Ellison syndrome   164
  peptic ulcers   67
zolmitriptan   701
zoonosis   814
zoster-immune immunoglobulin
      (ZIG)   14